Schwartz's

CLINICAL
HANDBOOK
OF PEDIATRICS

FIFTH EDITION

Schwartz's

CLINICAL HANDBOOK OF PEDIATRICS

FIFTH EDITION

EDITOR

Joseph J. Zorc

ASSOCIATE EDITORS

Elizabeth R. Alpern
Lawrence W. Brown
Kathleen M. Loomes
Bradley S. Marino
Cynthia J. Mollen
Leslie J. Raffini

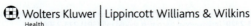
. Wolters Kluwer | Lippincott Williams & Wilkins
Health
Philadelphia · Baltimore · New York · London
Buenos Aires · Hong Kong · Sydney · Tokyo

Acquisitions Editor: Susan Rhyner
Product Manager: Stacey Sebring
Marketing Manager: Joy Fisher-Williams
Designer: Teresa Mallon
Compositor: Aptara, Inc.

Fifth Edition
Copyright © 2013, 2009, 2003, 1999, 1996 Lippincott Williams & Wilkins, a Wolters Kluwer business.

351 West Camden Street
Baltimore, MD 21201

Two Commerce Square
2001 Market Street
Philadelphia, PA 19103

Printed in China

9 8 7 6 5 4 3 2 1

Library of Congress Cataloging-in-Publication Data
Schwartz's clinical handbook of pediatrics / editor, Joseph J. Zorc ;
associate editors, Elizabeth R. Alpern ... [et al.]. – 5th ed.
    p. ; cm.
  Clinical handbook of pediatrics
  Includes bibliographical references and index.
  ISBN 978-1-60831-578-9 (alk. paper)
  I. Zorc, Joseph J. II. Alpern, Elizabeth R. III. Schwartz, M. William,
1935- IV. Title: Clinical handbook of pediatrics.
  [DNLM: 1. Pediatrics–Handbooks. WS 39]
  618.92–dc23
                                        2011050194

DISCLAIMER
Care has been taken to confirm the accuracy of the information present and to describe generally accepted practices. However, the authors, editors, and publisher are not responsible for errors or omissions or for any consequences from application of the information in this book and make no warranty, expressed or implied, with respect to the currency, completeness, or accuracy of the contents of the publication. Application of this information in a particular situation remains the professional responsibility of the practitioner; the clinical treatments described and recommended may not be considered absolute and universal recommendations.

The authors, editors, and publisher have exerted every effort to ensure that drug selection and dosage set forth in this text are in accordance with the current recommendations and practice at the time of publication. However, in view of ongoing research, changes in government regulations, and the constant flow of information relating to drug therapy and drug reactions, the reader is urged to check the package insert for each drug for any change in indications and dosage and for added warnings and precautions. This is particularly important when the recommended agent is a new or infrequently employed drug.

Some drugs and medical devices presented in this publication have Food and Drug Administration (FDA) clearance for limited use in restricted research settings. It is the responsibility of the health care provider to ascertain the FDA status of each drug or device planned for use in their clinical practice.

To purchase additional copies of this book, call our customer service department at **(800) 638-3030** or fax orders to **(301) 223-2320**. International customers should call **(301) 223-2300**.

Visit Lippincott Williams & Wilkins on the Internet: http://www.lww.com. Lippincott Williams & Wilkins customer service representatives are available from 8:30 am to 6:00 pm, EST.

PREFACE

For this fifth edition of the *Clinical Handbook of Pediatrics*, we have continued the pragmatic approach to assessment, differential diagnosis, and management of pediatric illness envisioned by Dr. M. William Schwartz in creating this text. We have also responded to recommendations from readers to continue to streamline and reduce the size of the book to make it easier to bring it to the bedside. I hope we have succeeded in these goals and look forward to receiving suggestions for the design of future editions.

Special thanks go to the associate editors, Elizabeth Alpern, Larry Brown, Kathy Loomes, Brad Marino, Cynthia Mollen, and Leslie Raffini, who worked closely with the authors and added much to the quality of this text. My thanks go to all of the authors who updated the evidence in their area and often brought on junior colleagues to add a fresh perspective. I would also like to thank the team at Lippincott/Wolters Kluwer, including Steve Boehm and Stacey Sebring. A book such as this resembles a quilt representing the efforts of many individuals, and I hope that we have successfully woven it together into a whole that will benefit the clinicians and the children for whom it was intended.

Nicholas S. Abend, MD

Assistant Professor of Neurology and
  Pediatrics
University of Pennsylvania School of
  Medicine
Philadelphia, PA

Attending Neurologist
Children's Hospital of Philadelphia
Philadelphia, PA

Elizabeth R. Alpern, MD, MSCE

Associate Professor
Department of Pediatrics
Perelman School of Medicine
University of Pennsylvania
Philadelphia, PA

Director of Research, Attending Physician
Division of Emergency Medicine
Children's Hospital of Philadelphia
Philadelphia, PA

Craig Alter, MD

Associate Professor of Clinical Pediatrics
Department of Pediatrics
University of Pennsylvania
Philadelphia, PA

Fellowship Director
Department of Pediatrics
Children's Hospital of Philadelphia
Philadelphia, PA

Jeffrey Anderson, MD, MPH

Assistant Professor of Pediatrics
Department of Pediatrics
University of Cincinnati
Cincinnati, OH

Electro Physiologist
Heart Institute
Cincinnati Children's Hospital Medical
  Center
Cincinnati, OH

Paul L. Aronson, MD

Instructor
Department of Pediatrics
University of Pennsylvania School of
  Medicine
Philadelphia, PA

Fellow
Division of Pediatric Emergency
  Medicine
Children's Hospital of Philadelphia
Philadelphia, PA

**Oluwakemi B. Badaki-Makun,
MD, CM**

Assistant Professor
Pediatrics and Emergency Medicine
George Washington University
Washington, DC

Attending Physician
Emergency Medicine and Trauma
  Services
Children's National Medical Center
Washington, DC, 20010

Fran Balamuth, MD, PhD

Lecturer
Department of Pediatrics
University of Pennsylvania School
  of Medicine
Philadelphia, PA

Fellow
Department of Pediatrics
Division of Emergency
  Medicine
Children's Hospital of Philadelphia
Philadelphia, PA

Christina Bales, MD
Assistant Professor of Clinical Medicine
Department of Pediatrics
Perelman School of Medicine
University of Pennsylvania
Philadelphia, PA

Attending Physician
Department of Pediatrics
Division of Gastroenterology, Hepatology,
and Nutrition
Children's Hospital of Philadelphia
Philadelphia, PA

Andrew J. Bauer, MD
Associate Professor
Department of Pediatrics
Uniformed Services University
Bethesda, MD

Senior Consultant
The Thyroid Center
Department of Endocrinology
Children's Hospital of Philadelphia
Philadelphia, PA

Suzanne E. Beck, MD
Associate Professor of Clinical Pediatrics
Department of Pediatrics
University of Pennsylvania
Philadelphia, PA

Attending Pediatric Pulmonologist and
Sleep Medicine Specialist
Department of Pediatrics
Children's Hospital of Philadelphia
Philadelphia, PA

Mercedes M. Blackstone, MD
Assistant Professor of Clinical Pediatrics
Department of Pediatrics
University of Pennsylvania School of
Medicine
Philadelphia, PA

Attending Physician
Division of Emergency Medicine
Children's Hospital of Philadelphia
Philadelphia, PA

Lawrence W. Brown, MD
Associate Professor
Departments of Neurology and Pediatrics
University of Pennsylvania School of
Medicine
Philadelphia, PA

Director, Pediatric Neuropsychiatry
Division of Neurology
Children's Hospital of Philadelphia
Philadelphia, PA

Diane P. Calello, MD
Staff Toxicologist
Department of Preventive Medicine
NJ Poison Information and Education
System
University of Medicine and Dentistry,
New Jersey
Newark, NJ

Faculty
Pediatric Emergency Medicine
Morristown Medical Center
Morristown, NJ

Leslie Castelo-Soccio, MD, PhD
Assistant Professor
Department of Pediatrics
Division of Dermatology
Children's Hospital of Philadelphia
Philadelphia, PA

Attending Physician
Division of Dermatology
Children's Hospital of Philadelphia
Philadelphia, PA

Christine S. Cho, MD, MPH
HS Assistant Clinical Professor
Department of Pediatrics
UCSF School of Medicine
San Francisco, CA

Attending Physician
Division of Emergency Medicine
Children's Hospital and Research Center
Oakland
Oakland, CA

Cindy W. Christian, MD

Professor
Department of Pediatrics
Perelman School of Medicine
University of Pennsylvania
Philadelphia, PA

Chair, Child Abuse and Neglect Prevention
Department of Pediatrics
Children's Hospital of Philadelphia
Philadelphia, PA

Esther K. Chung, MD, MPH

Associate Professor
Department of Pediatrics
Jefferson Medical College
Philadelphia, PA

Attending Physician
Department of Pediatrics
Thomas Jefferson University Hospital
Philadelphia, PA

Richard J. Czosek, MD

Assistant Professor
Pediatric Cardiology
Cincinnati Children's Hospital Medical Center
Cincinnati, OH

Jennifer A. Danzig, MD

Instructor
Department of Pediatrics
University of Pennsylvania School of Medicine
Philadelphia, PA

Fellow
Division of Endocrinology and Diabetes
Children's Hospital of Philadelphia
Philadelphia, PA

Katherine MacRae Dell, MD

Associate Professor
Department of Pediatrics
Case Western Reserve University
Cleveland, OH

Chief
Division of Pediatric Nephrology
Rainbow Babies and Children's Hospital
Cleveland, OH

Joel A. Fein, MD, MPH

Professor of Pediatrics and Emergency
  Medicine
University of Pennsylvania School of
  Medicine
Philadelphia, PA

Attending Physician
Emergency Department
Children's Hospital of Philadelphia
Philadelphia, PA

Alexander G. Fiks, MD, MSCE

Assistant Professor of Pediatrics
Department of Pediatrics
University of Pennsylvania
Philadelphia, PA

Attending Physician
Children's Hospital of Philadelphia
Philadelphia, PA

Kristin N. Fiorino, MD

Assistant Professor
Department of Pediatrics
University of Pennsylvania
Philadelphia, PA

Assistant Professor
Department of Gastroenterology,
  Hepatology, and Nutrition
Children's Hospital of Philadelphia
Philadelphia, PA

Susan A. Friedman, MD

Clinical Associate Professor
Department of Pediatrics
University of Pennsylvania School of
  Medicine
Philadelphia, PA

Associate Physician, Neonatal Follow-up
  Program

Medical Director, International Adoption
  Health Program
Division of Pediatrics
Children's Hospital of Philadelphia
Philadelphia, PA

Marc H. Gorelick, MD, MSCE
Professor
Department of Pediatrics
Medical College of Wisconsin
Milwaukee, WI

Jon E. Vice Endowed Chair
Emergency Medicine
Children's Hospital of Wisconsin
Milwaukee, WI

Monika Goyal, MD
Assistant Professor
Department of Pediatrics
University of Pennsylvania
Philadelphia, PA

Attending Physician
Pediatrics, Division of Emergency
  Medicine
Children's Hospital of Philadelphia
Philadelphia, PA

Adda Grimberg, MD
Associate Professor
Department of Pediatrics
University of Pennsylvania School
  of Medicine
Philadelphia, PA

Scientific Director
Diagnostic and Research Growth
  Center
Children's Hospital of Philadelphia
Philadelphia, PA

Toni Gross, MD, MPH
Attending Physician
Emergency Department
Phoenix Children's Hospital
Phoenix, AZ

Andrew Grossman, MD
Clinical Assistant Professor
Department of Pediatrics
Perelman School of Medicine
University of Pennsylvania
Philadelphia, PA

Attending Physician
Division of Gastroenterology, Hepatology,
  and Nutrition
Children's Hospital of Philadelphia
Philadelphia, PA

Andrew N. Hashikawa, MD, MS
Clinical Lecturer
Department of Emergency Medicine
Section of Children's Emergency Services
University of Michigan

Pediatric Emergency Medicine
Emergency Medicine
University of Michigan
Mott Children's Hospital
Ann Arbor, MI

Timothy M. Hoffman, MD
Associate Professor
Department of Pediatrics
Ohio State University College of Medicine
Columbus, OH

Medical Director
Heart Transplant and Heart Failure
  Program
The Heart Center
Nationwide Children's Hospital
Columbus, OH

Kan N. Hor, MD
Assistant Professor of Pediatrics
Department of Pediatric Cardiology
Cincinnati Children's Hospital Medical
  Center
Cincinnati, OH

Evelyn K. Hsu, MD
Assistant Professor
Department of Pediatrics
University of Washington Affiliated
    Hospitals
Seattle, WA

Assistant Professor of Pediatrics
Department of Pediatrics
Division of Gastroenterology, Hepatology,
    and Nutrition
Seattle Children's Hospital
Seattle, WA

Patty Huang, MD
Attending Physician
Division of Child Development,
    Rehabilitation, and Metabolic Disease
Children's Hospital of Philadelphia
Philadelphia, PA

Paul Ishimine, MD
Associate Clinical Professor
Departments of Emergency Medicine and
    Pediatrics
University of California, San Diego
San Diego, CA

Fellowship Director
Pediatric Emergency Medicine
Rady Children's Hospital
San Diego, CA

Beth Ann Johnson, MD, MA
Assistant Professor
Department of Pediatrics
University of Cincinnati
Cincinnati, OH

Heart Institute
Cincinnati Children's Hospital Medical
    Center
Cincinnati, OH

Sara Karjoo, MD
Fellow
Pediatric Gastroenterology
Children's Hospital of Philadelphia
Philadelphia, PA

Lorraine E. Levitt Katz, MD
Associate Professor
Department of Pediatrics
University of Pennsylvania School
    of Medicine
Philadelphia, PA

Associate Physician
Department of Pediatrics
Children's Hospital of Philadelphia
Philadelphia, PA

Leslie S. Kersun, MD
Assistant Professor
Department of Pediatrics
University of Pennsylvania School
    of Medicine
Philadelphia, PA

Attending Physician
Division of Oncology
Children's Hospital of Philadelphia
Philadelphia, PA

Timothy K. Knilans, MD
Professor
Department of Pediatrics
University of Cincinnati College
    of Medicine
Cincinnati, OH

Director, Cardiac Electrophysiology
Heart Institute
Cincinnati Children's Hospital Medical
    Center
Cincinnati, OH

Dorit Koren, MD
Instructor A
Department of Pediatrics
University of Pennsylvania
Philadelphia, PA

Attending Physician
Division of Endocrinology/Diabetes
Philadelphia, PA

Kate H. Kraft, MD
Fellow
Division of Urology
Children's Hospital of Philadelphia
Philadelphia, PA

Richard M. Kravitz, MD
Associate Professor of Pediatrics
Department of Pediatrics
Duke University School of Medicine
Durham, NC

Medical Director
Pediatric Sleep Laboratory
Department of Pediatrics
Duke University Medical Center
Durham, NC

Christopher J. LaRosa, MD
Clinical Assistant Professor
Department of Pediatrics
Jefferson Medical College
Philadelphia, PA

Attending Physician
Division of Nephrology
A.I. DuPont Hospital for Children
Wilmington, DE

Valerie Lewis, MD, MPH
Adolescent Medicine Specialist
Department of Pediatrics
Division of Pediatric Subspecialties
   in the Section of Adolescent
   Medicine
Lehigh Valley Health Network
Allentown, PA

Chris A. Liacouras, MD
Professor of Pediatrics
University of Pennsylvania School of
   Medicine
Philadelphia, PA

Attending Gastroenterologist
Division of Gastroenterology, Hepatology,
   and Nutrition
Children's Hospital of Philadelphia
Philadelphia, PA

Kathleen M. Loomes, MD
Associate Professor
Department of Pediatrics
University of Pennsylvania School of
   Medicine
Philadelphia, PA

Attending Physician
Division of Gastroenterology, Hepatology,
   and Nutrition
Children's Hospital of Philadelphia
Philadelphia, PA

Angela Lorts, MD
Assistant Professor
Department of Pediatrics
University of Cincinnati
Cincinnati, OH

Cardiac Interventionist
Department of Cardiology
Cincinnati Children's Hospital Medical
   Center
Cincinnati, OH

Bradley S. Marino, MD, MPP, MSCE
Associate Professor of Pediatrics
University of Cincinnati College of Medicine
Cincinnati, OH

Attending Physician
Pediatric Cardiac Intensive Care
Department of Pediatrics
Divisions of Cardiology and Critical Care
   Medicine
Cincinnati Children's Hospital Medical
   Center
Cincinnati, OH

Shoshana T. Melman, MD
Associate Professor
Department of Pediatrics
University of Medicine and Dentistry of
   New Jersey/SOM
Stratford, NJ

Medical Director
Foster Care Program
CARES Institute
Stratford, NJ

Kevin E. C. Meyers, MD

Associate Professor of Pediatrics
Department of Pediatrics/Nephrology
University of Pennsylvania
Philadelphia, PA

Assistant Division Chief
Department of Pediatrics/Nephrology
Children's Hospital of Philadelphia
Philadelphia, PA

Okeoma Mmeje, MD, MPH

Medical Resident
Department of Obstetrics and
  Gynecology
Philadelphia, PA

Medical Resident
Department of Obstetrics and
  Gynecology
Hospital of University of Pennsylvania
Philadelphia, PA

Cynthia J. Mollen, MD, MSCE

Assistant Professor
Department of Pediatrics
Perelman School of Medicine
University of Pennsylvania
Philadelphia, PA

Attending Physician
Division of Emergency Medicine
Children's Hospital of Philadelphia
Philadelphia, PA

Thomas Mollen, MD

Clinical Associate
Department of Pediatrics
University of Pennsylvania School of
  Medicine
Philadelphia, PA

Associate Medical Director
Intensive Care Nursery
Pennsylvania Hospital
Philadelphia, PA

Amanda Muir, MD

Fellow
Department of Gastroenterology,
  Hepatology, and Nutrition
Children's Hospital of Philadelphia
Philadelphia, PA

Frances Nadel, MD, MSCE

Associate Professor, Clinical Pediatrics
Department of Pediatrics
Perelman School of Medicine at the
  University of Pennsylvania
Philadelphia, PA

Attending Physician
Department of Emergency Medicine
Children's Hospital of Philadelphia
Philadelphia, PA

Sara Pentlicky, MD

OBGYN Fellow in Family Practice
Department of Obstetrics and Gynecology
University of Pennsylvania
Philadelphia, PA

Michael A. Posencheg, MD

Assistant Professor of Clinical Pediatrics
Division of Neonatology
Perelman School of Medicine at the
  University of Pennsylvania
Philadelphia, PA

Associate Medical Director, Intensive Care
  Nursery

Medical Director, Newborn Nursery
Hospital of the University of Pennsylvania
Philadelphia, PA

Jill C. Posner, MD, MSCE

Clinical Associate Professor
Department of Pediatrics
University of Pennsylvania
Philadelphia, PA

Attending Physician
Division of Emergency Medicine
Children's Hospital of Philadelphia
Philadelphia, PA

Madhura Pradhan, MD
Assistant Professor of Clinical Pediatrics
Department of Pediatrics
Perelman School of Medicine
University of Pennsylvania
Philadelphia, PA

Nephrologist
Department of Pediatrics
Children's Hospital of Philadelphia
Philadelphia, PA

Leslie J. Raffini, MD, MSCE
Assistant Professor
Department of Pediatrics
University of Pennsylvania
Philadelphia, PA

Director
Hemostasis and Thrombosis Center
Division of Hematology
Children's Hospital of Philadelphia
Philadelphia, PA

Rebecca Ruebner, MD
Fellow
Department of Pediatrics
Division of Nephrology
Children's Hospital of Pennsylvania
Philadelphia, PA

Andria Barnes Ruth, MD
Medical Director
Diabetes Resource Center of Santa Barbara
  County
Santa Barbara, CA

Pediatrician
Santa Barbara Neighborhood Clinics
Santa Barbara, CA

Matthew J. Ryan, MD
Assistant Professor
Department of Pediatrics
University of Pennsylvania
Philadelphia, PA

Attending Physician
Department of Pediatrics
Children's Hospital of Philadelphia
Philadelphia, PA

Jack Rychik, MD
Professor
Department of Pediatrics
University of Pennsylvania
Philadelphia, PA

Director
Fetal Heart Program
Children's Hospital of Philadelphia
Philadelphia, PA

Marta Satin-Smith, MD
Assistant Professor
Department of Pediatrics
Eastern Virginia Medical School
Norfolk, VA

Medical Director
Diabetes Center
Department of Pediatrics
Children's Hospital of the King's Daughters
Norfolk, VA

Esther M. Sampayo, MD, MPH
Assistant Professor
Department of Pediatrics
University of Pennsylvania School of
  Medicine
Philadelphia, PA

Attending Physician
Division of Emergency Medicine
Children's Hospital of Philadelphia
Philadelphia, PA

Matthew G. Sampson, MD

Clinical Instructor
Department of Pediatrics
Division of Nephrology
University of Pennsylvania School of
    Medicine
Philadelphia, PA

Fellow
Department of Pediatrics
Division of Nephrology
Children's Hospital of Philadelphia
Philadelphia, PA

Courtney Schreiber, MD, MPH

Assistant Professor
Department of Obstetrics and Gynecology
University of Pennsylvania
Philadelphia, PA

Attending Physician
Department of Obstetrics and Gynecology

Director
Penn Family Planning and Pregnancy Loss
    Center
Hospital of the University of Pennsylvania
Philadelphia, PA

Jeffrey A. Seiden, MD

Assistant Director
Pediatric Emergency Medicine/CARES
Virtua Hospital
Voorhees, NJ

Kara Shah, MD, PhD

Assistant Professor
Department of Pediatrics
University of Pennsylvania
Philadelphia, PA

Attending Physician
Department of General Pediatrics, Section
    of Pediatric Dermatology
The Children's Hospital of Philadelphia
Philadelphia, PA

Samir S. Shah, MD, MSCE

Assistant Professor
Department of Pediatrics and Epidemiology
University of Pennsylvania School of
    Medicine
Philadelphia, PA

Attending Physician
Divisions of Infectious Diseases and General
    Pediatrics
Children's Hospital of Philadelphia
Philadelphia, PA

Laura N. Sinai, MD, MSCE, FAAP

Pediatrician
Department of Pediatrics
Gaston Memorial Hospital
Gastonia, NC

Kim Smith-Whitley, MD

Associate Professor
Department of Pediatrics
University of Pennsylvania School of
    Medicine
Philadelphia, PA

Clinical Director of Hematology
Department of Pediatrics
Children's Hospital of Philadelphia
Philadelphia, PA

Philip R. Spandorfer, MD, MSCE

Associate Director of Research
Pediatric Emergency Medicine Associates
Atlanta, GA

Attending Physician
Department of Emergency Medicine
Children's Healthcare of Atlanta at Scottish
    Rite
Atlanta, GA

Katherine S. Taub, MD
Assistant Professor
Department of Neurology
University of Pennsylvania
Philadelphia, PA

Pediatric Epileptologist/Neurologist
Department of Neurology
Children's Hospital of Philadelphia
Philadelphia, PA

David T. Teachey, MD
Assistant Professor
Department of Pediatrics
University of Pennsylvania School
    of Medicine
Philadelphia, PA

Attending Physician
Pediatric Hematology–Oncology
Children's Hospital of Philadelphia
Philadelphia, PA

Lisa K. Tuchman, MD, MPH
Assistant Professor
Center for Clinical and Community
    Research
George Washington University
Washington, DC

Faculty
Adolescent and Young Adult Medicine
Children's National Medical Center
Washington, DC

René VanDeVoorde III, MD
Assistant Professor
Department of Pediatrics
University of Cincinnati
Cincinnati, OH

Medical Director, Dialysis
Pediatric Nephrology and Hypertension
Cincinnati Children's Hospital Medical
    Center
Cincinnati, OH

Brenda Waber, RD, CSP, CNSD, LDN
Neonatal Dietitian
Clinical Nutrition
Children's Hospital of Philadelphia
Philadelphia, PA

Stuart A. Weinzimer, MD
Associate Professor
Department of Pediatrics
Yale University
New Haven, CT

Attending Physician
Department of Pediatrics
Yale-New Haven Hospital
New Haven, CT

Amy L. Weiss, MD, MPH
Assistant Professor
Department of Pediatrics
Division of Adolescent Medicine
University of South Florida
Tampa, FL

Tampa General Hospital
Tampa, FL

Catherine C. Wiley, MD
Associate Professor
Department of Pediatrics
University of Connecticut School of
    Medicine
Farmington, CT

Chief, General Pediatrics
Connecticut Children's Medical Center
Hartford, CT

James F. Wiley II, MD, MPH
Clinical Professor of Pediatrics and
    Emergency Medicine/Traumatology
University of Connecticut School of
    Medicine
Farmington, CT

Attending Physician
Department of Pediatrics
Connecticut Children's Medical Center
Hartford, CT

Clyde J. Wright, MD

Assistant Professor
Department of Pediatrics
University of Pennsylvania School of
    Medicine
Philadelphia, PA

Assistant Professor
Department of Pediatrics, Division of
    Neonatology
Children's Hospital of Philadelphia
Philadelphia, PA

Donald Younkin, MD

Professor
Neurology and Pediatrics
University of Pennsylvania School of
    Medicine
Philadelphia, PA

Attending Physician
Department of Pediatrics
Division of Child Neurology
Children's Hospital of Philadelphia
Philadelphia, PA

Catherine S. Zorc, MD

Fellow, Academic General Pediatrics
Department of Pediatrics
Children's Hospital of Philadelphia
Philadelphia, PA

Joseph J. Zorc, MD, MSCE

Associate Professor of Pediatrics and
    Emergency Medicine
Perelman School of Medicine
University of Pennsylvania
Philadelphia, PA

Attending Physician
Emergency Department
Children's Hospital of Philadelphia
Philadelphia, PA

Kathleen Wholey Zsolway, DO

Clinical Associate Professor of Pediatrics
Department of General Pediatrics
University of Pennsylvania Medical School
Philadelphia, PA

Medical Director
General Pediatrics Faculty Practice
Children's Hospital of Philadelphia
Philadelphia, PA

CONTENTS

PART 3

Toxicology

PART 4

Cardiology Laboratory

PART 5

Surgical Glossary

PART 6

Syndromes Glossary

PART 1

Introduction

CHAPTER 1

Joseph J. Zorc
M. William Schwartz (3rd Edition)

Obtaining and Presenting a Patient History

This chapter presents a guide for obtaining a history of a pediatric patient and presenting a case on rounds or to an audience. Not every item described in this chapter is necessary in every write-up or presentation. The goal is to communicate key information about a patient; and the reader should not be overwhelmed with details that do not tell the patient's story.

HISTORY
Chief Complaint
Always ask the patient or the parents to describe their concerns, and record their actual words. Starting in an open-ended way may uncover concerns that can be missed if the clinician focuses too early on problem-oriented questions. The age and sex of the patient, as well as the duration of the problem, should be noted when presenting the chief complaint.

 HINT: Experienced pediatric clinicians state that most of the key evidence leading to a diagnosis is obtained through the history of the patient. Often, the physical examination and laboratory tests serve to confirm what the history suggests.

History of Present Illness

Indicate the person who provided the history (e.g., patient, parent, or guardian). Provide a clear, concise chronology of important events surrounding the problem—when did the problem start, how has it changed over time, and what tests and treatments were performed. Include key negative findings that may contribute to the differential diagnosis.

Medical History

- **Prenatal history**—mother's age and number of pregnancies; length of pregnancy; prenatal care, abnormal bleeding, illness, or exposure to illness; and medications or substances used (alcohol, drugs, tobacco) during pregnancy.
- **Birth history**—birth weight; duration of labor; mode of delivery, use of induction, anesthesia, or forceps; complications; and Apgar scores, if known.
- **Neonatal history**—length of stay, location (nursery vs. intensive care); complications such as jaundice, respiratory problems; and feeding history.

> **HINT:** Details about birth history are included in a write-up when they are relevant, but generally should be included for all children younger than 2 years.

- **Developmental history**—milestones for smiling, rolling over, sitting, standing, speaking, and toilet training; growth landmarks for weight gain and length. If delays are present, determine the approximate age at which the child functions for motor, verbal, and social skills.
- **Behavioral history**—proceed from less to more sensitive areas. The mnemonic SHADSSS can help structure the interview with an adolescent:
  School: grades, likes/dislikes, and plans for the future
  Home: others present and relationship with family
  Activities: friends and hobbies
  Depression: emotions, confidants, and suicidal thoughts/acts
  Substance abuse: exposure or use of drugs, tobacco, and alcohol
  Sexuality: partners, contraception use, and history of sexually transmitted diseases (STDs)
  Safety: violence and access to weapons
- **Immunization history**—immunizations by type and date, dates of recent boosters, and recent tuberculosis testing results.

> **HINT:** A statement in the patient's write-up that the patient's immunizations are "up to date" does not indicate whether recent changes in the recommendations were followed. Specific information should be provided when possible.

- **Past medical history**—childhood illnesses, estimated frequency of infections, and hospitalizations.
- **Surgical history**—procedures, complications, and dates of each.

Review of Systems

Do not duplicate the history of the present illness in this section of the write-up.

- **Head**—injuries, headaches, hair loss, and scalp infections.
- **Eyes**—acuity of vision; use of glasses; history of discharges, abnormal tearing, or injuries; and prior surgery.
- **Ears**—acuity of hearing and history of otitis, discharges, or foreign bodies.
- **Nose**—breathing difficulties, discharges, bleeding, and sinus infections.
- **Oral cavity and throat**—frequency of sore throats, dental problems, bleeding gums, herpes infections, and ulcers.
- **Lungs**—exercise tolerance (ability to keep up with peers during exercise), breathing difficulties, cough (day or night), history of pneumonia, wheezing, pains, hemoptysis, exposure to tuberculosis, and previous chest radiographs.
- **Heart**—exercise tolerance; history of murmurs; history of rheumatic fever in patient or family; history of Lyme disease or other infections that may affect the heart; feeling of heart racing, dyspnea, orthopnea, palpitations, or chest pain; cyanosis; and edema.
- **Gastrointestinal system**—appetite, weight changes, problems with food (e.g., allergy and intolerance), abdominal pain (location, intensity, precipitating events), bowel movements (number and character), jaundice, and rectal bleeding.
- **Genitourinary system**—history of infection, frequency of urination, dysuria, and hematuria, character of the urine stream, bedwetting, urethral or vaginal discharge, and age of menarche.
- **Extremities**—joint or muscle pain, muscle strength, swelling, and limitation of movement.
- **Neurologic system**—seizures, weakness, headaches, tremors, abnormal movements, development, school achievement, and hyperactivity.
- **Skin**—rashes and type of soap and detergent used.

Family History

- **Ages of parents and siblings**
- **Family history of illness**—seizures, asthma, cancer, behavior problems, allergies, cardiac disease, unexplained deaths, and lipid disorders
- **Deaths in family**—causes of death and age of the family member at the time of death
- **Social history**—other household members, sleeping arrangements, marital status of the parents, parents' employment status, and health insurance status

> **HINT:** In a patient with a suspected metabolic disorder, the most important question concerns early deaths of the patient's siblings or cousins. In a patient with a suspected infectious disease problem, the most important question concerns the patient's contact with others who are ill.

HINTS FOR PATIENT PRESENTATIONS

One of my images of hell is to be forced to spend a day listening to medical students' case presentations on rounds—both of them.

—Burt Sloane

Consider the Audience and Setting

The group members often have short attention spans, are usually standing, and often have other obligations. Make a **brief presentation,** no longer than 2 minutes, that provides highlights of the problem and leads the audience to the diagnosis. This is not the time to demonstrate your thoroughness or compulsive nature.

Also **consider the style** of the preceptor and those attending. Some may prefer a Socratic dialogue; while others want a more detailed presentation. Bear in mind that the Socratic style leads to interactive questions and answers. It is important, however, to appreciate the time pressures of audiences in inpatient rounds or clinics.

In contrast, **grand rounds** or formal case presentations may last as long as 10 minutes. These presentations focus on a diagnostic dilemma with many differential diagnoses, provide data for someone else to discuss with regard to findings and reaching a diagnosis or treatment, and include detailed histories, many negative findings, and most laboratory test results.

Decide What Information is Important to Include

It is important to **decide what negative information to include** in the presentation and what to rule out. The negative information should help exclude one or two of the major differential diagnoses. For example, you should mention respiratory distress in a case of cardiac failure but not in a case of urinary tract infection. Likewise, you should mention family history in a case of asthma or mental retardation but not in leg trauma.

After gathering information about the patient's problem, **select the highlights,** arranging them in an interesting and logical manner to lead to the diagnosis.

Organize the Presentation

The following format is suggested.

Chief Complaint

State in the patient's or the parent's words the reason for referral or admission. Mention the patient's age and the source of the referral. Avoid starting with a list of descriptors (e.g., "product of a gravida 1, para 1 full-term pregnancy" or "was well until 2 days before admission, when the following events occurred").

History of Present Illness

Give a summary of the pertinent events preceding admission and the changes in the patient's condition that precipitated the visit.

Review of the Patient History

Include only information that suggests the diagnosis or rules out major differential diagnoses. Consider the patient's developmental history, immunization history, past medical history, and family and social history.

Physical Examination Findings

Discuss how the child looked, but include only pertinent positive findings and a few negative findings that help eliminate major differential diagnoses or lead to the diagnosis.

Summary

Summarize the key facts that lead to the suspected diagnosis. Review other diagnoses that are in the differential. Outline your plan to complete the workup. Always think through your diagnosis and plan prior to a presentation, even if you are unsure, because this is the way to strengthen diagnostic skills.

Audience Questions

Be prepared for questions. They are compliments and mean that the audience was listening and thinking about the problem and the information you discussed. Questions are not criticisms of an incomplete presentation.

The Physical Examination

GENERAL CONSIDERATIONS
Performing the Physical Examination

The physical examination of a child is as much an art as a scientific procedure. The goal is to make the examination as productive and nontraumatic as possible.

To *minimize fear* in young children, conduct most of the physical examination with the child sitting on the parent's lap or nestled against his or her shoulder. If the child appears fearful, talk with the parent first so that the child has a chance to study you. Speak quietly, using a friendly tone of voice. Move gently and slowly, avoiding loud, sudden movements.

The physical examination is routinely presented and written in standard (adult) order, although it may not be carried out in that sequence. Children about 8 years and older can usually be examined easily in standard adult order, but with younger patients it is important to *examine the most critical areas first,* before the child cries. Always start with observation. Next, in a young child with a specific presenting complaint, it is often helpful to examine the corresponding organ system. In a young child with no specific complaints, palpate the fontanelles and then auscultate the heart and the lungs. Wait until the end of the examination to check the most threatening areas (e.g., the ears and the oral cavity).

Special Concerns
Mental Status

Since children often cannot vocalize their symptoms, their overall mental status is an essential clue to their degree of illness. Will the child smile or play? Observe interactions with parents or siblings. Be careful to differentiate a child who is simply tired from one who is lethargic (difficult to arouse). Similarly, distinguish the cranky child who comforts easily from one who is truly irritable and inconsolable.

> **HINT:** Cranky, febrile young children are often much more pleasant when their temperature has reduced. Children with meningitis are not easily comforted by being held; in fact, when picked up they may cry more.

Hydration Status

Physical findings consistent with dehydration include an increased heart rate, decreased blood pressure, sunken fontanelle, dry mucous membranes, decreased skin turgor, and increased capillary refill time (>2 seconds).

VITAL SIGNS AND STATISTICS

Temperature

Body temperatures are more labile in children than in adults and can be raised depending on the time of day (e.g., in the late afternoon) or following vigorous activity, excitement, or even eating.

A child's *normal oral temperature* is similar to an adult's, typically about 98.6°F. The rectal temperature is typically approximately 1° higher than the oral equivalent, and an axillary temperature (the least accurate method) is typically about 1° lower. Study results regarding the reliability of tympanic thermometers have been mixed; they are often used in low-risk older children.

 HINT: An infant or a young child can have a temperature of 103°F to 105°F, even with a minor infection. In contrast, a sick newborn may have a lower than normal temperature.

Pulse Rate

In an infant, palpate for pulse rate over the brachial artery. In an older child or adult, the wrist is generally the optimal location. Pulse rate is usually *120 to 160 beats per minute in the newborn* and steadily *declines as the child grows.* A typical teenager's pulse rate would be 70 to 80 beats per minute.

 HINT: In infants and children, the pulse rate responds much more distinctly to disease, exercise, or stress than it does in adults.

Respiration Rate

The most accurate measurements are obtained while the patient is asleep. In infants and young children, breathing is mostly diaphragmatic; the respiratory rate can be determined by *counting movements* of the abdomen. In older children and adolescents, chest movement should be *directly observed*. Table 2-1 summarizes the normal pediatric respiratory rates.

 HINT: Infants typically exhibit "periodic breathing," short periods of rapid breathing followed by several seconds without a breath. Pauses of 10 seconds or more are abnormal.

TABLE 2-1	Normal Pediatric Respiratory Rates (Respirations/min)		
Newborns	**Toddlers**	**School-Aged Children**	**Adolescents**
30–50	20–40	15–25	12

Blood Pressure

To obtain an accurate blood pressure measurement, *patient relaxation* is especially critical. Explain to a young child that the "balloon" will squeeze his arm and encourage him to watch the display.

Cuff width is also important. Choose a cuff width that covers 50% to 75% of the upper arm length. A too-narrow cuff may artificially increase the blood pressure reading.

If you are concerned about the possibility of heart disease, check blood pressure in *all four extremities*. Compare blood pressure measurements with standard norms for age and sex.

Length (Height)

To obtain a length measurement, place the infant on a firm table. Hold the baby's feet against a stationary board, keeping the knees straight, and bring a movable upright firmly against the baby's head to measure the infant's recumbent length.

Children >2 years can be measured with the child standing erect. The child should be positioned with feet flat, eyes looking straight ahead, and occiput, shoulders, buttocks, and heels against a vertical measuring board.

Figure 2-1 shows the National Center for Health Statistics percentiles for physical growth in girls and boys from birth through the age of 20 years. The Centers for Disease Control and Prevention recommends that health care providers for U.S. children use World Health Organization growth charts to monitor growth for infants and children aged 0 to 2 years and use Centers for Disease Control and Prevention growth charts to monitor growth for children aged 2 years and older.

Weight

Routinely *weigh infants unclothed*. For patients in whom small variations in weight are important, it is helpful to consistently use a single scale, preferably at the same time of day.

The growth charts in Figure 2-1 include body mass index (BMI) (wt/ht^2). This number is used in patients >2 years to determine whether weight is appropriate for height. By plotting BMI for age, health care providers can achieve early identification of patients at risk for being overweight/obese.

HEAD

Head Circumference

Start your examination of the head by measuring the head circumference at the maximum point of the occipital protuberance posteriorly and at the midforehead anteriorly. *Microcephaly* (small head size) could result from abnormalities such as craniosynostosis (premature fusion of the cranial sutures) or congenital TORCH (toxoplasmosis, other infections, rubella, cytomegalovirus, and herpes simplex) infection. *Macrocephaly* (large head size) could be caused by problems such as hydrocephalus or an intracranial mass. Figure 2-2 presents normal head circumferences.

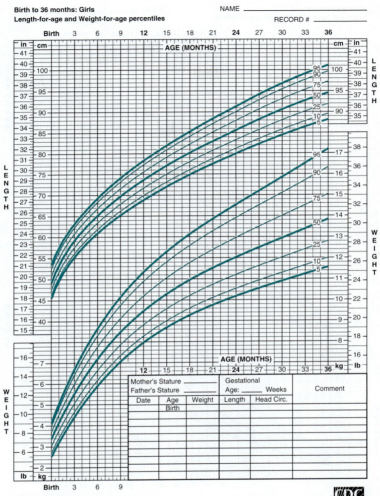

Birth to 36 months: Girls
Length-for-age and Weight-for-age percentiles

NAME _____

RECORD # _____

Published May 30, 2000 (modified 4/20/01).
SOURCE: Developed by the National Center for Health Statistics in collaboration
with the National Center for Chronic Disease Prevention and Health Promotion (2000).
http://www.cdc.gov/growthcharts

FIGURE 2-1   National Center for Health Statistics (NCHS). Clinical Growth Charts. A. Girls, birth to 36 months: Length-for-age and weight-for-age. (*continued*)

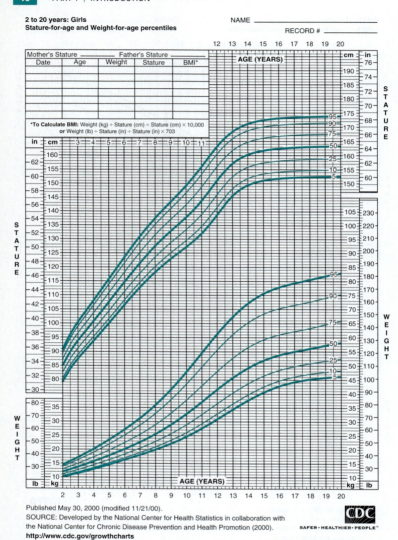

2 to 20 years: Girls
Stature-for-age and Weight-for-age percentiles

NAME _____

RECORD # _____

Published May 30, 2000 (modified 11/21/00).
SOURCE: Developed by the National Center for Health Statistics in collaboration with
the National Center for Chronic Disease Prevention and Health Promotion (2000).
http://www.cdc.gov/growthcharts

FIGURE 2-1 (*Continued*) **B.** Girls, 2–20 years: Stature for age and weight for age percentiles.

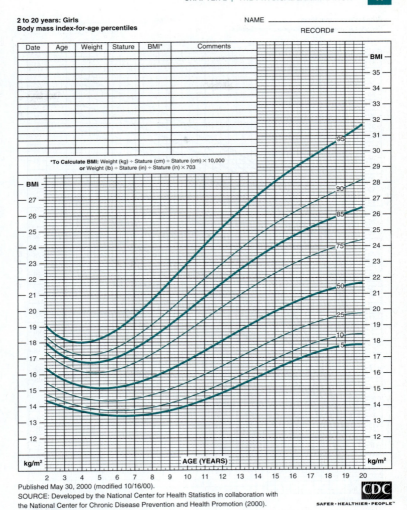

2 to 20 years: Girls
Body mass index-for-age percentiles

NAME _____

RECORD# _____

*To Calculate BMI: Weight (kg) ÷ Stature (cm) ÷ Stature (cm) × 10,000
or Weight (lb) ÷ Stature (in) ÷ Stature (in) × 703

Published May 30, 2000 (modified 10/16/00).
SOURCE: Developed by the National Center for Health Statistics in collaboration with
the National Center for Chronic Disease Prevention and Health Promotion (2000).
http://www.cdc.gov/growthcharts

FIGURE 2-1 (*Continued*) **C.** Girls, 2 to 20 years: Body mass index-for-age percentiles. (*continued*)

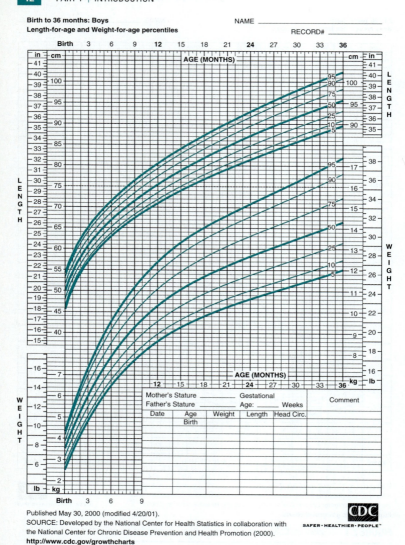

Birth to 36 months: Boys
Length-for-age and Weight-for-age percentiles

NAME _____

RECORD# _____

Published May 30, 2000 (modified 4/20/01).
SOURCE: Developed by the National Center for Health Statistics in collaboration with
the National Center for Chronic Disease Prevention and Health Promotion (2000).
http://www.cdc.gov/growthcharts

FIGURE 2-1 (*Continued*) **D.** Boys, birth to 36 months: length-for-age and weight-for-age percentiles.

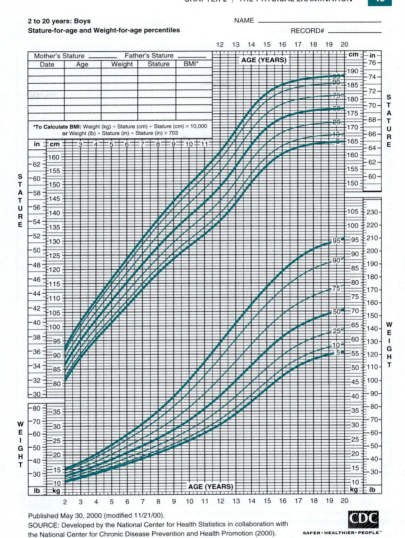

2 to 20 years: Boys
Stature-for-age and Weight-for-age percentiles

NAME _____

RECORD# _____

*To Calculate BMI: Weight (kg) ÷ Stature (cm) ÷ Stature (cm) × 10,000
or Weight (lb) ÷ Stature (in) ÷ Stature (in) × 703

Published May 30, 2000 (modified 11/21/00).
SOURCE: Developed by the National Center for Health Statistics in collaboration with
the National Center for Chronic Disease Prevention and Health Promotion (2000).
http://www.cdc.gov/growthcharts

FIGURE 2-1 (*Continued*) **E.** Boys, 2–20 years: Stature-for-age and weight-for-age percentiles. (*continued*)

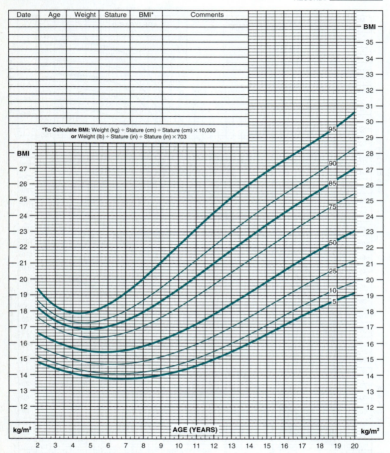

2 to 20 years: Boys
Body mass index-for-age percentiles

NAME _____

RECORD# _____

*To Calculate BMI: Weight (kg) ÷ Stature (cm) ÷ Stature (cm) × 10,000
or Weight (lb) ÷ Stature (in) ÷ Stature (in) × 703

Published May 30, 2000 (modified 10/16/00).
SOURCE: Developed by the National Center for Health Statistics in collaboration with
the National Center for Chronic Disease Prevention and Health Promotion (2000).
http://www.cdc.gov/growthcharts

FIGURE 2-1 (*Continued*) **F.** Boys, 2–20 years: Body mass index-for-age percentiles. (Centers for Disease Control and Prevention. http://www.cdc.gov/growthcharts/Default.htm. September 9, 2010). (Developed by the National Center for Health Statistics in collaboration with the National Center for Chronic Disease Prevention and Health Promotion [2000]. http://www.cdc.gov/growthcharts)

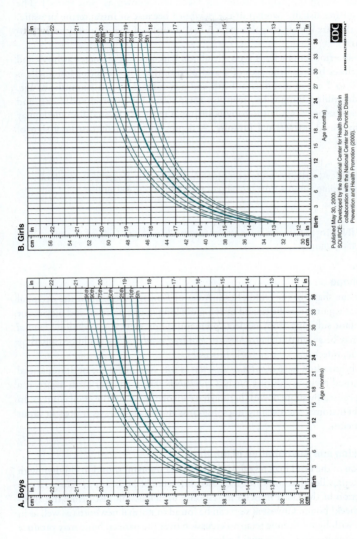

A. Boys

B. Girls

Age (months)

Published May 30, 2000.
SOURCE: Developed by the National Center for Health Statistics in collaboration with the National Center for Chronic Diseas Prevention and Health Promotion (2000).

FIGURE 2-2 Head circumference-for-age percentiles in **(A)** boys and **(B)** girls, birth to 36 months. (Developed by the National Center for Health Statistics in collaboration with the National Center for Chronic Disease Prevention and Health Promotion [2000])

15

Skull Depressions

Depressions of the skull may represent fractures but are most commonly *sutures* (i.e., membranous tissue spaces that separate the skull bones) and *fontanelles* (i.e., areas where the major sutures intersect; also known as "soft spots"). The cranial sutures usually overlap in the newborn because of intrauterine pressure. Sutures that are widely palpable after 5 to 6 months of age may indicate hydrocephalus.

The anterior fontanelle is typically about 1 to 4 cm in diameter at birth and usually closes between the ages of 4 and 26 months. The posterior fontanelle is usually 0 to 2 cm in diameter at birth and generally closes by 2 months of age. When describing fontanelles, mention their status (open or closed), size, and fullness. If palpated while the baby is sitting, a tense or elevated fontanelle may reflect increased intracranial pressure. A depressed fontanelle can be a sign of dehydration.

 HINT: At birth, the anterior fontanelle may appear closed as a result of overriding sutures from molding of the head during parturition.

 HINT: Try to examine the anterior fontanelle with the child calm and sitting upright.

Head Shape

Observe the shape of the child's head. Areas of *flatness,* especially in the occipital or parietal regions, may be caused by lying too long in one position and may occur in an infant suffering from neglect, prematurity, or mental retardation. *Frontal bossing* may be a sign of rickets. Areas of *localized head swelling* could be caused by neoplastic, infectious, or traumatic processes.

Newborns often have *caput succedaneum* (a soft swelling of the occipitoparietal scalp) caused by injury during birth. *Cephalohematoma,* another birth injury, is a swelling caused by subperiosteal hemorrhage involving one of the cranial bones. In cephalohematoma, the swelling does not cross the suture lines as it does in caput succedaneum.

Percussion and Auscultation of the Head

Percussion of the head may reveal *Macewen sign* (a resonant sound in children with closed fontanelles that indicates increased intracranial pressure) or *Chvostek sign* (contraction of the facial muscles in response to percussion just below the zygomatic [cheek] bone). Chvostek sign can be found in normal newborns as well as in children with hypocalcemic tetany. Percussion over the parietal bone may produce a "cracked-pot sound," a normal finding prior to suture closure.

Auscultation of the head for *bruits* is not particularly useful until late childhood. Systolic or continuous bruits may be heard in the temporal area until the age of 5 years. Abnormal conditions that may be associated with bruits include arteriovenous malformation, cerebral vessel aneurysms, brain tumors, and coarctation of the aorta.

Inspection of the Hair and Scalp

The child's hair should be assessed for quantity, color, texture, and infestations. Causes of *alopecia* include fungal infections (tinea capitis), stress (telogen effluvium), and excessive hair pulling (trichotillomania).

Dry, coarse hair may be a sign of hypothyroidism, and *fine, thin hair* may be seen in children with homocystinuria. In children with *pediculosis capitis* (head lice), close inspection reveals small adherent nits (eggs).

EYES

The eye examination is very important, providing information about the eyes and, in many cases, systemic problems. It is usually counterproductive (not to mention unkind) to try to pry a child's eye open. Instead, *distract the patient* with a toy or other object whenever possible to gain cooperation. A recalcitrant newborn can be encouraged to open his eyes by having an assistant gently rotate the baby from side to side while supporting him vertically (i.e., under the arms).

Assessment of the Eyes
Range of Motion and Orientation

Check for full range of motion by attracting the child's attention with a toy or piece of equipment. *Strabismus* (a condition in which the eyes do not move in a parallel manner) often manifests as *esotropia* (turning in of an eye) or *exotropia* (turning out of an eye). The following tests can be performed to test for strabismus:

- **Corneal light reflection.** Have the child focus on a small light. When the child is looking at the light, the reflection of the light from each cornea should be symmetrically placed. Asymmetries suggest the presence of strabismus.
- **Cover–uncover test.** The child focuses on a light, and one eye is covered and then uncovered. If either eye moves, strabismus may be present.

> **HINT:** Intermittent esotropia or exotropia in a young infant may be normal, but deviations beyond 6 months of age can cause permanent vision loss.

Distance Between the Eyes

Observe the distance between the eyes, which can be documented as either the inner canthal distance or the interpupillary distance. *Hypotelorism* (abnormal closeness of eyes) is frequently found with holoprosencephaly sequence, maternal phenylketonuria, trisomy 13, and trisomy 20p. *Hypertelorism* (increased distance between the eyes) is frequently associated with a wide number of syndromes, including Apert syndrome, DiGeorge sequence, fetal hydantoin effects, Noonan syndrome, trisomies 8 and 9p, and absence of the corpus callosum.

Nystagmus and "Setting Sun" Sign

Observe for nystagmus (rhythmical movements of the eyeballs) and "setting sun" sign (in which the eyes constantly appear to be looking downward). Nystagmus may be physiologic or it may be found with early loss of central vision, labyrinthitis, multiple sclerosis, intracranial tumors, or drug toxicity. "Setting sun" sign may be seen with hydrocephalus or intracranial tumor, but it may also be transiently noted in some healthy infants.

General Appearance

Check for an abnormal upward, outward *eye slant* and for *epicanthal folds* (vertical folds of skin over the medial portions of the eyes). Both can be associated with Down syndrome.

Assessment of the Individual Eyes
Visual Inspection

The following should be noted:

- **Pupil size and reaction to light**—both direct and consensual
- **Condition of the eyelids**—potential abnormalities include edema (swelling), erythema (redness), drooping, or the presence of masses
- **Hazy corneas**—causes include glaucoma and inborn errors of metabolism
- **Injected or inflamed conjunctivae**
- **Icteric sclerae**

> **HINT:** A jaundiced child has icteric sclerae, but a child with carotenemia (e.g., from excessively large feedings of carrots or sweet potatoes) has clear sclerae.

- **Brushfield spots on the irises**—small white spots frequently associated with Down syndrome
- **Excess tearing**—often caused by congenital obstruction of the nasolacrimal duct

Funduscopic Examination

In infants, a minimal funduscopic evaluation consists of evaluation of the *red reflex:* the ophthalmoscope is set at 0 diopters. At a distance of approximately 1 ft away from the patient, a reddish orange color (generally brightest in Caucasians) should be visible through the pupil. Leukocoria, a *white pupillary reflex,* can indicate serious disease, including cataracts, retinal detachment, or retinoblastoma. Inflammation or opacity of the *cornea* should be noted. Finally, if possible, the *optic disc and vessels* should be examined, ruling out fundal lesions and papilledema.

Vision Screening

The infant's vision should be screened using a brightly colored object. Note the infant's response and ability to track an object. Formal vision testing (often using the Snellen E Chart) can usually start at about 3 years of age (see Chapter 3, "Developmental Surveillance").

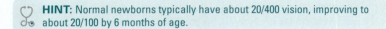

> **HINT:** Normal newborns typically have about 20/400 vision, improving to about 20/100 by 6 months of age.

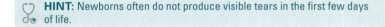

> **HINT:** Newborns often do not produce visible tears in the first few days of life.

EARS
External Examination
Rashes that favor the postauricular area include seborrheic dermatitis, measles, and rubella. *Pain* on gentle traction of the pinna or tragus can signal external otitis.

Otoscopic Examination
Before examining the tympanic membrane, ensure that any uncooperative child is *well restrained.* One simple method is to have the parent firmly hold the supine child's raised arms against either side of the head. This also allows easy access for the oral examination that follows.

> **HINT:** In an uncooperative child, press your otoscope hand against the patient's face. If the child suddenly moves despite proper restraint, the otoscope will move in tandem, decreasing the likelihood of injury.

It is also critical to *position the child's ear properly.* For an infant, pull the pinna down and back. For a school-aged child, pull straight back. For an adolescent, pull up and back.

- Check the tympanic membrane for *continuity.* Is it intact or perforated? Are there myringotomy tubes in place?
- Note the *color and degree of lucency.* Redness can indicate inflammation or merely be caused by a child's crying. A dull, purulent appearance indicates infection.
- Observe for *bulging* of the tympanic membrane, which suggests the presence of pus and fluid in the middle ear.
- Check for *visibility* of the bony landmarks and the cone of light reflex (which is absent with inflammation).
- Assess *mobility,* using a squeeze bulb. Poor movement can indicate the presence of fluid or purulent material in the middle ear.

Determining Hearing Acuity
Determining hearing acuity clinically is difficult in babies and young children. Watch the child's face as you make noise with a rattle or rustle paper behind each ear. Check to see whether the child is *startled* by the sound (usually by 1 month of age) or *looks toward the source* of the sound (by about 5 months of age).

HINT: One helpful approach to assessing hearing acuity in infants and young children is simply to ask the parents.

NOSE

Check the *nasal mucosae.* Pale, boggy mucosae with a watery discharge suggest allergy, whereas hyperemic mucosae with a mucopurulent discharge suggest infection. Be alert for the possibility of nasal *foreign bodies,* which often present with a unilateral, malodorous rhinorrhea. Examine the *nasal septum* for deviation, ulcerations, perforation, or bleeding. Check the *nasal turbinates* for bogginess or polyps.

 HINT: A newborn who is cyanotic when calm but pink when crying may have pulmonary disease with collapsed alveoli. Another possible diagnosis is choanal atresia (a congenital failure to develop openings between the nose and the nasopharynx).

ORAL CAVITY
Lips and Buccal Mucosa

Examine the lips for *asymmetry, fissures, clefts, lesions, and color.* Gray or purple lips may reflect cyanosis. Vigorous sucking can produce a callus on the lips. Small vesicles on an erythematous base can indicate herpes simplex infection.

Assess the buccal mucosae for *moistness* and check for *lesions.* For example, tiny blue-white dots on an erythematous base may be Koplik spots, an early sign of measles. Small white adherent plaques may be oral thrush (*Candida* infection). Note any *strange odors* to the breath (e.g., sweet [acetone], ammoniac [uremia]).

Tongue

Examine the tongue, checking for color, size, coating, and dryness. A bluish color to the tongue indicates central cyanosis, which reflects the presence of unsaturated hemoglobin. A "strawberry" *tongue* (characterized by large red papillae) may be seen with scarlet fever or Kawasaki disease.

Teeth and Oropharynx

Examine the *teeth* for number and condition. Observe the *tonsils* for color or exudate. Check the *palate* for a high arch, cleft, or mucosal lesions. The palates of newborns often have small whitish epithelial masses known as "Epstein pearls." Examine the *posterior pharynx* for exudate, vesicles, or bifid uvula.

NECK
Torticollis

Check for torticollis (fixed position of the head to one side), which may be *congenital or acquired.* Congenital torticollis may be caused by injury to the sternomastoid muscle. Acquired torticollis has many causes, including cervical spine disease, gastroesophageal reflux disease, posterior fossa or brainstem tumors, and infections within the head or the neck.

Range of Motion

Have the child touch the chin to the chest (to test the inferior cervical spine), look up and move the head side to side (to test the atlantoaxial joint), and bend the neck laterally ear to shoulder (to test the lower cervical spine). Always examine ill children for the presence of nuchal rigidity, which can signal the possibility of meningitis. To help rule out *nuchal rigidity* in a young child, encourage him to look up and down by shining a bright light or shaking noisy objects (e.g., keys).

> **HINT:** Children <2 years do not consistently develop nuchal rigidity with meningitis.

Palpation, Auscultation, and Visual Inspection of the Neck

Palpate the *thyroid gland,* evaluating both lobes for swelling, symmetry, consistency, and surface characteristics (e.g., smooth vs. nodular).

> **HINT:** Lymph nodes are relatively more prominent in children than in adults. Shotty cervical (as well as axillary and femoral) lymph nodes (up to 1 cm in diameter) are normal in children <10 years.

Auscultation may reveal a bruit, suggestive of thyrotoxicosis.

Examine the *neck* for other swellings or defects, including dermoid, branchial, and thyroglossal duct cysts. A thyroglossal duct cyst arises from a remnant of the embryonic thyroglossal duct. It is usually located in the midline, anywhere between the tongue and the hyoid bone. It should move up when the patient sticks out her tongue or swallows.

NEUROLOGIC SYSTEM

Assessment of Developmental Milestones

Assessment of a young child's developmental milestones is critical to the overall neurologic examination. Therefore, a *screening developmental examination,* such as Ages and Stages Questionnaires, should be a part of every well-child neurologic assessment from infancy to 6 years of age.

Assessment of Reflexes

Table 2-2 describes the examination of the infantile reflexes.

Test *deep tendon reflexes* using your finger, a reflex hammer, or the side of a stethoscope bell. Check for ankle or knee clonus (quick, repetitive muscle contractions). Bilateral clonus may be normal in an infant but can also reflect exaggerated muscle tone and deep tendon reflexes.

TABLE 2-2	Infantile Reflexes		
Reflex	**Usual Infant Age**	**Method of Elicitation**	**Description of Reflex**
Moro (startle) reflex	Birth to 4–6 mo	Lift the baby's head 15 and then let it fall gently into your hands	Arms suddenly extend and then flex; various movements of legs
Asymmetric tonic neck reflex	Birth to 4 mo	Place the baby supine, head turned to one side	Isolateral arm and leg extend; contralateral arm contracts like a fencer
Babinski reflex	Birth to 18 mo	Stroke the dorsum of the baby's foot	Toe dorsiflexion, fanning
Palmar grasp reflex	Birth to 4 mo	Place finger on the baby's palm	Involuntary grasping motion
Rooting reflex	Birth to 4 mo	Touch corner of the baby's mouth	Head turns to side, baby opens mouth
Parachute reflex	6–7 mo	Hold baby prone, move carefully downward	Extension of arms (to break fall)

Assessment of Cranial Nerve Function

Table 2-3 describes the examination of the cranial nerves.

Sensory Examination

Assess an infant's general sensation by checking for a response to light touch.

Assessment of Coordination

Assess the child's coordination as he reaches for a toy, crawls, or walks. Check for unusual muscle movements:

- **Fasciculations**—twitchings of groups of muscle fibers
- **Tremors**—trembling movements of the extremities
- **Chorea**—irregular, spastic, involuntary movements
- **Athetosis**—constant, slow, writhing movements, sometimes found in normal infants and in children with cerebral palsy and tuberous sclerosis
- **Spasmus nutans**—periodic head nodding, sometimes associated with gastroesophageal reflux disease, decreased intelligence quotient, or neuroblastoma, and often combined with nystagmus and head tilt

 HINT: The most critical part of the routine neurologic examination is your impression of the child's developmental abilities and general responsiveness. A reluctant toddler will often walk if her parent moves several steps away from her and offers encouragement. Entice the child to play with an interesting toy or other object.

TABLE 2-3 Examination of the Cranial Nerves

Cranial Nerve	Function	Elicitation Technique	Potential Abnormalities
I: Olfactory nerve	Smell	Cannot assess until child can speak	Absent responses
II: Optic nerve	Vision	In newborns, note response to objects brought from behind (peripheral vision) and ability to track objects in front (central vision)	Deviation from typical visual acuity vision testing (newborn = 20/400, improving to about 20/100 by 6 mo of age)
		Children >4 yr can undergo formal testing	
III: Oculomotor nerve	Elevation of upper eyelid, upward and downward gaze	Observe ocular movements and pupillary reflexes	Ptosis, pupil dilation, nystagmus
IV: Trochlear nerve	Upward gaze		
V: Trigeminal nerve	Chewing, sensation on face, forehead, lips, and tongue	Evaluate corneal reflexes; check facial sensation with a piece of gauze	Absent responses
VI: Abducens nerve	Lateral gaze		
VII: Facial nerve	Facial muscle control (eyelid closure, forehead wrinkling, asymmetry of face), taste (anterior two-thirds of tongue)	Check for facial symmetry at rest and when the child is smiling or crying	Asymmetry
VIII: Vestibulocochlear nerve	Hearing	In newborns, check for acoustic blink (in response to a loud noise); by 4 mo of age, baby should turn to sound	Absent responses
IX: Glossopharyngeal nerve	Taste (posterior two-thirds of tongue), elevation of palate, sensory gag reflex	Observe ability to handle secretions or beverages	Difficulty swallowing
X: Vagus nerve	Swallowing, movement of pharynx		
XI: Accessory nerve	Turning head, shrugging shoulders	Assess the child's posture	Head tilt or shoulder drop
XII: Hypoglossal nerve	Protrusion of tongue	Ask cooperative child to stick out tongue	Fasciculations or deviations from midline (tongue moves to side of lesion)

CHEST AND LUNGS
Shape of the Chest

A *barrel-shaped chest* in a child >6 years can be associated with acute asthma or a chronic pulmonary disease such as cystic fibrosis. *Pectus excavatum* (a funnel-shaped chest) is caused by a congenitally depressed sternum and costal cartilages. *Pectus carinatum* ("pigeon chest") is characterized by protrusion of the sternum and costal cartilages. Although this is often an idiopathic problem that is not associated with actual medical difficulties, pectus carinatum is sometimes caused by rickets or osteoporosis.

Assessment of Breathing

Check carefully for signs of *respiratory distress,* including nasal flaring, retractions, or grunting. Nasal flaring refers to a widening of the nostrils, which often occurs with each inspiration in respiratory distress. Retractions are movements of the spaces between the ribs, occurring with each breath in a child with respiratory distress. Grunting is an end-expiratory sound, most often heard in the newborn or infant with respiratory distress.

Percussion of the Lungs

Hyperresonance is usually caused by an increased amount of air in the chest (e.g., as in patients with asthma). *Dullness* is normally heard over the scapulae, liver, heart, and diaphragm.

Auscultation of the Lungs

In an infant, press the diaphragm of a small stethoscope firmly to the chest wall. Position the head in the midline, facing forward. Do not be reluctant to examine the lungs of a crying baby. Inspiratory sounds are actually enhanced by deep inspiration.

 HINT: Warm your stethoscope before auscultation.

Breath Sounds and Air Movement

Listen carefully for breath sounds, *comparing air movement* in the two lungs. Decreased breath sounds suggest decreased air exchange. It is important to evaluate air movement because a patient with severe asthma can have such overwhelming obstruction that no wheezing is heard. *The patient with severe asthma but no wheezing may be in impending respiratory failure!*

 HINT: Breath sounds tend to be harsher sounding (more bronchial) in children (as compared with adults) because the thinner chest wall of the child does not muffle the breath sounds as much.

Chest Sounds

Identify adventitious chest sounds:

- **Rales** are fine crackles, usually heard best at the end of inspiration, that generally reflect the presence of fluid or exudate in the alveoli. In patients with rales, consider bronchopneumonia, atelectasis, and congestive heart failure.
- **Rhonchi** are coarse inspiratory and expiratory sounds, caused by secretions in the upper airway. They are often caused by crying or upper respiratory infection.
- **Wheezes** are palpable and audible vibrations, often musical in character, produced when airflow is restricted. Expiratory wheezes are most common and typically reflect lower airway obstruction. Wheezes are most commonly found with asthma and bronchiolitis. Other causes include congestive heart failure and foreign body aspiration.

Extraneous Sounds

- **Peristalsis,** if heard in pulmonary examination, can suggest a diagnosis of diaphragmatic hernia (an abnormal opening of the diaphragm that allows the protrusion of abdominal contents into the chest).
- **A pleural friction rub** (a coarse grating sound with each breath) is occasionally present with pneumonia, lung abscess, or tuberculosis.

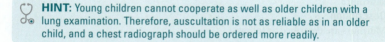

HINT: Young children cannot cooperate as well as older children with a lung examination. Therefore, auscultation is not as reliable as in an older child, and a chest radiograph should be ordered more readily.

CIRCULATORY SYSTEM

Many general physical examination clues can signal a child with cardiac disease. Typical observations include poor growth (weight affected more than length), developmental delay, cyanosis, clubbing of the fingers or toes, tachypnea, tachycardia, and peripheral edema. Routinely compare right-arm pulse strength with femoral pulse strength, which can be decreased in patients with coarctation of the aorta.

When examining the heart, first observe for *chest deformities* and *cardiac pulsations.* Palpate for the *point of maximum impulse (PMI).* In children <7 years, the heart's general horizontal position usually results in a PMI in the fourth intercostal space, to the left of the midclavicular line. In children >7 years, the PMI is usually in the fifth to sixth intercostal space within the midclavicular line. A PMI displaced down or lateral to these sites can indicate congestive heart failure.

The PMI may feel prominent in a thin child, in a child who has just finished exercising, or in a child who is anxious, febrile, in impending heart failure, or hyperthyroid. It is decreased in patients with pericardial or pleural effusions or pneumomediastinum (presence of gas or air in the mediastinal tissues). Thrills and pericardial friction rubs manifest as fine or coarse vibrations.

Listen with the child in both the *supine and sitting positions.* Listen over the whole precordium, especially at the apex, the pulmonic area (second interspace, left of the sternum), the aortic area (second interspace, right of the sternum), and the tricuspid valve (fourth interspace over the sternum). Listen for a split second heart sound (S_2), heard best over the pulmonic area during inspiration. (This finding is more obvious in school-aged children than in adults. It is usually only a potential problem if there is a large fixed split, such as that found with atrial septal defect.)

- **Are the heart sounds clear?** Distant sounds can suggest pericardial fluid.
- **Is there a third heart sound (S_3)?** (Usually heard at the apex, an S_3 may indicate mitral valve prolapse or atrial septal defect.)
- **Is there a gallop rhythm and other physical signs consistent with congestive heart failure?**

Rhythms

Sinus arrhythmia refers to the normal variation in pulse rate found with respiration. It is particularly prominent in young teenagers. Pulse rate increases with inspiration and decreases with expiration. *Premature ventricular contractions* are fairly common in the pediatric population. Generally, they should number less than six per minute at rest and decrease with exertion.

Murmurs
Description

Murmurs are described as follows:

- **Loudness**—reported as grades I to VI
- **Timing in the cardiac cycle**—described as diastolic or systolic, early or late
- **Pitch**—high or low
- **Quality**—blowing, musical, or rough
- **Location**—for example, apex, left lower sternal border
- **Transmission across the chest**—for example, radiating to the right lower sternal border

Innocent Murmurs

Nonpathologic murmurs typically heard in childhood include Still murmur and venous hum. Still murmur is the most common murmur in children between the ages of 2 years and adolescence. It is typically described as musical or vibratory, short, high pitched, early systolic, and grades I to III. It is usually heard best in the apical region. A venous hum is a continuous, low-pitched murmur heard under the clavicle and in the neck. It is caused by blood draining down the jugular vein (see Chapter 53, "Murmurs").

 HINT: The most important first step in assessing a murmur is to distinguish innocent from pathologic. Innocent murmurs are typically grade III or less, systolic in timing, and with no accompanying signs of cardiovascular disease.

ABDOMEN

A successful abdominal examination is especially reliant on having the *patient relaxed.* Place the patient in a supine position, with her knees bent and her arms at her sides. Warm your stethoscope and hands and then allow your hand to rest quietly for a moment on the patient's abdomen before making initial probing movements. To reduce ticklishness, place the child's hand on yours. Talking with the child about her siblings, friends, or school can be a useful distraction. It can also be helpful to allow children to examine your stethoscope while you examine them.

Abdominal Contour

Examine the abdominal contour. Is the abdomen flat, protuberant (common in toddlers), scaphoid (depressed, sometimes found with diaphragmatic hernia), or distended? Check for diastasis recti (vertical separation of the rectus abdominis muscles).

Abdominal Wall Motion

Respirations are generally abdominal in children <6 to 7 years. In young children, absence of abdominal wall motion may be caused by peritonitis, diaphragmatic paralysis, or large amounts of fluid or air in the abdomen. In older children, respirations that are mostly abdominal can indicate pneumonia or other pulmonary disorders.

Auscultation

Auscultation of the abdomen should be done *before palpation* to avoid altering the sounds of peristalsis. *Normal sounds* are short and metallic, occurring every 10 to 30 seconds. *Excessively frequent and high-pitched sounds* can indicate early peritonitis, gastroenteritis, or intestinal obstruction. *Absence of sounds* for >3 minutes can occur with paralytic ileus or peritonitis. Vascular obstruction may be indicated by a murmur over the aorta or renal arteries. It is especially important to check for vascular obstructions in any child with hypertension.

Percussion

Percussion can be useful to assess the liver (and occasionally the spleen) and to identify ascites, abdominal masses, or air in the gastrointestinal tract. Babies often have more swallowed air in their gastrointestinal tracts than adults do.

Percuss lightly in all *four quadrants* to assess general distribution of tympany and dullness. Tympany is generally the predominant sound. A distended abdomen with little tympany may contain fluid or solid masses. Dullness is typically found over the liver, over a full urinary bladder, or over masses.

To determine *liver span,* percuss the upper and lower borders in the right midclavicular line and measure the vertical distance. Normal spans are approximately 2 cm at 6 months, 4 cm at 3 years, 6 cm at 10 years, and 8 cm in adults. Causes of hepatomegaly include passive congestion, hepatitis, and tumor.

TABLE 2-4	Suggested Causes of Abdominal Tenderness According to Location
Location of Abdominal Tenderness	**Possible Causes**
Right upper quadrant	Acute hepatomegaly, hepatitis, intussusception
Left upper quadrant	Intussusception, splenic enlargement or rupture
Midline upper abdomen	Gastroenteritis, gastric or duodenal ulcer
Right lower quadrant	Appendicitis, abscess
Left lower quadrant	Constipation
Midline suprapubic area	Cystitis
Lower abdomen in general	Gastroenteritis, tumor, Meckel diverticulum, ovarian or testicular torsion
Poorly localized	Pneumonia, mesenteric adenitis, peritonitis, sickle cell crisis

Palpation

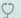 **HINT:** For crying children, palpate immediately on inspiration. The child often will relax his abdominal musculature for a moment.

Abdomen

Palpation of the abdomen is best done *on inspiration and on deep expiration.* Place one hand on the patient's back and the other on the abdomen. First palpate lightly, then deeply. Start in the left lower quadrant and continue in a clockwise manner. If any area seems tender, palpate that area last.

Rigidity (a tense abdomen) can indicate a surgical condition but is sometimes caused by voluntary muscle tightening in a frightened child.

Check for *tenderness,* trying to localize the point of maximum pain. The location of the tenderness can offer clues regarding the cause (Table 2-4). Rebound tenderness is associated with peritoneal inflammation.

 HINT: When checking for abdominal tenderness, ask a young child, "Does this feel OK?" Toddlers and preschoolers will often nod yes indiscriminately when asked whether something hurts. Facial expression is the most reliable sign of true tenderness.

Spleen

The spleen is often normally palpated in the first few years of life. It can be enlarged with infection (especially infectious mononucleosis), sickle cell or other hemolytic anemias, or leukemia (see Chapter 73, "Splenomegaly").

Liver

The liver generally can be palpated 1 to 2 cm below the right costal margin. Its edge is usually sharp and soft. A pathologically enlarged liver usually extends >2 cm below the right costal margin and has a rounded, firm edge (see Chapter 42, "Hepatomegaly").

Kidneys

In newborns, the kidneys can be gently trapped between the examiner's hands, allowing examination for masses. In all children, percussing gently over the costovertebral angles bilaterally can reveal tenderness over the kidneys.

GENITALIA

In infants, first assess the genitals for *ambiguity*. Is the baby "boy" really a virilized female with clitoromegaly and fused labial folds? Is the baby "girl" a male with a micropenis?

When examining children and teenagers, always respect the *patient's modesty*. Provide a gown and be sure to have a chaperone present.

Boys

- **Examine the glans penis and locate the meatus.** Is it ventrally displaced (hypospadias) or dorsally displaced (epispadias)? Observe for inflammation of the glans penis (balanitis) or of the prepuce (posthitis). Are there findings that may reflect injury (such as abrasions, bruising, or scarring) or infection (such as a penile discharge, vesicles, or verrucous lesions)?
- **Note whether the child has been circumcised.** In an uncircumcised boy, is there phimosis (i.e., an inability to retract the foreskin)? Normally, the foreskin is not retractable until 2 years of age.
- **Observe for scrotal masses.** Hydrocele is caused by an accumulation of fluid in the tunica vaginalis. You may demonstrate the fluid by shining a light to the scrotum. (Unlike inguinal hernias, hydroceles do not reduce.) Palpate for the testicles and note their location. In determining the presence of a retractile testis, it is helpful to have the boy sit cross-legged; the testes can then be "milked down" from the inguinal canal. Check for testicular masses.

Table 2-5 describes the Tanner staging of penis, testes, scrotum, and pubic hair development.

Girls

- **Observe the labia majora, labia minora, and clitoral hood/clitoris.** Are these structures well formed? Is there labial fusion? Are there signs of injury? Is the clitoris enlarged?
- **Examine the external genitalia by applying labial separation and traction to visualize the structures of the vaginal vestibule.** Observe the appearance of the hymenal orifice and note congenital variations and configuration of orifice. Are there acute or healed signs of injury or infection? Check for any abnormal degree of redness, vaginal discharge, or malodor. Also look for other signs of sexually transmitted diseases such as vesicles or verrucous lesions and for additional stigmata of trauma such as abrasions, bruising, or scarring. Consider the

TABLE 2-5	Tanner Staging of the Penis, Testes, Scrotum, and Pubic Hair

Tanner Stage	Penis	Testes	Scrotum	Pubic Hair
1	Immature	Small	Immature	None present
2	Immature	Initial enlargement	Initial rugae, reddening	Small amount near penile base
3	Initial enlargement	Continued enlargement	Increased rugae, reddening	Increased amount, distribution, coarseness, curl
4	Continued enlargement	Continued enlargement	Increased rugae, reddening	Increasing as above
5	Full adult	Full adult	Full adult	Adult amount and distribution (pubic area and medial thighs)

possibility of foreign bodies, which can present with particularly foul-smelling vaginal discharge.

- **Pelvic examinations** are done on females <21 years if a specific problem is suspected, and once yearly (to obtain cervical cytology) starting 3 years after the onset of sexual activity. In adolescent girls, the possibility of pregnancy should always be considered, even if the patient denies sexual experience.

Tanner staging of pubic hair in females is the same as in males (Table 2-5). Table 2-6 describes the Tanner staging of breasts.

RECTUM AND ANUS

Rule out fissures or anal prolapse. Check newborns for anal patency. A digital rectal examination is usually performed only if there are abdominal or rectal symptoms, a pelvic mass, or malformation. Check for sphincter tone, masses, and tenderness.

TABLE 2-6	Tanner Staging of Female Breasts

Tanner Stage	Breast	Areola
1	Prepubertal	Prepubertal
2	Small breast bud	Beginning enlargement
3	Continued development	Developing, continuous with breast
4	Continued development	Projection separate from breast
5	Full adult breasts	Flattened areola and protruding nipple

SKIN

- First, assess overall *skin color*. General erythema can reflect fever, sun exposure, or atropine toxicity. Pallor may be found in children with shock, anemia, or poor local circulation. Peripheral cyanosis (evidenced by bluish discoloration of the nail beds) can be caused by cold stress, local venous obstruction, or shock.

> **HINT:** In normal newborns, it is common for the hands and feet to be cyanotic, especially when they have been exposed to cold surroundings.

- Check for *skin pigmentation* (areas of generalized or localized color change). Hypopigmented lesions can be caused by tinea versicolor, vitiligo, tuberous sclerosis, or albinism. Bluish black lesions, especially over the lower back and buttocks in infants, are often Mongolian spots.
- **Vascular nevi** are commonly found in infants and children. Nevus flammeus lesions occur as flat, irregular pink patches. Strawberry hemangiomas are typically soft, compressible lesions. Port wine stains are flat markings embedded in the skin.
- **Burns** are classified as first degree (erythema only), second degree (erythema plus blister formation), and third degree (involving the subcutaneous tissue).
- **Skin puffiness** from edema (excess extracellular water and sodium) may be associated with renal, cardiac, or hepatic disease.

MUSCULOSKELETAL SYSTEM
Gross Deformities and Congenital Anomalies

Deformities are most commonly caused by *fractures* but can also be *congenital* (e.g., polydactyly [extra fingers or toes] or syndactyly [webbed or fused digits]).

> **HINT:** In evaluating injuries, consider child abuse if the damage is worse than accounted for by the history, if the child has multiple bruises, if there is a mixture of old and new injuries, or if there is a delay in seeking medical care.

Fingers and Toes

Observe the fingers and toes for *clubbing* (broadening and thickening of the terminal phalanges). Clubbing can be associated with many different systemic diseases, including congenital heart disease, pulmonary disease (e.g., cystic fibrosis), chronic hepatic disease, and gastrointestinal disorders (e.g., Crohn disease, ulcerative colitis).

Legs

Examine the shape of the leg bones:

- **Genu varum (bow-leggedness)** develops routinely in infants until about 18 months of age. Severe genu varum may be an indication of rickets or Blount disease (a growth disorder of the tibia).

- **Genu valgum (knock-knees)** is most often seen in children >2 years and often persists until adolescence.
- **Tibial torsion** is a twisting of the tibia thought to be caused by uterine pressure on the developing fetus. It often resolves spontaneously once the child begins walking.

Feet

In metatarsus adductus (inversion of the forefoot), the lateral border of the foot is "C" shaped instead of straight. The most serious congenital foot deformity is *clubfoot* (talipes equinovarus). This condition involves three major abnormalities: metatarsus adductus, fixed foot inversion, and equinus (or downward positioning of the foot).

 HINT: It is important to distinguish *rigid deformities,* which are more serious, from *flexible deformities*. With a flexible deformity, the foot can be brought to a normal position with gentle pressure.

Gait and Stance

Infants starting to walk typically have a wide-based gait that persists until approximately the age of 2 years.

- **Joints.** The joints should be examined for range of motion, warmth, redness, tenderness, and presence of effusion. In infants <6 months, always check for congenital hip dislocation using the Ortolani maneuver (Figure 2-3). Other useful signs of congenital hip dislocation are unequal leg length and asymmetric thigh skin folds.
- **Muscles.** Examine the muscles for tone by grasping the muscle and estimating its firmness during passive range of motion. Assess muscle strength, observing for weakness or paralysis. Look for contractures (fixed deformities that often have accompanying muscle atrophy). Check muscle mass, observing for atrophy or hypertrophy.
- **Spine.** Inspect the spine, observing for tufts of hair, dimples, abnormal coloration, masses, or cysts. Any of these can indicate spina bifida (a limited defect in the spinal column through which spinal membranes and spinal cord tissue may protrude). A small dimple anywhere in the midline can indicate a dermoid sinus (an epidermis-lined tract leading from the skin to the spinal cord that presents a risk of central nervous system infection). Check for spinal masses, including meningoceles, teratomas, or lipomas.
- **Posture.** Observe the child's posture, checking for abnormal spinal curvatures. In lumbar lordosis, the curve is anteroposterior, with the convexity anterior. Lumbar lordosis is usually normal for children but if severe can be a sign of rickets or abdominal wall weakness. In kyphosis, the anteroposterior curve of the spine has a posterior convexity. Scoliosis refers to a lateral curvature of the spine. All school-aged children and adolescents should be examined for scoliosis. Have the child bend forward, and look for unilateral elevation of the rib cage and hip.

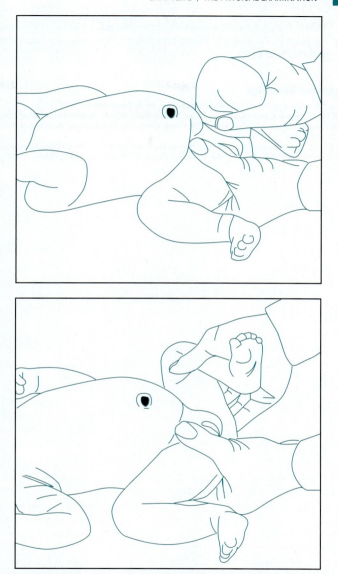

FIGURE 2-3   Ortolani maneuver to check for dislocated hip. With your index finger over the greater trochanter and your thumb over the inner thigh, flex the hip 90° and slowly abduct it from the midline. Feel for an abnormal "clunk" as a dislocated femoral head slips into the acetabulum.

HINT: The posture of the newborn often reflects the newborn's intrauterine position. For example, babies born breech often have very flexed hips and extended knees.

Suggested Readings

Barness LA. *Manual of Pediatric Physical Diagnosis.* 6th ed. St. Louis: Mosby; 1991.

Finkel M. The physical examination. In: Finkel M, Giardino's AP, eds. *Medical Evaluation of Child Sexual Abuse: A Practical Guide.* 3rd ed. Elk Grove Village, IL: The American Academy of Pediatrics; 2009;39–84.

Jones KL, ed. *Smith's Recognizable Patterns of Human Malformation.* 6th ed. Philadelphia: Saunders; 2005.

Zitelli BJ, Davis HW, eds. *Atlas of Pediatric Physical Diagnosis.* 5th ed. Philadelphia: Elsevier; 2007.

Developmental Surveillance

INTRODUCTION

Primary care physicians play a vital role in identifying children at risk for developmental disabilities and in referring them for appropriate early intervention services. Developmental surveillance involves using information obtained from the history, physical examination, and developmental screening tests to assess development on an ongoing basis. This ongoing monitoring of development is critical for two reasons. First, new circumstances (e.g., medical illness, family or environmental disruption, or injuries) may interfere with development. Second, as children develop, they gain new categories of skills that are difficult to assess at earlier stages (e.g., one cannot usually detect isolated language delays in children younger than 18 to 24 months, the point at which children begin to develop a good repertoire of language skills). In 2006, the American Academy of Pediatrics published guidelines recommending developmental surveillance at every well-child visit, as well as additional periodic developmental screening using a standardized test at the 9-, 18-, and 30-month-old visits.

HISTORY

The following information should be elicited:

- **Parental concerns regarding the child's development.** In most cases, parental concerns regarding the child's language development, articulation, fine motor skills, or global development are likely to be associated with true developmental delays. Parental concerns about behavior or personal–social skills are associated with developmental delays in some cases.
- **Risk factors for developmental disabilities** (Table 3-1).
- **Attainment of developmental milestones** (Table 3-2).

PHYSICAL EXAMINATION
Head Circumference

Brain growth is the principal stimulus for increasing head circumference. Therefore, a small head circumference may indicate abnormalities in brain growth that place a child at risk for developmental disabilities. A large head circumference may be a sign of hydrocephalus, a genetic syndrome, or a metabolic storage disease (see Chapter 51, "Macrocephaly"). However, before assuming pathology in a child, one should measure the head sizes of parents as a small or large head circumference may be a family trait.

TABLE 3-1	Risk Factors for Developmental Disabilities

Prenatal

Maternal illness, infection, or malnutrition

Maternal exposure to toxins, teratogens, alcohol, illicit drugs, anticonvulsants, antineoplastics, or anticoagulants

Decreased fetal movements

Intrauterine growth retardation

Family history of deafness, blindness, or mental retardation

Chromosomal abnormalities

Perinatal

Asphyxia: Apgar scores of 0–3 at 5 min

Prematurity, low birth weight

Abnormal presentation

Postnatal

Meningitis, encephalitis

Seizure disorder

Hyperbilirubinemia: bilirubin >25 mg/dL in full-term infant

Severe chronic illness

Central nervous system trauma

Child abuse and neglect

TABLE 3-2	Developmental Milestones from Birth to 5 Years of Age

Age (Months)	Adaptive/Fine Motor	Language	Gross Motor	Personal–Social
1	Grasp reflex (hands fisted)	Facial response to sounds	Lifts head in prone position	Stares at face
2	Follows object with eyes past midline	Coos (vowel sounds)	Lifts head in prone position to 45°	Smiles in response to others
4	Hands open Brings objects to mouth	Laughs and squeals Turns toward voice	Sits: head steady Rolls to supine	Smiles spontaneously
6	Palmar grasp of objects	Babbles (consonant sounds)	Sits independently Stands, hands held	Reaches for toys Recognizes strangers
9	Pincer grasp	Says "mama," "dada" non-specifically; comprehends- "no"	Pulls to stand	Feeds self Waves bye-bye
12	Helps turn pages of book	2–4 words Follows command with gesture	Stands independently Walks, one hand held	Points to indicate wants

(continued)

TABLE 3-2	Developmental Milestones from Birth to 5 Years of Age (*Cont.*)			
Age (Months)	Adaptive/Fine Motor	Language	Gross Motor	Personal–Social
15	Scribbles	4–6 words Follows command without gesture	Walks independently	Drinks from cup Imitates activities
18	Turns pages of book	10–20 words Points to four body parts	Walks up steps	Feeds self with spoon
24	Solves single-piece puzzles	Combines 2–3 words Uses "I" and "you"	Jumps Kicks ball	Removes coat Verbalizes wants
30	Imitates horizontal and vertical lines	Names all body parts	Rides tricycle using pedals	Pulls up pants Washes, dries hands
36	Copies circle Draws person with three parts	Gives full name, age, and sex Names two colors	Throws ball overhand Walks up stairs (alternating feet)	Toilet trained Puts on shirt, knows front from back
42	Copies cross	Understands "cold," "tired," and "hungry"	Stands on one foot for 2–3 sec	Engages in associative play
48	Counts four objects Identifies some numbers and letters	Understands prepositions (under, on, behind, in front of) Asks "how" and "why"	Hops on one foot	Dresses with little assistance Shoes on correct feet
54	Copies square Draws person with six parts	Understands opposites	Broad-jumps 24 in.	Bosses and criticizes Shows off
60	Prints first name Counts 10 objects	Asks meanings of words	Skips (alternating feet)	Ties shoes

> **HINT:** Microcephaly is defined as a head circumference <3rd percentile; macrocephaly is defined as a head circumference >97th percentile.

Congenital Anomalies or Dysmorphic Features

Congenital anomalies or dysmorphic features are associated with many genetic syndromes that may cause mental retardation or learning disabilities. Although a karyotype is a good initial screen, syndromes associated with small deletions

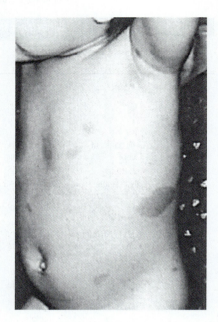

FIGURE 3-1   Patient with multiple café-au-lait spots. (Reprinted with permission from McMillan JA, et al., eds. *Oski's Pediatrics: Principles and Practice.* Philadelphia, PA: Lippincott Williams & Wilkins; 1999.)

(e.g., Williams syndrome, Prader–Willi syndrome, velocardiofacial syndrome) are not detected by a routine karyotype. Detecting these disorders requires the use of fluorescent in situ hybridization technology, using a probe for the specific region of the chromosome to be investigated. Genetics consultation is indicated when considering these tests.

Dermal Lesions of Neurocutaneous Syndromes

- **Ash leaf spots** are hypomelanotic macules found in 90% of patients with tuberous sclerosis. Ultraviolet light may be necessary to visualize the spots. One or two hypopigmented lesions may be seen in normal individuals. Approximately 50% of patients with tuberous sclerosis have mental retardation.
- **Café-au-lait spots** are light brown flat macules seen in patients with neurofibromatosis; they are also seen in 10% of the general population (Figure 3-1). They are more common on the trunk than on the extremities. Six or more lesions, >5 mm before puberty or >15 mm after puberty, should lead to investigation for other signs of neurofibromatosis. Patients with neurofibromatosis are at risk for hearing loss and learning disabilities.
- **Port wine nevus.** Ten percent of children with cutaneous angioma involving the upper face (forehead and eye) have an intracranial angioma (Sturge–Weber syndrome). Approximately 50% of patients with Sturge–Weber syndrome have mental retardation (Figure 3-2).

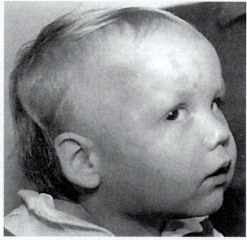

FIGURE 3-2   Patient with port wine nevus. (Reprinted with permission from McMillan JA, et al., eds. *Oski's Pediatrics: Principles and Practice.* Philadelphia, PA: Lippincott Williams & Wilkins; 1999.)

Muscle Tone
- **Hypertonia** (i.e., increased resistance of muscle groups to movement) may be a sign of cerebral palsy (CP), but in the first year of their life, children with isolated increases in muscle tone should not be diagnosed with CP as they may outgrow the problem.
- **Hypotonia** (i.e., decreased resistance of muscle groups to movement) occurs in infants with neuromuscular disorders or injury to the brain or spinal cord. Rarely, hypotonia is the only sign of a metabolic disorder (e.g., peroxisomal disorders, acid maltase deficiency). Hypotonia also occurs in some chromosomal disorders, such as Down syndrome, so obtaining a karyotype should be considered if the child is dysmorphic and hypotonic.

Primitive Reflexes
Asymmetries of primitive reflexes may help identify hemiplegias or other nerve injuries. Persistence of primitive reflexes beyond the time of usual disappearance (Table 3-3) or an obligate response may be signs of CP.

HEARING ASSESSMENT
Screening
Universal hearing screening during the newborn period is recommended because screening limited to infants with risk factors for hearing loss (Table 3-4) identifies

TABLE 3-3	Primitive Reflexes	
Primitive Reflex	**Age at Disappearance (Months)**	**Description**
Palmar grasp	3–4	Pressing against the palmar surface of the infant's hand results in flexion of all fingers.
Rooting	3–4	Stroking the perioral skin at the corners of the mouth causes the mouth to open and turn to stimulated side.
Galant	2–3	Stroking along the paravertebral area causes lateral flexion of the trunk with the concavity toward the stimulated side.
Moro	4–6	Sudden movement of the head causes symmetric abduction and extension of the arms followed by gradual adduction and flexion of the arms over the body.
Asymmetric tonic neck	4–6	Turning the head to one side leads to extension of extremities on that side and flexion on the contralateral side, putting the infant in the "fencing" position.
Tonic labyrinthine	2–3	In the supine position, neck extension leads to shoulder retraction and trunk and lower extremity extension that is reduced by neck flexion.
Positive support	2–3	Stimulation of the ball of the foot leads to cocontraction of opposing muscle groups, allowing weight to be borne.
Placing/stepping	Variable	When the dorsal surface of one foot touches the underside of a table, the infant places the foot on the tabletop.

TABLE 3-4	Risk Factors for Hearing Impairment

Family history of deafness
Congenital TORCH infections: toxoplasmosis, other infections, rubella, cytomegalovirus, and herpes simplex
Congenital malformation of the head and neck
Prematurity (<1,500 g at birth)
Extended stay in neonatal intensive care unit (>48 hr)
Hyperbilirubinemia requiring exchange transfusion
Meningitis or encephalitis
Anoxia

only half of infants with significant hearing impairment. Approximately three-quarters of the 50 states mandate this screening. The most cost-effective screening method is still the subject of some debate, but the currently available methods include otoacoustic emissions and auditory brainstem responses.

- **Otoacoustic emissions (OAEs).** OAEs refer to sounds that are thought to originate from the hair cells of the cochlea. Auditory threshold refers to the decibel (dB) level at which the response is no longer detected. In individuals with an auditory threshold of ≥20 dB, OAEs can be evoked by presenting clicking sounds to the ear. If the auditory threshold is above 30 to 40 dB, the evoked OAEs are absent. The test takes 2 to 5 minutes to administer and is relatively inexpensive. However, fluid in the middle ear or debris in the auditory canal may interfere with the test, leading to a false-positive rate as high as 10% in the newborn period.

- **Auditory brainstem response (ABR).** Electroencephalogram (EEG) electrodes attached to the forehead and behind the ears detect brain activity in response to 30 to 40 dB clicks presented to an ear. Absence of the expected brain activity suggests an abnormality of hearing. The test takes 5 to 15 minutes to perform and is significantly more expensive than OAE testing, but the false-positive rate is lower (2% to 3%).

In some locations, a two-step screening process is applied in which those who fail OAEs are screened by ABRs and only those who fail both screens are referred for further evaluation. This two-step process may have the lowest false-positive rate.

 HINT: Expressive language milestones (e.g., laughing, cooing, and babbling) can be misleading because deaf infants also exhibit these milestones in the first 4 to 6 months. By ~12 months of age, the babbling in deaf infants decreases but continues to increase in hearing infants and sounds more like baby talk.

Formal Hearing Testing

- **0–6 months: Auditory evoked responses (AERs).** The use of AERs as a screening test was described earlier. When the test is done by an audiologist, the intensity of the sound can be varied so the auditory threshold can be obtained. This test is highly sensitive (false-negative results are rare), but a false-positive result is also possible. Therefore, positive test results should be confirmed by audiometry when the child is old enough.

- **6–24 months: Visual reinforcement audiometry.** A sound is paired with a visual event (e.g., a doll's eyes light up). Once the child has learned the association, she looks toward the doll in anticipation of the visual event when a sound is heard.

- **2–5 years: Conditioned play audiometry.** The child is asked to engage in a play task every time a sound is heard.

- **Older than 6 years: Standard audiometry.**

VISION ASSESSMENT

The **detection of amblyopia** is the most important reason for early vision screening as early detection can prevent vision loss in the "neglected" eye. The most common causes of amblyopia are **strabismus** (see Chapter 2, "The Physical Examination") and **anisometropia** (an eye with a refractive error of ≥1.5 diopters than its pair).

Visual acuity improves with age. Newborns should be able to fixate on a face; by 1 to 2 months of age, infants should be able to follow an object horizontally across their visual field. By 6 months of age, visual acuity is about 20/100, and at 3 years it is 20/30 to 20/40. By 5 to 6 years of age, children should have 20/20 vision.

Office vision screening using the Snellen chart can be performed with children who know the letters of the alphabet. Variations of this test, such as the tumbling "E" chart and the Allen chart, have been developed for younger children. When using the tumbling "E" chart, the child is asked to point in the direction of the "legs" of the letter. The Allen chart contains pictures of toys, animals, and other familiar objects.

DEVELOPMENT SCREENING TESTS
General Development
Ages 0–5 Years: Ages and Stages Questionnaires

The Ages and Stages Questionnaires is a series of parent-completed questionnaires that assess the domains of communication, gross motor, fine motor, problem-solving, and personal adaptive skills. Norms are based on test administration to 2,008 children from diverse ethnic and socioeconomic backgrounds. Responses generate a pass/fail score; failing scores indicating possible need for further evaluation. Additional information about this questionnaire is available at www.brookespublishing.com/store/books/squires-asq/system.htm

Ages 0–8 Years: Parents' Evaluation of Developmental Status (PEDS)

This parent-completed questionnaire elicits parental concerns about aspects of the child's development and behavior. Based on the response of the parents to questions, an algorithm guides the clinician in determining whether the child needs referral, additional screening, or continued surveillance. Additional information on this test is available at www.pedstest.com

Autism Screening
Ages 16–30 Months: Modified Checklist for Autism in Toddlers (M-CHAT)

This parent-completed questionnaire is designed to identify children at risk of autism spectrum disorder. The screen is considered positive if the answer of the parent is "no" to any 3 of the 23 items or any 2 out of 6 critical items. Additional information on this test is available at www.firstsigns.org

Language Development
Age >2 Years 6 months: Peabody Picture Vocabulary Test-IV (PPVT-IV)

The PPVT-IV tests receptive language skills. From a group of four pictures, the patient must select a picture that best illustrates a specific word. A progressively

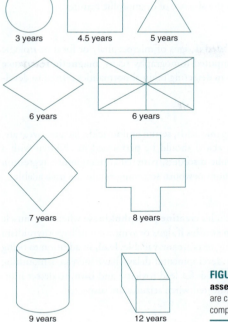

3 years	4.5 years	5 years
6 years	6 years
7 years	8 years
9 years	12 years

FIGURE 3-3   Gesell figures used to assess visual-motor skills. Children are capable of drawing progressively more complex shapes.

more difficult sequence of words and pictures is administered until the patient is no longer identifying the correct picture at a frequency higher than chance. Scores tend to correlate well with the verbal IQ. Additional information on this test is available at http://ags.pearsonassessments.com

Visual-Motor Skills
Ages 3–12 Years: Gesell Figures
Children develop the ability to draw progressively more complex figures in a predictable manner (Figure 3-3).

LABORATORY EVALUATION
Genetic Testing
In the etiologic workup of children with developmental delay or mental retardation, a **single nucleotide polymorphism (SNP) array analysis and Fragile X** testing should be performed. If SNP testing is normal, a **karyotype** may be considered to evaluate for balanced alterations. Additional genetic testing includes testing for the **MECP2** mutation in girls with severe delays (see Chapter 4, "Developmental

Disabilities"). ~5% to 10% of children with global developmental delays have abnormal genetic testing, even in the absence of dysmorphic features.

Neurologic Studies

Neuroimaging should be considered if signs of microcephaly or focal neurologic are present. Compared with computed tomography scans, **magnetic resonance imaging** scans are more sensitive in detecting brain abnormalities related to developmental delay.

Metabolic Studies

Metabolic testing (e.g., urine organic acids, serum amino acids, lactate, pyruvate, ammonia, very long chain fatty acids) should be performed in children with a positive family history of metabolic disorders, parental consanguinity, regression of developmental skills, or for whom newborn screening results are unavailable.

Additional Studies

Additional laboratory testing includes **creatine phosphokinase** when low muscle tone is present; **thyroid function studies** if signs or symptoms of hypothyroidism are present or if newborn screening tests are unavailable; **lead,** in addition to being a causative agent, children with developmental delays have increased mouthing behaviors, thereby increasing their risk for lead toxicity; and **iron,** to detect iron-deficiency anemia. An **EEG** is indicated when seizures are suspected.

Suggested Readings

American Academy of Pediatrics, Council on Children with Disabilities, Section on Developmental Behavioral Pediatrics, Bright Futures Steering Committee, Medical Home Initiatives for Children with Special Needs Project Advisory Committee. Identifying infants and young children with developmental disorders in the medical home: an algorithm for developmental surveillance and screening. *Pediatrics.* 2006;118(1):405–420.

Friendly DS. Development of vision in infants and young children. *Pediatr Clin N Am.* 1993;40:693–703.

Garganta C, Seashore MR. Universal screening for congenital hearing loss. *Pediatr Ann.* 2000;29:302–308.

Glascoe FP. Early detection of developmental and behavioral problems. *Pediatr Rev.* 2000;21:272–280.

Jones KL. *Smith's Recognizable Patterns of Human Malformation.* Philadelphia, PA: WB Saunders; 1997.

Liptak GS. The pediatrician's role in caring for the developmentally disabled child. *Pediatr Rev.* 1996; 17:203–210.

Developmental Disabilities

INTRODUCTION

When caring for children with developmental disabilities, the physician must consider possible causes for the disorder, screening for problems associated with the disorder, and interventions to minimize functional impairment and prevent long-term complications.

CEREBRAL PALSY

Definition and Etiology

Cerebral palsy (CP) is a nonprogressive disorder of motion and posture that results from injury to the developing central nervous system. It occurs in 1.5 to 2.5 children per 1,000 live births. **Prematurity** is the single most significant risk factor; approximately 8% to 10% of infants with a birth weight <1,500 g develop CP. Although **perinatal asphyxia** was once thought to be a major cause of CP, it is now thought to cause <10% of cases. A genetic abnormality can be identified in about 10% of cases and is more likely to be found in a term infant with CP than a preterm infant. In approximately 15% to 20% of patients, **no cause** can be identified.

Classification

- **Spastic.** This form of CP is characterized by increased deep tendon reflexes and increased muscle tone with a "clasp knife" quality (i.e., initially, resistance to movement is strong but then the muscle gives way suddenly). It can be further subclassified based on the limbs that are involved:
  - Hemiplegia: Involves both the arm and the leg on either the left or the right side of the body.
  - Quadriplegia: Significant impairment in all four extremities.
  - Diplegia: Bilateral leg involvement; arms may have mild impairment.
- **Extrapyramidal.** The most common form of extrapyramidal CP is choreo-athetoid CP, which is characterized by sudden involuntary movements of the extremities. Muscle tone is variable within the individual over time. The resistance to movement is described as "lead pipe" rigidity (i.e., persistent pressure results in slow movement of the limb).
- **Mixed.** Components of both spastic and choreoathetoid CP are present.

Associated Problems

- **Cognitive deficits**—mental retardation (50%) and learning disabilities.
- **Speech and language deficits**—communication disorders and dysarthria.
- **Sensory deficits**—visual impairment, strabismus, and hearing impairment.
- **Gastrointestinal problems**—oral-motor dysfunction, gastroesophageal reflex disease, and constipation.
- **Urinary tract problems**—spastic bladder and recurrent urinary tract infection.
- **Neurologic problems**—spasticity and seizures.
- **Musculoskeletal problems**—joint contractures, dislocated hips, and scoliosis.
- **Psychosocial and behavioral problems.**

 HINT: Multiple methods are available for managing spasticity and preventing or managing contractures for individuals with spastic CP, including physical therapy and positioning, oral medications (e.g., baclofen, dantrolene, and diazepam), botulinum toxin injections, intrathecal baclofen, and surgery (e.g., tendon lengthening and dorsal rhizotomy).

MYELOMENINGOCELE
Definition and Etiology

A myelomeningocele is a sac containing meninges and a malformed spinal cord that protrudes through defective vertebrae (in contrast, a meningocele is a sac containing only meninges; the spinal cord is normal).

Myelomeningoceles develop ~28 days after conception if the neural tube fails to close. The incidence varies with ethnicity and geography and ranges from one to five per 1,000 live births. The cause of this defect is not known, but both environmental exposures and genetic factors are important. **Maternal oral folic acid supplementation** prior to conception and throughout the first trimester reduces the risk of myelomeningocele by 50% to 70%. The risk of recurrence in the family of a child with a myelomeningocele is 15 to 30 times higher than in the general population; myelomeningocele may also occur in association with a chromosomal abnormality.

Classification

The level of the lesion is predictive of the degree of functional impairment. Difficulties with bowel and bladder function occur with virtually all lesions.

- **Thoracic lesions**—flaccid paralysis of both lower extremities with weakness of the trunk musculature
- **L1 to L2 lesions**—flaccid paralysis of the knees, ankles, and feet with voluntary hip flexion and adduction
- **L3 lesions**—same as L1 to L2 lesions, but knee flexion is present as well
- **L4 to L5 lesions**—knee flexion and extension and ankle dorsiflexion are present, but plantar flexion and hip extension are weak or absent
- **Sacral lesions**—mild weakness of ankles and toes

Associated Problems

The degree and type of associated problems are also related to the level of the lesion.

- **Cognitive deficits**—mental retardation (33%) and learning disabilities
- **Neurologic problems**—hydrocephalus (70% to 80%) and Arnold-Chiari deformity (type II)
- **Urinary tract problems**—incontinence, recurrent urinary tract infection, vesicoureteral reflex, and kidney damage
- **Bowel dysfunction**—incontinence and constipation
- **Musculoskeletal disorders**—scoliosis and hip dislocation
- **Sexual dysfunction**—partial erection and retrograde ejaculation
- **Ophthalmologic disorders**—strabismus
- **Dermatologic disorders**—decubitus ulcers

> **HINT:** At a few centers, fetal surgery to close the myelomeningocele is being done late in the second or early in the third trimester of the pregnancy. Although results are preliminary, this type of surgery seems to have the potential to decrease the neurologic impairment.

INTELLECTUAL DISABILITY (FORMERLY KNOWN AS MENTAL RETARDATION)

Definition and Etiology

Intellectual disability (ID) is defined as **"significant limitations in both intellectual functioning and adaptive behavior expressed in conceptual, social, and practical adaptive skills and age of onset before the age of 18"** (American Association on Intellectual and Developmental Disabilities, Washington, DC, 2010).

> **HINT:** Intellectual disability cannot be diagnosed from an intelligence test alone. The individual must also have a deficit in adaptive behavior.

The likelihood of identifying the cause of a patient's ID depends on the severity of the disability. A cause can be identified in ~50% of patients with mild ID, and in 80% of patients with severe or profound ID. **Chromosomal abnormalities** (e.g., Down syndrome and fragile X syndrome) are the most commonly identified causes of ID. Other causes of ID include perinatal or postnatal injury, teratogens (e.g., fetal alcohol syndrome), intrauterine infection, and inborn errors of metabolism.

Classification

Descriptions of an individual's strengths, weaknesses, and the level of support needed (intermittent, limited, extensive, or pervasive) are most helpful in planning for educational/vocational, social/recreational, and daily living needs.

IQ-based subclassifications are often used but are not as helpful for intervention planning.

- Mild ID: IQ 50–55 to ~70
- Moderate ID: IQ 35–40 to 50–55
- Severe ID: IQ 20–25 to 35–40
- Profound ID: IQ below 20–25

HINT: For IQ scores in the ranges that overlap between subclassifications, the individual's adaptive functioning should be used to determine the appropriate subclassification.

HINT: Developmental testing results in the toddler and preschool years are often described as a development quotient (DQ) as opposed to an IQ. A DQ equals the mental age divided by the chronological age, multiplied by 100. For example, a 4-year-old functioning at a 2-year-old level would have a DQ of 50.

Associated Problems

For children with a specific syndrome, the associated problems are related to the syndrome. In general, children with ID are at increased risk for **hearing or visual deficits,** which occur in up to 25% of children with mild ID and in >50% of children with severe ID. **Seizures and behavior problems** ranging from hyperactivity to self-injury occur with increased frequency in this population.

HINT: Physicians tend to underestimate the capabilities of children with ID. Many children diagnosed with mild ID function independently in the community as adults.

PERVASIVE DEVELOPMENT DISORDER
Definition and Etiology

Pervasive developmental disorder (PDD) encompasses a variety of disorders (e.g., autistic disorder, Asperger syndrome, Rett disorder) characterized by impairments in **reciprocal social interactions, communication skills, and a restricted range of interests and behaviors**. Many children engage in stereotyped behaviors and adhere inflexibly to nonfunctional routines. PDD is sometimes referred to as an "autism spectrum disorder" (ASD).

The prevalence of ASD has been rising over the past two decades and is currently estimated to be about 1 in 110 children with a male-to-female ratio of approximately 4:1. It is unclear whether this rise in prevalence is because of changing diagnostic criteria, a true increase in incidence, or a combination of both. These disorders are likely caused by damage to the brain or abnormal development of the brain. There is a strong genetic contribution; the incidence of ASD in siblings of affected children is 5 to 15 times higher than in the general population. Evidence does not support an association between immunizations and ASD.

Most cases of classic Rett syndrome have recently been discovered to be caused by mutations in a gene on the X chromosome that codes for methyl-CpG-binding protein 2 (MECP2). Interestingly, not all females with this mutation have Rett syndrome (perhaps related to X chromosome inactivation patterns). It was previously thought that this mutation was almost always lethal in males, but recent studies have described varying phenotypes of MECP2 mutations in males to include severe encephalopathies (leading to early infant death), a Rett-like syndrome, developmental delay with seizures, and nonspecific MR.

Classification
- **Autistic disorder**—severe impairments in reciprocal social interactions, communication skills, and restricted or repetitive interests and behaviors.
- **Asperger syndrome**—severe impairments in social interactions, frequent repetitive behaviors, and a restricted range of interests or activities but no significant delays in language skills or global cognitive skills.
- **PDD-not otherwise specified (PDD-NOS)**—problems such as those described for autistic disorder and Asperger syndrome but not of sufficient severity to meet criteria for one of these diagnoses.
- **Rett disorder**—characterized by loss of speech, loss of purposeful hand movements, acquired microcephaly, and atypical breathing patterns.
- **Childhood disintegrative disorder**—characterized by the loss of skills in multiple areas of functioning after at least 2 years of normal development; a diagnosis of exclusion after metabolic and neurodegenerative disorders are ruled out.

> **HINT:** Children with autistic disorder may learn a few words and then stop using them between 12 and 24 months of age. However, they should not lose more complex language skills or skills in other areas.

Associated Problems
- **Cognitive deficits**—mental retardation (60% to 70% of patients with autistic disorder) and learning disabilities.
- **Neurologic problems**—seizure disorder.
- **Psychosocial and behavioral problems**—hyperactivity, unusual responses to sensory input, self-injurious behaviors, and schizophrenia.

HEARING IMPAIRMENT
Definition and Etiology
Table 4-1 summarizes the causes of hearing loss.

- **Conductive hearing loss** is caused by damage to the external or middle ear. Hearing is decreased for sound conducted by air, but sounds conducted by bone are heard normally.
- **Sensorineural hearing loss** is caused by damage to the cochlea or auditory nerve. Both bone and air conduction of sound are abnormal.

TABLE 4-1	Causes of Hearing Loss

Congenital
Genetic syndromes (e.g., Waardenburg, Usher, and craniofacial)
Familial deafness (70–80% autosomal recessive)
Congenital toxoplasmosis, other infections, rubella, cytomegalovirus, and herpes simplex (TORCH) infection
Ototoxic drugs taken during first trimester

Acquired
Genetic syndromes (e.g., Alport syndrome, Alström syndrome, and neurofibromatosis)
Meningitis or encephalitis
Prematurity
Hyperbilirubinemia requiring exchange transfusion
Birth anoxia (Apgar score 0–3 at 5 min)
Ototoxic medications
Trauma

- **Central hearing loss** is characterized by absent or distorted auditory brainstem response, with intact otoacoustic and cochlear function.
- **Anacusis** is total hearing loss.

Classification

Table 4-2 summarizes the degrees of hearing loss. Individuals with moderate hearing loss miss most speech sounds at normal conversational levels.

Associated Problems

Associated problems largely depend on the cause of the hearing impairment and when the impairment develops. Difficulties with reading skills and behavioral disturbances are more common than in the general population.

VISION IMPAIRMENT
Definition and Etiology

Most classification schemes would consider an individual visually impaired if the corrected visual acuity in the best eye was 20/60 or worse. In the United States,

TABLE 4-2	Classification of Hearing Loss

Degree of Hearing Loss	Decibel Level at Which Sounds Become Inaudible
Slight	16–25
Mild	26–40
Moderate	41–65
Severe	66–95
Profound	≥96

TABLE 4-3	Causes of Vision Impairment

Congenital

Congenital toxoplasmosis, other infections, rubella, cytomegalovirus, and herpes simplex (TORCH) infections

Malformations of visual system (coloboma, aniridia, and retinal dysplasia)

Cataracts

Glaucoma

Acquired

Retinopathy of prematurity

Strabismus

Genetic syndromes (may be associated with either congenital or acquired vision loss)

Macular disease

Tumors (e.g., retinoblastoma)

Trauma

Infection

Anoxia (associated with cortical visual impairment)

the legal definition of blindness is a best corrected visual acuity of 20/200 or a peripheral visual field restricted to 20° or less. Table 4-3 summarizes the causes of vision impairment.

Associated Problems

- **Cognitive deficits**—mental retardation (20% to 25% of blind children).
- **Speech and language deficits**—developmental delays (imitation of mouth movements is an important component of speech development).
- **Psychosocial and behavioral problems**—stereotypic and self-injurious behavior.

 HINT: Blind children with normal intelligence have developmental delays. Gross motor skills (e.g., sitting) develop about 2 months later in blind children than in sighted children, and a blind child may begin to walk 3 to 7 months later than a sighted child. Signs of attachment may also occur at different times. Stranger anxiety occurs at approximately the same time as it does in sighted children, but separation anxiety does not develop until later.

SPEECH AND LANGUAGE DISORDERS
Definition and Etiology

Speech refers to the sounds used to communicate information, and language refers to the system by which the sounds are given meaning. Language disorders are present when a child's skills at using language are significantly below her nonverbal cognitive skills.

Language disorders may be acquired through a brain injury or they may be congenital. In some cases, differences in the processing of auditory information are thought to be the cause of congenital language disorders.

HINT: Always test the child's hearing.

 HINT: Assess verbal and nonverbal skills. For many children with MR, the initial concern is often about the child's language skills.

Classification

- **Expressive language disorder**—the child's ability to formulate ideas into words is below the ability to understand language and perform nonverbal skills.
- **Mixed receptive-expressive language disorder**—the child's ability to formulate ideas into words and to understand language is below the nonverbal cognitive skills.
- **Phonological disorder**—the child is not able to use speech sounds that are appropriate for age and dialect.

Associated Problems

- **Language-based learning disabilities**—for example, reading, spelling, and writing disorders.
- **Behavioral problems.**

LEARNING DISABILITIES
Definition and Etiology

The 2004 reauthorization of the Individuals with Disabilities Education Act continues to define a learning disability as "a disorder in one or more of the basic psychological processes involved in understanding language, spoken or written, which may manifest itself in an imperfect ability to listen, speak, read, write, spell, or do mathematical calculations." However, the law no longer requires that children with learning disabilities be identified on the basis of a severe discrepancy between actual and expected achievement. Instead, the law encourages schools to consider how the child responds to evidence-based instructional interventions in determining whether the child has a learning disability.

 HINT: One criticism of the discrepancy criteria in identifying learning disabilities is that it required children to be significantly behind peers before they could be diagnosed and receive interventions.

Learning disabilities may occur along with other conditions but are not the direct result of sensory impairments, mental retardation, social-emotional disturbance, cultural differences, or inappropriate instruction. Although the cause of learning disabilities is not known, **genetic factors** appear to play a vital role. Multiple members of a family often have learning disabilities, although the pattern does not follow classic Mendelian inheritance. In addition, learning disabilities occur with increased frequency in many **genetic syndromes**.

Classification

Dyslexia, reading and learning disability, is the most common learning disability. Learning disabilities may also occur in the areas of math, spelling, and written expression. Reading disability is usually related to deficits in phonemic awareness; thus, individuals with reading disability often have difficulty with other language-based skills such as spelling. Children with nonverbal learning disability often have problems with math, visual-perceptual, fine motor, organizational, and social skills.

Associated Problems

- **Psychosocial and behavioral problems**—attention deficit hyperactivity disorder (ADHD), low self-esteem, and school avoidance.

> **HINT:** Having a child repeat a grade is not an appropriate intervention for a learning disability. Physicians should insist that a psychoeducational evaluation be performed on any child having difficulty in school. There are few situations in which repeating a grade is an appropriate intervention.

ATTENTION DEFICIT HYPERACTIVITY DISORDER

Definition and Etiology

ADHD is characterized by developmentally inappropriate levels of **inattention, impulsivity, and hyperactivity**. In almost all cases, school functioning is impaired. Many children also have difficulties in meeting expectations at home and in social relationships.

Research suggests that individuals with ADHD may have decreased activity of basal ganglia and frontal lobe neurons involving the dopamine and norepinephrine neurotransmitter systems. Genetics is the strongest predictor of increased risk for ADHD. Other factors that increase the risk for ADHD include prenatal exposure to environmental toxins (e.g., cigarette smoke and alcohol) and postnatal brain injury (e.g., infections, inborn errors of metabolism, trauma).

> **HINT:** "Developmentally inappropriate" levels of inattention or activity are difficult to define. Clinically, standardized parent and teacher questionnaires are used to help make this assessment.

Classification

- **Primarily inattentive type**—the child is inattentive but does not have high levels of activity or impulsivity.
- **Primarily hyperactive-impulsive type**—the child has high levels of activity and impulsivity but not a high level of inattention.

- **Combined type**—the most common form of ADHD; the child has high levels of hyperactivity, impulsivity, and inattention.

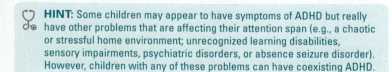

> **HINT:** The hyperactive-impulsive subtype is most often diagnosed in children younger than 7 years. Many of these children are diagnosed with the combined type when they get older.

Associated Problems
- Cognitive-learning disabilities.
- Neurologic problems—poor fine motor skills.
- Psychosocial and behavioral problems—oppositional defiant disorder, conduct disorder, anxiety disorder, depression, low self-esteem, and poor social skills.

> **HINT:** Some children may appear to have symptoms of ADHD but really have other problems that are affecting their attention span (e.g., a chaotic or stressful home environment; unrecognized learning disabilities, sensory impairments, psychiatric disorders, or absence seizure disorder). However, children with any of these problems can have coexisting ADHD.

Treatment
- Behavioral counseling and stimulant medications are the most effective treatments for ADHD.

Suggested Readings

Batshaw ML, Pellegrino L, Roizen NJ. *Children with Disabilities*. 6th ed. Baltimore, MD: Brookes; 2007.

Levine MD, Carey WB, Crocker AC. *Developmental-Behavioral Pediatrics*. 3rd ed. Philadelphia, PA: Elsevier; 1999.

Parker SJ, Zuckerman BS, Augustyn MC. *Developmental and Behavioral Pediatrics: A Handbook for Primary Care*. Philadelphia, PA: Lippincott, Williams & Wilkins; 2004.

Immunizations

IMMUNIZATION SCHEDULE

Figure 5-1 presents the recommended childhood immunization schedule for children and adolescents. The following are important general issues to consider:

- The simultaneous administration of multiple vaccines that are routinely recommended for infants, children, and adolescents is preferred. When available, combination vaccines are generally preferable to separate injections.
- A lapse in the immunization schedule does not require restarting a vaccine series. If a dose of vaccine is missed, it may be given at the next visit as long as it is still indicated. Many vaccines have upper age limits.
- Increasing numbers of vaccinations are required for teens. It is important to review the vaccine history at each adolescent visit.
- Immunizations, especially live virus vaccines, may be contraindicated in children with acquired or congenital immune deficiencies.
- Due to shortages and changing recommendations, the immunization schedule is continuously being updated. Be sure to consult the current schedule when making vaccine decisions.

ADMINISTRATION GUIDELINES
Procedures

Federal law requires providers to distribute information on vaccines, available from the Centers for Disease Control and Prevention (CDC), before each vaccination (www.cdc.gov/vaccines/pubs/vis/default.htm).

Sites

The preferred sites for the administration of vaccines are the **anterolateral aspect of the upper thigh** (subcutaneous or intramuscular), the deltoid area of the upper arm (intramuscular), or the upper, outer triceps area of the upper arm (subcutaneous). In **children <1 year,** intramuscular injections should be administered in the **anterolateral aspect of the thigh**. For **children >1 year,** the **deltoid muscle** is the preferred site of administration. Generally, the upper outer aspect of the buttocks should not be used for immunizing an infant.

Vaccine ▼ Age ▶	Birth	1 month	2 months	4 months	6 months	12 months	15 months	18 months	19–23 months	2–3 years	4–6 years
Hepatitis B[1]	HepB	HepB			HepB						
Rotavirus[2]			RV	RV	RV[2]						
Diphtheria, Tetanus, Pertussis[3]			DTaP	DTaP	DTaP	*See footnote*[3]	DTaP				DTaP
Haemophilus influenzae type b[4]			Hib	Hib	Hib[4]	Hib					
Pneumococcal[5]			PCV	PCV	PCV	PCV				PPSV	
Inactivated Poliovirus[6]			IPV	IPV	IPV						IPV
Influenza[7]					Influenza (yearly)						
Measles, Mumps, Rubella[8]						MMR		*See footnote*[8]			MMR
Varicella[9]						Varicella		*See footnote*[9]			Varicella
Hepatitis A[10]						HepA (2 doses)				HepA Series	
Meningococcal[11]										MCV	

Range of recommended ages for all children except certain high-risk groups

Range of recommended ages for certain high-risk groups

FIGURE 5-1 Recommended childhood immunization schedule United States, 2010. Immunization schedules courtesy of the Centers for Disease Control and Prevention, Atlanta, GA, 2010.

Vaccine ▼ Age ▶	7–10 years	11–12 years	13–18 years
Tetanus, Diphtheria, Pertussis[1]		Tdap	Tdap
Human Papillomavirus[2]	*See footnote 2*	HPV (3 doses)	HPV Series
Meningococcal[3]	MCV	MCV	MCV
Influenza[4]		Influenza (yearly)	
Pneumococcal[5]		PPSV	
Hepatitis A[6]		HepA Series	
Hepatitis B[7]		HepB Series	
Inactivated poliovirus[8]		IPV Series	
Measles, Mumps, Rubella[9]		MMR Series	
Varicella[10]		Varicella Series	

Range of recommended ages for all children except certain high-risk groups

Range of recommended ages for catch-up immunization

Range of recommended ages for certain high-risk groups

FIGURE 5-1 (*Continued*)

Diphtheria, Tetanus, and Acellular Pertussis (DTaP) Vaccine

IM: 0.5 mL. The Advisory Committee on Immunization Practices and the American Academy of Pediatrics (AAP) recommend four doses for primary immunization, with the first three administered at 4- to 8-week intervals starting at 2 months of age, and the fourth dose 6 months after the third dose and after 1 year of age. A fifth dose is recommended before school entry, at the age of 4 to 6 years. Subsequent boosters should be administered starting at 11 years of age using combined tetanus, diphtheria, and pertussis (Tdap) vaccine. Tdap should only be given once. Tetanus-diphtheria (Td) vaccine should be used for all subsequent boosters and given at 10-year intervals throughout life. An incomplete DTaP series is a common reason for vaccine delay in infants and toddlers.

Tetanus Immune Globulin

IM: 250 U (intramuscular) as a single dose for postexposure prophylaxis. The need for prophylaxis depends on wound cleanliness and severity, as well as prior tetanus toxoid (TT) vaccination history. TT is given along with immune globulin.

Contraindications

While adverse reactions are far less common than prior to the development of the acellular pertussis vaccine, contraindications for DTaP include the following:

- An immediate anaphylactic reaction
- Encephalopathy within 7 days
- A progressive neurological disorder (infantile spasms) until the condition has stabilized and the diagnosis clarified

Haemophilus influenza Type b Conjugate (Hib) Vaccine

IM: Three or four 0.5-mL doses are administered at 2 months, 4 months, 6 months, and 12 to 15 months of age. If a three-dose product is used, the third dose may be omitted. In situations in which the brand of vaccine used previously is not known, four doses are required. Hib vaccine is not required after 60 months of age.

Hepatitis A Vaccine (HAV)

IM: HAV 25U (VAQTA) or 720 EL.U (HAVRIX) in the deltoid muscle is recommended for the routine vaccine of all children beginning at 12 months of age. The second dose should be given 6 months later. For children and adolescents >23 months of age, HAV is recommended in areas where programs target older children, for those at increased risk, and for those desiring immunity.

Hepatitis B Vaccine (HBV)

IM: The first dose is ideally administered at birth in the neonatal nursery and must then be added to a child's primary care vaccination record. The next dose is administered 1 to 4 months later, most commonly at 1 to 2 months of age. The third dose is recommended beginning at 6 months of age and must be given 8 weeks after the second dose and 16 weeks after the first dose. It is acceptable to administer a fourth dose of HBV if combination products are used.

Hepatitis B Immune Globulin (HBIG)

Infants born to HBsAg-positive mothers: Both HBV (0.5 mL) and HBIG are recommended within 12 hours after birth. The second dose of HBV is then administered at 1 to 2 months of age and the third dose at 6 months of age. Hepatitis B surface antigen and hepatitis B surface antibody should then be checked starting at 9 months of age or the first preventive visit after completion of the series.

Infants born to mothers with HBsAg unknown: Mothers should be tested on admission for delivery. Administer HBV by 12 hours of age. HBIG should be administered as soon as possible and within 7 days of birth if the mother tests HBsAg positive.

Human Papilloma Virus (HPV) Vaccine

IM: 0.5-mL doses should be administered beginning at 11 to 12 years of age. The second dose is given 1 (HPV2) or 2 months (HPV4) after the first dose, and the third dose is administered 6 months after the first. Women may receive the vaccine up to 26 years of age if they have not completed the full series and are not pregnant. The vaccine may also be offered to males in this age group to help prevent genital warts. Of all adolescent vaccines, rates of completion are currently lowest for the HPV series.

Measles-Mumps-Rubella (MMR) Vaccine

SC: 0.5 mL at age 12 to 15 months. A booster dose is recommended at 4 to 6 years of age.

Contraindications

Contraindications to measles, mumps, and rubella vaccination include serious illness (not simple fever or upper respiratory infections), pregnancy, anaphylactic reaction to gelatin or neomycin, low platelets, recent injection of immune globulin, high-dose steroid use for at least 14 days, and compromised immunity (see discussion of HIV later). Autism is **not associated** with receipt of the MMR vaccine.

 HINT: In patients who have been exposed to the measles virus, the vaccine may be given within 72 hours of exposure to provide protection. Alternatively, if given within 6 days of exposure, immune globulin (0.25 mL/kg, IM) may prevent or modify measles in a susceptible person. Children and adolescents with symptomatic HIV infections who are exposed to measles should receive immune globulin prophylaxis (0.5 mL/kg) regardless of their immunization status. The maximum dosage for all patients is 15 mL.

Meningococcal Conjugate Vaccine (MCV4)

IM: Meningococcal vaccine is recommended beginning at 11 to 12 years of age for all teens. One 0.5-mL dose is currently required. The vaccine should be avoided in those with a history of Guillain-Barré syndrome. MCV4 is now recommended instead of meningococcal polysaccharide vaccine (MPS4) for children between 2 and 10 years of age at increased risk of meningococcal disease. In this age group, the primary recipients are children with terminal complement component deficiencies, those who have anatomic or functional asplenia, and those traveling to areas with especially high rates of disease. Based on developments at the time of publication, a booster dose for MCV4 is likely to be needed at age 16 years or 5 years after the first dose. Consult the current vaccine schedule.

Pneumococcal: Pneumococcal Conjugate Vaccine (PCV13)

IM: All children now vaccinated with PCV should receive the newer PCV13, instead of the older PCV7. Children who previously completed the series with PCV7 should receive a single dose of PCV13 between 14 and 59 months of age and at least 8 weeks after the last PCV dose. The routine schedule for PCV13 is as follows:

- **Infants and children:** 0.5 mL/dose given at 2, 4, and 6 months of age, with a booster dose given at 12 to 15 months of age
- **Previously unvaccinated older infants and children:**
  - **7 to 11 months of age:** Two doses are given at least 2 months apart. A third dose is given at 1 year of age
  - **12 to 23 months of age:** A total of two doses are given at least 2 months apart
  - **24 to 59 months with incomplete vaccination:** A single dose is given to healthy children. Children at high risk (sickle cell disease/hemoglobinopathies, asplenia, HIV, and cochlear implants) or presumed high risk (congenital immune deficiency, chronic cardiac disease, chronic pulmonary disease, cerebrospinal fluid leaks, chronic renal insufficiency, diabetes mellitus, or receiving immunosuppressive or radiation therapy) require two doses between 24 and 71 months of age if not previously vaccinated. In addition, children 6 to 18 years of age at increased risk may receive a single dose of PCV13 even if they have previously received PCV7 or the PPSV vaccine.

Pneumococcal Polysaccharide Vaccine, 23-Valent (PPSV23)

SC or IM: 0.5 mL. Recommended for those at high risk or presumed high risk of pneumococcal disease in addition to PCV13. Should be given at 24 months of age with an additional dose 5 years after the first only for children who are immunocompromised, have sickle cell disease, or functional asplenia. Doses must be given at least 8 weeks after the last dose of PCV13.

Poliovirus Vaccine

SC: Two 0.5-mL doses are administered at least 4 weeks apart, but preferably 8 weeks apart starting at 2 months of age. A third dose is administered at 6 to 18 months of age and a fourth dose should be given at school entry or at about 4 to 6 years of age. Oral poliovirus vaccine is no longer recommended in the United States.

Rotavirus Vaccine (Rota)

Oral: The rotavirus vaccine is recommended in a three-dose schedule at 2, 4, and 6 months of age. The first dose must be given between 6 and <15 weeks of age. If the first dose of rotavirus vaccine is not administered by 15 weeks of age, the series **should not** be initiated. In addition, rotavirus vaccination **must be completed**

before 8 months of age. Whenever possible, one product should be used for the entire series. Children who have had rotavirus disease should still complete the series.

Precautions for rotavirus vaccination include acute moderate to severe illness including gastroenteritis, moderate to severe illness, preexisting chronic gastrointestinal tract disease, intussusceptions, spina bifida, and bladder exstrophy. Of note, altered immunocompetence is a precaution, not a contraindication, to vaccination because the virus vaccine does not replicate well at the intestinal mucosal surface and wild-type virus infection is inevitable.

Varicella Vaccine

SC: Two 0.5-mL per dose are given, the first at 12 to 15 months and the second at 4 to 6 years of age. For children <13 years who are delayed, two doses may be administered at least 3 months apart. For previously unvaccinated teens ≥13 years, two doses are administered at least 28 days apart.

Special Note: To be considered immune without vaccination, individuals must have laboratory evidence of immunity or laboratory confirmation of disease, diagnosis, or verification of a history of varicella disease by a health care provider, or diagnosis or verification of herpes zoster by a health care provider.

Influenza Vaccine
Inactivated Trivalent Influenza Vaccines (TIV)
IM: TIV is recommended for the routine vaccination of all children **between** 6 months to 18 years of age annually. The dose is 0.25 mL for those <36 months of age and 0.5 mL for older children. While most children require a single dose, children <9 years of age receiving the vaccine for the first time or who only had one dose in the prior season require two doses at least 1 month apart. Recommendations also differ depending upon prior receipt of the H1N1 influenza vaccine. Vaccination of household contacts is a priority in preventing children from influenza.

Special Note: Severe egg allergy is a contraindication.

Live Attenuated Influenza Vaccine (LAIV)
Intranasal: LAIV may be substituted for TIV for healthy children >2 years of age. Those with high-risk conditions such as asthma or chronic pulmonary disease, hemodynamically significant cardiac disease, immunosuppressive disorders, HIV, sickle cell anemia and hemoglobinopathies, diseases requiring long-term salicylate therapy, chronic renal dysfunction, and chronic metabolic disease including diabetes should not receive LAIV.

Alternative Vaccine Schedules
Often citing scientifically unfounded concerns about vaccines, some have advocated delaying the administration of vaccines and following alternative schedules. Clinicians should work with families to discourage alternative vaccination schedules because these schedules:

- Increase the time individual children remain vaccine delayed and at risk for potentially life-threatening infection

- Decrease the rate of vaccination across populations of children causing an increased risk of an outbreak of a vaccine preventable disease
- Increase the risk of missed opportunities for vaccination that arise when children are not vaccinated according to standard protocols
- Increase the burden on medical offices which have to divert resources from routine preventive and acute care to attend to children who require more frequent visits.

Vaccine Refusal
Physicians and nurse practitioners are often the most trusted source of information on childhood immunizations. As a result, clinician recommendation is one of the strongest influences on vaccine decision making for families and is especially important when parents raise concerns that are not consistent with medical evidence. When concerns arise, clinicians should provide information tailored to the specific worries of parents or children. The resources listed at the end of this chapter provide scientifically valid information that can help address families' concerns. For families refusing vaccination, it is recommended that clinicians revisit the topic at future visits. In addition, clinicians should request that parents sign a refusal to vaccinate form documenting vaccines that are accepted or declined. This form can be accessed through the AAP website (www.aap.org/immunization/pediatricians/pdf/RefusaltoVaccinate.pdf).

SPECIAL CIRCUMSTANCES
Premature Infants and Infants with Medical Problems
Premature infants should be immunized **at the usual age** with the usual dose. Reducing or dividing doses of vaccines are not recommended.

Infants who have had an **intraventricular hemorrhage** or other neurologic event soon after birth but are **stable at age 2 months** should also be **immunized**. Infants who are still in the hospital at 2 months of age can also receive immunizations. The **influenza vaccine** (TIV) should be administered at 6 months of age and household contacts and caretakers should also be vaccinated. Premature infants born prior to 32 weeks of age, those with chronic lung disease, as well as those with certain cardiac conditions may also benefit from respiratory syncytial virus monoclonal antibody (palivizumab).

Immunodeficient and Immunosuppressed Children
Patients being **treated with corticosteroids** may need to be considered immunocompromised depending on the dose, route, and duration of treatment. In general, live vaccines **should not be given** to patients with congenital or secondary disorders of immune function.

Asplenic Children
Children who have undergone splenectomy, children with functional asplenia (sickle cell disease), and children with congenital asplenia have an increased risk of fulminant bacteremia, which is associated with a high mortality rate. Important

pathogens in asplenic children include *Streptococcus pneumoniae, Neisseria meningitidis, Haemophilus influenzae* type B, *Staphylococcus aureus, Salmonella species,* and *Escherichia coli.*

In addition to routine childhood vaccines including Hib and PCV13, the PPSV23 and the MCV4 should be given to all asplenic children at 2 years of age. Daily antimicrobial prophylaxis is often recommended for asplenic children regardless of their vaccination status.

Children with Personal or Family History of Seizures
A family history of convulsive disorders is neither a contraindication to immunization with DTP nor other vaccines and is not a reason to postpone immunization.

Children with Chronic Disease
Overall, children with chronic disease should receive the same immunizations recommended for healthy children.

However, children with immunologic disorders in general should not receive live vaccines. However, patients who are **HIV positive** and not severely immunocompromised should receive the MMR and varicella vaccines. Immunocompromise is a precaution, not a contraindication, to rotavirus vaccination.

As mentioned above, certain chronic conditions are contraindications to the LAIV. Children with these conditions, who are also at high risk of complications from influenza, should receive inactivated TIV.

Those with chronic liver disease are at high risk for complications from acute hepatitis. Clinicians should be sure that they are up-to-date for both HAV and HBV.

Children awaiting transplants should be immunized prior to the start of immunosuppressive therapy.

Children with Wounds
The treatment of a wound depends on the nature of the wound and on the patient's immunization history. Table 5-1 lists the guidelines for tetanus prophylaxis in older children and adolescents. DTaP is recommended when wound prophylaxis is needed among children <7 years of age.

COMMON MISCONCEPTIONS REGARDING CONTRAINDICATIONS TO IMMUNIZATION
Many misconceptions exist regarding contraindications to immunization. According to the AAP, the following are *not* appropriate contraindications to immunization:

- A mild acute illness characterized by a low-grade fever or mild diarrhea in an otherwise well child
- Antimicrobial therapy or being in the convalescent phase of an illness
- A reaction to a previous dose that involved only soreness, redness, or swelling in the immediate vicinity of the vaccination site or a temperature <105°F (40.5°C)
- A household contact who is pregnant

TABLE 5-1	Guide to Tetanus Prophylaxis in Routine Wound Management: Children 7 Years of Age and Older and Adolescents			
History of Absorbed Tetanus Toxoid (Doses)	**Clean, Minor Wounds**		**All Other Wounds**[a]	
	Td or Tdap[b]	**TIG**[c]	**Td or Tdap**[b]	**TIG**[c]
Unknown or <3	Yes	No	Yes	Yes
≥3[d]	No[e]	No	No[f]	No

Adapted from American Academy of Pediatrics. In Pickering LK, Baker CJ, Kimberlin DW, Long SS, eds. *Red Book: 2009 Report of the Committee on Infectious Diseases,* 28th ed. Elk Grove Village, IL, American Academy of Pediatrics, 2009.

Td, adult-type tetanus and diphtheria toxoids; Tdap, booster tetanus toxoid (TT), reduced diphtheria toxoid, and acellular pertussis; TIG, tetanus immune globulin (human).

[a]Includes wounds contaminated with dirt, feces, soil, or saliva; puncture wounds; avulsions; and wounds resulting from missiles, crushing, burns, or frostbite.

[b]Tdap is preferred to Td for adolescents who never have received Tdap. Td is preferred to TT for adolescents who received Tdap previously or when Tdap is not available.

[c]Immune Globulin Intravenous should be used when TIG is not available.

[d]If only three doses of fluid toxoid have been received, a fourth dose of toxoid, preferably an absorbed toxoid, should be given.

[e]Yes, if ≥10 years since the last dose.

[f]Yes, if ≥5 years since the last dose. (More frequent boosters are not needed.)

- Recent exposure to an infectious disease
- Prematurity
- Breast-feeding
- A history of nonspecific allergies or relatives with allergies
- Allergies to penicillin (none of the vaccines licensed in the United States contains penicillin)
- Family history of convulsions (it is permissible to administer pertussis and measles vaccinations to patients with a family history of convulsions)
- Family history of sudden infant death syndrome (DTP vaccination is permissible in these patients)
- Family history of an adverse event following a vaccination
- Malnutrition

OTHER SOURCES OF INFORMATION

The **schedule** for the immunization of children is **constantly changing**. The following publications are excellent sources of up-to-date information and have informed the information presented in this chapter:

- **2009 Red Book: Report of the Committee on Infectious Diseases,** 28th ed. This reference is published at 3-year intervals by the Committee on Infectious Diseases of the AAP.
- **Morbidity and Mortality Weekly Report.** http://www.cdc.gov/mmwr/. This report is published weekly by the CDC and contains current vaccine recommendations and updates.

- **Vaccine Schedules.** These are available online through the CDC at www.cdc.gov/vaccines/recs/schedules/child-schedule.htm.
- **Health Information for International Travel.** Information is available online from the CDC at www.cdc.gov/travel/contentVaccinations.aspx.
- **Vaccine Information Sheets for Families.** Information is available online from the CDC at www.cdc.gov/vaccines/pubs/vis/default.htm.
- **General Information on Vaccines with Answers to Frequently Asked Questions.** See The Children's Hospital of Philadelphia Vaccine Education Center at www.chop.edu/service/vaccine-education-center/home.html.

Feeding Infants

NUTRITIONAL NEEDS OF HEALTHY FULL-TERM INFANTS

Table 6-1 summarizes the nutritional needs of a healthy full-term infant.

> **HINT:** Contraindications to both breast- and bottle-feeding:
> - Respiratory rate >80 breaths/min
> - Infant with poor suck/swallow
> - Absent gag reflex
> - Symptoms of sepsis or asphyxia

BREAST-FEEDING

Breast-feeding is the optimal choice for feeding almost all infants, and breast milk is the gold standard on which most routine infant formulas are based.

RISKS OF FORMULA FEEDING

- Increased incidence and severity of infectious diseases, including diarrhea, respiratory tract infections, bacterial meningitis, otitis media, urinary tract infections, necrotizing enterocolitis, and bacteremia
- Increased incidence of sudden infant death syndrome
- Increased incidence of childhood obesity
- Increased incidence of type 1 and type 2 diabetes mellitus
- Increased incidence of leukemia, lymphoma, and Hodgkin disease
- Possible increased incidence of hypercholesterolemia
- Possible reduced cognitive development
- Maternal outcomes, including increased postpartum bleeding, slower return to pre-pregnancy weight, increased risk of breast cancer and ovarian cancer, increased risk of postmenopausal osteoporosis, and increased risk of postpartum depression.

CONTRAINDICATIONS TO BREAST-FEEDING

- Some inborn errors of metabolism (e.g., classic galactosemia)
- Maternal HIV-positive status
- Active (untreated) tuberculosis

TABLE 6-1	Nutritional Needs of Healthy, Full-Term Infants
Nutritional Element	**Daily Requirement**
Calories	~110 kcal/kg/d[a]
Fluids	~160 mL/kg/d[b]
Carbohydrates	37–44% of cal
Protein	10–12% of cal
Fat	40–50% of cal; 3% from linoleic acid

[a]Calories decrease over first year as follows:
EER kcal/d
0–3 mo 89 × wt (kg) − 100 + 175
4–6 mo 89 × wt (kg) − 100 + 56
7–12 mo 89 × wt (kg) − 100 + 22
[b]Of formula or breast milk, to provide adequate calories.

- Maternal alcohol abuse and certain maternal illicit drug use. Significant cigarette smoking (more than four cigarettes per day) should be evaluated on a case-by-case basis
- Herpes simplex lesions on a breast
- Breast cancer (currently under treatment)
- Maternal prolactinoma (in most cases)
- History of breast reduction surgery involving ligation of many/most of the milk ducts (may breast-feed if supplements are provided as needed)
- Maternal use of medications and/or radioactive materials that are contraindicated with breast-feeding, as per the findings of the American Academy of Pediatrics Committee on Drugs, 2001

 HINT: Maternal hepatitis B infection is not a contraindication to breast-feeding, provided the infant receives hepatitis vaccination and hepatitis immunoglobulin shortly after birth. Maternal hepatitis C infection is not a contraindication to breast-feeding.

PATIENT COUNSELING
Drug Use During Lactation
The nursing mother should be counseled to **avoid all drugs,** including over-the-counter and herbal medications, **until she has consulted her physician.** The reference by Hale (see Suggested Readings) is an excellent resource for evaluating maternal medication use. Alcohol intake should be limited. If the mother does have an occasional small drink (up to 6 oz beer or 4 oz wine), she should wait at least 2 to 3 hours before breast-feeding. Cigarette smoking should be discouraged but is no longer considered an absolute contraindication to breast-feeding because its benefits outweigh the risks for light smoking. The mother should be counseled regarding the dangers of decreased milk supply and the effects of nicotine on the infant if smoking exceeds four cigarettes per day.

Nutrition and Rest

Nursing mothers need greater amounts of most vitamins, protein, zinc, and fluid. Calcium needs, along with most other minerals, are not increased during lactation. Iron requirements are reduced due to lack of menses. It is recommended that mothers eat a well-balanced diet with a variety of foods including high-quality protein foods, fruits, vegetables, dairy products, and whole grains. A multivitamin is recommended. Mothers who have lost all their pregnancy weight gain may need to consume additional calories. **Adequate rest** is also important (it is ideal if the mother can nap when the infant naps).

Breast-Feeding Technique

It is neither necessary nor desirable to wash the nipples, but **clean hands are important**. The mother should be comfortable—it may be helpful to place extra pillows under her elbows and on her lap. The baby should be positioned on his side in the mother's arms, facing the mother, with his nose lined up across from the nipple so the head is in the "neutral" position (i.e., the infant should not have to turn the head to latch on) and tipped back with the chin up.

The mother should support the breast, taking care to keep her fingers away from the areola. Stroking the lips downward from the nose toward the chin will induce him to open his mouth wide, at which point he should be drawn close to the mother's body, encouraging latching on to as much of the alveolar tissue as possible. Both breasts should be offered at each feeding and the infant allowed to remain on each breast as long as suckling continues. One breast may be sufficient, especially during the first few days of life. The starting breast should be alternated. **Nipples should be allowed to air-dry** or be patted dry before covering them at the end of the feeding.

Feeding Frequency and Intake

The healthy infant should be encouraged to latch on within the first hour after birth. Continuous rooming-in facilitates breast-feeding. Feedings for the first few weeks should take place on demand **at least every 2 to 3 hours, ideally 8 to 12 times per 24 hours**. **No supplemental water or formula** should be given to the baby **during the first 2 weeks,** unless medically indicated. Table 6-2 summarizes nutrition supplementation for full-term breast-fed infants. An adequate latch-on and suckling should be assured and documented prior to hospital discharge.

TABLE 6-2	Nutrition Supplementation for Full-Term, Breast-Fed Infants
Formula	Not recommended during the first 2 wk unless medically indicated
Fluoride	0.25 mg/d, after 6 mo (if water is not fluoridated). Avoid fluoridated toothpaste until after 2 yr of age
Vitamin D	400 IU/d, starting ASAP after birth
Iron	Elemental iron (1 mg/kg/d starting @ 4 mo) Starting at 6 mo pureed meat as first food

MANAGEMENT OF PROBLEMS
Engorgement
Engorgement may occur on the third or fourth postpartum day and can cause significant discomfort for the mother. It is important to reassure the mother that a high level of engorgement typically lasts only 24 to 48 hours. Management strategies include the following:

- Continuing to nurse frequently
- Application of hot compresses or taking a hot shower before nursing to alleviate discomfort
- Application of ice packs to the breasts after nursing. Chilled cabbage leaves are also effective
- Administration of acetaminophen or ibuprofen
- Pumping only a small amount of milk to avoid increased milk production (if a breast pump is being used)

Sore, Cracked, or Hemorrhagic Nipples
- The infant's position on the nipple should be reevaluated by a medical professional or lactation consultant; an infant that latches on to an inadequate amount of the nipple is the most common cause of sore nipples. The mother should be sure the infant's lower lip is furled outward.
- Exposure of the nipples to air is important. In addition, applying expressed breast milk to cracked nipples and allowing them to air-dry has resulted in dramatic healing in some patients. Lansinoh cream and ComfortGel pads may also be helpful.
- Mothers should be advised to nurse the baby on the least affected side first. Prefeeding with milk that has been manually expressed may appease the overly vigorous nurser. In severe cases, breast-feeding on the affected side should be temporarily discontinued and a breast pump used.
- Administration of acetaminophen 20 minutes before nursing (not to exceed recommended dosing) may alleviate discomfort.

Plugged Milk Ducts
A **plugged milk duct or galactocele** presents as a persistent hard, round, or linear lump, usually in the lateral and inferior quadrants of the breast. **Warm moist heat** should be applied to the breast for 20 minutes before each nursing, and the **breast should be massaged** from the body toward the nipple, concentrating on the involved area. Mothers should be advised to **nurse the baby frequently** (i.e., every 1 to 2 hours) for at least 10 minutes on each side. The **affected side should be offered first,** and the infant should be positioned with his chin toward the affected area, which will facilitate emptying of the affected quadrant. It may take several nursing sessions to empty the plugged duct. Complete emptying of the breast is advised; this may require the use of a breast pump after nursing. Rarely, a galactocele will become large enough to require surgical aspiration.

Mastitis

Lactating mothers with mastitis present with **fever, shaking chills, and malaise,** followed by **localized breast erythema and pain**. Mothers should be advised to continue to nurse frequently. Treatment is with oral ampicillin, the application of warm compresses, rest, and pain medication (if necessary).

Poor Early Weight Gain

Breast-fed full-term infants may **lose as much as 10% of their birth weight** during the first several days of life, but they should regain it by 7 to 10 days of age. Weight loss of ≥10% of birth weight should prompt a reevaluation of the infant and breast-feeding technique, with improvement documented prior to discharge.

Follow-Up of the Breast-Fed Infant

An evaluation by a pediatrician or health professional at 3 to 5 days of age is important to catch any problems early. This visit should include an infant weight and physical examination, with emphasis on hydration status and jaundice. The mother should be questioned regarding:

- The frequency and duration of nursing sessions.
- Signs of established lactation (i.e., diminished breast fullness after nursing, leaking, cessation of nipple discomfort after latching on, and uterine cramps during nursing).
- Normal infant voiding (minimum of four to six times per day, pale urine). Note: The baby may void twice between diaper changes, so the number of voidings may vary.
- Normal infant defecation (3 to 4 loose stools/day on days 3 to 4, 4 to 6 loose stools/day on days 4 to 6, 8 to 10 loose stools/day during weeks 2 to 4). Note: continued meconium stooling after day 5 may indicate low milk supply.
- Infant response to feeding (e.g., sleepy and satisfied).

According to Lawrence (6th ed., 2005), these are the most common factors associated with poor early weight gain:

- Ineffective breast-feeding technique
- Infrequent or inappropriately short feedings (e.g., excessive nighttime intervals)
- Water supplementation
- Maternal problems that inhibit milk letdown

BOTTLE-FEEDING
Patient Counseling
Bottle-Feeding Technique

The bottle should be held so that no air enters the nipple, and the bottle should never be propped. Prop feeding is associated with a significantly higher risk of otitis media.

Feeding Frequency and Intake

Formula can be given **every 3 to 4 hours**. A small-for-gestational-age infant may require small frequent feedings until his gastric capacity increases, whereas a large-for-gestational-age infant of a mother with diabetes should be given early and frequent feedings, and his blood sugar should be monitored carefully to reduce the risk of hypoglycemia.

The typical full-term neonate drinks only 15 to 30 mL (0.5 to 1 oz) per feeding during the first few days of life. The mother should be assured that this is sufficient because of stores acquired in utero. She should be told to expect an **intake of 2 to 4 oz per feeding** (approximately every 3 to 4 hours) **by the end of the first week**.

Formula Types

Tables 6-3 and 6-4 list the specific compositions for and indications for many commonly available infant formulas. Cow's milk should not be introduced until 1 year of age. Manufacturers frequently change formula names and composition. Check websites (listed at end of this chapter) for most current accurate information.

Cow's Milk-Based Formulas

Full-term (standard) formulas, which provide 20 kcal/oz, are generally suitable for infants with **birth weights >2,000 g,** and most **full-term small-for-gestational-age** infants.

Soy-Based (Lactose-Free) Formulas

Soy-based formulas are indicated for infants with **temporary or chronic lactose intolerance** and for infants with **galactosemia**. They are also often used when intolerance to cow's milk protein is suspected. However, the use of soy-based formula in this situation is not generally recommended because of a significant antigenic crossover between cow's milk protein and soy protein. Soy-based formulas are **not recommended for prolonged use in preterm infants** because the phytate content may lead to hypophosphatemia and rickets.

Preterm Formulas

The advantages of breast milk are even more significant for preterm infants because of the anti-infectious properties and easy digestibility of breast milk. If breast milk is not available, preterm formulas should be used. These formulas, available as 20, 24, or 30 kcal/oz, are specially designed to meet the needs of preterm infants. These can be mixed in different caloric concentrations to meet the nutritional needs of individual infants. They should be used until the infant reaches 40 weeks post-conception (or longer, if the infant's birth weight is <1,000 g). Transitional formulas providing 22 kcal/oz are available and should be used for preterm infants until 9 to 12 months of adjusted age.

Dietary Calorie Supplementation

Caloric supplements are often required for infants with higher-than-usual caloric needs, decreased oral intake, decreased fluid tolerance, or a combination of these factors (e.g., preterm infants, infants with bronchopulmonary dysplasia, and

TABLE 6-3 Composition of Select Infant Formulas (Note: Names and Composition Frequently Change. Please Check Company Website for Latest Information)

A: Breast Milk/Term Formulas

Product (Manufacturer)	kcal/oz	Carbohydrate (g/100 mL)	Protein (g/100 mL)	Fat (g/100 mL)	Fe mg/ 100 mL	mOsm kg Water
Mature human milk	20	Lactose (7.2)	Mature human milk (whey, casein) (1.1)	Mature human milk (3.9)	0.3	290
Enfamil Premium (Mead Johnson)	20	Lactose (7.5)	Whey Nonfat milk (1.4)	Palmolein, coconut, soy, high-oleic sunflower oils DHA/ARA (3.6)	1.2	300
Similac Advance (Abbott)	20	Lactose Galactooligosaccharides (7.3)	Nonfat milk Whey concentrate (1.4)	High-oleic safflower, soy and coconut oils DHA/ARA (3.7)	1.2	310
Similac Advance Organic (Abbott)	20	Organic corn maltodextrin, organic Lactose, organic sugar (7.1)	Organic Nonfat milk (1.4)	Organic high-oleic sunflower, organic soy and organic coconut oils DHA/ARA (3.7)	1.2	225
Good Start Gentle Plus (Gerber/Nestle)	20	Lactose 70% Maltodextrin 30% (7.8)	Whey protein concentrate hydrolysate (1.5)	Palmolein, coconut, soy, high-oleic sunflower oils, DHA/ ARA (3.4)	1.0	250
Good Start Protect Plus probiotics (Gerber/Nestle)	20	Lactose 70% Maltodextrin 30% (7.5)	Whey protein concentrate hydrolysate (1.5)	Palmolein, coconut, soy, high-oleic sunflower oils DHA/ ARA (3.4)	1.0	250
Bright Beginnings Premium (Bright Beginnings)	20	Lactose (7.4)	Whey concentrate and nonfat milk (1.4)	High-oleic sunflower, safflower, palmolein, and coconut oils (3.6)	1.2	300
Bright Beginnings Organic (Bright Beginnings)	20	Lactose (7.1)	Whey concentrate and nonfat milk (1.5)	High-oleic sunflower, safflower, palmolein, and coconut oils (3.6)	1.2	274

B: Soy Formulas

Product (Manufacturer)	kcal/oz	Carbohydrate (g/100 mL)	Protein (g/100 mL)	Fat (g/100 mL)	Fe mg/100 mL	mOsm kg Water
Similac Sensitive Isomil Soy (Abbott)	20	Corn syrup and sucrose (7.0)	Soy protein isolate, L-methionine (1.7)	High-oleic safflower, coconut, and soy oils DHA/ARA (3.7)	1.22	200
Enfamil ProSobee (Mead Johnson)	20	Corn syrup solids (7.1)	Soy protein isolate, L-methionine (1.7)	Palmolein, coconut, soy, and high-oleic sunflower oils DHA/ARA (3.6)	1.2	170
Bright Beginnings Soy (Bright Beginnings)	20	Corn syrup (7.1)	Soy protein isolate, L-methionine (1.7)	Palmolein, coconut, soy, and high-oleic safflower/sunflower oils DHA/ARA (3.6)	1.2	162
Good Start Soy Plus (Gerber/Nestle)	20	Corn Maltodextrin (7.5)	Enzymatically hydrolyzed Soy protein isolate (1.7)	Palmolein, coconut, soy, high-oleic sunflower oils DHA/ARA (3.4)	1.2	180

C: Additives

Product (Manufacturer)	kcal per Additive	Carbohydrate (g/100 mL)	Protein (g/100 mL)	Fat (g/100 mL)	Fe mg/100 mL	mOsm kg Water
Similac Human Milk Fortifier (Abbott)	4 kcal/oz fortifier (per 4 pkts)	Corn syrup solids (1.8)	Nonfat milk and whey protein concentrate (1.0)	MCT oil and lecithin (0.36)	0.35	Adds 90
Prolact + H2MF + 4 (20:80 to maternal BM) (Prolacta)	4 kcal/oz fortifier (per 20 mL)	Human milk concentrate (2.0)	Human milk (1.2)	Human milk (1.8)	0.2	Adds 76
MCT oil (Nestle)	7.6 kcal/mL	None	None	MCT oil		
Microlipid (Nestle)	4.5 kcal/mL	None	None	Safflower oil emulsion		

(continued)

73

TABLE 6-3 Composition of Select Infant Formulas (Note: Names and Composition Frequently Change. Please Check Company Website for Latest Information) (Cont.)

C: Additives (Cont.)

Product (Manufacturer)	kcal per Additive	Carbohydrate (g/100 mL)	Protein (g/100 mL)	Fat (g/100 mL)	Fe mg/ 100 mL	mOsm kg Water
Beneprotein (Nestle)	25 kcal per scoop = 1.5 Tbsp	None	Whey protein isolate lecithin (6.0)	None		
Polycose (Abbott)	23 kcal per 6 g powder = 1 Tbsp	Glucose polymers (5.6)	None	None		
Duocal (Nutricia)	42 kcal/Tbsp	Hydrolyzed cornstarch (6.2)	None	Corn, coconut, MCT oil (1.9)		
Rice cereal (per Tbsp)	9 kcal/Tbsp	Rice starch (1.9)	None	None		

D: Preterm Breast Milk/Premature Formulas

Product (Manufacturer)	kcal/oz	Carbohydrate (g/100 mL)	Protein (g/100 mL)	Fat (g/100 mL)	Fe mg/ 100 mL	mOsm kg Water
Preterm Human Milk	20	Human milk (6.6)	Human milk (whey and casein) (1.4)	Human milk (3.9)	0.12	290
Enfamil Premature 20 (Mead Johnson)	20	Corn syrup solids and lactose (7.4)	Whey and nonfat milk (2.0)	MCT, soy, hi oleic sunflower/ safflower oils DHA/ARA (3.4)	1.2	240
Enfamil Premature 24 (Mead Johnson)	24	Corn syrup solids and lactose (8.7)	Whey and nonfat milk (2.4)	MCT, soy, hi oleic sunflower/ safflower DHA/ARA (4.1)	1.4	300
Good Start Premature 24 (Gerber/Nestle)	24	Corn maltodextrin. lactose (8.4)	Hydrolyzed whey (2.4)	MCT, soy oil, hi oleic safflower oil DHA/ARA (4.2)	1.44	275

		Carbohydrate			Fe mg/	mOsm kg
Similac Special Care 20 (Abbott)	20	Corn syrup solids and lactose (7.0)	Nonfat milk and whey protein concentrate (2.0)	MCT, soy, and coconut oils DHA/ARA (3.7)	1.22	235
Similac Special Care 24 (Abbott)	24	Corn syrup solids and lactose (8.4)	Nonfat milk and whey protein concentrate (2.4)	MCT, soy, and coconut oils DHA/ARA (4.4)	1.46	280
Similac Special Care 30 (Abbott)	30	Corn syrup solids and lactose (7.8)	Nonfat milk and whey protein concentrate (3.0)	MCT, soy, and coconut oils DHA/ARA (6.7)	1.83	325
Enfamil Enfacare (Mead Johnson)	22	Corn syrup solids and lactose (7.7)	Whey concentrate and nonfat milk (2.1)	Soy, high-oleic sunflower, MCT, and coconut oils DHA/ARA (3.9)	1.33	250
Similac Expert Care Neosure (Abbott)	22	Corn syrup solids and lactose (7.5)	Whey concentrate and nonfat milk (2.1)	Soy, coconut and MCT oils DHA/ARA (4.1)	1.34	250

E: Formulas with Protein Alterations

Product (Manufacturer)	kcal/oz	Carbohydrate (g/100 mL)	Protein (g/100 mL)	Fat (g/100 mL)	Fe mg/ 100 mL	mOsm kg Water
Similac Expert Care Alimentum (Abbott)	20	Sucrose, modified tapioca starch (6.9)	Casein hydrolysate, L-Cysteine, L-Tyrosine, L-Tryptophan, L-Methionine (1.9)	Safflower, MCT, and soy oils DHA/ARA (3.7)	1.2	370
Nutramigen with Enflora LGG (Mead Johnson)	20	Corn syrup solids, modified cornstarch (6.9)	Casein hydrolysate, L-Cysteine, L-Tyrosine, L-Tryptophan (1.9)	Palmolein, soy, coconut, and high-oleic sunflower oils DHA/ARA (3.6)	1.22	300
Pregestimil (Mead Johnson)	20	Corn syrup solids, modified cornstarch (6.8)	Casein hydrolysate, L-Cysteine, L-Tyrosine, L-Tryptophan (1.9)	MCT, soy, and high-oleic safflower/sunflower oil, corn oil DHA/ARA (3.8)	1.28	290

(continued)

TABLE 6-3 Composition of Select Infant Formulas (Note: Names and Composition Frequently Change. Please Check Company Website for Latest Information) (Cont.)

E: Formulas with Protein Alterations (Cont.)

Product (Manufacturer)	kcal/oz	Carbohydrate (g/100 mL)	Protein (g/100 mL)	Fat (g/100 mL)	Fe mg/ 100 mL	mOsm kg Water
EleCare (Abbott)	20	Corn syrup solids (7.2)	L-Amino acids (2.1)	High-oleic safflower oil, MCT, soy oil DHA/ARA (3.3)	1.0	350
Nutramigen AA (Mead Johnson)	20	Corn syrup solids (6.9)	L- Amino acids (1.9)	Palmolein, soy coconut and high-oleic sunflower oil, DHA/ARA (3.6)	1.2	350
Neocate Infant with DHA/ARA (Nutricia)	20	Corn syrup solids (7.8)	L-Amino acids (2.1)	Palm and or coconut, hi oleic safflower, soy oil DHA/ARA (3.0)	1.24	375

F: "Gentle" Formulas

Product (Manufacturer)	kcal/oz	Carbohydrate (g/100 mL)	Protein (g/100 mL)	Fat (g/100 mL)	Fe mg/ 100 mL	mOsm kg Water
Enfamil Gentlease (Mead Johnson)	20	Corn syrup solids, lactose 25% (7.2)	Partially hydrolyzed nonfat milk, whey protein concentrate solids (1.5)	Palmolein, coconut, soy, and high-oleic sunflower oils DHA/ARA (3.6)	1.2	220
Enfamil AR Also known as Enfamil Restful (Mead Johnson)	20	Rice starch, lactose, and maltodextrin (7.4)	Nonfat milk (1.7)	Palmolein, coconut, soy, and high-oleic sunflower oils source DHA/ARA (3.4)	1.2	240
Similac Sensitive for Spit up (Abbott)	20	Corn syrup, rice starch, sugar (7.2)	Milk-protein isolate (1.5)	High-oleic safflower, soy and coconut oil, DHA/ARA (3.7)	1.22	180

TABLE 6-4	Indications for Infant Formulas

Maternal breast milk:
- Best choice for most term infants

Term Infants (If Breast Milk Not Used)

Cow's Milk-based Standard Formulas
- Enfamil PREMIUM Newborn (prebiotics) (0–3 mo)

Enfamil Premium (prebiotic)

- Enfamil PREMIUM Infant (prebiotics) (0–12 mo)
- Similac Advance (prebiotic) or Similac Organic
- Good Start Gentle Plus or Good Start Protect Plus (probiotics)
- Bright Beginnings Premium (prebiotics) or Bright Beginnings Organic

Lactose-free Cow's Milk-based Formulas

For short-term diarrhea or lactose intolerance:

Lactose reduced OR partially hydrolyzed protein:

- Enfamil Gentlease
- Similac Sensitive
- Bright Beginnings Gentle

For term infants with uncomplicated reflux:
- Enfamil AR (added rice)
- Similac Sensitive for Spit Up (rice starch)

Soy Formulas

For infants with primary or secondary lactose intolerance or galactosemia:

- Bright Beginnings Soy
- Similac Sensitive Isomil Soy
- Similac Expert Care for Diarrhea (>6 mo has added fiber–soy formula)
- Enfamil ProSobee

Altered Protein Formulas: Casein hydrolysates
Altered Protein Formulas Without MCT

For infants sensitive to casein and soy protein/milk-protein allergy:

- Nutramigen and Nutramigen with Enflora LGG

Altered Protein Formulas with MCT

For infants with abnormal absorption, digestion and transport, and intractable diarrhea:

- Pregestimil
- Similac Expert Care Alimentum

Altered Protein Formulas: Elemental
- Amino acid formulas

Altered Protein Formulas: Elemental with Low MCT

For severe allergy:

- Nutramigen AA

Altered Protein Formulas: Elemental with High MCT

For severe allergy also with abnormal absorption, digestion and transport, intractable diarrhea:

- EleCare
- Neocate Infant DHA and ARA

(*continued*)

TABLE 6-4	Indications for Infant Formulas (*Cont.*)

Preterm Formulas

For preterm infants with need for increased protein, calcium, and phosphate needs:

- Enfamil Premature 20
- Similac Special Care 20

For preterm infants with need for increased calories, protein, calcium, and phosphate needs:

- Enfamil Premature 24

Good Start Premature 24 (whey hydrolysate)

- Similac Special Care 24 and Similac Special Care High Protein 24

Fluid-restricted preterm infants with need for increased calories, protein, calcium, and phosphate:

- Similac Special Care 30

Preterm Transitional Formulas

Nutrient enriched for preterm infants after hospital discharge (22 cal/oz):

- EnfaCare
- Similac Expert Care NeoSure

Preterm Fortifiers

For preterm infants on breast milk with need for increased calories, protein and electrolytes:

- Similac Human Milk Fortifier
- Enfamil Human Milk Fortifier (Liquid commercially sterile form in 2011)
- Prolact + H2MF (Liquid frozen pasteurized human product in various caloric aliquots)

infants with congestive heart failure). Care should be taken to maintain the **correct balance of nutrients**. In general, the first step to increase calories should be to increase the concentration of the formula by adding less water to the powder or liquid concentrate. **Careful instructions must be given to the parents to ensure the correct amount of water is added.**

Multinutritional Supplements

These supplements include calories from a combination of sources (e.g., fat and carbohydrate). Examples include Human Milk Fortifier (Mead Johnson and Abbott), Duocal, formula concentrates, and concentrated human milk (Prolact + H2MF) is available in +4, +6, +8, and +10 formulations—adding specific kcal/oz (Note: this is extremely expensive).

Carbohydrate

Carbohydrate supplements (e.g., Polycose and corn syrup) are generally **well tolerated and inexpensive** but **low in caloric and nutrient density**. These supplements may cause diarrhea. Polycose provides 23 kcal/6 g powder.

Fat

Fat supplements are **high in caloric density**. The best-tolerated form, **microlipids** (1 mL/oz of formula), is **more expensive and lower in caloric density** than inexpensive, less well-tolerated vegetable oil, which may cause diarrhea. Vegetable oil is also harder to keep mixed with the formula. Medium chain triglycerides (MCT) oil, another option, should be reserved for specific indications, such as short-bowel syndrome and malabsorption. It is expensive and can cause diarrhea. Microlipids supply 4.5 kcal/mL, MCT oil supplies 7.6 kcal/mL, and vegetable oil supplies 9 kcal/mL. Increasing fat in the formula may slow gastric emptying time.

Protein
Protein supplements are usually well tolerated but of relatively low caloric density. They are generally indicated only for patients with unusually high protein needs. Beneprotein (whey protein) provides 25 kcal/scoop powder or 1.5 Tbs (6 g protein).

VITAMIN-MINERAL SUPPLEMENTS
Vitamins
Breast-fed and most formula-fed infants may require vitamin D supplementation to meet the current 400 international units/day recommendation. Infants with fat malabsorption may require additional vitamin supplementation. ADEK is often used for this purpose. **It is recommended that all infants receive 400 IU/day of vitamin D/day.** Baby D drops (Carlson Labs) provide 400 units per drop in a well tolerated, cost-effective form (http://www.carlsonlabs.com/p-162-baby-ddrops-400-iu.aspx) Table 6-5.

Fluoride
Fluoride supplementation (0.25 mg/day) is recommended **after 6 months** of age for **breast-fed infants,** as well as for **formula-fed infants** who are given formula that is reconstituted using nonfluoridated water or who are fed ready-to-feed formula. Nonfluoridated toothpaste should be used for children until at least 2 years of age to avoid excessive fluoride intake.

Iron
Formula-fed infants (<1 year of age) should be fed an iron-fortified formula, which should meet their iron needs. These formulas should also be used for the breast-fed infant <1 year of age needing a milk supplement. For exclusively breast-fed infants, supplementation of 1 mg/kg/day of elemental iron is recommended beginning at 4 months of age until the babies are eating iron-fortified foods. Partially breast-fed infants who receive more than half of their daily feedings as human milk should also be managed according to this guideline: Preterm breast-fed infants generally require iron supplements of 2 mg/kg/day from 1 month to 1 year of age. Iron intake of 11 mg daily is recommended for full-term infants from 6 months to 12 months of age. Early foods with higher iron content, such as meats and high iron vegetables, should be introduced at 6 months to help meet this need. Liquid iron supplements should be used as needed if the recommended iron intake is not met by diet.

TABLE 6-5	Vitamin D Formulations (Subject to Change—check Manufacturers Website) for Healthy Infants			
Supplement	**Indication**	**Standard Dose**	**Vitamin Content/Dose**	**Of Interest**
Baby D drops (Carlson Labs)	Vitamin D supple-ment	1 drop/d (0.03 mL/ drop)	400 IU vit D	One bottle = 365 doses Cost varies ($15–26/yr) No flavoring added Not covered by insurance
Tri-Vi-Sol (Mead Johnson)	Vitamin D supple-ment	1 mL/d	400 IU vit D 1500 IU vit A 35 mg vit C	One bottle = 50 doses Cost $10–15/bottle or $73 = 110/ yr
Tri-Vi-Sol w/ Iron	Vitamin with iron		Above + 10 mg Iron	Flavoring added-> high osmolality Insurance may cover
Poly-Vi-Sol (Mead Johnson)	Vitamin supple-ment	1 mL/d	400 IU vit D 1500 IU vit A	One bottle = 50 doses
Poly-Vi-Sol w/Iron	Vitamin with iron	1 mL/d	35 mg vit C 5 IU vit E 0.5 mg Thiamin 0.6 mg Riboflavin 8 mg Niacin 0.4 mg vit B_6 2 mcg vit B_{12} Above + 10 mg Iron	Cost $10–15/bottle or $73 = 110/ yr Flavoring added-> high osmolality Insurance may cover
D-Vi-Sol (Mead Johnson)	Vit D supple-ment	1 mL/d	400 IU vit D	One bottle = 50 doses Cost ~ $10/bottle or ~ $73/yr Flavoring added-> high osmolality

Solid Foods

Solid foods are typically introduced to the infant's diet at **6 months of age**. Foods can be introduced earlier (4 to 5 months of age) if the infant seems to require >32 oz/day of formula and shows developmental readiness for solids (able to sit well with support and to turn head away when no longer hungry).

Initially, small volumes of solid foods are provided once daily. The volume is gradually increased, and the frequency is increased to three times daily with some snacks. **Formula or breast milk** remains the basis of the infant's diet **throughout the first year of life** and should be maintained at 24 to 32 oz/day.

The order in which foods are introduced varies widely across cultural groups and is based more on tradition than on science. Table 6-6 offers a suggested schedule for introducing solid foods. **Parents who opt to make their own baby food should be counseled to use the food within 24 hours or freeze it to avoid the danger of a high nitrite content. This is particularly relevant for carrots and beets.**

TABLE 6-6	Suggested Schedule for Introducing Solid Foods
Baby's Age	**Appropriate Solid Foods**
6–8 mo	Iron-fortified infant cereal[a] mixed with breast milk, water, or juice to a mustard-like consistency and offered on a small spoon (not in a bottle); rice, oatmeal, and barley varieties should be introduced before the mixed type Pureed meats,[a,b] fruits, and vegetables Note: Meats first for breast-fed infants and cereal first for formula-fed infants
7–9 mo	Plain yogurt and cottage cheese Well-cooked vegetables and pasta Soft "finger foods" (e.g., banana chunks and pancakes) Cheerios, fruit and veggies "puffs" and crackers Tofu and refried beans Introduce cup: water; limit juice to 4 oz/d Eat together as a family
9–12 mo	Decrease pureed foods and increase soft table foods
>12 mo	Switch from formula to whole cow's milk (OK to use reduced fat milk in overweight toddlers over 12 mo age) Can introduce foods with higher allergenic potential (e.g., egg whites, citrus fruits, chocolate, and berries); Continue to avoid peanut products until 3 yr of age (This recommendation currently under review) Continue breast-feeding; wean from bottle Avoid soda or sweetened drinks

[a]Fomon S. Feeding normal infants: Rationale for recommendations. *JADA*. 2001;(101):1002–1005.
[b]Krebs N. Meat as complementary food for breast fed infants: Feasibility and impact on zinc intake and status. *JPGN*. 2006;(42):207–214.

 HINT: Certain foods (e.g., raisins, nuts, popcorn, hard candy, hot dogs, raw carrots, hard teething biscuits, and grapes) should be avoided because of the risk of choking. No honey should be given for the first year of life because of the increased risk of infant botulism.

SPECIAL CONSIDERATIONS FOR PRETERM INFANTS
Calorie Requirements
Healthy preterm infants usually grow well with a diet that provides **110 to 130 kcal/kg/day**. Infants with **complications** (e.g., pulmonary bronchodysplasia and congestive heart failure) frequently require **130 to 180 kcal/kg/day,** titrated to achieve adequate growth.

Increasing Caloric Density
To increase caloric intake, it is necessary to increase the feeding volume (if fluid restriction is not a concern), the caloric density of the feedings, or both. If it is necessary to increase the feeding volume but the infant is unable to consume the

increased volume, supplemental feedings can be provided through a nasogastric or orogastric tube.

Prior to discharge, most preterm infants initially require a caloric density of at least 24 kcal/oz (the density of most preterm formulas). Increased caloric density can be achieved by mixing 30 kcal/oz preterm formula 1:1 with 24 kcal/oz preterm formula to result in 27 kcal/oz. After discharge, formula caloric density can be increased by adding less water. Additional increases in caloric density can be achieved by adding caloric supplements (see section on "Dietary Calorie Supplementation").

Breast Milk

Breast milk provides a low renal solute load and excellent digestibility and absorption. **In smaller preterm infants, supplementation of breast milk is necessary for long-term growth.** Breast-milk fortifiers developed for supplementation include Enfamil Human Milk Fortifier (Mead Johnson) and Similac Human Milk Fortifier (Ross). Both increase the calories, protein, minerals (particularly calcium and phosphorus), and vitamins of human milk to the levels required for preterm infants. These fortifiers are expensive and difficult to obtain outside of the hospital. If bovine fortifier is not tolerated by the infant, Prolact + H2MF fortifier can be used. This is concentrated, pasteurized human milk. Note that the cost of this fortifier is ~50 times that of the bovine fortifiers!

 HINT: An inexpensive alternative for the infant who still requires a caloric density of 24 kcal/oz after hospital discharge is to supplement breast milk with preterm formula (1 tsp formula powder to 3 oz breast milk) or with transitional formula (Neosure or Enfacare) powder (1 tsp powder to 3 oz breast milk). Breast-milk feedings can also be alternated with 24 or 27 kcal/oz formula feedings.

Formula

Preterm infant formulas (see Table 6-3) should be used for **all preterm infants with a birth weight <2,000 g who are not breast-fed** until the infant reaches the 40-week postconception mark. EnfaCare (Mead Johnson) or Neosure, special formulas designed to be consumed by the preterm infant from the time of hospital discharge until the postconceptional (adjusted) age of 9 months, in order to provide the extra calories and minerals these infants need.

Solid Foods

Assuming the baby's oral motor skills are normal, solid foods can be introduced to the preterm infant following the **same recommendations as those for full-term infants,** using the corrected (adjusted) age. Abnormal oral motor skills and other feeding disorders are relatively common in the preterm population; therefore, the baby's **feeding skills should be assessed** carefully for both liquid and solid feedings.

Suggested Readings

American Academy of Pediatrics, Committee on Fetus and Newborn, and The American College of Obstetricians and Gynecologists, Committee on Obstetric Practice. *Guidelines for Perinatal Care.* 6th ed. Elk Grove Village, IL/Washington DC; 2007.

American Academy of Pediatrics/The American College of Obstetricians and Gynecologists. *Breastfeeding Handbook for Physicians* (Editor-in-Chief RJ Schanler). Elk Grove Village, IL/Washington DC; 2006.

American Academy of Pediatrics, Committee on Nutrition. Effects of nutritional interventions on the development of atopic disease in infants and children. *Pediatrics.* 2008;121(1):183–191.

American Academy of Pediatrics, Committee on Nutrition. Lipid screening and cardiovascular health in children. *Pediatrics.* 2008;122(1):198–208.

American Academy of Pediatrics, Committee on Nutrition. *Pediatric Nutrition Handbook.* 6th ed. Elk Grove Village, IL: American Academy of Pediatrics; 2008.

American Academy of Pediatrics, Committee on Nutrition. Prevention of rickets and vitamin D deficiency in infants, children and adolescents. *Pediatrics.* 2008;122(5):1142–1152.

American Academy of Pediatrics, Committee on Nutrition. Use of soy protein based formulas in infant feeding. *Pediatrics.* 2008;121(5):1062–1068.

American Academy of Pediatrics, Committee on Nutrition. Clinical Report: Diagnosis and prevention of iron deficiency and iron deficiency anemia in infants and young children (0–3 years of age). *Pediatrics.* 2010;126(5):1040–1050.

American Academy of Pediatrics, Section on Breastfeeding. Breastfeeding and the use of human milk. *Pediatrics.* 2005;115(2): 496–506.

Groh-Wargo S, ed. *ADA Pocket Guide to Neonatal Nutrition.* Chicago, IL: American Dietetic Association; 2009.

Hale T. *Medications and Mothers' Milk.* 14th ed. Amarillo, TX: Hale Publishing; 2010.

Huggins K. *The Nursing Mother's Companion: Revised Edition.* Boston, MA: Harvard Common Press; 2005.

Lawrence RA. *Breastfeeding: A Guide for the Medical Profession.* 7th ed. St. Louis, MO: Mosby; 2011.

Meek JY. *New Mother's Guide to Breastfeeding.* Elk Grove Village, IL: American Academy of Pediatrics; 2002.

Mohrbacher N, Kendall-Tackett K. *Breastfeeding Made Simple.* Oakland, CA: New Harbinger Publication, Inc; 2010.

Newman J, Pitman T. *The Latch and Other Keys to Breastfeeding Success.* Amarillo, TX: Hale Publishing; 2006.

Wiessing D, West D, Pitman T. La Leche League International: The Womanly Art of Breastfeeding. New York, Ballantine Books; 2010.

Useful Websites

http://www.cdc.gov (growth charts: WHO charts for 0–2 years)
http://www.eatright.org (The American Dietetic Association)
http://www.infantrisk.org/ (evidence-based information on the use of medications during pregnancy and breastfeeding)
http://www.hmbana.org (Human Milk Banking Association of North America)
http://www.mjn.com
http://www.abbottnutrition.com
http://medicalgerber.com

Well-Newborn Care

INTRODUCTION

The birth of a new baby is a marvelous time for a family, full of excitement as well as some uncertainty as the amazing journey of child-rearing begins. The well-newborn visits are an opportunity for parents to ask questions regarding the health and development of their baby. These visits enable the physician to **assess the baby's health, growth, and development** and offer guidance to parents throughout their baby's early years. It is also an important time for the pediatrician to assess the infant's temperament, to evaluate the adequacy of maternal and paternal bonding with their infant, and to be sensitive to any family stressors. The physician's role may involve encouraging parents to be sensitive to the cues that their normal newborn will give them regarding their need to feed, sleep, be changed, be held, or even to cry. Parents are often given **reassurance** about many aspects of normal newborn physical findings and development. This chapter describes the concerns most frequently encountered during the well-newborn visits.

SKIN
Generalized Rashes

Neonatal rashes are a common cause of concern for parents. A full discussion of rashes occurring in infancy is provided in Chapter 64, "Rashes."

Diaper Dermatitis (Diaper Rash)

Diaper dermatitis is a common problem presenting in infancy. Multiple conditions can predispose an infant to diaper rash, including sensitive skin, moisture trapped by a diaper, and the acid–base balance of stool and urine. Parents should be advised that **prevention is the best cure**. The diaper area should be kept as dry as possible; frequent diaper changes decrease the occurrence of diaper dermatitis. Parents should also be instructed to leave the perineal area open to air as much as possible and apply a barrier cream to protect against local irritation.

Physical examination allows for the diagnosis of some of the more common skin irritations in the diaper area:

- **Irritant contact dermatitis** appears as erythema with shallow ulcerations predominantly located on the buttocks, thighs, abdomen, and perianal area, sparing the creases. The diagnosis is made clinically, and treatment involves elimination of the irritant, use of a barrier cream, and exposure of the area to air as much as possible.

- **Candida diaper dermatitis** can appear at any age and is characterized by beefy red, scaly plaques with satellite lesions, papules, and pustules. Diagnosis is most often made clinically on the basis of the characteristic appearance of the skin; however, a potassium hydroxide preparation would demonstrate the presence of yeast. Treatment involves application of a topical antifungal agent (e.g., nystatin or clotrimazole ointment) and exposure of the perineal area to air.

 HINT: Candida diaper dermatitis can be easily differentiated from irritant diaper dermatitis by its involvement of the creases (which are spared in irritant diaper dermatitis) and by the presence of satellite lesions.

Mongolian Spots (Congenital Dermal Melanocytosis)
Mongolian spots are **blue-gray macules** that are most commonly seen in Asian, Hispanic, and African American infants. They are typically a few centimeters in diameter and located on the buttocks and lumbosacral area; less commonly, they may be much larger or located on the face or extremities. They typically disappear by 7 to 13 years of age, but some lesions (particularly the larger ones) persist into adulthood.

Salmon Patch (Nevus Simplex and Telangiectatic Nevus)
A salmon patch is a congenital capillary malformation that involves the eyelids, glabella, forehead, or occiput. It consists of **smooth pink or red macular lesions,** often accompanied by telangiectasia. Salmon patches on the glabellar region or upper eyelids usually disappear by 1 year of age, whereas those on the nape of the neck persist ~50% of the time.

Port Wine Stain
A port wine stain or nevus flammeus is present in 0.1% to 0.3% of newborns. They are low flow capillary malformations which are pink or red and generally are unilateral. They persist in 40% to 60% of affected patients. **Sturge–Weber syndrome** is a rare syndrome in which infants with a facial capillary malformation involving the first or second division of the trigeminal nerve have associated ocular and neurologic abnormalities, including glaucoma and seizures.

Café-au-Lait Macules
Café-au-lait macules are **pale brown macules with irregular margins** that range in size from 2 mm to 2 cm. They may appear at birth or in early childhood. Isolated café-au-lait macules occur in 10% to 20% of the normal population. The presence of six or more café-au-lait macules >5 mm prior to puberty in combination with one of the following additional criteria are diagnostic of neurofibromatosis: two or more neurofibromas, axillary or inguinal freckling, optic glioma, Lisch nodules (iris hamartoma), osseous lesions, or a first-degree relative with neurofibromatosis.

CRANIUM
Fontanelles

There are commonly two palpable fontanelles: the **anterior fontanelle** and the **posterior fontanelle**. The anterior fontanelle may minimally increase in size immediately after birth but then gradually decreases in size and is generally closed by 6 to 18 months of age. The posterior fontanelle is generally smaller than the anterior fontanelle and usually closed to palpation by 4 months of age.

Caput Succedaneum

A caput succedaneum is a **diffuse swelling of the soft tissue of the scalp,** usually involving the presenting portion of the head during a vertex delivery. The edema, which is evident during the first few hours of life, crosses suture lines and may cross the midline. In uncomplicated cases of caput succedaneum, no specific treatment is needed; the swelling resolves during the first few days of life. In rare instances, a hemorrhagic caput may occur and cause shock secondary to loss of circulating blood volume. In this instance, blood transfusion and circulatory support are needed. Extensive ecchymoses may result in hyperbilirubinemia, necessitating phototherapy. Molding of the head and overriding of the parietal bones is often associated with a caput succedaneum; however, these conditions resolve during the first few weeks of life.

Cephalohematoma

A cephalohematoma is a **subperiosteal hemorrhage** that results in swelling limited in distribution to one cranial bone (i.e., the swelling does not cross suture lines). Subperiosteal bleeding is a slow process; therefore, the cephalohematoma may not be evident until several hours after birth. A skull fracture, usually linear, may be an associated finding. Most cephalohematomas are resorbed between the ages of 2 weeks and 3 months. In some cases, a bony protuberance remains. Despite this residual calcification, no specific treatment is recommended.

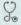 **HINT:** Cephalohematoma may be differentiated from caput succedaneum by the fact that the swelling in cephalohematoma does not cross suture lines.

Molding

Asymmetry in the appearance of the cranium, known as molding or positional plagiocephaly, results from the gentle application of asymmetric pressure on the cranial bones, which occurs when an infant spends a significant portion of time in the same position. The incidence of this condition has increased markedly since implementation of the recommendation to place infants to sleep in a supine position. Infants with asymmetric plagiocephaly should be examined carefully for the presence of **torticollis,** which manifests as decreased range of motion of the neck and head tilt to one side. Affected infants may have a characteristic mass in the affected sternocleidomastoid muscle. Positional plagiocephaly can be managed by environmental manipulation and repositioning the infant to eliminate asymmetric pressure. In cases where torticollis is present, passive stretching is also recommended. In severe cases, cranial molding helmet therapy may be prescribed to diminish the asymmetry.

Craniosynostosis (premature closure of a suture) is another cause of progressive cranial asymmetry. Positional plagiocephaly can generally be differentiated from craniosynostosis by clinical features. When the diagnosis is not apparent clinically, radiographic studies may be performed. Computed tomography (including three-dimensional surface reconstruction) can be used to delineate the extent of craniosynostosis as well as to evaluate intracranial structures. In the event of craniosynostosis, neurosurgical intervention is indicated because of the possibility of asymmetric brain growth and compression of intracranial structures.

 HINT: It is important to differentiate craniosynostosis from positional plagiocephaly early to improve clinical outcome.

EYES
Eye Color
Eye color is a frequent question posed by parents. Eye color is usually established by 3 to 6 months of age; however, additional iris pigmentation continues throughout the first year of life. Depth of eye color may not be evident until the first birthday.

Strabismus
During the newborn period, the eyes frequently wander. However, the **wandering should diminish** (until it eventually disappears) within the first 2 to 3 months of life. Intermittent or persistent esotropia or exotropia after the age of 3 months warrants an evaluation by an ophthalmologist.

 HINT: True strabismus must be differentiated from pseudostrabismus with the use of the corneal light reflex and the cover/uncover test.

Nasolacrimal Duct Obstruction
The lacrimal system develops fully over the first 3 to 4 years of life. The lacrimal glands begin to produce tears by week 3 or 4 of life. In ~6% of newborns, one or both of the lacrimal ducts is blocked, preventing drainage of tears.

Affected children appear to have **excessive tearing**. Therapy entails gentle massage of the lacrimal duct in a downward direction and the use of a warm wet cloth to wipe the collection of tears and mucus from the eye. Most (~90%) blocked lacrimal ducts open spontaneously by 6 months of age. Of those that are still blocked at 1 year of age, <1% open spontaneously. Thus, children with persistent lacrimal duct obstruction beyond 6 to 12 months of age should be evaluated by an ophthalmologist. Parents should be cautioned to call the pediatrician if the conjunctiva becomes red, if the eye discharge becomes purulent, or if the area surrounding the eye or the medial aspect of the nose becomes swollen. These physical findings may indicate conjunctivitis, ophthalmia neonatorum, or dacryocystitis (see Chapter 65, "Red Eye").

EARS
Hearing
Significant bilateral hearing loss (>35 dB) is present in 1 to 3 per 1,000 well-newborns, and in 2 to 4 per 1,000 infants in the intensive care unit. Because auditory stimulation during the first 6 months of life is very important for the development of speech and language skills, significant hearing loss that goes undetected can impede speech, language, and cognitive development. **Universal hearing screening** should occur prior to discharge from the hospital, with appropriate rescreening for those who do not pass the initial test. For infants with significant hearing loss, audiologic and medical evaluations should be performed before 3 months of age, and intensive interventions should be implemented before 6 months of age.

ORAL CAVITY
Teeth
Primary teeth eruption typically occurs at the age of 6 months (range, 3 to 16 months). Natal teeth are teeth present at or shortly after birth. These teeth are generally poorly formed with thin enamel and poor attachments and often located at the end of a stalk of uncalcified tissue. The **natal teeth often are primary teeth that have erupted early**. If removed, spacing of the secondary teeth may be affected; therefore, removal of the natal teeth is recommended only if they are a significant irritant to the tongue, if they present a danger of aspiration secondary to their poor attachment, or if they interfere with feeding.

Dental Lumina Cysts, Bohn Nodules, and Epstein Pearls
Dental lumina cysts are clear or bluish fluid-filled sacs located bilaterally or quadrilaterally on the gum surfaces. These cysts are generally not painful, do not interfere with feeding, and are not associated with surrounding erythema. They disappear within a few weeks and do not require any intervention.

Yellowish white cysts composed of islands of epithelial cells are termed **Bohn nodules** when they are located on the alveolar ridge and **Epstein pearls** when they are located near the midpalatal raphe at the junction of the hard and soft palate. These cysts require no treatment and commonly disappear within a few weeks.

Thrush
White patches in the mouth of an infant may indicate the presence of thrush, a fairly common infection caused by *Candida albicans*. Unlike residual breast

milk or formula, these white patches cannot be easily wiped from the oral mucosa or tongue surface. When thrush is removed from the oral mucosa, the exposed mucosa is typically red and raw and may bleed. Treatment consists of the use of a topical antifungal agent (e.g., nystatin oral suspension). Care should be taken to avoid reinfection from nipples and pacifiers by resterilizing or replacing these items.

> **HINT:** Differentiation between thrush and residual breast milk on a tongue surface is easily made by attempting gentle scraping with a tongue depressor.

CHEST
Breast Hypertrophy and Galactorrhea
Breast buds are present in most infants (both male and female) born after 36 weeks of gestation.

- **Breast hypertrophy** results from the passage of maternal hormones across the placenta during gestation.
- **Galactorrhea** occurs in up to 6% of normal-term infants and typically occurs in infants with larger breast nodules. The thin milky discharge may be caused by maternal estrogen or neonatal prolactin.

Generally, both breast hypertrophy and galactorrhea resolve within several weeks, but occasionally they can persist for several months.

Mastitis
Mastitis, which can manifest as cellulitis or an abscess, occurs in newborns when bacteria invade the already hypertrophied breast tissue. *Staphylococcus aureus* is the most frequently involved organism, but 5% to 10% of infections are caused by gram-negative enteric bacteria.

Typically, the breast bud is erythematous, enlarged, warm, and tender; purulent drainage from the nipple may be present. Infants usually appear well, with only 25% presenting with fever or ill appearance. After obtaining appropriate cultures (including culture of the purulent nipple drainage), the infant should be treated with intravenous antibiotics. Occasionally, a fluctuant abscess forms, requiring surgical drainage.

UMBILICUS
Normal Umbilicus
The umbilical cord is composed of two umbilical arteries and one umbilical vein, which are surrounded by Wharton's jelly, a gelatinous tissue. After birth, the cord is clamped and cut. The trend of dry cord care, without the application of antimicrobial agents, has become common practice in many areas. The remnant of the cord is then left exposed to dry.

The cord generally falls off on its own in 7 to 21 days, but it may take longer. Delayed cord separation can be associated with urachal abnormalities, infection, or underlying immunodeficiency, particularly leukocyte adhesion deficiency syndromes. Parents should be reassured that the presence of **oozing, a few drops of blood, or a mild odor are normal**. Indications for concern are significant redness of the skin (especially circumferential), significant malodorous discharge, or bleeding that is not stopped by gentle pressure.

Umbilical Hernia

An umbilical hernia, which is an outpocketing of layers of skin, fascia, and/or peritoneum, is caused by failure of the fascial opening to close completely. This presents as a **bulge at the umbilicus**. Umbilical hernias are more common in African American infants, premature infants, and infants with certain medical conditions: congenital hypothyroidism, Ehlers–Danlos syndrome, Beckwith–Wiedemann syndrome, trisomy 18, and Down syndrome.

Most defects close spontaneously by the age of 5 years and incarceration or strangulation rarely occurs, so reassurance is most appropriate. Generally, the **likelihood of closure is inversely related to the size of the hernia,** with most small- to moderate-size hernias closing spontaneously. Hernias with a diameter >2 cm are less likely to close spontaneously. Repair is usually indicated if the hernia persists beyond 5 years. Traditional remedies (e.g., umbilical bands, taping coins over the umbilicus) do not hasten closure of the hernia, may irritate the surrounding skin, and are not recommended.

Omphalitis

Omphalitis is an **infection of the umbilical cord and/or surrounding tissues** resulting when bacteria colonize and invade the umbilical cord stump. Once a major cause of neonatal mortality, omphalitis is now **rare in developed countries**.

The condition typically presents with purulent, foul-smelling drainage from the umbilical cord and erythema (frequently circumferential) that progresses to induration and erythema of the abdominal wall. Systemic signs of lethargy, irritability, fever, and poor feeding may suggest more severe infections. Pathogens typically include *Staphylococcus aureus, Streptococcus pyogenes, Escherichia coli, Klebsiella pneumoniae, Proteus mirabilis,* and occasionally anaerobic bacteria. Complications include sepsis, necrotizing fasciitis, hepatic abscess, peritonitis, and portal vein thrombosis.

Appropriate cultures of the purulent umbilical discharge, as well as blood and cerebrospinal fluid, if indicated, should be obtained before initiating therapy. Treatment consists of the intravenous administration of an antistaphylococcal penicillin or vancomycin (in communities with a high incidence of methicillin-resistant *Staphylococcus aureus*) and an aminoglycoside agent.

Umbilical Granuloma

Umbilical granuloma results when an **excessive amount of granulation tissue,** which is not covered by epithelium, accumulates after the separation of the umbilical cord. A small pink mass with persistent weeping and crusting is found at the base of the umbilicus. It is important to differentiate this relatively common and benign condition from umbilical polyps which are firm masses, patent omphalomesenteric ducts, or urachal embryological remnants (see the following section).

Treatment consists of the application of silver nitrate to the granulation tissue once or twice per week for several weeks, but generally only a few applications are required. Care should be taken to avoid the normal surrounding skin, which can be burned by the silver nitrate.

Patent Omphalomesenteric Duct and Patent Urachus

The **omphalomesenteric duct** is a connection between the intestinal tract and the yolk sac during fetal development that normally regresses by the ninth week of gestation. If it remains completely patent, a tubular attachment persists between the ileum and the umbilicus through which intestinal contents can drain. A patent omphalomesenteric duct may be demonstrated by inspection and probing of the tract that is visible at the surface of the umbilicus. Varying degrees of persistent patencies may result in umbilical polyp, Meckel diverticulum, or omphalomesenteric duct cyst. These require further evaluation and surgical referral.

If the **urachus** persists with complete patency after birth, there is a free connection between the urinary bladder and the abdominal wall through which urine may pass. The patient with this condition may present with a constantly wet umbilicus or with a urinary tract infection. Incomplete patency and persistent tissues may result in an umbilical polyp, bladder diverticulum, or urachal cyst. For these conditions, the treatment is prompt evaluation and surgical repair as indicated.

GENITALIA

Boys

Normal Care of the Penis

In **uncircumcised** boys, the foreskin is generally not retractable at birth. Parents should attempt to keep the foreskin clean, avoiding attempts at forcible retraction of the prepuce, which may result in scarring and in true surgical phimosis. The foreskin gradually becomes retractable over time with growth and with the gentle stretching involved with washing. In newborn **circumcised** boys, the exposed glans should be coated with petroleum jelly with each diaper change until it is epithelialized.

Hypospadias and Epispadias

In **hypospadias,** the urethral meatus is abnormally located ventral to the tip of the glans. Classification of the type of hypospadias is based on the anatomic location of the urethral meatus (i.e., glanular, coronal, midshaft, distal shaft, penoscrotal, or perineal). There is frequently an associated abnormality of the foreskin (absence of the ventral portion of the foreskin) as well as associated chordee (ventral curvature of the penis). The abnormality of the foreskin is usually a clue that hypospadias or chordee may be present. In patients with suspected hypospadias, circumcision should be deferred because the presence of the foreskin facilitates the subsequent repair of hypospadias.

Epispadias, in which the urethra opens on the dorsum of the penis, is a more severe but far less common abnormality that is part of a spectrum of anomalies that includes, in its most severe form, bladder exstrophy. Incontinence is a commonly associated finding.

Cryptorchidism (Undescended Testicle)

Cryptorchidism is found in 3.4% to 5.8% of full-term boys and may be unilateral or bilateral. Most testes that are not descended at birth spontaneously descend during the first 3 to 6 months; few testes descend after this time. The incidence of cryptorchidism at the age of 1 year is ~0.8%.

The treatment for cryptorchidism is **orchiopexy,** which can be performed at any age after 4 months and is optimally performed before 1 year of age to decrease the risk of infertility, malignancy, and testicular torsion. Because timing is very important, all infants with unilateral or bilateral undescended testes at the 4- or 6-month visit should be referred to a urologist for evaluation.

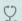 **HINT:** In phenotypically male infants with bilateral nonpalpable testes, the clinician should rule out congenital adrenal hyperplasia and intersex abnormalities immediately to improve clinical outcome.

Inguinal Hernia and Hydrocele

Both hernias and hydroceles result from failure of the processus vaginalis to undergo fusion and obliteration during fetal life.

- **Inguinal hernia** occurs in 1% to 5% of children, is 10 times more common in boys than in girls, and may occur in up to 30% of premature infants born before 36 weeks of gestation.
- **Indirect inguinal hernia** presents as a bulge in the inguinal canal that may be present at rest or may only be appreciated during straining or crying as a loop of intestine descends into the hernia sac. Appropriate therapy consists of referral for surgical repair within a short time of diagnosis to minimize the risk of incarceration or strangulation.
- A **hydrocele** represents persistence of the processus vaginalis with partial closure proximally, which allows fluid to pass into the scrotal sac. The condition is evidenced by the presence of scrotal swelling, which transilluminates in the absence of a hernia. Hydroceles in infants may communicate with the peritoneal cavity, or they may be noncommunicating. Hydroceles are often associated with inguinal hernias or they may be an isolated finding. Most infants with isolated hydrocele undergo spontaneous closure of the processus vaginalis with resolution of the hydrocele, so reassurance is most appropriate. Referral to a surgeon is indicated for patients with hydroceles that persist beyond the age of 6 months to 1 year (surgeons have different preferences for timing of surgery) or that wax and wane in size, indicating communication with the peritoneal cavity and the associated risk of hernia.

Girls
Vaginal Discharge and Bleeding

Normal newborn girls have well-estrogenized vaginal mucosa because of the trans-placental passage of maternal hormones; therefore, a thick white vaginal discharge is a normal finding in a newborn girl. Many newborns also have a scant amount of vaginal bleeding in the first week of life owing to the withdrawal of maternal estrogen. Parents should be reassured that both findings are normal.

HIP EXAMINATION

Infants are examined in the newborn period and at all subsequent visits for the presence of developmental dysplasia of the hip (DDH), which includes unstable, subluxed, or dislocated hips. These conditions have an incidence of 1 in 1,000 newborns with instability and 1 to 1.5 in 1,000 infants with dislocation. The incidence is higher in girls, infants with a family history of DDH, infants with breech presentation, and infants with other risk factors which limit mobility such as neuromuscular conditions and oligohydramnios. The Ortolani and Barlow maneuvers are used to assess hip stability in the newborn (see Chapter 2, "The Physical Examination"). The Ortolani maneuver detects a dislocated femoral head that is reduced into the acetabulum, and the Barlow maneuver detects a hip that can be dislocated posteriorly by gentle adduction and posterior pressure. They are only present for the first 2 to 3 months of age. Other signs that are suggestive of hip dislocation are asymmetry of thigh folds or buttock creases, a positive Galeazzi sign (relative shortness of the femur with the hips and knees flexed), discrepancy of leg lengths, and limited hip abduction.

If a true positive Ortolani or Barlow sign is found, the infant should be referred to an orthopedist. Infants with other equivocally positive signs such as a soft click should have a follow-up examination in 2 weeks. If findings persist, infants may be referred to an orthopedist or have ultrasonography of their hips by 3 weeks of age. For infants detected with concerns who are >4 months of age, plain radiography of the hips is the preferred imaging modality. Because of the high risk of DDH in girls who are born breech (absolute risk of DDH is 12 of 1,000) and girls with a positive family history of DDH (absolute risk of 44 of 1,000), imaging with ultrasonography at 6 weeks of age or plain radiography of the pelvis and hips at 4 months of age is recommended in these select groups.

URINATION AND DEFECATION
Urate Crystals ("Pink Diaper Syndrome")

Parents may notice a **pink crystalline substance** in the diaper or a **salmon-pink residue** on the surface of the diaper, resulting from the deposition of urate crystals. Urate crystals are usually easily distinguished from blood on the basis of appearance, but occult blood testing can also be performed. Urate crystals are typically found in the setting of concentrated urine and **may indicate dehydration,** so a careful assessment for hydration status is warranted (including frequency of wet diapers, vital signs, and presence of a sunken fontanelle or dry mucous membranes). Parents should be counseled to increase the frequency and amount of feedings if there are concerns about an infant's hydration.

Meconium, Transitional Stool, and Typical Stool

Passage of some amount of **meconium** usually occurs within the first 12 hours of life, with 99% of all term infants and 95% of preterm infants passing meconium within the first 48 hours of life. **Transitional stools** follow the passage of meconium until the passage of the typical stool of the newborn is established. Typically, the stool is described as yellow and seedy in breast-fed infants and yellow or brown in formula-fed infants.

Failure to pass meconium can occur as a result of imperforate anus, functional intestinal obstruction (i.e., Hirschsprung disease), illness, or hypotonia. Failure to pass transitional stools following the passage of meconium may be indicative of a volvulus or malrotation. Any newborn who fails to pass meconium or fails to progress to passing **typical stools** should be evaluated in a timely fashion to rule out the presence of intestinal obstruction.

Establishment of a Bowel Pattern and Constipation

In each newborn, the establishment of a **normal bowel pattern** occurs over time and varies as the newborn grows. The typical breast-fed baby passes a bowel movement after each feeding initially, but normal patterns vary from a bowel movement after each feeding to one every 1 to 7 days. The typical formula-fed baby has a bowel movement every 1 to 3 days.

Constipation is the infrequent passage of hard or painful bowel movements or a decrease in the frequency of bowel movements from an established pattern. Constipation can occur at any age. It is important to discuss with the parents of a newborn the fact that the consistency and regularity of the passing of stool varies over time. Parents should be advised to contact the physician if the infant develops abdominal distention, vomiting, refusal to eat, bloody stools, or extremely hard stools. These clinical signs and symptoms may indicate pathology, including many of the entities discussed in Chapter 22, "Constipation."

ROUTINE CARE

Vitamin K should be administered after delivery via intramuscular injection to reduce the risk of hemorrhagic disease of the newborn. Erythromycin or tetracycline ophthalmic ointment is recommended to prevent neonatal ophthalmic infections due to gonorrhea.

 HINT: Topical ophthalmic ointment is not effective in preventing chlamydia conjunctivitis, presumably because it does not eliminate nasopharyngeal carriage. Screening of all pregnant women with appropriate treatment of exposed infants with oral antibiotics, usually erythromycin, is recommended.

Hepatitis B Immunization

All newborns should be vaccinated before hospital discharge against Hepatitis B regardless of maternal Hepatitis B surface antigen (HBsAg) status. For infants born to HBsAg-positive mothers, the initial dose of hepatitis B vaccine should be administered within 12 hours of birth and hepatitis B immune globulin 0.5 mL should be administered at the same time but at a different anatomic site. For infants born to mothers with unknown HBsAg status, the initial dose of hepatitis B vaccine should be administered within 12 hours of birth while awaiting maternal results. If the mother is found to be HBsAg positive, term infants should receive hepatitis B immune globulin as soon as possible, but within 7 days of birth.

Newborn Screening Tests

Capillary blood from a heelstick is obtained from every infant after 24 hours of age and prior to discharge from the hospital, with the ideal age being between 2 and 4 days of age. This blood is sent for newborn screening tests, which look for a variety of **metabolic and genetic disorders**. The specific tests vary by state, but all states test for congenital hypothyroidism, phenylketonuria, hemoglobinopathies (sickle cell disease, sickle C disease, and thalassemia), and galactosemia. The *majority* of states screen for biotinidase deficiency and congenital adrenal hyperplasia. New techniques in mass spectroscopy have enabled a majority of states to test for fatty acid disorders (such as medium-chain acyl-coenzyme A dehydrogenase deficiency), organic acid disorders (including methylmalonic academia), and amino acid disorders such as tyrosinemia and homocystinuria. Selected states also screen for glucose-6-phosphatase deficiency, toxoplasmosis, and cystic fibrosis.

Follow-up of abnormal newborn screening tests, with appropriate and timely confirmatory testing, referral, and care, requires close cooperation among the primary pediatrician and the birth hospital, state newborn screening laboratory, and appropriate subspecialists in endocrinology, metabolism, or hematology.

Recommended Sleeping Position

The American Academy of Pediatrics recommends placing healthy term infants to sleep in a nonprone position. **Sleeping supine confers the lowest risk of sudden infant death syndrome (SIDS)** and is preferred. This recommendation is based on analysis of a number of studies from around the world that demonstrate an association between the prone sleeping position and an increased risk of SIDS. In the United States, there has been a reduction in prone sleeping from 70% to 20% of infants since 1992, with a concomitant 40% reduction in the rate of SIDS.

In addition, parents should be instructed not to put infants to sleep on waterbeds, sofas, or soft mattresses. They should not place any soft objects (such as pillows, quilts, sheepskins, or stuffed toys) in an infant's sleeping environment, and they should recognize that loose bedding may also present a hazard to a small infant. Overheating and over-bundling should be avoided.

COMMON PARENTAL CONCERNS

There are many common concerns shared by new parents. The following discussion may aid in reassuring parents. Many babies **hiccup**. The precise cause is unknown, although many feel it is a reflection of an immature nervous system. If hiccups persist for 5 to 10 minutes and are distressing to those caring for the baby, nursing or a few sucks on a bottle of sugar water may relieve the hiccups.

In babies, **sneezing and coughing** can be a protective mechanism to clear material from the respiratory passages. Therefore, intermittent sneezing or coughing should not be of concern. Persistent coughing or sneezing may be a sign of a problem and requires evaluation by a physician. In addition, perceived **nasal congestion** can be a concern of new parents. Most of the time this is related to normal narrow newborn nasal passages or fluids, which may pass intranasally during delivery. Persistent nasal congestion or blockage can be a sign of choanal stenosis or choanal atresia, which should be evaluated.

A baby's **chin** may intermittently **quiver**. This motion is a reflection of an immature nervous system, and it does not indicate that the infant is cold. This quivering stops as the nervous system matures.

Suggested Readings

American Academy of Pediatrics, Committee on Quality Improvement, Subcommittee on Developmental Dysplasia of the Hip. Clinical Practice Guideline: Early detection of developmental dysplasia of the hip. *Pediatrics.* 2000;105:896–905.

Barthold TS, Gonzalez R. The Epidemiology of congenital cryptorchidism, testicular ascent and orchiopexy. *J Urology.* 2003;170:2396.

Gill B, Kogan S. Cryptorchidism. Current concepts. *Pediatr Clin N Am.* 1997;44(5):1211–1227.

Joint Committee on Infant Hearing. Year 2007 Position Statement: principles and guidelines for early hearing detection and intervention. *Pediatrics.* 2007;120(4):898–921.

Kaye CI and the Committee on Genetics: Introduction to the newborn screening fact sheets. *Pediatrics.* 2006;118:1304–1312.

Komotar RJ, Zacharia BE, Ellis JA, et al. Pitfalls for the pediatrician: positional molding or craniosynostosis? *Pediatr Ann.* 2006;35(5):365–375.

MacDonald MG, Mullett MD, Seishia MM. *Avery's Neonatology: Pathophysiology and Management of the Newborn.* Philadelphia, PA: Lippincott, Williams & Wilkins; 2005.

Paller AS, Mancini AJ. *Hurwitz Clinical Pediatric Dermatology: A Textbook of Skin Disorders of Childhood and Adolescence.* Philadelphia, PA: Elsevier Saunders; 2006.

Scheinfeld N. Diaper dermatitis: a review and brief survey of eruptions of the diaper area. *Am J Clin Dermatol.* 2005;6(5):273–281.

Scheree LR, Grosfels JL. Inguinal hernia and umbilical anomalies. *Pediatr Clin N Am.* 1993;40(6):1121–1131.

Shusterman S. Pediatric dental update. *Pediatr Rev.* 1994;15:311–319.

Stellwagen L, Boies E. Care of the well newborn. *Pediatr Rev.* 2006;27:89–98.

PART 2

Problems

CHAPTER 8

Marc H. Gorelick

Abdominal Mass

INTRODUCTION

In children, abdominal masses present in variable ways. **Some produce symptoms or signs; others remain silent** even when large. An abdominal mass may be discovered by a parent or caregiver, or it may be an incidental finding during physical examination. The **age of the child is an important factor** in the differential diagnosis. Most masses discovered in neonates are benign, whereas up to 50% of masses in older children are malignant (Table 8-1). Table 8-2 lists the most common sites of origin of abdominal masses according to the age of the patient.

 HINT: In newborns, the bladder is an abdominal organ.

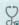 **HINT:** An abdominal mass in a neonate is usually renal in origin—hydronephrosis and multicystic kidney are the most common causes of abdominal mass in neonates.

TABLE 8-1	Common Abdominal Masses	
Neonates	**Infants**	**Older Children**
Hydronephrosis	Hydronephrosis	Constipation
Ureteropelvic obstruction	Wilms tumor	Wilms tumor
Multicystic kidney	Neuroblastoma	Neuroblastoma
Distended bladder	Distended bladder	Hydronephrosis
Ectopic kidney	Multicystic kidney	Appendiceal abscess
Hydrometrocolpos	Pyloric stenosis	Ovarian cyst
Gastrointestinal duplication	Intussusception	
Posterior urethral valves	Hydrometrocolpos	
Mesonephric blastoma		

 DIFFERENTIAL DIAGNOSIS LIST

Infectious Causes
- Appendiceal abscess
- Tubo-ovarian abscess
- Hepatic abscess
- Perinephric abscess

Neoplastic Causes
Malignant
- Wilms tumor (nephroblastoma)
- Neuroblastoma
- Lymphoma
- Rhabdomyosarcoma
- Rhabdoid tumor
- Hepatoblastoma
- Sarcomas (retroperitoneal and embryonal)
- Ovarian tumor
- Metastatic disease

Benign
- Ovarian teratoma
- Sacrococcygeal teratoma
- Mesonephric blastoma

Traumatic Causes
- Perinephric hematoma
- Pancreatic pseudocyst
- Adrenal hematoma
- Duodenal hematoma

Congenital or Vascular Causes
- Cysts—ovarian, choledochal, hepatic, mesenteric, urachal
- Hydrometrocolpos or hematocolpos
- Anterior myelomeningocele
- Renal vein thrombosis
- Hepatic hemangioma

Gastrointestinal System Causes
- Gastrointestinal (bowel) duplication
- Constipation
- Pyloric stenosis
- Hepatitis
- Intestinal distention—intussusception, imperforate anus, Hirschsprung disease, volvulus, meconium ileus
- Gallbladder hydrops

TABLE 8-2	Sites of Origin of Abdominal Masses			
	Renal	**Retroperitoneal**	**Gastrointestinal**	**Genital**
Neonates	20%	15%	55%	10%
Infants and older children	55%	23%	18%	4%

Genitourinary System Causes

- Hydronephrosis
- Polycystic or multicystic kidney
- Ectopic or horseshoe kidney
- Posterior urethral valves
- Distended bladder
- Pregnancy (intrauterine or ectopic)

 HINT: The patient's age is an important key in helping narrow down the possible differential diagnosis of an abdominal mass because its causes differ among neonates, infants, and children.

DIFFERENTIAL DIAGNOSIS DISCUSSION
Constipation

Constipation is discussed in Chapter 22, "Constipation."

Intussusception

Intussusception is discussed in Chapter 9, "Abdominal Pain, Acute."

Appendiceal Abscess
Etiology

Untreated acute appendicitis leads to perforation with abscess formation.

Clinical Features

A child with an appendiceal abscess appears generally ill. **Fever and abdominal pain** are common symptoms. Although many children have a history highly suggestive of appendicitis (see Chapter 9, "Abdominal Pain, Acute"), others have an atypical history characterized by a subacute course, with symptoms present for days to weeks.

 HINT: Patients (especially young children) with appendiceal abscess may not show typical abnormalities associated with appendicitis, such as anorexia and peritoneal signs.

Evaluation

A **tender mass** is located in the **right lower quadrant,** and signs of peritoneal irritation are often, but not invariably, present. The mass may be palpable on rectal examination. In **postpubertal females, a pelvic examination** is important to exclude pelvic inflammatory disease.

Leukocytosis with a left shift is a helpful supportive finding. If the diagnosis of appendicitis is clear, additional studies are unnecessary. In difficult cases, an abdominal radiograph may provide confirmatory evidence (e.g., a fecalith, present in <10% of cases, free intraperitoneal air, or a right lower quadrant mass effect with ileus); however, **ultrasound** is the diagnostic study of choice.

Treatment

Urgent surgical consultation is necessary. Preoperatively, patients should receive broad-spectrum parenteral **antibiotics** to cover gram-negative and anaerobic organisms.

Distended Bladder

Etiology

A palpably distended bladder results from **obstruction** (e.g., posterior urethral valves in boys, extrinsic mass, and stricture), **neurologic dysfunction** (e.g., spinal cord injury, myelomeningocele, and anticholinergic medication), or **voluntary retention** (as a result of dysuria).

Evaluation

The history should include questions about urinary frequency, dysuria, and the quality of the stream, as well as bowel function, which may also be affected in cases of neurogenic bladder.

Palpation of the abdomen reveals a **smooth suprapubic mass,** which may be somewhat tender if the abdomen is grossly distended. The mass is cystic to percussion. Look for evidence of urethral or vaginal irritation and evaluate **neurologic function**. The innervation of the bladder is S2-S4, the same area as the sacrum, so **testing the anal wink** identifies those patients with disruption of bladder innervation.

An **ultrasound** confirms that the mass is the bladder, and a **voiding cysto-urethrogram** may help identify the cause of the distention. **Urinalysis** should be performed if dysuria suggests cystitis.

Treatment

Urethral catheterization relieves the distention. Definitive treatment depends on the underlying cause of the obstruction, but usually referral to a urologist is required.

Hydronephrosis

Etiology

Hydronephrosis **(dilation of the renal collecting system)** results from **partial or complete obstruction of urine flow**. Causes include ureteropelvic junction obstruction, posterior urethral valves, vesicoureteral reflux, ureterocele, and duplication of the collecting system. Hydronephrosis can be unilateral or bilateral.

Clinical Features

Many children with hydronephrosis are **asymptomatic;** others present with **abdominal pain** (often chronic or recurrent) or, in rare cases, evidence of **renal failure**. Hydronephrosis tends to be more common in males and more commonly involves the left kidney.

Evaluation

Abdominal examination reveals a palpable unilateral or bilateral smooth flank mass, especially in infants. Any palpable kidney in a child >3 years of age is suspicious, as is asymmetry in younger children.

Ultrasound is diagnostic. It shows a dilated renal pelvis surrounded by several cystic structures (calyces).

Treatment

Most causes of hydronephrosis are treated with **surgical repair**.

Wilms Tumor (Nephroblastoma)

Etiology

Wilms tumor, the **second most common intra-abdominal malignancy in children,** accounts for virtually all pediatric renal neoplasms. Wilms tumor is associated with certain **congenital anomalies:** genitourinary malformations, hemihypertrophy, sporadic aniridia, cryptorchidism, Beckwith–Wiedemann syndrome, Denys–Drash syndrome, and the Wilms (tumor), aniridia, genitourinary (abnormalities), and (mental) retardation (WAGR complex). There is also a **familial form** of Wilms tumor.

Clinical Features

Peak incidence is at **3 years** of age. Most patients present with an **asymptomatic abdominal mass or abdominal distention**. It can go unnoticed owing to the tumor's retroperitoneal location and painless quality. This diagnosis should be considered in any young child with a large abdomen. Occasional symptoms include abdominal pain, vomiting, hematuria, and hypertension.

Evaluation

The mass is **smooth and firm,** rarely crossing the midline; in 5% to 10% of patients, masses are **bilateral**. In some cases, the mass is so large (mean diameter of 11 cm at the time of diagnosis in one study) that **diffuse distention,** rather than a discrete mass, is felt.

Although it may show microscopic hematuria, urinalysis is too nonspecific to be helpful. An **abdominal sonogram or computed tomography (CT) scan** shows a solid intrarenal mass.

Treatment

Wilms tumor is treated with a combination of **surgical resection (nephrectomy) and chemotherapy**. Success rates depend on the extent of disease and the clinical stage at the time of diagnosis. Approximately 15% are metastatic at diagnosis, most commonly to the lungs.

HINT: The most common solid renal tumor in a neonate is congenital mesoblastic nephroma. This is different from Wilms tumor in that it is benign and usually occurs in the first 3 months of life, whereas Wilms tumor usually presents after 6 months of life.

Neuroblastoma

Etiology

A malignancy arising from neural crest cells, neuroblastoma is the **second most common solid tumor of childhood and the most common extracranial solid**

tumor in childhood. In approximately two-thirds of patients, the primary site is in the **abdomen** (usually adrenal); the **thoracic region** is the next most common site.

Clinical Features

Like Wilms tumor, neuroblastoma may present as an **asymptomatic mass**. However, patients tend to be somewhat **younger** (median age, 2 years) and they appear **more ill**—an indication of the high incidence of metastatic disease at diagnosis (~60%).

Associated symptoms may include **abdominal pain, urinary obstruction, flushing, sweating, diarrhea** (caused by tumor secretion of vasoactive intestinal peptide), **anorexia, malaise, and site-specific symptoms** from metastases to the bone, skin, liver, or central nervous system. Although most tumors produce catecholamines, rapid metabolism makes symptoms of hypertension and irritability rare.

 HINT: Opsomyoclonus, consisting of myoclonic jerks, ataxia, and jerky eye movements ("dancing eyes and dancing feet"), is a unique paraneoplastic syndrome associated with neuroblastoma. Findings suggestive of opsomyoclonus should prompt a search for an occult neuroblastoma, even in the absence of an abdominal mass.

Evaluation

A firm, irregular, nontender mass is palpable in the abdominal region. Other physical examination findings include pallor, subcutaneous nodules, and hepatomegaly.

 HINT: Neuroblastoma is one of the few causes of massive hepatomegaly.

Urinary levels of catecholamine metabolites, which are elevated in 90% to 95% of patients (i.e., vanillylmandelic acid, homovanillic acid, and metanephrine), were used for screening in the past, but abdominal ultrasound or CT is the current diagnostic procedure of choice. Identification of a solid adrenal or paraspinal mass, which is calcified in 80% of patients, strongly suggests neuroblastoma. Findings usually produce biliary tract obstruction with jaundice and acholic stools. Bone scan and skeletal radiographs are helpful to delineate bony involvement.

Treatment

Treatment may include **bone marrow transplantation, chemotherapy, radiation therapy, and surgical debulking or resection**. The prognosis depends on the stage of the disease, the age of the patient, the site of the primary tumor, and the findings on histologic evaluation. N-myc oncogene amplification is associated with a poorer prognosis and occurs in about 20% of patients. Patients with stage IV-S disease, which often presents in the first few months of life, may experience spontaneous regression of the primary tumor.

Cysts
Etiology
Cysts may arise as **developmental variants** from any number of structures.

Clinical Features
Symptoms are **variable** and depend on the site of the cyst; **nonspecific abdominal pain** is most common. An ovarian cyst may cause cyclic pain in menarchal girls; a choledochal cyst usually produces biliary tract obstruction with jaundice and acholic stools.

Evaluation
Many cysts are palpable on abdominal or pelvic examination as a **smooth, soft, or firm mass** at the site of the organ of origin.

A **sonogram** is the optimal diagnostic tool.

Treatment
Ovarian or mesenteric cysts discovered as an incidental finding may be followed because they spontaneously regress much of the time; cysts causing **significant symptoms** require **excision**.

Renal Cystic Disease
Types of Renal Cystic Disease
- **Multicystic dysplastic renal disease.** This is one of the most common causes of abdominal masses in neonates. The affected kidney consists of a mass of cysts with little or no identifiable renal tissue ("grape cluster" appearance on ultrasound). These are usually unilateral and sporadic with symptoms that may include abdominal pain, hematuria, and urinary tract infections; bilateral cases are associated with renal failure.
- **Polycystic renal disease.** In polycystic renal disease, one or both kidneys contain multiple cortical and medullary cysts consisting of dilated tubules. The more common autosomal dominant form usually presents in adulthood but is sometimes diagnosed in children. The autosomal recessive form, which is more severe and more likely bilateral, usually manifests itself in infancy. Both forms are uncommon in children. Ultrasound findings show many small cysts in the collecting ducts with no intrinsic renal dysplasia.

 HINT: The majority of infants with autosomal recessive polycystic kidney disease also have hepatic cysts, sometimes leading to severe liver disease.

Clinical Features
Except for those with bilateral involvement, infants with multicystic dysplastic kidney present with an **asymptomatic flank mass** that is irregular and nontender. Infants with bilateral cystic kidneys may have a history of **oligohydramnios** and, in severe cases, findings of **Potter syndrome**. Children with multicystic dysplastic kidney have a high incidence of **associated urinary tract anomalies** and require **complete urologic evaluation**.

Patients with polycystic kidney disease often have concomitant **hematuria** (gross or microscopic) or **hypertension,** but renal failure is rare. Again, a **unilateral or bilateral flank mass** is palpated.

Evaluation
In all cases, **ultrasound** confirms the diagnosis.

Treatment
Patients with renal cystic disease require close follow-up to monitor signs of **renal insufficiency or hypertension**. These patients are usually on dialysis until transplantation can occur.

Gastrointestinal (Bowel) Duplication
Etiology
Occurring in any part of the gastrointestinal tract, but most commonly in the **region of the ileocecal valve,** duplication cysts result from a **morphogenetic defect**. The cyst varies in size, has a tubular or spherical shape, and may or may not communicate with the true intestinal lumen, producing a closed cystic mass. These can present as asymptomatic abdominal distension or with signs of obstruction, bleeding, or perforation. Gastrointestinal (bowel) duplication is the **most common cause of neonatal gastrointestinal masses**.

Evaluation
Bowel duplications may be **asymptomatic** or they may cause **intestinal obstruction**. They are typically compressible and mobile, and either round or tubular. The diagnosis is made by **ultrasound** or a **gastrointestinal contrast study**.

 HINT: The mucosa of the cyst may arise from any part of the gastrointestinal tract, regardless of location; when gastric mucosa is included, ulceration or perforation may result. A Meckel scan may be useful in cases where gastric mucosa may be present.

Treatment
Surgical resection is generally curative.

Hydrometrocolpos and Hematocolpos
Etiology
Imperforate hymen leads to accumulation of secretions in the vagina; if undetected until puberty, accumulated menstrual blood causes hematocolpos.

Clinical Features
The distended vagina may **interfere with voiding or defecation,** but infants are otherwise **asymptomatic**.

Evaluation
The **mass is smooth, suprapubic, and frequently palpable** on rectal examination. The imperforate hymen may also be seen bulging externally.

An **ultrasound** shows the dilated, fluid-filled vagina.

Treatment
Resection of the imperforate hymen is required.

EVALUATION OF ABDOMINAL MASS
Patient History
The following items should be noted:

- In neonates: maternal pregnancy complicated by oligohydramnios/polyhydramnios, or any interventions (such as amniocentesis)
- Symptoms (e.g., fever, abdominal pain, vomiting, or jaundice)
- Stooling pattern (frequency and consistency)
- Voiding pattern (frequency and hematuria)
- History of trauma
- Menstrual history
- History of abdominal surgery or umbilical catheterization

Physical Examination
The following should be noted or sought on physical examination:

- Size and location of mass (asymmetry, position of the umbilicus)
- Presence of tenderness
- Findings on percussion
- Texture (solid or cystic)
- Blood pressure
- Presence of scleral icterus
- Evidence of dehydration

Laboratory Studies
The choice of laboratory studies is guided by the type of symptoms and signs that are involved. Studies to be considered include:

- Urinalysis
- Complete blood cell count
- Blood urea nitrogen and creatinine
- Electrolytes
- Hepatic transaminases and bilirubin

Diagnostic Modalities
- **Ultrasound.** The diagnostic study of choice in most cases of abdominal mass is ultrasound. Exceptions include clinically diagnosed constipation, intrauterine pregnancy, and appendicitis, where further studies are generally unnecessary. Ultrasound examination provides information regarding the location and character (cystic vs. solid, homogeneous vs. heterogeneous, calcified) of the abdominal mass and should be the initial study in most cases.
- **Abdominal radiographs.** Although these are frequently obtained, they provide little information in a relatively asymptomatic child. Some exceptions are the use

TABLE 8-3	Abdominal Masses Commonly Associated with Calcification

Neuroblastoma
Teratoma
Ovarian
Sacrococcygeal
Adrenal hematoma
Hepatic hemangioma
Meconium peritonitis

of radiographs to detect calcifications in a mass, organomegaly, or displacement of the intestines, all of which may help narrow the differential diagnosis (Table 8-3).
- **Abdominal CT.** CT provides more detailed anatomic information than ultrasound. However, due to the substantial radiation exposure, it should be reserved for further delineation of certain masses; may be a substitute as the initial study when ultrasound is unavailable.
- **Magnetic resonance imaging (MRI).** MRI provides the best anatomic information, but rarely used as the initial imaging study due to limited availability and cost. In many centers, this is replacing the CT as the definitive study of choice.
- **Intravenous urography.** Once the initial study of choice, has now been supplanted by the preceding methods.

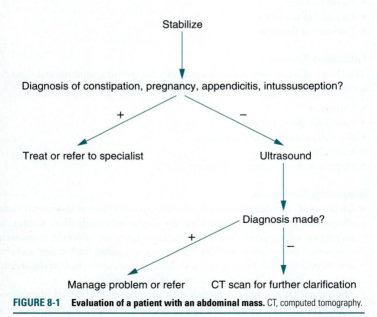

FIGURE 8-1 **Evaluation of a patient with an abdominal mass.** CT, computed tomography.

APPROACH TO THE PATIENT

The workup of an abdominal mass should be accompanied by **supportive care and resuscitation** in an ill-appearing child, including **fluid therapy** in the presence of dehydration, **supplemental oxygen and assisted respiration** in patients with respiratory compromise, and **control of blood pressure** in patients with symptomatic hypertension (Figure 8-1). The initial study in these patients is an **abdominal series** (flat and upright) to evaluate for obstruction or perforation. Once the child is stabilized, additional studies may be undertaken.

Suggested Readings

Cass DL, Hawkins E, Brandt ML, et al. Surgery for ovarian masses in infants, children, and adolescents: 102 consecutive patients treated in a 15-year period. *J Pediatr Surg.* 2001;36(5):693–699.

Caty MG, Shamberger RC. Abdominal tumors in infancy and childhood. *Pediatr Clin N Am.* 1993; 40:1253–1271.

Chandler JC, Gauderer MW. The neonate with an abdominal mass. *Pediatric Clin N Am.* 2004;51:979–997.

Golden CB, Feusner JH. Malignant abdominal masses in children: quick guide to evaluation and diagnosis. *Pediatr Clin N Am.* 2002;49:1369–1392.

Hoffer FA. Magnetic resonance imaging of abdominal masses in the pediatric patient. *Semin Ultrasound CT MRI.* 2005;26:212–223.

Kim S, Chung DH. Pediatric solid malignancies: neuroblastoma and Wilms tumor. *Surg Clin N Am.* 2006;86:469–487.

Merten DF, Kirks DR. Diagnostic imaging of pediatric abdominal masses. *Pediatr Clin N Am.* 1985; 32:1397–1425.

Morrison SC. Controversies in abdominal imaging. *Pediatr Clin N Am.* 1997;44(3):555–574.

Olsen OE. Imaging of abdominal tumors: CT or MRI? *Pediatr Radiol.* 2008;38(Suppl 3):S452–S458.

Ota FS, Maxson RT, Abramo TJ. Ominous findings in toddlers with increasing abdominal girth: two unusual cases and a review of the clinical evaluation. *Ann Emerg Med.* 2005;45(5):517–523.

Abdominal Pain, Acute

INTRODUCTION

The evaluation of acute abdominal pain in a child presents a challenge to any clinician. A common chief complaint, the causes of abdominal pain range from benign to life-threatening processes. Furthermore, abdominal pain can originate from both intra-abdominal organs and sources outside the abdomen (see Chapter 59, "Pelvic Pain" and Chapter 70, "Sexually Transmitted Diseases"). An ordered approach to evaluation is required and is guided by the age and sex of the patient, the history and physical examination, and selected laboratory and imaging studies. In many cases, a definitive diagnosis may not be made on a single patient encounter, and repeated evaluation is required.

DIFFERENTIAL DIAGNOSIS LIST

Gastrointestinal
- Constipation
- Appendicitis/appendiceal abscess
- Peptic ulcer disease/gastritis
- Gastroenteritis
- Esophagitis/gastroesophageal reflux
- Foreign body ingestion
- Cholecystitis
- Pancreatitis/pancreatic pseudocyst
- Hepatitis
- Bowel obstruction
- Incarcerated hernia
- Intussusception
- Abdominal trauma
- Hirschsprung disease
- Inflammatory bowel disease
- Peritonitis
- Necrotizing enterocolitis
- Mesenteric adenitis
- Malrotation/volvulus
- Infectious colitis
- Antibiotic-associated (pseudomembranous) colitis
- Food allergy (e.g., milk or soy protein)
- Malabsorption syndromes

Genitourinary
- Urinary tract infection (e.g., cystitis, pyelonephritis)
- Renal calculus
- Pregnancy (e.g., intrauterine, ectopic)
- Pelvic inflammatory disease
- Ovarian cyst
- Adnexal torsion
- Mittelschmerz
- Dysmenorrhea
- Endometriosis
- Hematocolpos/hydrometrocolpos
- Testicular torsion/torsion of the appendix testis

- Orchitis
- Epididymitis

Respiratory
- Pneumonia
- Streptococcal pharyngitis
- Asthma

Malignancy
- Wilms tumor
- Neuroblastoma
- Leukemia
- Lymphoma
- Hepatoblastoma
- Ovarian tumor
- Teratoma
- Typhlitis
- Rhabdomyosarcoma

Systemic Disorders
- Diabetic ketoacidosis
- Vasculitis (e.g., Henoch-Schönlein purpura)

- Collagen vascular disease (e.g., lupus, polyarteritis nodosa, juvenile dermatomyositis, scleroderma)
- Kawasaki disease
- Hemolytic uremic syndrome
- Infectious mononucleosis
- Sickle cell disease
- Cystic fibrosis
- Porphyria

Miscellaneous
- Functional
- Colic
- Myocarditis
- Pericarditis
- Toxins (e.g., caustic ingestion, black widow spider bite)
- Orthopedic (e.g., septic arthritis/osteomyelitis/diskitis)
- Abdominal migraine
- Familial Mediterranean fever
- Herpes zoster
- Heat cramps

Any of the causes of chronic abdominal pain can present with acute exacerbations of pain (see Chapter 10, "Abdominal Pain, Chronic")

DIFFERENTIAL DIAGNOSIS DISCUSSION
Acute Gastroenteritis
Acute gastroenteritis is discussed in Chapter 27, "Diarrhea, Acute."

Adnexal Torsion
Adnexal torsion is discussed in Chapter 59, "Pelvic Pain."

Appendicitis
Etiology
Appendicitis is a common cause of abdominal pain, occurring in children of all ages. Appendicitis is typically caused by obstruction of the appendiceal lumen, resulting in appendiceal distention, inhibition of lymphatic and vascular drainage, edema, and perforation.

Clinical Features
The classic symptoms of appendicitis are periumbilical abdominal pain, followed by fever, anorexia, and vomiting. As the disease progresses, pain localizes to the right lower quadrant (i.e., McBurney's point). However, patients with appendicitis

often present atypically and with nonspecific symptoms. An appendix situated in the lateral colonic gutter may cause flank pain, while an appendix positioned more medially may irritate the bladder and cause dysuria and suprapubic pain. Alternatively, an appendix positioned in the pelvis may cause diarrhea if the inflamed appendix irritates the sigmoid colon. Patients may prefer to lie still because of the peritoneal irritation caused by an inflamed appendix, and children may report increasing pain with coughing or jumping.

 HINT: Patients with appendicitis are frequently misdiagnosed because of misleading symptoms, such as diarrhea, constipation, dysuria, or lethargy, that suggest other diagnoses.

Unfortunately, making the diagnosis of appendicitis can be challenging, especially in preverbal children in the early stages of the disease process. As a result, young patients frequently present after the appendix has perforated. These patients may report transient improvement of their pain immediately after perforation but soon complain of diffuse abdominal pain from peritonitis. Patients with appendiceal perforation may go on to develop intra-abdominal abscesses (see Chapter 8, "Abdominal Mass").

Evaluation

The physical examination frequently reveals a fever and tenderness in the right lower quadrant, although fever may be absent and tenderness may be found in the flank or elsewhere in the abdomen, depending on the location of the appendix. The Rovsing sign (pain in the right lower quadrant with palpation of the left lower quadrant), the psoas sign (pain in the right lower quadrant with extension of the right thigh while the patient is lying on his or her left side), and the obturator sign (pain in the right lower quadrant when the flexed thigh and knee are held and the hip is rotated internally) are all signs that may be seen with appendicitis. A rectal examination may reveal irritation of the rectal wall by an inflamed appendix. If the appendix has perforated and the child has developed peritonitis, he or she may have diffuse abdominal tenderness, rebound tenderness, and abdominal wall rigidity. These children frequently also have signs of systemic toxicity, such as a high fever, tachycardia, and tachypnea.

Laboratory studies can be helpful in cases where the history and physical examination are equivocal. A peripheral white blood count often reveals a mild leukocytosis with an increasing left shift as the appendix becomes more gangrenous or ruptures; however, a normal white blood cell count does not rule out appendicitis. Electrolytes are usually not abnormal unless significant dehydration exists. A few white blood cells in the urine may be found if the appendix lies near the bladder or the ureter. Plain radiographs of the abdomen may occasionally reveal an appendicolith. More commonly, however, the x-ray findings are nonspecific. Diagnostic accuracy is enhanced in patients with equivocal presentations for appendicitis by the use of either abdominal ultrasound and/or abdominal computed tomography (CT) scan. Ultrasound spares the child from ionizing radiation but more frequently results in indeterminate results than CT. CT scans are better at identifying other diagnoses that might cause abdominal pain and are generally more easily obtainable than ultrasound studies, but young patients frequently require sedation.

 HINT: Appendicitis is primarily a clinical diagnosis, and normal lab values and imaging studies may be found in some patients with this disease. If a child has normal studies but a worrisome history or examination, he or she should undergo a period of close observation with serial abdominal examinations.

Treatment
The treatment for appendicitis is appendectomy, and therefore surgical consultation should be requested promptly once the diagnosis of appendicitis is suspected. Pain management and supportive care should be provided while awaiting operative intervention. Antibiotic therapy should be initiated prior to surgery in patients with appendicitis.

Constipation
Constipation is discussed in Chapter 22, "Constipation."

Henoch-Schönlein Purpura
Henoch-Schönlein purpura is discussed in Chapter 18, "Bleeding and Purpura."

Intussusception
Etiology
Intussusception occurs when a proximal segment of bowel telescopes into a distal portion of intestine, causing edema, lymphatic obstruction, and vascular compromise. Intussusception is typically ileocolic but can also be ileoileal or colocolic. If a diagnosis is not made in a timely fashion, this ischemic portion of bowel becomes gangrenous and eventually perforates, leading to peritonitis. While most cases are idiopathic, intussusception may arise from an intestinal lead point, especially in older children. In infants, hypertrophied Peyer patches may create lead points, whereas in older children tumors, polyps, Meckel diverticula, duplications, or intestinal lesions associated with Henoch-Schönlein purpura are most often identified as lead points. The first oral rotavirus vaccine (RotaShield®) was associated with an increased risk of intussusception and withdrawn from use in 1999. Newer rotavirus vaccinations have not been found to be associated with an increased risk of intussusception.

Intussusception is the most common cause of intestinal obstruction in young children and occurs most commonly in patients 4 to 12 months of age. The classic symptoms of intussusception are episodic abdominal pain, vomiting, and stools with the appearance of "currant jelly." Periods of severe pain, often causing the child to pull up his legs, are followed by periods of no obvious discomfort. Occasionally, however, the child appears lethargic between the painful episodes. Eventually, the child begins to vomit and develops more consistent pain as the intestine becomes more edematous and ischemic. This circulatory compromise causes sloughing of the intestinal mucosa, which results in passage of "currant jelly" stools, and represents a late finding in intussusception.

 HINT: The history of intermittent abdominal pain provider by a caretaker is of critical importance, as this should raise the concern for intussusception. These children will often appear deceptively well in between episodes of pain.

Evaluation

Patients with intussusception may look well or may be quite ill appearing with unstable vital signs. Abdominal examination may reveal distention because of either partial or complete obstruction. Occasionally, a sausage-like mass can be palpated, most often in the right upper quadrant. Rectal examination may reveal heme-positive stool. Laboratory studies are generally unhelpful in the diagnosis of intussusception. An abdominal radiograph may show varying degrees of small-bowel obstruction, a paucity of gas in the right lower quadrant, and an intracolonic mass. Rarely, free air may be noted because of intestinal perforation. These radiographic findings are helpful if present, but frequently, the plain radiographs show nonspecific gas patterns. A contrast enema is the imaging study of choice for patients with suspected intussusception because it is also potentially therapeutic. Intussusception can also be seen with both CT and ultrasound (although the patient will require an additional therapeutic intervention if intussusception is diagnosed with one of these noninvasive methods). Ultrasound, in particular, is a reasonable option when the clinical suspicion of intussusception is low, given the radiation exposure and frequent need for sedation associated with CT.

Treatment

Intravenous fluids should be provided for presumed dehydration and a nasogastric tube placed to decompress the stomach and intestines. An air or barium emesis contrast enema can be both a diagnostic and a therapeutic maneuver in suspected intussusception. If barium enema or air insufflation is unsuccessful, or if the child appears systemically toxic prior to the enema, intraoperative reduction is necessary. Because of the potential for failure of enema reduction, and because contrast enemas can occasionally cause perforation, early surgical consultation is advised when intussusception is suspected. Broad-spectrum antibiotics are sometimes given just prior to attempted reduction because of the risk of perforation. The recurrence rate after successful nonoperative reduction is reported to be 5% to 10%; recurrence is more common in an older child with a lead point.

Malrotation with Volvulus
Etiology

Intestinal malrotation is a consequence of abnormal embryonic development, resulting in abnormal fixation of the mesentery of the intestines. Although malrotation can be asymptomatic, this predisposes children to volvulus, the twisting of loops of bowel around its mesenteric base, leading to bowel obstruction. Furthermore, because the vascular supply to the intestines is carried within this mesenteric stalk, this twisting leads to ischemia and abdominal pain and can cause intestinal necrosis within hours. Malrotation with volvulus is most commonly seen in young infants, but more indolent forms of malrotation can present later in childhood. Patients who present at an older age more commonly have symptoms such as feeding difficulties with intermittent bilious emesis, or with failure to thrive because of feeding intolerance.

Young infants with volvulus commonly present with the sudden onset of emesis and abdominal pain. The emesis is usually bilious, and the abdominal pain is constant. The patient appears ill and in distress and may present with unstable vital signs if necrosis has already occurred. The abdomen is tender on examination, and there may be varying degrees of abdominal distension, depending on the location of the malrotation. The presence of blood on rectal examination implies that ischemic injury to the intestinal mucosa has already occurred and is a late finding with volvulus.

Evaluation

Patients with clinical findings suggestive of volvulus need to be evaluated immediately. Plain radiographs may reveal air-fluid levels and dilated loops of bowel. There may also be a paucity of air in the lower gastrointestinal (GI) tract. Both the "double-bubble" sign, dilation of the stomach and the proximal duodenum, and the presence of loops of small bowel overlying the liver shadow can be found in volvulus. However, plain radiographs may be normal. An upper GI series is the diagnostic study of choice and may reveal a corkscrew-like appearance of the contrast within the twisted intestinal loops. The role of ultrasound in the diagnosis of malrotation is not well defined. Ultrasonography may detect an abnormal position of the superior mesenteric vessels or a "whirlpool" sign (twisting of the mesentery around the mesenteric vessels), but accuracy of ultrasound is inferior to the accuracy of the upper GI series.

 HINT: Bilious emesis in a young infant should be presumed to be malrotation with volvulus and evaluated emergently until this diagnosis is disproven.

Treatment

Malrotation with volvulus is a surgical emergency. Both patient survival and intestinal viability are directly related to the timeliness of making this diagnosis. As a consequence, a young infant with bilious emesis and abdominal pain should be presumed to have malrotation with volvulus until this diagnosis is excluded. Immediate surgical consultation is mandatory and should not be delayed for the results of abdominal imaging. A child with suspected malrotation with volvulus should have a nasogastric tube and intravenous access. Patients who are unstable need to undergo fluid resuscitation and should receive antibiotics. Plans should be made for emergent surgery because the only definitive treatment for volvulus is operative intervention.

Respiratory Tract Infections

Group A Streptococcal Pharyngitis

Patients with group A streptococcal pharyngitis sometimes present with abdominal pain in addition to throat pain, fever, and cervical adenopathy (see also Chapter 72, "Sore Throat"). A child with abdominal pain and suspected strep throat should have his or her posterior pharynx swabbed and evaluated either by a rapid streptococcal antigen detection test or by throat culture. Patients with streptococcal pharyngitis should be treated with antibiotics.

Lower Lobe Pneumonia

Children with lower lobe pneumonia can present with respiratory symptoms and abdominal pain. Evidence for pneumonia can be as subtle as an increased respiratory rate or unexplained high fevers. Lower lobe pneumonias are sometimes discovered incidentally on abdominal radiographs taken for evaluation of abdominal pain. Treatment consists of appropriate antibiotics for pneumonia.

Testicular Torsion

Testicular torsion is discussed in Chapter 67, "Scrotal Pain, Acute."

Toxin Exposures and Foreign Body Ingestions

Although many substances can cause nausea and vomiting when ingested, some toxins are more commonly associated with abdominal pain. Examples include iron, aspirin, caustics, lead, and other heavy metals. Specific antidotes (e.g., deferoxamine for iron toxicity) can be given in addition to activated charcoal and other GI decontamination measures. Treatment of the patient who has a toxic ingestion should be coordinated with a poison control center or a toxicologist. Many swallowed foreign bodies may not result in symptoms, but some, such as needles or disc batteries, can cause abdominal pain by irritating or perforating the GI mucosa. Most swallowed foreign bodies travel through the GI tract without difficulty, but foreign bodies that cause symptoms or are at high risk of causing perforation or other complications should be removed by a gastroenterologist, otolaryngologist, or surgeon, depending on the location of the foreign body and institutional practice patterns. A unique toxic exposure causing abdominal pain is a black widow spider bite. Venom from the black widow spider (*Latrodectus mactans*) can cause severe abdominal cramping as well as cardiovascular collapse in young children. Black widow spider antivenin may be indicated in the presence of systemic symptoms.

Trauma
Etiology

The history is an important consideration in evaluating a child with abdominal trauma. Abdominal trauma is categorized as either blunt or penetrating, and most children with abdominal trauma have blunt trauma. Common mechanisms of injury include falls, motor vehicle-related injuries, and child abuse. Although the history is crucial in evaluating children with abdominal trauma, children injured because of child abuse may have inaccurate or deceptive histories.

 HINT: Consider child abuse in patients with more severe or multiple injuries if the reported mechanism of injury does not seem to correlate with physical findings, or if the caretakers provide inconsistent histories.

Clinical Features and Evaluation

Abdominal symptoms may be subtle immediately after an injury and may be further limited by distracting injuries and alterations in mental status. A high index of suspicion for abdominal injury is appropriate in the evaluation of the patient with trauma. Patients with abdominal trauma must be thoroughly examined. Children with blood loss present initially with tachycardia; hypotension is a late sign, developing only after significant bleeding. Children may present with tachypnea and shallow respirations in an attempt to minimize abdominal pain associated with breathing. Pain and tenderness may be focal because of a solid organ injury or diffuse because of peritoneal irritation from a perforated viscus or intraperitoneal blood. Bruising on the abdominal wall from a seat belt increases the risk of intra-abdominal injury in children who have been involved in motor vehicle crashes. The presence of gross blood on rectal examination suggests a hollow viscus injury.

Further evaluation of the patient's abdominal pain depends on the results of the history and physical examination. In a child in whom the suspicion of injury is low, observation and repeated physical examinations are appropriate. However, in patients with worrisome findings, additional evaluation is warranted. Laboratory studies commonly include complete blood counts, liver function tests, pancreatic enzymes, blood type and screen, and urinalysis. These tests may suggest intra-abdominal injury if abnormal; however, normal values do not rule out intra-abdominal injury and thus, should not supplant imaging studies if the clinical suspicion for intra-abdominal injury is high. With the exception of the pelvis radiograph to look for fracture, radiographs are of limited value in the evaluation of abdominal trauma. The imaging studies of choice are CT scans of the abdomen and pelvis, frequently with intravenous and oral contrast. The sensitivity of the CT scan for detecting solid organ injury is excellent, but CT scans are less sensitive in detecting hollow viscus and pancreatic injury. Diagnostic peritoneal lavage (DPL) is performed in rare circumstances (e.g., when a patient is too unstable to go to the CT scanner). Although DPL is even more sensitive than CT scan in detecting intra-abdominal blood, the DPL is less specific for injuries that need surgical repair because many solid injuries that cause a positive DPL are managed nonoperatively. Abdominal ultrasound is used more extensively in adult trauma patients, but its role in the evaluation of the pediatric trauma patient is less clear. Immediate surgical consultation is indicated for patients with significant abdominal trauma.

Treatment

A patient with abdominal trauma should have his or her life-threatening conditions addressed first. After the patient's airway, breathing, circulation, and cervical spine have been stabilized, the patient's abdominal injuries can then be addressed. Penetrating trauma of the abdomen is a surgical emergency, and wounds that violate the peritoneal cavity are generally explored in the operating room. Patients with solid organ injuries are frequently managed nonoperatively, but these management decisions should be directed by a trauma surgeon. For those patients who do not have any obvious injuries after initial evaluation with persistent posttraumatic abdominal pain, close observation is indicated.

Evaluation of Acute Abdominal Pain

The differential diagnosis of acute abdominal pain in a child is extensive, and determining the etiology of a patient's abdominal pain often taxes a physician's diagnostic abilities.

History
Type and Location of Pain

- Visceral pain is caused by stretching of the nerve fibers surrounding an abdominal organ and is a poorly localized (although typically midline), aching pain.
  - Epigastric pain originates from structures derived from the foregut (e.g., the stomach, duodenum, pancreas, liver, and biliary tree).
  - Periumbilical pain arises from involvement of the midgut structures (e.g., the jejunum, ileum, and large intestine up to the splenic flexure).
  - Suprapubic pain is produced by hindgut structures (e.g., the distal colon and rectum).
- Somatic pain occurs when pain fibers in the parietal peritoneum are irritated either by inflammation of the peritoneum itself or by an adjacent inflamed organ. Somatic pain is better localized than visceral pain and typically worsened by movement.

- Referred pain to the lower neck and shoulders is associated with phrenic nerve irritation from pancreatitis, splenic pathology, or hepatobiliary disease.

Characteristics of Pain
- Sudden onset suggests perforation of a visceral organ or ischemia.
- Gradual onset suggests inflammation, such as pain associated with appendicitis.
- Colicky pain suggests pain from a hollow viscus, such as intussusception, kidney stones, or gallstones.

Associated Symptoms
- Fever or chills.
- Nausea or vomiting (specifically if there is bile or blood in the emesis).
- Abdominal distention.
- Stool irregularities (e.g., constipation, diarrhea, hematochezia, melena, or mucus in the stools).
- Other complaints, such as sore throat, dyspnea, cough, dysuria or urinary frequency, and extra-abdominal pain.
- Adolescents should be asked about their sexual history. Ask adolescent girls about menstrual history, vaginal bleeding, or vaginal discharge.
- Previous episodes of similar pain.
- Previous surgeries.
- Past medical history and medications.

Physical Examination
A complete physical examination should be performed on patients with abdominal pain prior to examining the abdomen itself, with emphasis on:

- Vital signs and general appearance.
- Head, ears, eyes, nose, and throat: Eyes and mucous membranes should be checked for icterus, and the pharynx should be inspected.
- Lungs and heart: Focal findings on lung auscultation may suggest pneumonia. Distant heart sounds, a gallop, or a friction rub may be found on cardiac examination in patients with myocarditis or pericarditis.
- Lower extremities: Inspection of the legs may reveal purpura seen with Henoch-Schönlein purpura.
- Inspection: Look for scars, bruising, masses, distension, and peristalsis.
- Auscultation: May reveal high-pitched bowel sounds typical of bowel obstruction or the absence of bowel sounds as seen in a patient with an ileus.
- Palpation: In a verbal child, ask the patient which part of his or her abdomen hurts the most; this should be the last area palpated. Palpation may reveal masses or guarding.
- A rectal examination including testing for occult blood should be considered in patients with unexplained abdominal pain. A genital examination is important

for both males and females. A pelvic examination should be considered in all postpubertal females. In prepubertal females, the external genitalia should be inspected.

 HINT: Patients often have pain radiating to the abdomen because of genitourinary pathology and are reluctant to volunteer this information.

Laboratory Studies

The following laboratory tests may be helpful:

- A peripheral white blood count, erythrocyte sedimentation rate, or C-reactive protein may be abnormal in the setting of infection but are neither sensitive nor specific.
- Electrolytes, blood urea nitrogen, and creatinine are of limited diagnostic utility but may help in the management of fluid repletion.
- A glucose level is helpful in patients suspected of having diabetic ketoacidosis.
- Liver function tests and amylase and lipase levels should be sent when hepatic or pancreatic disease is suspected.
- Blood type and crossmatch should be sent if transfusion is a possibility.
- Urinalysis may reveal infection or hematuria.
- Urine pregnancy test should be performed in all pubertal females with abdominal pain.
- Throat, stool, cervix, and urine cultures should be ordered if infection is suspected.

Imaging Modalities

Various imaging studies can be used in the evaluation of the patient:

- Plain abdominal radiographs: a two-view abdominal obstruction series is more helpful than a single film of the abdomen and may reveal a bowel obstruction, ileus, fecalith, free air, or abdominal masses. A chest radiograph may reveal thoracic pathology causing abdominal pain.
- Radiographic studies with contrast can be helpful when looking for malrotation (upper GI series) or intussusception (air or contrast enema).
- Ultrasound can help evaluate right upper quadrant pain, the kidneys, gynecologic causes of abdominal pain, suspected appendicitis, and intussusception. Ultrasound can also be used to detect free fluid in the peritoneal cavity.
- Abdominal and pelvic CTs are helpful in the evaluation of abdominal masses and solid organ injury. CT is commonly used in the evaluation of patients with suspected appendicitis.

Approach to the Patient

See Figure 9-1.

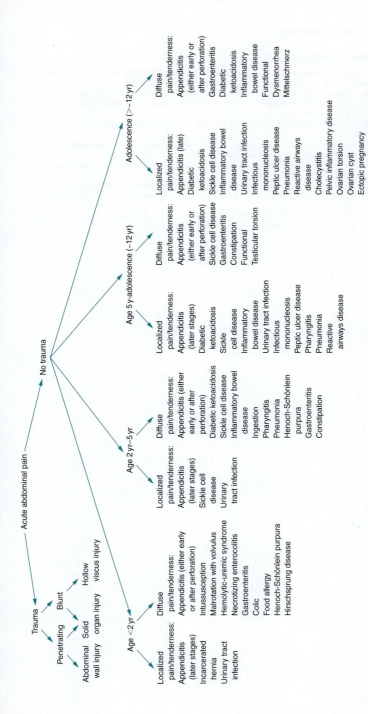

FIGURE 9-1 Approach to the patient with acute abdominal pain.

Suggested Readings

Bhatt M, Joseph L, Ducharme FM, et al. Prospective validation of the pediatric appendicitis score in a Canadian emergency department. *Acad Emerg Med.* 2009;16:591–596.

Bundy DG, Byerley JS, Liles EA, et al. Does this child have appendicitis? *JAMA.* 2007;298(4):438–451.

Doria AS, Moineddin R, Kellenberger CJ, et al. US or CT for diagnosis of appendicitis in children and adults? A meta-analysis. *Radiology.* 2006;241(1):83–94.

Gaines BA. Intra-abdominal solid organ injury in children: diagnosis and treatment. *J Trauma.* 2009; 67:S135–S139.

Hryhorczuk AL, Strouse PJ. Validation of US as a first-line diagnostic test for assessment of pediatric ileocolic intussusception. *Pediatr Radiol.* 2009;39:1075–1079.

Justice FA, Auldist AW, Bines JE. Intussusception: trends in clinical presentation and management. *J Gastroenterol Hepatol.* 2006;21:842–846.

McCollough M, Sharieff GQ. Abdominal pain in children. *Pediatr Clin N Am.* 2006;53:107–137.

Milar AJW, Rode H, Cywes S. Malrotation and volvulus in infancy and childhood. *Semin Pediatr Surg.* 2003;12(4):229–336.

Neuman MI. Pain—abdomen. In: GR Fleisher, S Ludwig, eds. *Textbook of Pediatric Emergency Medicine.* 6th ed. Philadelphia, PA: Lippincott, Williams & Wilkins; 2010:421–428.

Abdominal Pain, Chronic

 DIFFERENTIAL DIAGNOSIS LIST

Neonate/Toddler
Functional
- Infant colic
- Infant dyschezia
- Infant regurgitation
- Eosinophilic gastroenteritis
- Gastroesophageal reflux disease
- Milk-protein allergy

Child/Adolescent
Functional
- Abdominal migraine
- Appendiceal colic
- Childhood functional abdominal pain
- Childhood functional abdominal pain syndrome
- Functional dyspepsia
- Intestinal pseudo-obstruction
- Irritable bowel syndrome
- Functional constipation

Inflammatory Causes
- Chronic cholecystitis
- Chronic pancreatitis, with or without pseudocyst
- Inflammatory bowel disease (IBD)
- Non-*Helicobacter pylori*-mediated esophagitis, gastritis, and peptic ulcer disease (reflux, nonsteroidal anti-inflammatory drugs, corticosteroids, etc.)

Infectious Causes
- *Giardia lamblia* enteritis and other parasitic infections
- *H. pylori*-mediated esophagitis, gastritis, and peptic ulcer disease
- Vertebral infection—diskitis and osteomyelitis

Anatomic/Mechanical Causes
- Abdominal muscle strain
- Choledochal cyst
- Cholelithiasis
- Chronic nephrolithiasis
- Hematoma, intra-abdominal
- Hernia, internal
- Intestinal duplication
- Malrotation with or without volvulus
- Musculoskeletal
- Slipping-rib syndrome
- Ureteropelvic junction obstruction

Gynecologic Causes
- Cystic teratoma
- Dysmenorrhea
- Endometriosis
- Hematometrocolpos
- Mittelschmerz

Toxic Causes
- Lead poisoning

Systemic Causes
- Abdominal tumor—Wilms tumor and neuroblastoma

- Acute intermittent porphyria
- Carbohydrate intolerance/malabsorption
- Celiac disease
- Chronic Henoch-Schönlein purpura
- Collagen vascular disease
- Hepatitis
- Hereditary angioedema
- Leukemia

- Lymphoma, including gastrointestinal (GI) tract lymphomas
- Sickle cell disease
- Spinal column tumor (e.g., leukemia, osteosarcoma)

Neurologic/Psychiatric
- Conversion reaction
- Depression
- Factitious

DIFFERENTIAL DIAGNOSIS DISCUSSION

Chronic abdominal pain is one of the **most commonly encountered symptoms** in pediatrics. The definition has evolved since the 1950s when Apley described it as intermittent abdominal pain in children between the ages of 4 and 16 that is present for >3 months and affects daily activity. In clinical practice, pain lasting >**2 months** is considered to be chronic. Prevalence studies indicate that as many as 20% of middle and high school students experience frequent abdominal pain. Approximately 90% of these children have **functional or nonorganic abdominal pain,** pain without demonstrable evidence of a pathologic condition, such as an infectious, inflammatory, anatomic, or biochemical mechanism. The remaining children have **organic abdominal pain,** whose most common causes are described in detail here.

Abdominal Pain in Infants/Toddlers
Infant Colic
Infant colic is a **functional GI** disorder in an infant <4 to 5 months without a clear organic basis. While the term "colic" implies abdominal pain secondary to obstruction of blood flow from an organ such as the kidney, gallbladder, or intestine, **"infant colic"** is a behavioral syndrome incorporating bouts of **crying and difficult-to-soothe behavior** that is usually influenced by psychosocial issues in a family. No clear evidence indicates that colic pain is from GI organs or from any other body part. Nonetheless, it is often assumed that the cause of the excessive colic is GI in origin.

Etiology
Colic, when referring to the prolonged crying seen in infancy, is technically defined as colic syndrome. The definition of infantile colic has evolved from the seminal definition by Wessel in the 1950s to include paroxysms of crying, irritability or fussiness **lasting >3 hours/day and occurring at least 3 days/week for >1 week**. Organic etiologies such as failure to thrive need to be excluded. The **etiology of colic is not well understood,** and the mechanisms proposed to cause it are at best vague. The **immaturity of the infant nervous system** may play a role, particularly the transitioning to a more awake state. The gradual decrease in colic symptoms coincides with the acquisition of skills that enable the infant to more adequately maintain a calm awake state. Behavioral factors such as burping abnormalities or crying while feeding leading to ingested air **(aerophagia)** are suggested; however, it

is argued that intestinal gas is a result of colic rather than a cause. Baseline **motilin** levels are raised, suggesting that increased gastric emptying increases small-bowel peristalsis leading to perceived intestinal pain. Other proposed etiologies include **intolerance to cow's milk,** although little evidence indicates that children with colic have true milk protein intolerance, and the symptoms of that disorder do not include colic-like symptoms.

Evaluation

The **crying** noted in colic typically **peaks in the evening** at the **age of 6 weeks,** generally tapering off by 3 to 4 months of age. Other features include movements and facial features interpreted as being consistent with pain, as well as **GI symptoms** such as gas and abdominal distention. Clearly, these criteria are loose and may fall within the realm of normal infant behavior, albeit at one end of the curve. Physical and laboratory examinations of children with colic are uniformly normal.

Treatment

Treatment of colic is designed to **relieve the parents' stress**. Infants in this age range are targets of abuse, and preventing overstressed parents from harming these children is an important goal. Advice to parents of an infant with colic should always include suggestions on how to manage the stress, such as taking a brief break from caregiving. **Reassurance** that the crying will eventually stop is helpful. **Environmental changes** that facilitate the awake state and reduce crying, such as increasing rhythmic rocking, using a pacifier, increasing background white noise with a vacuum cleaner or washing machine, or taking a ride in the car or stroller, may be helpful. Antispasmodics and anticholinergics are not indicated for use in infants because they are associated with **respiratory distress and apnea**. Changing from breast- to formula-feeding is not indicated, and switching formulas should only be done if there is a suggestion of true milk-protein intolerance.

Infant Dyschezia
Etiology

Infant dyschezia is defined as a **functional** GI disorder. It is characterized by otherwise healthy infants <6 months of age experiencing at least **10 minutes of straining and crying** before successful passage of soft stools. Infant dyschezia is secondary to failure to coordinate increased intra-abdominal pressure with pelvic floor relaxation. Crying is analogous to creating increased abdominal pressure (Valsalva maneuver) prior to learning how to coordinate and bear down more effectively.

Evaluation and Treatment

Parents describe screaming, crying, and turning red or purple in the face with effort prior to defecation. **Physical examination,** which should be performed in the presence of the parents to help promote effective reassurance, is **normal,** inclusive of rectal examination. Diagnostic tests are not required. **Avoidance of rectal stimulation** is advised to negate artificial sensory experiences. Infant dyschezia rarely lasts >1 to 2 weeks and responds spontaneously.

Infant Regurgitation

Etiology

Uncomplicated regurgitation of food in otherwise healthy infants aged 3 weeks to 12 months is a **functional** GI disorder. It is defined as regurgitation **two or more times per day for >3 weeks** without evidence of pathologic symptoms such as apnea, failure to thrive, aspiration, feeding difficulties, retching, or hematemesis. When regurgitation contributes to tissue damage or inflammation of the esophagus, it is known as **gastroesophageal reflux disease**.

Evaluation and Treatment

Parents usually describe **irritability or arching of the back** after feeds. Regurgitation occurs in more than two-thirds of healthy 4-month-old infants. Daily regurgitation decreases with age to 5% of infants 10 to 12 months of age. Risk factors include abnormalities of the chest, lungs, central nervous system, oropharynx, heart, or GI tract. Milk allergy may be present, especially if associated with eczema or wheezing and may require switching of infant formula. The natural history of infant regurgitation suggests **spontaneous improvement**. Left-sided positioning and thickening of feeds may help reduce symptoms. Improving the parent–child relationship and decreasing familial stress are ways to help provide effective reassurance. Gastroesophageal reflux in infants is treated with **acid blockade,** most commonly a **histamine$_2$-receptor antagonist**.

ABDOMINAL PAIN IN CHILD/ADOLESCENT

Children with functional GI disorders typically exhibit one of the three clinical presentations, including isolated paroxysmal abdominal pain, abdominal pain associated with dyspepsia, and abdominal pain associated with irritable bowel syndrome as specified by the **Rome III criteria** and described here and in Table 10-1. Also included in functional disorders are abdominal migraine, appendiceal colic, and functional constipation. Chronic intestinal pseudo-obstruction is a defect in bowel intestinal motility. Approximately 20% of school-age children, most commonly **4 to 16 years of age,** are believed to have some variety of functional abdominal pain. The mean age of onset is **between 4 and 8 years of age,** with boys and girls affected equally until 9 years of age, at which point more girls are affected. Onset **>14 years** is usually associated with symptoms more consistent with **irritable bowel syndrome,** whereas onset **<4 years** has a greater chance of an **organic etiology**. Although psychological factors are important, there is no correlation of functional abdominal pain with personality traits such as perfectionism or chronic worrying.

Etiology

The factors that produce functional abdominal pain are not entirely clear. Pathophysiologic studies have focused on the autonomic nervous system and GI motility, suggesting a role for **altered gastric motility and heightened visceral sensitivity** to intestinal contractions in individuals with functional abdominal pain. Although psychological factors do not distinguish organic from nonorganic

TABLE 10-1	Rome Criteria for the Diagnosis of Functional Abdominal Pain in Children with Pain at Least Once per Week for at Least 2 Months Prior to Diagnosis		
Childhood Functional Abdominal Pain	**Childhood Functional Abdominal Pain Syndrome**	**Functional Dyspepsia**	**Irritable Bowel Syndrome**
Episodic or continuous abdominal pain	Episodic or continuous abdominal pain 25% of the time	Persistent or recurrent pain or discomfort in the upper abdomen (above the umbilicus)	Abdominal pain or discomfort at least 25% of the time with two or more of the following: relief with defecation, onset associated with a change in frequency, or onset associated with a change in stool consistency
No structural or biochemical abnormalities to explain the symptoms	Some loss of daily functioning	Symptoms not relieved by defecation or associated with the onset of a change in stool frequency or stool form	Associated with abnormal stool frequency (≤2 times/wk or ≥4 times/d), alternating stool character, straining, urgency, passing mucus, bloating, and distension
The child does not satisfy criteria for another type of functional abdominal pain	Somatic systems such as headache, limb pain, or difficulty sleeping. No structural or biochemical abnormalities to explain the symptoms	No structural or biochemical abnormalities to explain the symptoms	No structural or biochemical abnormalities to explain the symptoms

etiology, correlation with various psychosocial factors, such as **family stress,** are described. Often there is a family history of alcoholism, behavioral problems, abdominal pain, or migraine headaches. The **family dynamic in response to the pain** is important as well, as often there is positive reinforcement for having abdominal pain, ranging from emotional support to excusing from school or household chores.

Childhood Functional Abdominal Pain

Childhood functional abdominal pain is defined as episodic or continuous pain that occurs **at least once per week for at least 2 months prior to diagnosis** without a clear organic etiology. Childhood functional abdominal pain syndrome includes functional abdominal pain **at least 25% of the time and either some loss of daily functioning or somatic symptoms** such as headaches, limb pain, or difficulty sleeping. Pain is usually generalized or periumbilical, lasts <1 hour, and does not have a temporal relation to meals.

Functional Dyspepsia

Functional dyspepsia is defined as persistent or recurrent abdominal pain or discomfort centered **above the umbilicus and not relieved by defecation or associated with changes in stool frequency or consistency**. There is no evidence of an underlying etiology including an inflammatory, anatomic, metabolic, or neoplastic process that can explain the symptoms that need to be present at least once per week for at least **2 months** prior to diagnosis. Often there is a temporal relation between meal ingestion and symptoms. Commonly associated symptoms include nausea, early satiety, postprandial abdominal distention, and excess gas.

Irritable Bowel Syndrome

Irritable bowel syndrome is characterized by abdominal discomfort or pain occurring at least 25% of the time without an underlying etiology and two of the following: **improvement with defecation, a change in stool frequency, or a change in stool consistency**. The symptoms are present at least once per week for at least **2 months** prior to diagnosis. Irritable bowel is usually associated with autonomic-type symptoms and environmental stress, as is isolated functional abdominal pain.

Evaluation

Functional abdominal pain is categorized by the different constellation of symptoms. The pain of functional abdominal pain is **recurrent and paroxysmal**. There is typically **a clustering of the pain episodes** within days or weeks that waxes and wanes over the course of months. The pain is often difficult for the child to describe and often not associated with eating or other activities but frequently occurs at the **same time of day** and usually lasts **<1 hour**. The presence of alarming symptoms such as weight loss, melena, and other red flags listed in Table 10-2 suggests the presence of an organic etiology to the pain.

As with all diagnoses in medicine, **a thorough and careful history** is the most helpful tool in the diagnosis of functional abdominal pain because it reveals the absence of alarming signals. The **physical examination** of the child with functional abdominal pain is **normal,** including rectal exam and stool guaiac. Although indiscriminate testing of these children is unwarranted, **normal screening laboratory tests** will reassure the clinician and family there is no organic cause of the abdominal pain. **Laboratory testing** suggested includes complete blood cell count, erythrocyte sedimentation rate, liver function tests including aminotransferases and albumin, urinalysis, and examination of the feces for ova and parasites.

TABLE 10-2	**Clinical Features of Abdominal Pain of Organic Etiology**

Age <4 yr
Pain localized to the right upper quadrant
Pain referred to the back, chest, shoulder, or lower extremities
Associated joint pain or swelling
Dysuria, flank pain, hematuria, or dark-colored urine
Dyspareunia or vaginal discharge
Constitutional symptoms such as fever, weight loss, growth deceleration, rash, or night sweats
Significant vomiting
Significant diarrhea
Gross or occult blood in the stool
Intermittent fecal incontinence
Perianal disease (tags, fissures, and fistulae)
Decreased energy or sleepiness after pain attacks
Abnormal physical examination (i.e., hypotonia)
Abnormal screening laboratory studies, including elevated white blood count or erythrocyte sedimentation rate, hypoalbuminemia, anemia

Upper endoscopy is indicated in patients with **dyspepsia pain** if response to treatment is poor or if symptoms recur after a 4- to 6-week course of medication. **Lactose breath test** is helpful if lactose intolerance is a concern, and **abdominal ultrasound** may be helpful if the child is difficult to examine or if there is concern for an anatomic problem.

In addition to screening for organic causes, the clinician should work with the family to track the course of the pain and to attempt to gain a psychosocial understanding of the child and the family. A **pain diary** kept by the family is often a useful diagnostic and even occasionally therapeutic tool. Despite the clear influence of stress and other psychosocial factors in this disease, it is important that this diagnosis not be arrived at as a last resort, after "more serious" causes of abdominal pain have been "ruled out." As an adjunct in managing the situation, a **psychologist or psychiatrist** may be helpful because abdominal pain of any nature causes stress on the child and the family. Clearly, the clinician should use the tools available to identify the cause of abdominal pain while attempting to avoid overreliance on elaborate tests and unnecessary referrals to specialists.

Treatment

The treatment of functional GI disorders begins with making the diagnosis and letting the family understand this is a **genuine entity**. The goal of therapy is to restore **normality** to the patient's lifestyle and reduce or eliminate the pain. Generally, this involves **explaining that the pain is real,** most likely caused by altered intestinal motility or visceral hypersensitivity. In addition, **addressing the stressors** that seem to be contributing to the pain and **reversing the positive reinforcement** the child may be receiving are important. **School attendance is critical** to breaking the cycle, and school health officials must be instructed of the need for negative reinforcement. Involvement of **mental health professionals** may be helpful for many families in particularly stressful situations. Drug therapy for functional paroxysmal abdominal pain is generally not indicated, and hospitalization should be avoided. For functional dyspepsia, **avoidance** of nonsteroidal anti-inflammatory agents and foods that aggravate symptoms is recommended. The mainstay of treatment for irritable bowel syndrome in adults is a high-fiber diet; results in children, however, are less convincing. Peppermint oil and antispasmodics such as hyoscyamine may be helpful. Calcium channel antagonists and antimuscarinic agents, as well as biofeedback and psychotherapy have also been used. Much of the therapy for irritable bowel syndrome in children relies on **reassurance and education,** with psychological or behavioral support added if necessary.

Chronic Intestinal Pseudo-obstruction
Etiology
Chronic intestinal pseudo-obstruction refers to a heterogeneous set of **functional GI motility disorders** resulting in **symptoms consistent with obstruction** but **without an actual mechanical blockage**. These diseases appear to result from **decreased contractility of the intestinal smooth muscle** and are generally caused by a multitude of conditions that result in **myopathy or neuropathy,** either localized to the viscera or in systemic diseases such as muscular dystrophy.

Evaluation and Treatment
Symptoms include pain similar to the pain of true obstruction: **vomiting, abdominal distention, constipation, and early satiety**. Diagnosis is difficult and requires exclusion of the causes of obstruction but may be suggested by **plain radiographs or scintigraphic studies of motility**. **Intestinal manometry** is helpful, although these tests are not done frequently in children. Treatment is often **supportive** and may include supplemental **enteral feeding or intravenous nutrition**. Pharmacological treatment is not consistently advantageous.

Peptic Disease
Etiology
"Chronic peptic disease" is a term that encompasses **ulcers in the small bowel and duodenum** as well as **esophagitis, gastritis, and duodenitis**. In children, gastroesophageal reflux, nonsteroidal anti-inflammatory drugs, COX-2 inhibitor or corticosteroid exposure, extensive burns, or head trauma are common etiologies for peptic disease. In older children and adolescents, *H. pylori* infection becomes relatively more common and duodenitis becomes more prevalent, although the other conditions still persist but at a much lower incidence. Often this group has a positive family history of ulcer disease.

Evaluation
The **symptoms** of chronic peptic disease **vary with age**. In **younger children, pain** is generally present in the **mid- to upper abdomen** and has no temporal relation to eating. In contrast, peptic disease in the **older child** is characterized by **epigastric pain,** occasionally associated with vomiting, occurring after meals and in the early morning.

Relief of pain during eating is not a characteristic sign of peptic disease in children. In any age child, **blood loss** from inflammation may lead to melena or occult blood in the stool. Diagnosis is established by **endoscopy and biopsy,** although milder cases may be inferred as positive by a successful therapeutic trial of medication. A **pH probe** may be helpful to document reflux-associated pain. **Urea breath tests,** *H. pylori* **serology, and stool polyclonal antigen** testing are various methods to detect *H. pylori.*

Treatment

Peptic disease is treated with acid blockade, by either a histamine$_2$-receptor antagonist or a proton pump inhibitor. If reflux is a concern, a prokinetic agent such as metoclopramide or erythromycin ethylsuccinate may be tried after an upper GI series has been obtained to rule out an anatomic cause of reflux such as malrotation. Treatment for *H. pylori* infection involves acid blockade using a proton pump inhibitor as well as double antibiotic therapy with amoxicillin plus clarithromycin or metronidazole.

Carbohydrate Intolerance
Etiology

Dietary carbohydrates serve as the substrates for bacterial fermentation, resulting in nausea, abdominal distention, and excessive flatulence with resultant abdominal pain and cramps. **Malabsorption of lactose** is by far the **most common type of carbohydrate intolerance**. Intolerance of lactose is caused by deficiency of the enzyme lactase, an inhabitant of the small intestinal brush border. Congenital lactase deficiency is extraordinarily rare, and the **most common causes of true lactase deficiency** are a **genetic late-onset lactase deficiency or mucosal injury**. The genetic form of late-onset lactase deficiency is least common in those of Scandinavian and Northwest European descent and most common in those of Native American, Southeast Asian, Turkish, Italian, and African descent. Mucosal injury may occur after gastroenteritis, particularly that caused by rotavirus, parasitic infections such as *Giardia,* celiac disease, Crohn disease (CD), and radiation or drug exposure. **Sorbitol and fructose** are two carbohydrates that are frequent offenders. **Sorbitol** is found in **many sugar-free items, and fructose** is the primary sweetener in **most foods,** including soda and juices.

Evaluation

Ingestion of lactose-containing food usually results in abdominal distention, **excessive flatulence,** and nausea progressing to **periumbilical abdominal pain, cramps,** and finally **watery diarrhea**. Occasionally in adolescents there may be vomiting. Diagnosis may be made by history alone, although the gold standard of diagnosis is a **lactose breath test**. In this test, patients are fed lactose and breath is tested for hydrogen gas produced by fermentation of undigested lactose by colonic bacteria.

Treatment

Treatment involves **avoidance** of the offending sugar. Multiple dairy products, including formula, do not contain lactose. In addition, **dietary supplements of lactase** can predigest the lactose before consumption. Avoidance of other carbohydrates is more difficult, although there are special formulas and nutritional supplements for many types of carbohydrate intolerance. Complete resolution of symptoms with removal of the offending agent confirms the diagnosis.

Celiac Disease
Etiology
Celiac disease is an inheritable disorder of the small intestine. It is characterized by an inflammatory T-cell response to proteins in **wheat, rye, and barley** (collectively known as **gluten**). Although it has been demonstrated that the use of oats as part of a gluten-free diet in adults does not have unfavorable results, a few celiac patients show intolerance to oats. If untreated, celiac disease can lead to **anemia, infertility, osteoporosis, and intestinal lymphoma**. Celiac disease is most common in **whites,** frequent in Asians from India, Pakistan, and Iran, and rare in Native Americans, Japanese, and Chinese.

Evaluation
The most common presenting symptoms include chronic diarrhea, steatorrhea, **iron deficiency anemia,** abdominal distention, muscle wasting, **short stature,** and **failure to thrive**. Abdominal pain usually accompanies other symptoms and is frequently associated with irritable bowel syndrome. Diagnosis is based on history, laboratory, and endoscopy findings. Serological markers include the **IgA antibodies to tissue transglutaminase and endomysium IgA antibodies**. **IgA levels** are obtained to rule out selective IgA deficiency, which occurs more frequently in children with celiac disease. Anti-gliadin antibodies have a poor positive predictive value. **Upper endoscopy** is the gold standard of diagnosis with biopsies taken from the distal duodenum or proximal jejunum while the patient is on a diet containing gluten, with resolution when gluten is removed from the diet. Endoscopic findings include total or subtotal villous atrophy, crypt elongation, surface cell damage, an increase in intraepithelial lymphocytes, and infiltration with inflammatory cells. Celiac disease is also associated with genetic factors encoded by the HLA complex, specifically **HLA-DQ2 and HLA-DQ8**.

Treatment
Treatment involves **removing gluten from the diet**. Wheat, rye, and barley are the predominant grains containing the peptides. A gluten-free diet should result in a rapid clinical response, with histological recovery over 2 years. Strict adherence to the diet is difficult for many patients, especially among adolescents. Minute amounts of gluten in the diet induce change in the small bowel.

Inflammatory Bowel Disease
Etiology
IBD commonly refers to **Crohn disease (CD) and ulcerative colitis (UC),** inflammatory conditions of the GI tract that cause chronic abdominal pain in children and adolescents. The etiology is unclear but thought to be multifactorial. A multitude of environmental, genetic, and immune factors leads to the development of IBD. Both CD and UC are more prevalent in the northern hemisphere and in industrialized nations.

Evaluation

History and physical examination are imperative in evaluating patients with IBD because the symptoms depend on the site and extent of mucosal inflammation and include extraintestinal manifestations in a subset of patients. Family history and growth charts are necessary. The most common presentations include abdominal pain, weight loss, bloody or nonbloody diarrhea, skin lesions, fevers, arthralgias, and growth failure. In CD, **abdominal pain** is most commonly in the **right lower quadrant** because most patients have disease in the terminal ileum and ascending colon, whereas in UC the **abdominal pain** is usually limited to **times of defecation** because most have rectosigmoid disease. Perirectal disease is most commonly associated with CD. **Laboratory testing** suggested includes evaluation of iron deficiency anemia, inflammatory markers, and nutritional status with albumin and prealbumin. *Anti-Saccharomyces cerevisiae* antibody and perinuclear antineutrophil cytoplasmic antibody assays are associated with CD and UC, respectively. **Upper GI series with small bowel** follow through is essential for evaluating the small bowel, which may be affected in CD. Diagnosis is by **endoscopy with biopsies**. UC usually involves the rectum and extends proximally, whereas CD may involve any portion of the GI tract and may have skip lesions. The presence of granulomas on histology is diagnostic of CD.

Treatment

The goals of therapy are aimed at **decreasing bowel inflammation and preventing recurrent or worsening disease**. Initial therapy for mild symptoms is 5-aminosalicylates and, if the symptoms are severe, corticosteroids. Patients with severe disease may need immunomodulatory or biologic therapy. Nutritional support with oral supplements or nasogastric or gastrostomy feedings may be critically important in addressing growth failure. Patients who fail to respond to medical therapy may require surgery. Colonic cancer and sclerosing cholangitis are associated risk factors.

Chronic Pancreatitis

Etiology

Chronic pancreatitis, usually preceded by **recurrent acute pancreatitis,** is typified by **recurrent bouts of abdominal pain with periods of intervening wellness** that **may progress to pancreatic insufficiency**. The etiology of chronic pancreatitis in children is often unclear. The differential includes hereditary pancreatitis, congenital or acquired pancreatic duct anomalies, cystic fibrosis, trauma, hypercalcemia, organic acidemias, and various hyperlipidemia syndromes. Occasionally, chronic pancreatitis is associated with pseudocyst formation.

Evaluation

Symptoms of chronic pancreatitis include **midepigastric pain** that may be **associated with stress or a large fatty meal**. Pain may radiate to the back, and **nausea and vomiting** are frequently associated. The episode usually **resolves within 1 week**. Occasionally, symptoms are associated with pancreatic insufficiency or diabetes mellitus. Diagnosis is based on history and laboratory findings of **elevated amylase and lipase,** although the levels may not correlate with the intensity of the pain. Amylase typically peaks 3 days after the onset of pancreatitis; the timing of the elevation of lipase is variable. With pancreatic insufficiency, serum amylase and lipase can be normalized. Late in the disease, fat-soluble vitamin deficiency, hypoalbuminemia, glucose intolerance, and abnormalities in liver enzymes can be seen. **Abdominal ultrasound or computed tomography (CT) scan** may show enlargement or inflammation of the pancreas. Endoscopic retrograde cholangio-pancreatography and noninvasive magnetic resonance cholangiopancreatography are useful in patients in whom gallstones are suspected (unusual in children) or in whom there is a concern for anatomic abnormalities.

Treatment

Treatment of acute pancreatitis involves **bowel rest and pain control**. Chronic pancreatitis may require **parenteral nutrition**. For those children in whom pancreatic insufficiency is suspected, **pancreatic enzyme supplementation** may be helpful. **Drainage or removal of a pseudocyst** may be indicated to prevent possible infection or rupture.

Ureteropelvic Junction Obstruction and Other Genitourinary Disorders

Ureteropelvic junction obstruction refers to a **kink in the ureter at the outlet from the renal pelvis**. Ureteral obstruction leads to abdominal pain and occasional renal damage in children. The condition is **more common in males,** more often **left sided,** and frequently associated with **vomiting**. Symptoms vary with age. **Infants** often present with a **palpable abdominal mass or pyelonephritis,** whereas in **children** the presentation is more frequently **abdominal pain**. The pain is crampy and intermittent, occasionally as infrequent as twice per week, and may radiate to the groin or flank. **Older children** may have a **palpable abdominal mass or abnormalities on urinalysis** such as hematuria, but the absence of these findings does not rule out an obstruction. The diagnosis is made by **renal ultrasound or CT scan** of the abdomen; testing should be performed while symptoms are present. Treatment involves **surgical repair** of the obstruction.

Other genitourinary disorders may cause abdominal pain as well. **Chronic nephrolithiasis** may present as recurrent bouts of abdominal and/or groin pain, usually associated with hematuria. **Cystic teratoma of the ovary** may lead to chronic or recurrent abdominal pain, generally in the lower quadrants or pelvic region. As with ureteropelvic junction obstruction, **ultrasound** is the diagnostic method of choice for both of these entities. Treatment of nephrolithiasis in children is **supportive,** although further diagnostic evaluation for a cause may be indicated, especially in young children.

Parasitic Infections
Etiology

The most common parasitic infection associated with chronic abdominal pain is **giardiasis,** caused by the protozoan *Giardia lamblia*. This infection is most frequently associated with **drinking contaminated fresh water,** although **day care** may be a source in children.

Evaluation and Treatment

Symptoms usually **resolve over weeks,** but **occasionally children develop chronic symptoms** of diffuse, crampy abdominal pain, nausea, abdominal distention, increased flatulence, watery diarrhea, and weight loss from malabsorption. Diagnosis may be made by **collecting the stool** specifically to **look for the cysts or trophozoites,** or if these are negative and the suspicion is high, examination of **duodenal aspirates or biopsy specimens** may be revealing. Treatment is with **metronidazole**.

Infection with other parasites such as *Ascaris lumbricoides, Trichuris trichiura,* which is more common in the tropics, *Blastocystis hominis, or Dientamoeba fragilis* may lead to abdominal pain. Associated symptoms include anorexia, diarrhea, rectal prolapse, and occasionally small-bowel obstruction. The diagnosis is made by screening the **stool for ova and parasites**. Peripheral eosinophilia may be observed in *D. fragilis*. **Treatment** of these helminths is mebendazole or albendazole for *Ascariasis or Trichuriasis*. Iodoquinol is the drug of choice for *D. fragilis;* metronidazole, iodoquinol, and trimethoprim-sulfamethoxazole are effective in eradicating *B. hominis*. Improvement of sanitation is necessary for population-wide eradication.

History: Important Questions

- Duration and location of the pain?
- Association of the pain with menses?
- Any ingestion of toxins such as lead?
- Any medications: prescribed, herbal, or over the counter?

History: Alarming Points

- Associated fever, weight loss, joint pain, or rash
- Associated vomiting, especially bilious, or bloody emesis
- Associated change in stool pattern, especially diarrhea, bloody stool, or melena

History: Does not Distinguish Between Functional and Organic

- Pain quality is altered by eating or stooling.
- Pain wakes patient up at night.
- Family history of IBD, peptic ulcer disease, functional abdominal pain, and migraines.

Physical Examination: Important Clues

- Vital signs, general appearance, and interactions with others
- Weight and height percentile patterns
- Mouth: Ulcers? Destruction of tooth enamel?
- Abdominal exam: Distended? Tender? If so, location? Rebound? Mass or stool palpable? Hepatosplenomegaly?
- Rectal examination: Tone of rectum? Size of rectal vault? Perianal disease? Hard stool? Grossly bloody or occult blood?
- Skin: Jaundice? Rash?
- Musculoskeletal: Joint swelling, redness, or tenderness?

TABLE 10-3 Distinguishing Characteristics of Various Causes of Chronic Abdominal Pain

Diagnosis	Historical Clues	Physical Examination Clues	Lab/Diagnostic Study Clues
Infant colic	• Irritability or fussiness for >3 hrs/d, at least 3 d/wk, for at least 1 wk • Occurs sporadically and usually in the evening	Normal examination	Normal lab findings.
Childhood functional abdominal pain	• Episodic or continuous • Duration >2 mo • Pain not associated with eating or stooling • Functional abdominal pain syndrome includes some loss of daily functioning or somatic symptoms	Normal examination	Normal lab findings.
Functional dyspepsia	• Abdominal pain above the umbilicus • Duration >2 mo • Pain not associated with stooling	Normal examination	Normal labs and studies, including endoscopy.
Irritable bowel syndrome	• Duration >2 mo • Associated with straining, urgency, passing mucus, bloating, and distension • Pain relieved by defecation or associated with a change in bowel pattern	Normal examination	Normal lab findings.
Abdominal migraine	• Intense paroxysmal periumbilical pain that interferes with normal activity • Intervening periods of usual health • May be associated with headache, vomiting, photophobia, pallor, anorexia, or nausea • Family history of migraine	Normal examination	• May respond to antimigraine medications. • Trigger avoidance.
Chronic intestinal pseudo-obstruction	• Intermittent crampy pain, vomiting, and decreased flatus • Vomiting may be bilious • May have history of previous abdominal surgery	• Abdominal distension and tenderness • May have scars from previous surgery on abdomen	• Abdominal radiograph frequently shows fixed air-fluid levels with decreased air distally.

Functional constipation	• Diffuse and vague pain • Decreased stool frequency; hard or voluminous stool • Large-diameter stools that may obstruct toilet • May have withholding or encopresis	• Often large fecal mass on rectal examination • Often dilated rectal vault	• Normal lab findings. • Abdominal radiograph may show abundant stool, dilated colon.
Peptic disease	• Epigastric pain • Pain often, but not always, after meals • Family history of ulcers possible	• May have epigastric tenderness • Heme-positive stools possibly present	• Anemia possible. • A pH probe may be helpful. • Endoscopy shows esophagitis, gastritis, duodenitis, or ulcers. • *Helicobacter pylori* studies may be positive.
Carbohydrate intolerance	• Diffuse, crampy pain after meals • Watery diarrhea typical • May have poor weight gain • May be postinfectious • More common in certain ethnic groups	• Usually normal	• Breath tests for the offending sugar are the tests of choice.
Celiac disease	• May have chronic diarrhea • May have failure to thrive • May have abdominal distention	• Tooth discoloration/loss of enamel possible • Rash possible	• Iron-deficiency anemia. • Abnormal anti-tissue transglutaminase and anti-endomysial antibodies. • Endoscopy and histology show flattened villi in duodenum/jejunum.

(continued)

TABLE 10-3 Distinguishing Characteristics of Various Causes of Chronic Abdominal Pain (*Cont.*)

Diagnosis	Historical Clues	Physical Examination Clues	Lab/Diagnostic Study Clues
Inflammatory bowel disease	• Pain diffuse or localized • Constitutional symptoms such as fever, weight loss, rash, joint pain common • Diarrhea or bloody stool possibly present • Vomiting possible • Mouth ulcers or perianal disease possibly present	• Fever and tachycardia • Abdominal tenderness • Heme-positive stools frequent • Rash or joint findings possible	• Elevated erythrocyte sedimentation rate, anemia, and hypoalbuminemia are common. • Upper GI-small-bowel series may show strictures in Crohn disease. • Endoscopy and biopsy needed for diagnosis.
Chronic pancreatitis	• Midepigastric pain • May radiate to back • May have vomiting or loss of appetite • May have malabsorptive symptoms	• May be ill appearing or cachectic • Midepigastric tenderness common	• Elevated amylase and lipase. • May have enlargement of pancreas or pseudocyst by ultrasound or CT.
Ureteropelvic junction obstruction	• Diffuse intermittent pain that may radiate to groin or flank • May have hematuria • Frequently associated with vomiting	• May have palpable abdominal mass • May have costovertebral angle tenderness	• Ultrasound or CT scan shows anomaly.
Nephrolithiasis	• Severe intermittent crampy pain in abdomen and/or flank, occasionally radiating to groin • Often associated with hematuria • Often associated with nausea and vomiting	• May have abdominal or costo-vertebral angle tenderness	• Ultrasound or CT scan may show presence of stone.
Giardiasis	• Diffuse, crampy pain • Weight loss or poor weight gain • Nausea, watery diarrhea, bloating, increased flatulence common • Exposure through day care or contaminated fresh water	• Abdominal distention common	• Stool examination may show cysts or trophozoites. • May need to perform duodenal aspirates or endoscopy.

Biliary colic	• RUQ or midepigastric crampy pain after meals, especially fatty foods • May have vomiting • May be obese or have concurrent illness	• RUQ or midepigastric tenderness possible	• May have elevated bilirubin or transaminases. • Ultrasound shows gallstones or thickened gallbladder wall.
Ovarian teratoma	• Intermittent lower quadrant pain, often one sided • Vomiting possible	• Lower-quadrant fullness, and tenderness	• Ultrasound or CT scan will show anomaly. • Ultrasound can also determine blood flow.
Dysmenorrhea	• Crampy lower abdominal pain, occurring during menses • Often a family history of dysmenorrhea	• Normal examination	• Normal studies, although some may have endometriosis.
Lead poisoning	• Diffuse pain • Often a history of pica • In high-risk exposure area	• Usually normal	• Elevated serum lead level. • Microcytic anemia. • May see basophilic stippling.

CT, computed tomography; EEG, electroencephalogram; GI, gastrointestinal; RUQ, right upper quadrant; WBC, white blood cell.

Supportive Laboratory Studies

- Complete blood cell count
- Erythrocyte sedimentation rate
- Liver function tests: aminotransferases, albumin, and bilirubin
- Amylase and lipase
- Urinalysis and culture
- Electrolytes, blood urea nitrogen, and creatinine
- Stool ova and parasites

Diagnostic Tests: Based on Clinical Suspicion

- Abdominal two-view radiograph
- Abdominal ultrasound
- Lactose or other breath tests
- Endoscopy and biopsy

Table 10-3 displays distinguishing characteristics of the different causes of chronic abdominal pain. The determination of the exact cause of a child's abdominal pain may require multiple visits. Occasionally, referral to a specialist is indicated. It is critical that all those involved work as a team and address all of the factors that have produced chronic abdominal pain in the child.

Suggested Readings

Diefenbach KA, Breuer CK. Pediatric inflammatory bowel disease. *World J Gastroenterol.* 2006; 12(20):3204–3212.

DiLorenzo C, Colletti RB, Lechmann HP, et al. Chronic abdominal pain in children: a clinical report of the American Academy of Pediatric and the North American Society for Pediatric Gastroenterology, Hepatology and Nutrition. *J Pediatr Gastroenterol Nutr.* 2005;40:245–248.

Drossman DA. The functional gastrointestinal disorders and the Rome III process. *Gastroenterology.* 2006;130:1377–1390.

Gold BD, Colletti RB, Abbott M, et al. *Helicobacter pylori* infection in children: recommendations for diagnosis and treatment. *J Pediatr Gastroenterol Nutr.* 2000;31:490–497.

Hyman PE, Milla PJ, Benninga MA, et al. Childhood functional gastrointestinal disorders: neonate/toddler. *Gastroenterology.* 2006;130:1519–1526.

Mahajan LA, Kaplan B. Chronic abdominal pain of childhood and adolescence. In: R Wyllie, JS Hyams, M Kay, eds. *Pediatric Gastrointestinal and Liver Disease.* 4th ed. Philadelphia, PA: WB Saunders; 2011.

Markowitz J. Ulcerative colitis in children and adolescents. In: R Wyllie, JS Hyams, M Kay, eds. *Pediatric Gastrointestinal and Liver Disease.* 4th ed. Philadelphia, PA: WB Saunders; 2011.

Mearin ML. Celiac disease among children and adolescents. *Curr Probl Pediatr Adolesc Heath Care.* 2007;7(3):86–105.

Megraud F. Comparison of non-invasive tests to detect *Helicobacter pylori* infection in children and adolescents: results of a multicenter European study. *J Pediatr.* 2005;146:198–203.

Rabizadeh S, Hyams JS, Dubinsky M. Crohn's Disease. In: R Wyllie, JS Hyams, M Kay, eds. *Pediatric Gastrointestinal and Liver Disease.* 4th ed. Philadelphia, PA: WB Saunders; 2011.

Rasqion A, DiLorenzo C, Forbes D, et al. Childhood functional gastrointestinal disorders: child/adolescent. *Gastroenterology.* 2006;130:1527–1537.

Vandenplas Y, Rudolph CD, Di Lorenzo C, et al. Pediatric gastroesophageal reflux clinical practice guidelines: joint recommendations of NASPGHAN and ESPGHAN. *J Pediatr Gastroenterol Nutr.* 2009;49(4):498–547.

Alopecia

INTRODUCTION

Tinea capitis, trichotillomania, alopecia areata, and telogen effluvium account for >95% of cases of alopecia in children. The growth cycle of hair consists of an active growth phase (anagen), a transition phase (catagen), and a resting phase (telogen). After the telogen phase, the hair is shed and replaced by a new anagen bulb. On a normal scalp, approximately 85% to 90% of the hair is in the anagen phase. There are 100,000 hairs on the normal scalp. Hair loss is only clinically apparent when a person has lost 25% to 50% of his hair.

DIFFERENTIAL DIAGNOSIS LIST

Infectious Causes
Tinea capitis
Secondary syphilis

Toxic Causes
Cytotoxic agents
Anticonvulsants
Radiation
Hypervitaminosis A
Anticoagulants

Neoplastic Causes
Histiocytosis

Traumatic Causes
Trichotillomania
Traction alopecia
Friction alopecia

Congenital Causes
Aplasia cutis congenita
Nevus sebaceous
Epidermal nevus
Hemangioma

Loose anagen syndrome
Ectodermal dysplasia
Hair shaft defects

Metabolic or Genetic Causes
Androgenic alopecia
Acrodermatitis enteropathica
Anorexia nervosa
Malnutrition
Hypo- or hyperthyroidism
Hypopituitarism
Diabetes mellitus

Inflammatory Causes
Alopecia areata
Systemic lupus erythematosus
Scleroderma

Miscellaneous Causes
Atopic dermatitis
Seborrheic dermatitis
Psoriasis
Telogen effluvium
Anagen effluvium

DIFFERENTIAL DIAGNOSIS DISCUSSION

Tinea Capitis

Etiology

Caused by dermatophyte infection of the scalp hairs, tinea capitis is responsible for **<50% of cases of hair loss** in children. Currently, the most prevalent fungus causing tinea capitis is *Trichophyton tonsurans* in the United States.

Clinical Features

Tinea capitis is seen most commonly in school-aged **children**. The infection causes **patchy hair loss** that may or may not be accompanied by **scale**. Some areas may seem completely bald and indistinguishable from alopecia areata, but on closer examination the scalp contains **very short hairs,** called **"black-dot" tinea capitis. There may be posterior cervical or occipital lymphadenopathy.**

Evaluation

Unlike *Microsporum canis,* which caused epidemic outbreaks of tinea capitis during the 1940s, *T. tonsurans* does not show immunofluorescence under Wood lamp examination. Diagnosis can be confirmed using a **potassium hydroxide (KOH) preparation** and by **fungal culture** of the hair and scale. A KOH preparation reveals organisms inside the hair shaft.

Treatment

Oral griseofulvin dosed at 20 to 25 mg/kg/day microsize (or 10 to 15 mg/kg/day ultramicrosize) once daily for 6 to 8 weeks is the standard therapy for tinea capitis in children. It is best absorbed when taken with **fatty foods**. The medication is **safe in children;** it is not necessary for the patient to undergo laboratory testing before initiating drug therapy. Newer antifungal medications such as **fluconazole, itraconazole, and terbinafine** may also be effective and require a shorter course of therapy. An **antifungal or selenium shampoo** may hasten resolution in combination with systemic antifungal medication. An effort should be made to identify and treat infected household contacts to avoid reinfection.

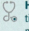 **HINT:** The infection may be accompanied by a hypersensitivity reaction called a "kerion," which is a boggy, inflammatory mass. The surface may contain pustules, and cervical lymphadenopathy is usually present. Although it may appear to be superinfected, the lesion can usually be treated successfully with griseofulvin and oral prednisone.

 HINT: Tinea capitis mimics many other conditions, which should be considered prior to treatment.

Alopecia Areata

Etiology

Alopecia areata is the **second most common cause** of alopecia in children and may appear insidiously in an otherwise healthy school-aged patient. Multiple factors are implicated in the pathophysiology, including genetic, organ-specific autoimmune, and nonspecific immune components.

Clinical Features

The hair loss occurs in **variably sized patches** completely **devoid of hair**. Hairs surrounding the area of alopecia may demonstrate a narrow waist on microscopic examination ("exclamation point" hairs). The **entire scalp** is **involved in alopecia totalis,** and the **entire body** is **involved in alopecia universalis**. Accompanying features may include **pitting** or a **scotch-plaid pattern** on the **nails**. Other autoimmune disorders may occur in these patients, such as Hashimoto thyroiditis, diabetes mellitus, vitiligo, Addison disease, and inflammatory bowel disease.

Evaluation

Hair pluck with microscopy should be performed to look for classic **"exclamation point" hairs,** which confirm the diagnosis of alopecia areata. Routine screening for autoimmune disease is not generally indicated.

Treatment

Treatment for this disorder is less than straightforward. Modalities such as topical and systemic steroids, minoxidil, and anthralin have been used; unfortunately, none have proved effective in reversing the course of disease. In **one-third of patients,** the **condition regresses spontaneously** within 6 months. More extensive cases are less likely to resolve. A frank discussion with the patient and family and **close follow-up** are mandatory. A **wig or hairpiece** may be necessary to counteract the psychological trauma of this disease. **Referral to a pediatric dermatologist** should be considered in all cases in which aggressive therapy seems warranted.

Trichotillomania

Etiology

Seen more commonly in children than in adults, trichotillomania is an **uncontrollable urge to pull out one's own hair**. Adolescent girls are most commonly afflicted; however, in children <6 years, it is more common in boys.

Clinical Features

The hair-pulling results in **ill-defined areas of baldness** in **unusual distributions**. The diagnosis is usually made clear by the presence of **many broken hairs of various lengths**. The sites involved are varied, although a predilection for the side of handedness may be seen. The periphery of the scalp is usually spared. Other body hair may also be involved in severe cases. Often nail biting, thumb sucking, and **other compulsive behaviors** are also present.

Evaluation

Hair pluck should be performed to rule out alopecia areata. A **scalp biopsy** may be necessary to confirm the diagnosis.

Treatment

This diagnosis may be difficult for the family to accept. Treatment strategies include **cognitive behavior therapy**. Severe cases should be **referred to a psychiatrist** for adjuvant pharmacotherapy.

Telogen Effluvium

Telogen effluvium occurs when a **large percentage of scalp hairs enter the resting phase** after a **stressful event** and are shed 2 to 4 months later. The precipitant may be childbirth, major surgery, anesthesia, febrile illness, crash dieting, or psychological trauma. The hallmark of telogen effluvium is **diffuse acute hair loss** that **spontaneously resolves** over several months. Hair pluck reveals a disproportionate number of hair follicles in the telogen phase. Eventually, **full recovery** of hair growth ensues and no treatment is necessary.

Traction Alopecia and Friction Alopecia

Tension on the hair shaft can cause hair loss in areas most affected (traction alopecia). Tight braiding of the hair, ponytails, cornrows, and hot combs are the worst culprits. In a similar fashion, hair in **areas of pressure,** such as the occiput in a supine infant, may exhibit hair loss, although the scalp is functionally normal (friction alopecia). Hair loss occurs in a **classic distribution**. Diagnosis is made on a clinical basis. If the alopecia fails to respond to conservative management, the diagnosis should be reevaluated. The hairstyle or positioning should be altered. Normal hair growth should follow.

Anagen Effluvium

Like telogen effluvium, anagen effluvium is characterized by **diffuse acute hair loss**. In anagen effluvium, hair loss results from **disruption of the normal hair growth cycle** following a toxic insult to the hair follicle. The causes are usually cytotoxic agents such as vincristine and cyclophosphamide. Heavy metal toxicity, hypothyroidism, and severe malnutrition are also implicated. If the cause is not apparent, hair pluck differentiates anagen effluvium from telogen effluvium. The **hair regrows following removal of the offending agent,** although the color and texture of the new hair may be different.

EVALUATION OF ALOPECIA

Patient History

The elements of the history most crucial to the diagnosis of alopecia disorders are as follows:

- **Time of onset**—congenital versus acquired
- **Associated stressors**—childbirth, recent surgery, toxic exposures, seizures, and febrile illnesses
- **Any abnormal behaviors**—for example, thumb sucking and nail biting

Physical Examination

Physical examination should focus on **distribution of hair loss, presence of scale, presence of broken hairs, and nail findings**. A magnifying glass and good lighting aid in detection of subtle scalp findings.

Laboratory Studies

A **KOH preparation** is important when the diagnosis of tinea capitis is suspected, and **fungal culture** should be obtained. A **hair pluck** is used to diagnose telogen

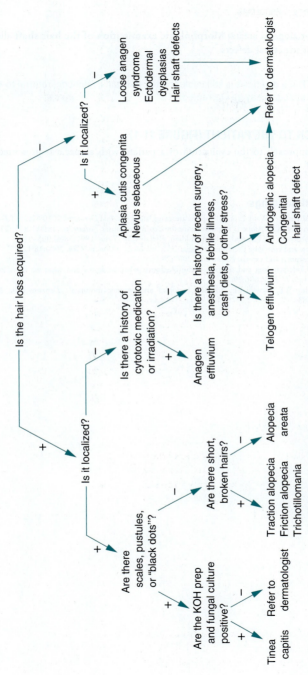

FIGURE 11-1 Evaluation of a patient with alopecia. KOH prep, potassium hydroxide preparation.

effluvium or alopecia areata. **Morphologic examination of the hair shaft** allows detection of structural defects.

 HINT: If a diagnosis is still unclear after an initial evaluation, referral to a dermatologist may be warranted.

APPROACH TO THE PATIENT (FIGURE 11-1)

A general approach to the evaluation of a patient with alopecia is presented in Figure 11-1.

Suggested Readings

Alkhalifah A, Alsantali A, Wang E, et al. Alopecia areata update. *J Am Acad Dermatol.* 2010;62(2):177–188.

Atton AV, Tunnessen WW. Alopecia in children: the most common causes. *Pediatr Rev.* 1990;12(25):25–30.

Levy ML. Disorders of the hair and scalp in children. *Pediatr Clin N Am.* 1991;38(4):905–919.

Raimer SS. New and emerging therapies in pediatric dermatology. *Dermatol Clin.* 2000;18:1.

Shy R. Tinea corporis and capitis. *Pediatr Rev.* 2007;28:164–174.

Woods DW. Understanding and treating trichotillomania: what we know and what we don't know. *Psychiatr Clin N Am.* 2006;29:2.

Zhang AY, Camp WL, Elewski BE. Advances in topical and systemic antifungals. *Dermatol Clin.* 2007; 25:165–183.

Ambiguous Genitalia

INTRODUCTION

Genitalia are defined as ambiguous when it is not possible to categorize the gender of the child based on outward appearances. Abnormalities in external genitalia that require endocrine evaluation occur in 1 out of every 4,500 births. Ambiguous genitalia may be associated with genotypic **females who are virilized,** genotypic **males who are undermasculinized,** problems of **gonadal differentiation, and congenital embryopathy**.

Sexual Differentiation

Management of patients with sexual ambiguity requires an understanding of normal sexual differentiation. The primitive gonad is bipotential, containing both ovarian (cortical) and testicular (medullary) components. Sexual differentiation is determined by the genetic information contained in the sex chromosomes, as well as by hormonal factors. Pseudohermaphroditism occurs when the external genitalia do not correspond to the chromosomal or gonadal sex (i.e., an XX female who is masculinized or an XY male who is inadequately masculinized). The internal genitalia develop normally.

Male Sexual Differentiation

The SRY gene (i.e., the sex-determining region) on the short arm of the Y chromosome is the **primary testis-determining factor**. Additional genetic factors important to sexual differentiation include DAX-1, SOX-9, and Wnt-4. The transcription factors WT1 and SF-1 are necessary for gonadal development. Testis-determining factor induces the bipotential gonads to develop as testes by 6 to 7 weeks of gestation. At 7 to 8 weeks of gestation, Sertoli cells in the testes secrete anti-müllerian hormone (AMH), also called müllerian-inhibiting substance (MIS), which causes regression of the müllerian ducts in the male fetus.

Human chorionic gonadotropin (HCG) and fetal pituitary gonadotropin stimulate the Leydig cells in the fetal testes to secrete **testosterone,** which causes the wolffian structures to develop into the vas deferens, epididymis, and seminal vesicles. Testosterone is converted locally to dihydrotestosterone (DHT) by 5α-reductase. DHT is necessary for the development of the scrotum and phallus from the labial scrotal folds and the genital tubercle.

Although the formation of the male genitals is complete by 12 weeks of gestation, MIS stimulates abdominal descent of the testes in the second trimester.

During the second and third trimesters, further testicular descent and penile growth are stimulated by testosterone.

Female Sexual Differentiation

The differentiation of the bipotential gonad into an ovary by 10 weeks of gestation requires that two X chromosomes be present and that the Y chromosome (i.e., the SRY gene) be absent. Because MIS is not produced, the müllerian ducts develop into the uterus, the fallopian tubes, and the upper two-thirds of the vagina. In the **absence of androgens,** the wolffian ducts degenerate, the external genitalia differentiates as the clitoris and labia, and the urogenital sinus becomes the lower third of the vagina and urethra.

 DIFFERENTIAL DIAGNOSIS LIST

 HINT: The most common cause of virilization in a female is 21-hydroxylase deficiency. The most common cause of undervirilization in a male is androgen insensitivity syndrome (AIS).

Virilized Genetic Female (Female Pseudohermaphroditism)

Congenital adrenal hyperplasia (CAH)—21-hydroxylase deficiency, 3β-hydroxysteroid dehydrogenase deficiency, 11β-hydroxylase deficiency

Exogenous androgen exposure—exogenous, excess androgen production

Aromatase Deficiency

Undervirilized Genetic Male (Male Pseudohermaphroditism)

Androgen Insensitivity Syndrome (AIS) and partial androgen receptor defects

CAH—Steroidogenic acute regulatory protein (StAR)

deficiency, 17, 20-desmolase deficiency, 3β-hydroxysteroid dehydrogenase deficiency, 17α-hydroxylase deficiency

Other androgen synthesis defects—17-lyase deficiency, 17-ketosteroid reductase deficiency, **5α-reductase deficiency,** Smith-Lemli-Opitz syndrome

Persistent müllerian duct syndrome

Leydig cell hypoplasia

Gonadal Dysgenesis

Partial Gonadal Dysgenesis

Mixed Gonadal Dysgenesis— Chromosomal Aberrations (XO/XY, XX/XY)

True Hermaphroditism

Congenital Embryopathy

DIFFERENTIAL DIAGNOSIS DISCUSSION
Virilized Genetic Female
Etiology

Virilization of the genotypic female fetus is usually caused by **androgens** produced by the fetus or transferred across the placenta. Androgen exposure before 12 weeks of gestation results in interference of septation of the urogenital sinus and some degree of labial scrotal fusion. After 12 weeks of gestation, androgen exposure can cause clitoral enlargement but not labial scrotal fusion. The following are sources of androgen exposure:

- **Congenital Adrenal Hyperplasia (CAH).** This is the most common cause of virilization in genetic females and 21-hydroxylase deficiency represents 90% of cases of CAH. CAH is an autosomal recessive disorder caused by enzymatic defects in cortisol synthesis. Deficient cortisol causes a rise in corticotropin releasing hormone and adrenocorticotropic hormone (ACTH), which stimulates adrenal hyperplasia. As a result, adrenal androgen and steroid precursors prior to the enzyme defect accumulate. 21-Hydroxylase deficiency causes impaired production of cortisol and aldosterone and infants are susceptible to adrenal crisis. 11β-Hydroxylase deficiency is the second most common cause of CAH and has similar clinical features except elevated 11-deoxycortisol and 11-deoxycorticosterone result in hypertension. 3β-Hydroxysteroid dehydrogenase deficiency results in impaired cortisol, aldosterone, and testosterone biosynthesis. Affected females have mild virilization due to peripheral conversion of elevated DHEA to androgens.

Clinical Features
The external genitalia are virilized. Patients with 21-hydroxylase or 3β-hydroxysteroid dehydrogenase deficiencies may present with salt-losing crises within a few weeks of birth.

Evaluation
The diagnosis of CAH can be made by obtaining baseline steroid measurements and steroid measurements following ACTH administration (Tables 12-1 through 12-3). Baseline and stimulated steroid levels are elevated.

Treatment
Patients with CAH should receive cortisol and mineralocorticoid replacement as needed. Cosmetic surgical repair may be appropriate for all patients.

TABLE 12-1	Clinical and Biochemical Features of Congenital Adrenal Hyperplasia (CAH)			
	Sexual Ambiguity		**Additional Clinical**	
Enzyme Defect	**Female**	**Male**	**Manifestations**	**Predominant Steroids**
StAR, Desmolase	–	+	Salt wasting	—
3β-Hydroxysteroid Dehydrogenase	+	+	Salt wasting	17-OH-Pregnenolone, DHEA
21-Hydroxylase	+	–	Salt wasting	17-OH-Progesterone, androstenedione
11-Hydroxylase	+	–	Hypertension	11-Deoxycortisol
17-Hydroxylase	–	+	Hypertension	DOC, corticosterone

DHEA, dehydroepiandrosterone; DOC, deoxycorticosterone.

TABLE 12-2	Normal Serum Adrenal Steroid Levels in Newborn Infants			
Steroid	**Preterm Sick 24–28 wk**	**Preterm Well 31–35 wk**	**Full Term 31–35 wk**	
Cortisol (μg/dL)	7.5 ± 4	6 ± 2.7	6.9 ± 3.8	6.2 ± 3.9
17-OH-Preg (ng/dL)	1794 ± 1818	1395 ± 694	942 ± 739	245 ± 291
17-OH-Pro (ng/dL)	651 ± 661	373 ± 317	169 ± 95	36 ± 13[a]
11-deoxycortisol (ng/dL)	662 ± 548	294 ± 239	111 ± 62	87 ± 42
DHEA (ng/dL)	1872 ± 4038	675 ± 502	920 ± 1227	286 ± 238
DHEAS (μg/dL)	467 ± 312	459 ± 209	341 ± 93	162 ± 88
Androstenedione (ng/dL)	479 ± 1032	206 ± 86	215 ± 134	149 ± 67

Data based on information in Lee MM, Rajagopalan L, Berg G, et al. Serum adrenal steroid concentrations in premature infants. *J Clin Endocrinol Metab* 69:1133–1136, 1989, and in Wiener D, Smith J, Dahlem S, et al. Serum adrenal steroid levels in healthy term 3-day-old infants. *J Pediatr* 110(1):122–124, 1987.
17-OH-Preg, 17-OH-pregnenolone; 17-OH-Pro, 17-OH-progesterone; DHEA, dehydroepiandrosterone; DHEAS, dehydroepiandrosterone sulfate.
[a]17-OH-Pro values in full-term sick newborns may be double or triple the baseline values. No data are available for other steroid hormones in sick full-term infants.

- **Exogenous Androgen Exposure.** Examples of exogenous androgens include progestational agents for prevention of spontaneous abortion and maternal use of androgenic drugs. The production of androgens by the mother as a result of poorly controlled CAH or androgen-secreting ovarian or adrenal tumor may also cause virilization of the female fetus.
- **Aromatase Deficiency.** Aromatase deficiency is a rare autosomal recessive disorder. Aromatase in the fetus and placenta converts adrenal androgens to estrogens in utero, so a deficiency results in elevated androgens and virilization. In placental aromatase deficiency, the mother also becomes virilized during the pregnancy.

TABLE 12-3	Serum Adrenal Steroid Levels in Infants 1-Hour Post-ACTH Administration		
		Well Infants (2–12 mo)[a]	
Steroid	**Preterm Sick (24–28 wk)**	**Female**	**Male**
Cortisol (μg/dL)	18.3 ± 6.8	40 ± 8.1	38.2 ± 4.4
17-OH-Preg (ng/dL)	5730 ± 4461	1610 ± 800	1242 ± 753
17-OH-Pro (ng/dL)	968 ± 876	142 ± 50	196 ± 85

Data based on information in Hingre RV, Gross SJ, Hingre KS, et al.: Adrenal steroidogenesis in very low birth weight preterm infants. *J Clin Endocrinol Metab* 78(2):266–270, 1994, and in Lashansky G, Saenger P, Fishman K, et al.: Normative data for adrenal steroidogenesis in a healthy pediatric population: age- and sex-related changes after adrenocorticotropin stimulation. *J Clin Endocrinol Metab* 73:674–686, 1991.
ACTH, adrenocorticotropic hormone; 17-OH-Preg, 17-OH-pregnenolone; 17-OH-Pro, 17-OH-progesterone.
[a]No post-ACTH steroid data are available for full-term newborns.

Undervirilized Genetic Male
Etiology
Inadequate masculinization of the genotypic male fetus can be caused by enzyme disorders of testosterone synthesis or a lack of responsiveness to testosterone action (androgen resistance syndromes).

Clinical Features
Patients with male pseudohermaphroditism may show micropenis, hypospadias, a poorly developed scrotum, or undescended testes. Alternatively, a normal female phenotype may be present.

- **AIS.** This is the most common cause of undervirilization in a genetic male and is caused by X-linked mutations or deletions of the androgen receptor or post-receptor defects. **Partial androgen insensitivity** results in a spectrum of phenotypes with varying degrees of androgen resistance. Individuals with **complete AIS** appear phenotypically female with female external genitalia and a blind vaginal pouch with absent wolffian and müllerian structures. It may be diagnosed in infancy if gonads are palpated in the labia or inguinal canal of a phenotypic female, but is often diagnosed in adolescent girls with primary amenorrhea. There is no virilization at puberty and breasts develop as a result of peripheral conversion of high levels of testosterone to estradiol.

Evaluation
Patients have an XY karyotype, no müllerian structures, and elevated testosterone and luteinizing hormone (LH) levels in the newborn period. The typical phenotype for partial androgen insensitivity is hypospadias, micropenis, a bifid scrotum, and undescended testes, but there is a broad spectrum of presentations based on the degree of response to androgens.

- **CAH.** This can result in undervirilization of the male fetus when the adrenal enzymes necessary for testosterone synthesis are also deficient in the testes. **17α-Hydroxylase deficiency** is a rare disorder that results in the inability to produce sex steroids. Congenital lipid adrenal hyperplasia associated with defects in **StAR,** and **cholesterol desmolase deficiency** result in insufficient mineralocorticoid, glucocorticoid, and androgen synthesis.

Evaluation and Treatment
See Evaluation and Treatment of CAH in Virilized Female explained above.

- **Other Androgen Synthesis Defects.** 17-Ketosteroid reductase deficiency in the testes prevents the conversion of androstenedione to testosterone; 17-lyase is necessary for the conversion of C21 steroids to C19 androgenic steroids in the testes. Both cause varying degrees of undervirilization.

Evaluation
17-Ketosteroid reductase deficiency can be diagnosed by an abnormal ratio of androstenedione to testosterone, either at baseline or after stimulation with HCG. 17-Lyase deficiency is suggested by low androgen levels and increased gonadotropin levels.

TABLE 12-4	Penile and Clitoral Length in the Newborn Infant
Gestational Age	**Length**
Males[a]	
30 wk	2.5 ± 0.4 cm
34 wk	3.0 ± 0.4 cm
Term	3.5 ± 0.4 cm
Females[b]	
Term[c]	4.0 ± 1.24 mm

Data based on information in Feldman KW, Smith DW: Fetal phallic growth and penile standards for newborn male infants. *J Pediatr* 86:395, 1975, and in Oberfield S, Mondok A, Shanrivar F, et al.: Clitoral size in full-term infants. *Am J Perinatol* 6(4):453, 1989.

[a]Measure from the pubic ramus to the tip of the glans with gentle pressure applied.
[b]Measure with the labia majora separated and the prepuce skin retracted.
[c]The clitoris achieves full size by 27 wk of gestation and may appear more prominent in premature infants relative to the labia.

- **5α-Reductase Deficiency** prevents conversion of testosterone to DHT, which is necessary for the development of the male external genitalia. Patients have a blind vaginal pouch, small phallic structure, and severe hypospadias. Because the testis produces both MIS and testosterone, regression of the müllerian ducts and normal development of wolffian structures occur. With increasing testosterone concentrations at puberty, individuals develop penile enlargement, testicular descent of inguinal testes into the labial scrotal folds, and secondary sexual characteristics (e.g., pubic hair, increased muscle mass).

Evaluation

The testosterone-to-DHT ratio is normally <16 basally and following HCG stimulation; a ratio >30 suggests the diagnosis of 5α-reductase deficiency (Table 12-4). The diagnosis is confirmed by finding reduced 5α-reductase activity in fibroblasts in genital skin samples.

- **Leydig Cell Hypoplasia** is a rare autosomal recessive disorder caused by an inactivating mutation of the LH receptor. Patients have female external genitalia, undescended gonads, complete müllerian regression, and absent wolffian structures.

Evaluation

Serum testosterone is low and does not increase with HCG stimulation. Precursor steroids are not elevated.

Gonadal Dysgenesis

Etiology and Clinical Features

- In **pure gonadal dysgenesis,** dysgenesis of the genital ridges results in gonads that are hypoplastic. The condition may be inherited or caused by teratogenic agents. The phenotype is that of a normal female.
- In **partial gonadal dysgenesis,** teratogenic factors or vascular accidents may damage the gonads following differentiation into testes (in genetic males). AMH has been secreted and the müllerian structures have degenerated, but

the development of male external genitalia (which depends on the conversion of testosterone to DHT) does not occur. External genitalia are phenotypically female or ambiguous, but there are no gonads or müllerian structures. Testicular damage that occurs during the second and third trimesters may be less severe and may result in micropenis or cryptorchidism.

- In **mixed gonadal dysgenesis,** individuals with the mosaic genotypes XO/XY and XX/XY have gonads that contain both medullary and cortical elements. External genitalia may be normal female, intersex, or normal male. Patients with XO/XY mosaicism often have many of the classic features of Turner syndrome. The presence of testicular tissue in patients with mixed gonadal dysgenesis increases the likelihood of androgenic hormonal function and the presence of Wolffian duct structures.

True Hermaphroditism

True hermaphrodites possess both ovarian and testicular elements and include patients with mixed gonadal dysgenesis, 46,XX, and less commonly 46,XY. They may have a separate ovary and a testis on the contralateral side or a combination of the two gonads ("ovotestes"). The differentiation of the internal duct structures corresponds to the amount of testicular tissue present in the gonad on the same side. Müllerian duct structures may develop on the side of an ovary with contralateral Wolffian duct structures.

Clinical Features

The degree of functional testicular tissue determines the appearance of the external structures.

Evaluation

The diagnosis is made by chromosomal analysis. In some cases, gonadal biopsy is indicated.

Treatment

Individuals with mixed gonadal dysgenesis have an increased risk of malignant degeneration of gonadal tissues, and gonadectomy is recommended.

Congenital Embryopathy

Abnormalities of the development of the urogenital tract can occur independently and are frequently associated with other congenital abnormalities.

Anomalies of the gastrointestinal and urinary tract may be associated with virilization of the female external genitalia without exposure to androgens.

- **Hypospadias** may be a finding in various intersex disorders. Although isolated first-degree hypospadias is usually not associated with endocrine abnormalities, the incidence of associated intersex disorders increases as the severity of the hypospadias increases and with the presence of bilateral undescended testes.
- **Micropenis** describes a normally formed, appropriately positioned phallus with a length <2.5 standard deviations below the appropriate mean for the patient's age and may occur with congenital hypopituitarism, isolated gonadotropin deficiency (Kallmann syndrome), testicular dysfunction, or partial androgen resistance.

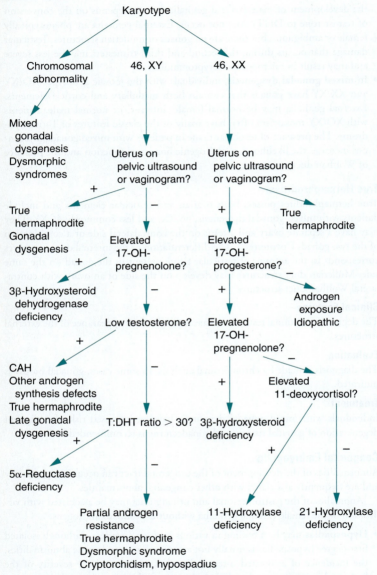

FIGURE 12-1 Approach to the patient with ambiguous genitalia.

APPROACH TO THE PATIENT

Ambiguous genitalia in the neonate should be treated as a **medical emergency** and the diagnostic evaluation undertaken as soon as possible (Figure 12-1). A team approach with consultations from endocrinology, genetics, urology, and psychiatry is useful.

Often, it is advisable for parents to delay naming or announcing the birth of their child until the definitive gender is assigned. The parents should be informed that the definitive gender will be determined within 48 to 72 hours. **Gender assignment** usually can be made on the basis of the physical examination, karyotype, and internal pelvic structures while awaiting the results of serum studies; however, karyotype should not be the only factor in gender determination because gonadal function and future sexual function are also important. In addition, the size of the phallus and the degree of hypospadias need to be considered. For families known to carry CAH mutations, prenatal diagnosis and treatment may help reduce virilization of the female fetus.

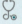 **HINT:** Females with CAH, even when severely virilized, should be raised as females because cosmetic repair can be managed surgically, and patients have good future potential for sexual function and reproduction.

Patient History
- Maternal obstetric history that focuses on drug ingestion and exposure to teratogens or infections during the pregnancy, particularly during the first trimester
- Family history, focusing on any androgenic changes in the mother or anything suggestive of CAH in other family members (e.g., neonatal death, virilization, or precocious adrenarche)

Physical Examination
A complete physical examination should be performed, and the following information needs to be noted:

- Palpable gonads
- The length and diameter of the phallus, the position of the urethra, the degree of fusion of the labioscrotal folds and the existence of a vagina (Table 12-5)
- Other dysmorphic features, especially those involving the urinary tract and anus

 HINT: The presence of palpable gonads implies the presence of Y chromosome material.

Laboratory Studies
- **Karyotyping.** Blood and bone marrow samples should be submitted for karyotyping. Some laboratories can have a karyotype result from a bone marrow specimen available within 6 hours. A standard chromosome analysis should be performed as well because bone marrow karyotyping can miss mosaicism.

TABLE 12-5	Normal Laboratory Values for Serum Testosterone and Dihydrotestosterone (DHT)			
	Testosterone (ng/dL)		DHT (ng/dL)	
	Male	**Female**	**Male**	**Female**
Cord blood	13–55	5–45	<2–8	<2–8
26–28 wk of gestation	59–125	5–16	. . .	. . .
31–35 wk of gestation	37–198	5–22	10–53	2–13
Full term	75–400[a]	20–64[b]	5–60[c]	<2–15[d]

Data provided by the Esoterix Endocrinology Laboratory, Los Calabasas Hills, California.
[a]Levels decrease to 20–50 ng/dL during week 1 and then increase to 60–400 ng/dL at 20–60 days. Levels decrease to prepubertal values by 7 months.
[b]Levels decrease to 10 ng/dL during the first month and remain at that level until puberty.
[c]Levels decrease during week 1 and then increase to 12–85 ng/dL by 30–60 days. Levels decrease to prepubertal values by 7 months.
[d]Levels decrease to 3 ng/dL during the first month and remain at that level until puberty.

- **AMH** levels are a marker for testicular tissue.
- **Serum levels** of **17-hydroxyprogesterone, 17-hydroxypregnenolone, dehydroepiandrosterone, testosterone, DHT, 11-deoxycortisol, and androstenedione** should be obtained. Table 12-4 lists the normal values for serum testosterone and DHT. Recall that adrenal steroid levels are elevated in premature infants, particularly when the child is ill and under stress (see Tables 12-2 and 12-3).
- **Serum levels** of **LH and maternal androgens** may be appropriate to obtain.
- **Biopsy samples.** A gonadal or skin biopsy to evaluate testosterone metabolism may be indicated.
- **DNA** analysis for specific disorders following the initial evaluation.

Diagnostic Imaging Studies
- **Pelvic ultrasound** can demonstrate a uterus and gonads.
- **Vaginogram.** The injection of contrast dye into urethral or vaginal openings demonstrates müllerian ducts (if any are present). The absence of a müllerian system implies functioning testicular tissue early in gestation and the secretion of MIS.

Suggested Readings
Hughes IA. Androgen resistance. *Best Pract Res Clin Endocrinol Metab.* 2006;20:577–598.
Lee PA, Houk CP, Ahmed SF, et al. International Consensus Conference on Intersex organized by the Lawson Wilkins Pediatric Endocrine Society and the European Society for Paediatric Endocrinology. Consensus statement on management of intersex disorders. *Pediatrics.* 2006;118:488–500.
McLaughlin DT, Donahoe PC. Sex determination and differentiation. *N Engl J Med.* 2004;350:367–378.
New MI. Inborn errors of adrenal steroidogenesis. *Mol Cell Endocrinol.* 2003;211:75–83.
Ogilvy Al, Brani CE. Early assessment of ambiguous genitalia. *Arch Dis Child.* 2004;89:401–407.
Speiser PW, White PC. Congenital adrenal hyperplasia. *N Engl J Med.* 2003;349:776–788.
Vaiman D, Pailhoux E. Mammalian sex reversal and intersexuality: deciphering the sex-determination cascade. *Trends Genet.* 2000;16(11):488–494.
Yong EL, Lim J, Qi W, et al. Molecular basis of androgen receptor diseases. *Ann Med.* 2000;32(1):15–22.

Amenorrhea

INTRODUCTION

Amenorrhea, defined as the **absence of menses,** is common during adolescence. Determining the underlying cause of amenorrhea necessitates an understanding of the normal menstrual cycle. Although the broad differential diagnosis includes genetic, endocrine, structural, environmental, and psychological disorders, **pregnancy should always be considered**. Evaluation should begin soon after amenorrhea is noted because underlying pathological conditions can cause tremendous physical and emotional sequelae.

Menarche, a pivotal event of puberty, requires intact and functioning interactions between the hypothalamus, pituitary, ovaries, and uterine endometrial lining. Successful menstrual cycles also require the presence of an unobstructed uterus, cervix, and vagina. The body must have an adequate amount of fat and not be under any extremes of stress (e.g., excessive exercise, emotional stress). Normal (regular) cycles indicate the presence of ovulation. **Menarche is one of the latest signs of puberty in females,** occurring at Tanner stage (or sexual maturity rating) IV in the majority of adolescents. Menarche generally occurs ~3 years after the growth spurt, 2 to 2.5 years after thelarche, and 1 year after peak height velocity. In the United States, 12.5 years is the average age of menarche (the average age is lower for black females, intermediate for Mexican American females, and later for white females). Race, nutritional status, body fat, and maternal age at menarche all influence an individual's age of menarche. The majority of cycles are anovulatory for the first year and remain so for an average of ≥2 years. Normal menstrual cycles are 21 to 45 days, have flow lasting 2 to 7 days, and have an average blood loss of between 30 and 40 mL.

> **HINT:** Although the arbitrary age of primary amenorrhea is 16 years, if a girl 13 years or older presents with absence of breast budding, diagnostic evaluation should be performed immediately, because it is unlikely that she will menstruate within the next 2 years.

The menstrual cycle begins with pulsatile release of gonadotropin-releasing hormone from the hypothalamus, causing secretion of follicle-stimulating hormone (FSH) and luteinizing hormone from the pituitary. Ovarian follicles grow and develop under the influence of FSH. Theca cells produce androgens that are converted to estrogen by granulosa cells. This increased estrogen not only inhibits the pituitary release of FSH, causing follicles to involute, but also stimulates uterine development and endometrial growth. In the first part of the cycle, increased estrogen leads to decreased FSH release. Midcycle, FSH results in a luteinizing hormone surge and ovulation. In **early adolescence,** although estrogen levels are high, the feedback patterns are not mature, and **menses may be anovulatory,** representing sloughing of a proliferative endometrium rather than shedding secondary to the luteal phase of an ovulatory cycle. Clinically, this may be characterized by irregular or heavy bleeding (dysfunctional uterine bleeding) and lack of dysmenorrhea.

Primary amenorrhea is the absence of menarche by 16 years of age (with normal pubertal development), 13 years of age (without normal pubertal development), or within 2 years after completion of sexual maturation. Secondary amenorrhea is the absence of menstruation for at least three consecutive cycles (if regular cycles), or for 6 months (if irregular cycles). Although primary and secondary amenorrhea are helpful in describing menstrual cycle interruption in terms of timing, the terms do not indicate an underlying cause or offer information about treatment or prognosis. In addition, because several of the processes that cause amenorrhea can present as primary or secondary, a more informative evaluation and diagnostic strategy is to distinguish whether normal pubertal and sexual development have occurred or not.

 DIFFERENTIAL DIAGNOSIS LIST

Amenorrhea with Delayed Puberty
Hypergonadotropic Hypogonadism

Gonadal Failure
Congenital causes:
>   *Genetic:* Turner syndrome (45, XO)
>   *Ovarian:* Pure or mosaic karyotype gonadal dysgenesis
>   *Receptor Defect:* Androgen insensitivity or complete testicular feminization

Acquired causes:
>   Medications, chemotherapy/ radiation
>   Gonadotropin-resistant ovary syndrome; autoimmune oophoritis
>   Infiltrative, ischemic, or destructive disorders

Hypogonadotropic Hypogonadism

Disorders of the Hypothalamus and/or Pituitary
Congenital causes:
>   Abnormal hypothalamic development (e.g., Kallmann syndrome)

Acquired causes:
>   Central nervous system (CNS) lesions/tumors (e.g., pituitary adenoma); head trauma; medications, chemotherapy/ radiation; infiltrative, ischemic, or destructive disorders; chronic illness; weight loss (anorexia nervosa); exercise, stress; marijuana use

Endocrine:
>   *Chronic disease:* Thyroid disease, diabetes mellitus, Addison disease

Hyperprolactinemia: Pituitary adenoma, renal failure, psychoactive drugs (e.g., Haldol)

Others:

Constitutional delay

Structural genital tract defects: Congenital absence of the uterus

Amenorrhea with Normal Puberty

Hypergonadotropic Hypogonadism

Gonadal Failure

Acquired causes:

Medications, chemotherapy/radiation; premature ovarian failure; autoimmune oophoritis; infiltrative, ischemic, or destructive disorders

Hypogonadotropic Hypogonadism

Acquired causes:

CNS lesions/tumors (e.g., pituitary adenoma); head trauma; medications, chemotherapy/radiation; infiltrative, ischemic, or destructive disorders; chronic illness; weight loss (anorexia nervosa); exercise, stress; marijuana use

Endocrine:

Chronic disease: Thyroid disease, diabetes mellitus, Addison disease

Hyperprolactinemia: Pituitary adenoma, renal failure, psychoactive drugs (e.g., Haldol)

Hyperandrogenism: Polycystic ovary syndrome, late-onset congenital adrenal hyperplasia, Cushing disease, ovarian or adrenal tumors, hyperthecosis (hypertrophy of ovarian stroma)

Anovulatory cycles: Immature hypothalamic–pituitary–ovarian axis

Others:

Pregnancy

Lactation

DIFFERENTIAL DIAGNOSIS DISCUSSION

 HINT: Pregnancy is the most common cause of secondary amenorrhea in women of reproductive age, and this possibility should always be ruled out first.

Gonadal Failure

Etiology

Gonadal failure (i.e., **lack of ovarian estrogen production**) is the **most common cause of primary amenorrhea,** accounting for almost 50% of cases. Sometimes, it is a consequence of therapies (chemo or radiation) or disease processes, but it is usually caused by a **chromosomal disorder or deletion of all or part** of an **X chromosome**. The chromosomal disorders that cause gonadal failure are usually the result of a **random** meiotic or mitotic **abnormality** (i.e., they are not inherited). If the chromosomes are normal (46,XX or 46,XY [pure gonadal dysgenesis]), a gene disorder may be the cause of the primary amenorrhea. Because two X chromosomes are necessary for normal ovarian development, patients with **Turner syndrome** (45,XO), **mosaicism** involving an X chromosome, **or an abnormal X chromosome** may develop **streak ovaries,** which are masses of fibrous tissue located in the normal anatomic position of the ovary. These streak ovaries **do not produce estrogen;** therefore, estrogen-induced negative feedback inhibition of the hypothalamic-pituitary axis fails to occur, and gonadotropins remain elevated.

Evaluation

An **FSH level > 40 mIU/mL** suggests a lack of functioning ovarian follicles, confirming the diagnosis of gonadal failure.

Complete Androgen Insensitivity (Testicular Feminization)
Etiology

Complete androgen insensitivity is a syndrome caused by a **mutation in the androgen receptor gene,** which is located on the long arm of the **X chromosome**. It is inherited in an **X-linked recessive** or sex-limited autosomal dominant fashion with transmission **through the mother.** Patients are **genetically normal males** with a 46,XY karyotype and properly functioning testes that produce appropriate levels of testosterone and dihydrotestosterone. However, during embryogenesis, because of receptor insensitivity to androgens and increased estrogen production, a **female habitus and external genitalia develop**. The fetal testes produce müllerian-inhibiting substance, which causes müllerian-duct regression (explaining the absence of the fallopian tubes, uterus, and upper vagina).

Clinical Features

Patients have normal female external genitalia and a short or absent vagina. Pubic and axillary hair is absent or scant because of the lack of androgen receptors, but breast development is normal or excessive because there is no androgenic opposition to the small amounts of estrogen produced by the testes and adrenals. The gonads in these patients are abnormal, and 20% develop a malignancy (gonadoblastoma or dysgerminoma).

> **HINT:** Patients with testicular feminization can be differentiated from patients with uterine agenesis by the absence of normal pubic hair.

Treatment

Patients with complete androgen insensitivity are **phenotypically female** and have been raised as such. They should be informed that they are **sterile** and that their **gonads must be removed** because they are at risk of developing a malignancy. These malignancies rarely occur before the age of 20 years; therefore, it is recommended that the gonads be left in place until after puberty to allow normal sexual maturation.

Hypothalamus and Pituitary Disorders
Etiology

Patients with **normal female internal genitalia** but **absent secondary sex characteristics** as a result of a CNS-hypothalamus-pituitary disorder have **low levels of gonadotropin and estrogen**. In addition, any **anatomic lesion** of the hypothalamus or pituitary gland can cause low gonadotropin production. These lesions can be **congenital** (e.g., aqueductal stenosis or absence of the sellar floor) or **acquired** (e.g., tumors). The most common tumors are **pituitary adenomas,** which result in **elevated levels of prolactin.** (Most, but not all, pituitary tumors secrete prolactin; chromophobe adenomas are the most common non-prolactin-secreting pituitary tumors.)

Evaluation

Patients with suspected CNS-hypothalamic-pituitary disorders should undergo **magnetic resonance imaging** (best modality) or **computed tomography** or of the hypothalamic–pituitary region to rule out the presence of a lesion. Pituitary adenoma can be detected by finding an elevated **serum prolactin level**.

Structural Genital Tract Defects
Etiology

Congenital absence of the uterus (uterine agenesis, uterovaginal agenesis, and Rokitansky-Kuster-Hauser syndrome) is the **second most common cause of primary amenorrhea,** after gonadal failure. **Congenital** absence of the uterus accounts for ~15% of cases of primary amenorrhea, and occurs in 1 of every 4,000 to 5,000 female births. Congenital absence of the uterus is typically a sporadic event and is only rarely genetically inherited. Patients have no underlying endocrine abnormality, but are amenorrheic because of absence of the end organ.

Clinical Features

Patients have normal breasts and pubic and axillary hair, but the **vagina is shortened or absent** and the **uterus is absent**. The ovaries are present and function normally, with ovulation occurring cyclically. Approximately 33% of patients with congenital absence of the uterus have **congenital renal abnormalities,** and 12% have **skeletal abnormalities. Cardiac and other congenital abnormalities** occur with increased frequency.

EVALUATION OF AMENORRHEA
Patient History

Delayed or absent menstruation can be very anxiety provoking. Be sensitive to the parent and adolescent's level of concern during the history. Review of growth and development, detailed menstrual history (e.g., menarche, dysmenorrhea, duration, and flow), history of illnesses, and medications can all be discussed with the patient and the parent. To obtain accurate information, the **sexual history, psychosocial assessment, and substance use** history should be **obtained privately with the patient**. Questions regarding diet, physical activity (duration and intensity), weight change, and body image can give an indication if there is an eating disorder. Review of symptoms should focus on:

- New-onset virilizing symptoms: acne, hirsutism, and clitoromegaly
- Vasomotor symptoms (e.g., hot flashes, associated with low circulating estrogens)
- Galactorrhea (hyperprolactinemia)
- Cyclic abdominal pain, bloating or breast changes (vaginal outlet obstruction)
- Palpitations, fatigue, or nervousness (hyperthyroidism)

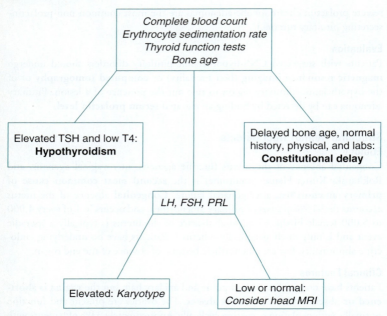

Complete blood count
Erythrocyte sedimentation rate
Thyroid function tests
Bone age

Elevated TSH and low T4:
Hypothyroidism

Delayed bone age, normal
history, physical, and labs:
Constitutional delay

LH, FSH, PRL

Elevated: *Karyotype*

Low or normal:
Consider head MRI

FIGURE 13-1 **Amenorrhea with delayed puberty.** (Modified from Pletcher JB, Slap GB. Menstrual disorders. Amenorrhea. *Pediatr Clin N Am* 46(3):505–518, 1999.)

Physical Examination

Height, weight, body habitus, and vital signs (**hypertension** may indicate the presence of a condition associated with hyperandrogenicity such as Cushing disease) should be measured. Signs of **anorexia nervosa** include bradycardia, hypotension, and hypothermia. Thorough funduscopic and neurologic examinations can help to rule out **pituitary or other CNS lesions**. Other areas of focus should include the **thyroid**, the **breasts** (for Tanner staging and galactorrhea), and the **genital area** (for Tanner staging and signs of hyperandrogenism, virilization, or imperforate hymen; consider pelvic examination to rule out an ovarian mass). **Pelvic examination** is not necessary if the patient has never been sexually active and genital anomalies are not suspected. Otherwise, pelvic examination can help evaluate for imperforate hymen and the presence of uterus and ovaries. Laboratory work-up is dependent on the pubertal development (see Figures 13-1 through 13-3 for step-wise work-up).

TREATMENT OF AMENORRHEA

Apart from specific therapies with regard to the diagnoses listed in the differential diagnosis list, the principles behind management of amenorrhea are the same regardless of the etiology:

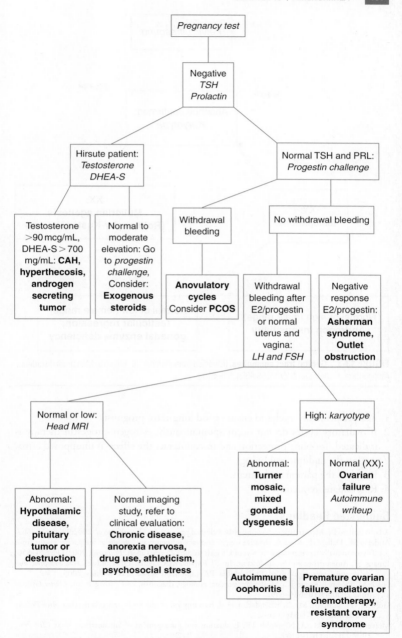

FIGURE 13-2   Amenorrhea with otherwise normal puberty. (Modified from Pletcher JB, Slap GB. Menstrual disorders. Amenorrhea. *Pediatr Clin N Am* 1999;46(3):505–518.)

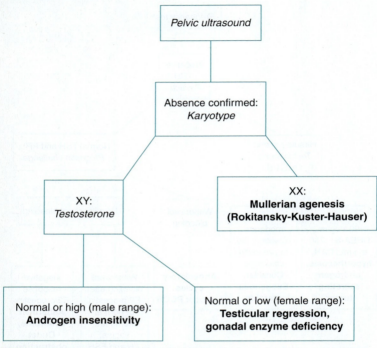

FIGURE 13-3 **Genital tract anomalies.** (Modified from Pletcher JB, Slap GB. Menstrual disorders. Amenorrhea. *Pediatr Clin N Am* 1999;46(3):505–518.)

1. Restore ovulatory cycles to ensure good long-term prognosis.
2. If ovulatory cycles do not occur spontaneously, estrogen–progestin therapy is indicated (for bone protection and to counteract the effects if unopposed estrogen on the endometrial lining).
3. Reassure the patient and parent.
4. Re-evaluate frequently.

Suggested Readings

Adams Hillard PJ. Menstruation in young girls: a clinical perspective. *Obstet Gynecol.* 2002;99(4):655–662.

Anderso SE, Dallal GE, Must A. Relative weight and race influence average age at menarche: results from two nationally representative surveys of US girls studied 25 years apart. *Pediatrics.* 2003;111:844–850.

Emans SJ. Amenorrhea in the adolescent. In: SJ Emans, MR Laufer, DP Goldstei, eds. *Pediatric and Adolescent Gynecology.* 5th ed. Philadelphia, PA: Lippincott Williams & Wilkins; 2005.

Folch M, Pigem I, Konje JC. Mullerian agenesis: etiology, diagnosis, and management. *Obstet Gynecol Surv.* 2000;55(10):644–649.

Golden NH, Jacobson MS, Schebendach J, et al. Resumption of menses in anorexia nervosa. *Arch Pediatr Adolesc Med.* 1997;151(1):16–21.

McIver B, Romanski SA, Nipploldt TB. Evaluation and management of amenorrhea. *Mayo Clin Proc.* 1997;72(12):1161–1169.

Pletcher JR, Slap GB. Menstrual disorders. Amenorrhea. *Pediatr Clin N Am.* 1999;46(3):505–518.

Animal Bites

INTRODUCTION

Humans have contact with animals in a variety of occupational and recreational settings, and over half of households in the United States have at least one pet. Animal and human bite wounds are frequent in the pediatric population and are treated in primary care offices and emergency departments. As a result, all pediatric practitioners should be familiar with evaluation and management of the most common animal bite wounds. The complex microbiology of animal bite wounds makes management a challenging clinical problem, and therapy is often empiric.

DIFFERENTIAL DIAGNOSIS LIST

- Lacerations, fractures, crush injuries, and tendon and nerve injuries
- Local bacterial wound infection—mouth flora vary by species (Table 14-1)
- Rabies—many animals, especially dogs, cats, bats, foxes, raccoons, and skunks
- Tularemia—many animals, especially rabbits, cats, squirrels, pigs, sheep, coyotes, and ticks
- Rat-bite fever
- Cat-scratch disease (CSD)
- Crotalinae envenomation

DIFFERENTIAL DIAGNOSIS DISCUSSION
Dog and Cat Bites

Dog and cat bites make up the **majority of bite wounds,** accounting for 85% and 10%, respectively. Because of their inquisitive nature and decreased protective mechanisms, children are bitten by dogs and cats three times more frequently than adults, with most bites occurring in the 5- to 9-year-old age group. Their size relative to an animal causes children to sustain **more facial bites,** resulting in greater severity of **laceration, infection, disability, and death,** especially when large dogs are involved. **Cat bite wounds** are typically **puncture wounds** that involve the hand or extremity. The sharp and slender nature of cat's teeth can **penetrate bones,** which may lead to greater morbidity from complicated wounds.

TABLE 14-1	Organisms Commonly Associated with Bite Wounds	
Animals	**Organism**	**Special Considerations**
Dog and cat	*Pasteurella* species *Streptococcus* species *Staphylococcus aureus* *Neisseria* species Anaerobes: *Bacteroides, Fusobacterium, Porphyromonas, Prevotella*	Rabies prophylaxis based on immunization status, ability to observe animal, local epidemiology
Horse	Similar to dog and cat	Crush injury, osteomyelitis
Pig and sheep	Dog and cat flora + *Francisella tularensis* and others	
Rat	Dog and cat flora + *Streptobacillus moniliformis, Leptospira*	Rabies prophylaxis generally not needed
Ferret and gerbil	Rat flora + *Acinetobacter anitratus*	Antipseudomonal penicillin
Raccoon, bat, fox	High risk for rabies	RIG, HDCV
Squirrel	*Francisella tularensis*	Gentamicin
Aquatic	*Aeromonas hydrophila, Vibrio, Enterobacter, Pseudomonas*	
Avian	*Staphylococcus, Clostridium, Aspergillus, Bacteroides, Pseudomonas*	
Human	*Streptococcus* species *Staphylococcus* species *Eikenella corrodens* Anaerobes: *Prevotella, Fusobacterium, Veillonella, Peptostreptococcus*	Hand injuries high risk
Monkey	Human flora + *Herpes B*	Antiviral therapy

This table is not an exhaustive list of organisms.
HDCV, human diploid cell vaccine; *RIG*, rabies immune globulin.

Dog bites have an infection rate of approximately 5% to 15%, the lowest of all mammalian bites. **Cat bites become infected more frequently** (~50%). Wound characteristics and initial wound care determine the risk of infection. Puncture wounds, wounds on the hands or feet, those involving joints, tendons, or other deep structures and those in hosts with comorbid illness or immunosuppression are at higher risk for infection. Wounds treated more than 12 hours after the injury and those not properly irrigated and debrided are more likely to become infected. The microbiology of infected dog and cat bite wounds has been well studied (see Table 14-1). Most bite wound infections are **polymicrobial** and include anaerobic organisms.

Human Bites

Following dog and cat bites, **human bites** are the **next most common** type of mammalian bite injuries. Human bites are most commonly seen in **teenage or young adult males** and are often related to **aggressive behavior, sports, and sexual activity**. **Wound infections** occur in about 15% to 50% of human bites.

Delays in care, which are common as a result of the circumstances of injury, **have a direct effect on infection rates and prognosis**. **Simple bites** that occur from occlusion of the teeth on skin, such as bites occurring in daycare, **rarely become infected**. Human bite infections are **polymicrobial** with a mixture of anaerobes and aerobes (see Table 14-1). ***Eikenella corrodens*** deserves special mention, as it is present in 25% of isolates from clenched fist injuries. It has also exhibited synergistic growth with other aerobic organisms.

> **HINT:** When a bite occurs as the result of a direct blow of the victim's hand into the biter's mouth, there is typically a puncture wound overlying one of the metacarpal–phalangeal joints on the dorsum of the hand (clenched-fist syndrome). Penetration of the joint capsule may occur with tendon, nerve, or bone damage. These wounds may appear mild at first, but are deceiving and can result in extensive infection that requires surgical exploration, debridement, and intravenous antibiotics.

Other significant infectious diseases like *Herpes* virus, syphilis, tuberculosis, actinomycosis, tetanus, and hepatitis B and C have also been documented as occurring through human bites. Although there have been no definitive cases of HIV transmission from this route, detection of HIV in saliva makes this an unlikely but possible way to acquire HIV infection.

Complications
Local Wound Infection
Characteristics of infected bite wounds include **erythema, warmth, fluctuance, purulent drainage, and/or tenderness** at the site, and can include **surrounding edema and regional adenitis**. Local wound infections can also be accompanied by **mild systemic symptoms,** such as **fever, chills, and malaise,** and may be associated with **serum leukocytosis**.

Various clinical syndromes may help differentiate the type of organism that predominates in a bite-wound infection. Infection caused by *Pasteurella* species may evolve rapidly with intense cellulitis and lymphangitis within 24 hours. Cellulitis caused by *Staphylococcus or Streptococcus* species usually evolves more slowly and may be associated with abscess formation. More **serious infections,** such as **osteomyelitis or septic arthritis,** may present with increased pain and decreased movement of the affected part. Deep infections may occur after direct inoculation into deeper tissues or by localized extension of cellulitis. **Immunocompromised hosts** can present with local or systemic infections and are at **higher risk for invasive disease,** specifically with *Capnocytophaga canimorsus,* which is associated with a 25% mortality rate.

Rabies
Individuals often seek medical care after an animal bite wound because of the concern for rabies. Rabies is caused by a rhabdovirus and is **transmitted via the saliva**

of an infected animal, **usually through a bite or scratch**. Cases usually result from an unrecognized exposure or from failure to administer prophylaxis. In the United States, the Centers for Disease Control and Prevention (CDC) reported four cases of human rabies in 2009. **Rabies prophylaxis recommendations vary by the geographic area and the type of animal** involved. In the United States, bats, skunks, raccoons, foxes, dogs, and coyotes serve as the primary reservoirs of rabies, and bats are responsible for the majority of cases. Individuals who awake to find a bat in the room should be considered exposed. Treatment is discussed below.

> **HINT:** In 2004, a teenage girl became the first known person to survive rabies infection. Timely postexposure prophylaxis remains the only reliable strategy to prevent the development of clinical disease. Once rabies develops, the outcome is almost always fatal.

The clinical syndrome of rabies is characterized by **fever, malaise, headache, and anxiety** in the early stages. This is followed by **progressive neurologic symptoms,** including muscle spasm, autonomic instability, altered mental status with hallucinations, respiratory muscle paralysis, lacrimation, salivation, perspiration, and coma. Infection can be confirmed with **specific serologic testing**.

Tularemia

Tularemia, caused by infection with *Francisella tularensis,* is primarily a **tick-borne disease** but may be transmitted by **bites from animals** such as rabbits, cats, squirrels, pigs, sheep, and coyotes. The classic ulceroglandular syndrome is characterized by a **painful ulcer** associated with **tender regional lymph nodes** that can drain spontaneously. The clinical syndrome is characterized by an **abrupt onset of fever, chills, headache, anorexia, malaise, and fatigue**. The diagnosis can be confirmed with **serologic testing,** and treatment is usually with **streptomycin, gentamicin, or amikacin**.

Rat-Bite Fever

Rat-bite fever is caused by *Streptobacillus moniliformis.* The organism is found in the oral flora of **wild, pet, and laboratory rats** and is transmitted by **bites, scratches, and handling dead rats**. There is a 3- to 10-day incubation period after exposure, followed by **sudden onset of fever, chills, arthritis, muscle pain, and maculopapular rash,** which often involves **palms and soles**. The rash may take on other forms such as petechiae, purpura, vesicles, or desquamation. They may also be associated with **septic polyarthritis,** and more rarely with endocarditis, pericarditis, and brain abscess. **Fatality** occurs in 7% to 10% of untreated patients.

The organism can be **cultured from blood, synovial fluid, and vesicle fluid,** and the receiving laboratory should be informed that *Streptobacillus moniliformis* is the organism of interest. Cultures should be held up to 3 weeks. *Streptobacillus* is **sensitive to penicillin,** and therapy should be initiated with this drug. Alternative drugs are ampicillin, cefuroxime, cefotaxime, and doxycycline. **Recovery is excellent**.

Cat-Scratch Disease

Cat-scratch disease (CSD) is caused by *Bartonella henselae,* a gram-negative bacillus. It is transmitted primarily through **bites or scratches** to individuals who have close contact with cats.

Patients with uncomplicated CSD will develop a **nontender papule** at the site of inoculation followed by **regional lymphadenopathy** that **persists for weeks to months**. The most common involved nodes are axillary, cervical, submandibular, and inguinal. Nodes may suppurate and be accompanied by symptoms such as **fever, malaise, anorexia, and headache**. Complicated CSD is more common in **immunosuppressed patients** and may cause **neurologic symptoms** such as encephalopathy, peripheral neuropathy, or vision loss, as well as **pneumonia, endocarditis, and osteomyelitis**.

Diagnosis is by serology. Many cases of CSD **resolve spontaneously** without specific therapy. Painful suppurative nodes can be treated with needle aspiration. **Incision and drainage should be avoided**. Antimicrobial therapy with macrolides, ciprofloxacin, trimethoprim–sulfamethoxazole, or rifampin can hasten recovery. **Routine antimicrobial treatment is not recommended** for otherwise healthy individuals with regional lymphadenitis.

Crotalid Envenomation

Approximately one-half of the **8,000 annual venomous snake bites in the United States** occur in children, and most commonly are caused by **rattlesnakes and copperheads**. Pain, swelling, and fang marks are common local signs, and **compartment syndrome** may ensue. Systemic complications may include **thrombocytopenia, coagulopathy, renal failure, and neuropathy** that can lead to **respiratory failure**.

All snakebite victims warrant **admission to the hospital for at least 8 hours**. **Immobilization** of the affected extremity **below the level of the heart** is advocated until emergency care can be administered. Compression dressings are not recommended. **Crotalidae polyvalent immune Fab** should be given **within 6 hours** to all patients with minimal or moderate crotalid envenomation.

EVALUATION OF ANIMAL BITES

Patient History

Unstable patients should be **evaluated immediately for massive blood loss and wounds that interfere with a patent airway** (tracheal or laryngeal location) **or breathing** (pneumothorax). Important facts to elicit when taking a history from a bitten individual include **type of animal, provoking factors** for the bite, **allergies, medications, and comorbid conditions,** especially those associated with immune suppression. Obtain a history of **tetanus immunization** as well as any previous bites or rabies immunizations.

Physical Examination

The following items should be noted during examination of a bite wound:

- Body location
- Depth of the wound

- Range of motion of the affected part
- Type of wound—puncture, crush, laceration, abrasion
- Involvement of deeper structures—tendon, nerve, vessel, bone
- Function of tendons and nerves
- Signs of inflammation or infection—edema, erythema, warmth, induration, fluctuance, exudates, adenopathy
- Foreign bodies or debris

The **physical examination** may need to take place **after local anesthesia** to maximize the ability to explore the wound. **Photographs or diagrammatic drawings** of wounds are helpful.

Imaging

When **fractures or foreign bodies** such as tooth fragments are suspected, a radiograph should be obtained.

Laboratory Evaluation

Routine wound cultures are not needed for animal or human bites that do not have any signs of infection. As a general rule, cultures from most bite wounds at or near the time of injury will be more likely to reflect the indigenous flora of the animal's mouth and are not predictive of future infection. **Older wounds** or those with **evidence of infection** should be cultured for both **aerobic and anaerobic organisms** after superficial crusts are removed. It is imperative to **notify the laboratory of the source of a bite wound culture** and of any suspected organisms.

TREATMENT OF ANIMAL BITES
Wound Management

Experts advocate **copious irrigation** of bite wounds as well as **surface cleaning**. The fluid of choice is **normal saline** (1% povidone–iodine may be added) using a volume of at least 250 mL. Irrigation should be performed **under pressure** with an 18- or 19-gauge catheter attached to a syringe, and **devitalized tissue should be débrided**. **Puncture and other small wounds should never be injected** as this may inoculate bacteria into deeper structures, increasing tissue trauma and the risk of infection.

The decision to primarily suture a bite wound is made on a case-by-case basis and depends on many factors, including the length of time between the bite and the presentation, the location of the wound, the appearance of the wound, and comorbidities of the patient. Studies have suggested that carefully selected bite wounds are safe for primary closure. **Wounds that are candidates for primary closure** are those to the **head and face** and those in other **low-risk areas** such as the proximal extremities and the trunk.

It is generally agreed that all **bites older than 24 hours, bites to the hand, and bites with evidence of infection should not be sutured**. Delayed primary **closure** 72 hours after antimicrobial prophylaxis has begun is a consideration for high risk wounds. Aftercare should consist of explicit **instructions for wound** cleansing, dressing changes, and antibiotic use (topical or oral as indicated), as well as **signs and symptoms of possible infection**. **Large wounds or those over joint surfaces** should be **splinted and elevated**. Appropriate **analgesics** should be prescribed for several days. **Close follow-up** should be arranged for all bite wounds.

Antimicrobial Prophylaxis

Prophylactic antimicrobial therapy is generally recommended for the following:

- All bites to the hand
- Wounds with moderate-to-severe tissue destruction (crush)
- Puncture wounds
- Cat bites
- Injuries involving bone or joint
- Wounds to patients with comorbid conditions or immunosuppression.

Amoxicillin–clavulanate is the drug of choice for prophylaxis of an animal bite wound, with an appropriate spectrum of activity against common flora in the mouths of dogs, cats, and humans. An alternative regimen for penicillin-allergic patients is **a second-/third-generation cephalosporin or trimethoprim/sulfamethoxazole *plus* clindamycin**. Post-pubertal, nonpregnant patients may receive **doxycycline or tetracycline**.

Antimicrobial Treatment for Infected Wounds

Infected wounds that have **failed outpatient therapy** require **hospitalization**. *Pasteurella multocida* should be considered in any patient with a wound infection **following a dog or cat bite**. **Ampicillin/sulbactam** is appropriate empiric intravenous therapy. Alternatives for penicillin-allergic patients are **a second-/third-generation cephalosporin or trimethoprim/sulfamethoxazole *plus* clindamycin; or ciprofloxacin or tetracycline,** if appropriate for age.

Tetanus Prophylaxis

Tetanus immunization should be given according to standard CDC recommendations when patients are **deficient in immunization status** or in cases of **high-risk wounds**.

Rabies Prophylaxis

Immediate active and passive prophylaxis is indicated for wild animals known to carry rabies and domestic animals with symptoms of rabies; these **animals should be euthanized and the brain examined** in a qualified laboratory. Passive immunization with **rabies immune globulin (RIG)** in a dose of 20 IU/kg should be given as follows: **half of the dose at the site of the bite wound and the other half at a separate intramuscular location**. In **children,** the recommended site is the **anterolateral thigh**. Active immunization with the **human diploid cell vaccine (HDCV)** must be initiated **(day 0)** and **repeated on days 3, 7, and 14 after the injury in immunocompetent children** and also on day 28 in immunosuppressed children. The dose of the vaccine is 1.0 cc intramuscularly given at a site distant from the immune globulin.

Domestic animals with an unknown rabies immune status may be **observed for 10 days**. RIG and HDCV should be initiated at the first sign of rabies symptoms in the animal. Cases in which the animal is unavailable should be treated as recommended by local health officials.

 HINT: Animal bites should be reported to the local health department for surveillance as indicated by local jurisdiction. The risk of rabies differs geographically and appropriate treatment may vary. Reports to law enforcement agencies may also be necessary to facilitate observation of animals for rabies.

HIV Prophylaxis for Human Bites

The risk of HIV transmission from a human bite is controversial but **thought to be rare**. **Bites from a person infected with HIV** or bites from a person in whom there was **visibly blood-tainted saliva** should be **treated prophylactically** with **oral antiviral agents** according to standard CDC recommendations. In all other instances, postexposure prophylaxis should be determined on a case-by-case basis, but **baseline and 6-month HIV testing** of the victim is prudent. All human bite wounds should be **thoroughly cleansed with a virucidal agent** as soon as possible to lessen any risk of HIV transmission.

PREVENTION OF ANIMAL BITES

Since bites frequently lead to infection, efforts to reduce the risk of infection should be aimed primarily at prevention. Adults, especially pet owners, should become familiar with the behavior of cats and dogs and teach children to avoid provoking behaviors. Children should not be left alone with a dog and they should be instructed not to approach an unknown dog without the owner's permission or any dog while its food is present. When handling other animals, appropriate precautions, such as **wearing gloves** and other **protective garments,** should be taken.

Suggested Readings

American Academy of Pediatrics. Pediculosis capitis. In: Pickering LK, Baker CJ, Long SS, McMillan JA, eds. *Red Book: 2006 Report of the Committee on Infectious Diseases.* 27th ed. Elk Grove Village, IL: American Academy of Pediatrics. 2006;648–653.

Chen E, Hornig S, Shepherd SM, et al. Primary closure of mammalian bites. *Acad Emerg Med.* 2000;7:157–161.

Committee on Infectious Diseases. Rabies-prevention policy update: new reduced-dose schedule. *Pediatrics.* 2011;127:785–787.

Glaser C, Lewis P, Wong S. Pet-animal,- and vector-borne infections. *Pediatr Rev.* 2000;21(7):219–232.

Goldstein EJ. Current concepts on animal bites: bacteriology and therapy. *Curr Clin Top Infect Dis.* 1999;19:99–111.

Griego RD, Rosen T, Orengo IF, et al. Dog, cat, and human bites: a review. *J Am Acad Dermatol.* 1995;33:1019–1029.

Lion C, Conroy MC, Carpentier AM, et al. Antimicrobial susceptibilities of pasteurella strains isolated from humans. *Int J Antimicrob Agents.* 2006;27:290–293.

Medeiros I, Saconato H. Antibiotic prophylaxis for mammalian bites. *Cochrane Database Syst Rev.* 2001;(2):CD001738.

Moore DA, Sischo WM, Hunter A, et al. Animal bite epidemiology and surveillance for rabies postexposure prophylaxis. *J Am Vet Med Assoc.* 2000;217:190–194.

Talan DA, Abrahamian FM, Moran GJ, et al. Clinical presentation and bacteriologic analysis of infected human bites in patients presenting to emergency departments. *Clin Infect Dis.* 2003;37:1481–1489.

Talan DA, Citron DM, Abrahamian FM, et al. Bacteriologic analysis of infected dog and cat bites. *N Engl J Med.* 1999;340(2):85–92.

The Centers for Disease Control and Prevention—Rabies surveillance data in the United States. http://www.cdc.gov/rabies/location/usa/surveillance/index.html. Accessed November 23, 2011.

Apnea

INTRODUCTION

The *1986 Consensus Statement on Infantile Apnea and Home Monitoring* from the National Institute of Health (NIH) describes an apparent life-threatening event (ALTE) as "an episode that is frightening to the observer and is characterized by some combination of apnea (central or occasionally obstructive), color change (usually cyanotic or pallid but occasionally erythematous or plethoric), marked change in muscle tone (usually marked limpness), choking, or gagging ... [I]n some cases, the observer fears that the infant has died ... [P]reviously used terminology such as 'aborted crib death' or 'near-miss SIDS' should be abandoned because it implies a possibly misleading close association between this type of spell and SIDS."

 DIFFERENTIAL DIAGNOSIS LIST

Infectious Causes
- Sepsis
- Pneumonia
- Respiratory syncytial virus (RSV) infection
- Viral upper respiratory tract infections
- Meningitis
- Pertussis

Gastrointestinal Causes
- Gastrointestinal reflux (gastroesophageal reflux disease [GRD])

Traumatic Causes
- Intracranial hemorrhage (subdural, subarachnoid)
- Munchausen by proxy syndrome
- Child abuse

Cardiovascular Causes
- Cardiac arrhythmias
- Congenital heart disease

- Cardiomyopathy
- Vascular ring

Respiratory Causes
- Reactive airway disease
- Laryngomalacia
- Other airway anomalies
- Structural lung malformation

Neurologic Causes
- Seizure
- Intracranial mass
- Cerebral dysgenesis
- Structural or cerebrovascular anomalies

Metabolic Causes
- Inborn errors of metabolism
- Hypoglycemia
- Electrolyte imbalance

Miscellaneous Causes
- Apnea of prematurity
- Idiopathic apnea of infancy or ALTE

- Physiologic periodic breathing
- Central hypoventilation syndromes
- Breath-holding spells
- Anemia
- Hypothermia
- Vocal cord paralysis
- Tracheoesophageal fistula
- Choking event
- Upper airway obstruction
- Drug- or toxin-induced apnea

DIFFERENTIAL DIAGNOSIS DISCUSSION

Infection

Clinical Features

Although apnea can be the only initial symptom of infection, untreated sepsis progresses rapidly and the infant develops other signs and symptoms that suggest this diagnosis. **Pneumonia or bronchiolitis** caused by RSV can be **associated with life-threatening apnea** and is a **significant cause of infant mortality** among **premature infants** after hospital discharge, especially during the **winter months**.

Evaluation

In an infant who presents with acute apnea, a **careful history and physical examination** should be performed in an attempt to elucidate the presence of an acute infection. Depending on the history and physical examination findings, appropriate **tests** should be ordered.

Treatment

Treatment depends on the underlying infection. Effective antibacterial therapies, as well as some antiviral therapies, are available. Prompt diagnosis and treatment are essential.

Obstructive Apnea

Etiology

Obstructive apnea is the **inability to effectively oxygenate, ventilate, or both,** despite adequate central respiratory drive. The most common causes include the following:

- **Gastrointestinal reflux (GRD).** The most common cause of obstructive apnea is GRD; as many as 20% of premature infants with apnea have an obstructive component.
- **Prematurity.** The incomplete development of cartilaginous structures in a premature infant's airway can lead to kinking of the airway and obstructive apnea.
- **Laryngeal webs or laryngomalacia** can also present as obstructive apnea.

Clinical Features

The parents describe that their baby **regurgitate formula or milk,** either during or after the feedings. Infants may have **"awake apnea,"** which is most commonly caused by GRD. Alternatively, infants may **struggle during feeding**, with **exaggerated respiratory effort**.

Evaluation

If GRD is suspected, a **barium swallow with video** capabilities allows the radiologist and the speech therapist to assess both reflux and swallowing function to determine appropriate therapy. Other causes of obstructive apnea require evaluation by an **otolaryngologist**.

Treatment
Thickened feeds and metoclopramide are used to treat GRD. **Upright positioning** after feeds, with the infant's head elevated to a 45-degree angle, has also been effective. Home monitoring devices may not detect obstructive apnea because they measure chest wall movement but not airflow.

Trauma
Etiology
Birth trauma (e.g., intracranial or subgaleal hemorrhage, rather than a caput or cephalohematoma) and **child abuse** (including physical abuse and Munchausen by proxy syndrome) can be associated with apnea.

 HINT: Munchausen by proxy syndrome is among the differential diagnoses for recurrent apnea; parents with this psychological disorder can interfere with the proper functioning of home monitoring. In addition, parentally induced suffocation can lead to true apnea; the associated hypoxia can be detected with a monitor capable of storing and downloading the data for physician interpretation.

Evaluation
A **careful history and imaging studies** help in confirming the diagnosis of child abuse or birth trauma. Often, the information stored in the **home apnea monitor** can help in determining if events at home are real and the time of their occurrence.

Neurologic Disorders
Seizures, central nervous system (CNS) structural abnormalities (e.g., arteriovenous malformation, Arnold–Chiari malformation), CNS tumors, and **intracranial hemorrhage** can be associated with an ALTE initially. **Persistent idiopathic apnea** is the **hallmark of central hypoventilation disorders,** the most well known of which is Ondine curse.

Clinical Features
The apnea may be associated with **seizures** or symptoms of **increased intracranial pressure.** If a neurologic diagnosis is suspected, then appropriate **CNS imaging studies,** an **electroencephalogram (EEG), and laboratory blood tests** are indicated.

Treatment
Treatment depends on the underlying cause. Either **anticonvulsant therapy** or **surgical intervention** may be necessary. Patients with central hypoventilation syndromes may require **nighttime mechanical ventilation**.

Cardiac Disease

 HINT: An infant with an ALTE rarely has cardiac disease.

The most common life-threatening cardiac abnormality is **cardiac arrhythmia**. A prolonged QT interval has been noted in infants who have died of sudden infant death syndrome (SIDS). On rare occasions, **congenital heart disease** presents as an ALTE.

Clinical Features

In addition to apnea, infants with heart disease usually have more obvious signs of heart failure, such as **failure to thrive or cyanosis**. A **vascular ring** can be associated with **inspiratory stridor**.

Evaluation

When congenital heart disease is suspected, the initial evaluation usually includes an **electrocardiogram (ECG), chest radiograph,** and an **echocardiogram**.

Treatment

Treatment depends on the underlying pathological condition; **medical therapy** is useful for some arrhythmias, and **surgical therapy** may be required by patients with structural heart disease.

Respiratory Abnormalities

Clinical Features

An infant with apnea caused by a structural lung abnormality is often **tachypneic and cyanotic** and may show signs of respiratory distress preceding the apnea. An **abnormal cry or inspiratory stridor** is present in infants with vocal cord paralysis. **Choking during feeding** is seen with tracheoesophageal fistula.

Evaluation

A chest radiograph is helpful initially. Flexible laryngoscopy or bronchoscopy is often needed.

Treatment

Some structural lung abnormalities (e.g., cystic adenomatoid malformation, diaphragmatic hernia) are **surgically correctable**. Vocal cord paralysis may improve **spontaneously**.

Apnea of Prematurity

Premature infants have a much **higher risk for ALTE and SIDS** than infants who were born at or near-term gestation (~37 weeks).

Clinical Features

Apnea of prematurity is characterized by **pauses in respiration** that last >**20 seconds**. Accompanying **bradycardia** may also be present.

Only some of these episodes are detected by hospital personnel or parents. In a study involving tracings of asymptomatic premature infants' respiratory patterns, heart rates, nasal airflow, and oxyhemoglobin saturations, almost 50% of the infants had prolonged apnea and other findings defined as abnormal.

Treatment

Several strategies are proposed to address **home monitoring** of premature infants. The NIH consensus report to the American Academy of Pediatrics recommends against the routine evaluation of premature infants before discharge with a standard two-channel pneumogram (thoracic impedance and heart rate monitoring) because this test has a high rate of both false-positive and false-negative results and is not a reliable predictor of infants who will suffer an ALTE or succumb to SIDS.

One accepted approach is to monitor **all premature infants up to and beyond the postnatal age associated with the highest rate of SIDS** (i.e., 2 to 4 months). If the infant is stressed (e.g., by an upper respiratory tract illness), it is speculated that the "normal" pauses in respiration can become pathological and present as an ALTE.

> **HINT:** Periodic breathing (i.e., short intervals of apnea interspersed between short intervals of respirations) can appear pathologic to the parent. However, *isolated periodic breathing* in a premature infant is *not predictive* of ALTE or SIDS.

> **HINT:** Many premature infants have mild GRD and a history of choking during feeding. It can be extremely difficult to determine when these episodes are truly ALTEs and when they are merely normal variations. If the episode is associated with the factors listed in the NIH's definition of ALTE (i.e., apnea, color change, marked and change in muscle tone), then the infant should be admitted for a more complete evaluation.

EVALUATION OF APNEA

There are several approaches to evaluating an infant who has experienced an ALTE. A thorough **history and physical examination** is the most important component of an apnea evaluation. The event should be described in detail by the witness including **events immediately preceding and subsequent to the event**. A careful history may, in many cases, narrow the focus of the investigation and should include the following:

- Duration of the event
- Relationship to feeding
- Choking, gagging, and vomiting
- Muscle tone prior to and after the event
- Level of consciousness prior to and after the event
- Presence of seizure activity or a postictal state
- Recent trauma
- Fever, coryza, or any upper respiratory infection symptoms
- Sleep position
- Resuscitation required
- Household medications
- Prior history of similar events

Once the history and physical examination narrows the list of differential diagnoses, the appropriate tests will then be decided upon which may include the following:

- EEG
- ECG
- Chest radiograph
- Complete blood cell count
- Serum electrolyte panel
- Serum calcium level
- Serum glucose level
- Blood urea nitrogen and creatinine level
- Multichannel recordings of the heart rate
- Thermistor nasal airflow
- Respiratory rate
- Pulse oximetry
- Esophageal pH
- Brain scan
- Viral studies

TREATMENT OF APNEA

Treatment of an apneic event or ALTE is immediate **cardiopulmonary resuscitation**. However, most infants present to a clinician for evaluation after the event has resolved and when no further resuscitation is required. Treatment thus involves addressing the **underlying cause**. Although **hospitalization is not required for all infants** who present with an ALTE, prolonged cardiovascular monitoring may aid in diagnosis by allowing evaluation of any recurrences. Hospitalization also provides reassurance to caregivers while allowing time for **education in cardiopulmonary resuscitation and SIDS risk factors**.

The **role of home cardiorespiratory monitors remains controversial**. A 2003 policy statement by the Committee on the Fetus and Newborn of the American Academy of Pediatrics suggests that home monitoring may be useful to alert caregivers to a recurrent event when predisposing factors are present but **recommends against routine use**. Caregivers should be counseled that the use of home monitors does not prevent SIDS. If caregivers are involved in the decision and elect to use a home monitor, it is recommended that it be discontinued after 2 months without any apnea alarms.

Suggested Readings

Al Khushi N, Cote A. Apparent life-threatening events: assessment, risks, reality. *Pediatr Respir Rev.* 2011;12:124–132.

American Academy of Pediatrics Committee on Fetus and Newborn. Apnea, sudden infant death syndrome, and home monitoring. *Pediatrics.* 2003;111(4):914–917.

Claudius I, Keens T. Do all infants with apparent life-threatening events need to be admitted? *Pediatrics.* 2007;119(4):679–683.

DeWolfe CC. Apparent life-threatening event: a review. *Pediatr Clin N Am.* 2005;52:1127–1146.

National Institutes of Health. Consensus development conference on infantile apnea and home monitoring. *Pediatrics.* 1987;79:292–299.

Ascites

INTRODUCTION

Ascites is the pathologic accumulation of fluid in the peritoneal cavity. It can be caused by decreased plasma oncotic pressure, obstructed lymphatic or venous drainage, or irritation of the peritoneum (e.g., as a result of infection, trauma, or neoplasia).

DIFFERENTIAL DIAGNOSIS LIST

Gastrointestinal/Hepatic Causes
- Chronic liver failure/cirrhosis
- Protein-losing enteropathy (PLE) (see Table 16-1 for differential diagnosis)
- Pancreatitis

Infectious Causes
- Bacterial peritonitis
- Chronic tuberculous peritonitis
- Congenital TORCH infection: toxoplasmosis, other, rubella, cytomegalovirus, and herpes simplex virus

Neoplastic Causes
- Hodgkin disease
- Intraperitoneal tumor

Congenital or Vascular Causes
- Hepatic vein occlusion (Budd–Chiari syndrome, veno-occlusive disease)
- Portal vein obstruction/portal hypertension
- Renal vein thrombosis

- Congestive heart failure
- Thoracic duct obstruction (chylous ascites)

Metabolic or Congenital Causes
- Lysosomal storage disease

Inflammatory Causes
- Chronic adhesive pericarditis
- Peritonitis—rheumatic, meconium, bile

Renal Causes
- Nephrotic syndrome
- Perforation of the urinary tract
- Obstructive uropathy
- Acute glomerulonephritis
- Chronic renal failure

Miscellaneous Causes
- Systemic lupus erythematosus
- Familial Mediterranean fever
- Maternal diabetes
- Enlarged lymph node
- Pulmonary lymphangiectasia
- Malnutrition

EVALUATION OF A PATIENT WITH ASCITES

Paracentesis is an essential tool for determining the cause of new-onset ascites, and is also recommended to detect bacterial peritonitis in the setting of abdominal pain

TABLE 16-1	Diseases Associated with Enteric Protein Loss

Loss from Intestinal Lymphatics
Intestinal lymphangiectasia
Primary
Secondary (i.e., resulting from cardiac disease)
- Constrictive pericarditis
- Congestive heart failure
- Cardiomyopathy
- Fontan physiology

Obstructive lymphatic disorders
- Malrotation
- Lymphoma
- Tuberculosis
- Sarcoidosis
- Radiation therapy and chemotherapy
- Retroperitoneal fibrosis or tumor
- Arsenic poisoning

Loss from an Abnormal or Inflamed Mucosal Surface
Ménétrier disease
Eosinophilic gastroenteritis
Milk- and soy-induced enterocolitis
Celiac disease
Tropical sprue
Ulcerative jejunitis or colitis
Radiation enteritis
Graft-versus-host disease
Necrotizing enterocolitis
Crohn disease
Hirschsprung disease
Systemic lupus erythematosus
Bacterial overgrowth
Giardiasis
Bacterial and parasitic infections
Common variable immunodeficiency

Modified from Proujansky R. Protein-losing enteropathy. In: Walker WA, Durie PR, Hamilton JR, et al., eds. *Pediatric Gastrointestinal Disease*, 2nd ed. Philadelphia, PA: BC Decker; 1996.

or fever. **Fluid should be obtained for cell count and differential, gram stain and culture, and albumin concentration. Serum–ascites albumin gradient (SAAG),** the difference in albumin concentration between serum and ascitic fluid, is a useful measurement that dividing ascites into two categories—**high gradient (>1.1 g/dL) and low gradient (<1.1 g/dL)**. High gradient SAAG is suggestive of portal hypertension, most suggestive of cirrhosis, heart failure, fulminant hepatic failure, and hepatic venous outflow obstruction (Budd–Chiari or veno-occlusive disease). Low-gradient ascites suggests conditions without portal hypertension, such as pancreatic ascites, tuberculous ascites, peritoneal carcinomatosis, and nephrotic syndrome. The SAAG is a superior measure compared to total protein of the fluid in differentiating cases of portal hypertension.

DIFFERENTIAL DIAGNOSIS DISCUSSION
Cirrhosis

In children other than neonates, cirrhosis is the **most common cause** of ascites. Cirrhosis is a process characterized by **increased fibrous tissue and nodule formation following necrosis of hepatocytes** within the liver. It represents **irreversible distortion** of the intrahepatic vascular and biliary structures. Cirrhosis may develop in association with chronic viral hepatitis, autoimmune hepatitis, cystic fibrosis, Wilson disease, and structural abnormalities of the biliary system (biliary atresia, sclerosing cholangitis). The differential diagnosis of cirrhosis is extensive and varies with the age at presentation.

The ascites of hepatic cirrhosis is a consequence of **hypoalbuminemia** (secondary to failure of protein synthesis), **portal hypertension and excess salt and water retention (secondary to activation of the renin–angiotensin system)**. Cirrhosis is commonly associated with **peripheral edema** after the presence of ascites has become evident. The physical examination may demonstrate a **firm liver with irregular margins (hepatomegaly)** or a **small liver, spider angioma, palmar erythema, and splenomegaly,** depending on the degree of cirrhosis.

The two major sequelae of cirrhosis are **portal venous hypertension and hepatocellular failure**. The main signs of portal hypertension are **splenomegaly and hematemesis** (as a result of bleeding from esophageal varices). **Hepatic coma** may also occur. **Serum transaminases, serum albumin levels, prothrombin time, and blood ammonia levels** are often ordered to assess hepatic inflammation and synthetic function. A **complete blood cell count** may reveal anemia, thrombocytopenia, and leukopenia as a result of hypersplenism. Various imaging options are available: **Abdominal ultrasound** may reveal increased echogenicity; **radioisotope scanning** may reveal decreased uptake, increased flow to the spleen, and irregular hepatic texture; and magnetic resonance cholangiopancreatography is useful to assess the biliary system and hepatic texture. A **liver biopsy** is often needed to identify the cause of the cirrhosis.

Dietary and drug regimens should be initiated in a controlled hospital environment. The diet should provide adequate calories for growth and be supplemented with **calcium and vitamins D, E, and K. Diuretics and decreased sodium** content in the diet may improve the ascites and edema. Albumin infusions are commonly used to reverse ascites.

Additional management of cirrhosis entails the **prevention and treatment** of **life-threatening complications,** such as variceal bleeding. **Liver transplantation** is considered the standard therapy for patients with advanced and decompensated cirrhosis.

Infectious Peritonitis

Primary peritonitis is an infection in the peritoneal cavity secondary to microorganism invasion via the blood or lymphatics. Causative organisms include pneumococci, group A streptococci, and, less commonly, Gram-negative bacilli and viruses.

Secondary peritonitis is an infection in the peritoneal cavity that occurs through the rupture of an intra-abdominal viscus or extension of an abscess. In children, the most common cause of secondary peritonitis is appendicitis. Other causes include gangrenous bowel, necrotizing enterocolitis, and idiopathic gastric or bowel perforation. The causative organisms are the normal flora of the gastrointestinal tract. Secondary peritonitis may also occur as a complication of a ventriculoperitoneal shunt and in patients receiving peritoneal dialysis. *Staphylococcus epidermidis* can be the causative agent in these patients.

Typically, the history includes the **rapid onset of abdominal pain, fever, and vomiting** (e.g., over the course of **48 hours**). Physical examination reveals either diffuse or lower quadrant **severe abdominal tenderness**. **Bowel sounds are hypoactive or absent, and abdominal rigidity** may be present. The **patient prefers** to lie in a **supine position** and experiences severe discomfort with movement or palpation.

Abdominal radiographs of patients with peritonitis often reveal intestinal dilation, edema of the small intestine, peritoneal fluid, and absence of the psoas shadow. Patients with intestinal perforation have radiographic evidence of free air in the peritoneal cavity.

Diagnostic needle aspiration of the peritoneal fluid should be performed if peritonitis is suspected or if the patient has an unexplained fever and fluid in the abdomen. Analysis of the peritoneal fluid from a patient with **spontaneous bacterial peritonitis (SBP)** typically reveals an **elevated protein level** and an **elevated white blood cell count** (i.e., >300 cells/mm^3), of which >25% are polymorphonuclear leukocytes. A **Gram stain and culture** of the fluid should be performed to help guide antimicrobial therapy.

In patients with SBP, careful attention must be paid to **fluid and electrolyte status**. In addition, parenteral **antimicrobial therapy** should be initiated. Combination therapy with ampicillin, gentamicin, and clindamycin provides appropriate initial coverage. Antimicrobial therapy should be modified based on culture and Gram stain results. **Surgical evaluation** should occur early because surgical exploration may be necessary to evaluate for a perforated viscus.

Protein-Losing Enteropathy

Protein-losing enteropathy (PLE), the **loss of proteins across the gastrointestinal mucosa,** occurs in a variety of disease states (Table 16-1). The patient's **history** reflects the underlying disease state. Edema may be the presenting symptom, but a careful history may identify a disturbance in bowel function as the underlying cause.

The primary method of diagnosing enteric protein loss is the **detection of elevated a_1-antitrypsin** (a_1-AT) **in the stool,** a protein that is not actively secreted, absorbed, or digested by the gastrointestinal tract. Quantification can be performed on a spot stool sample or on stool samples collected over several days. Spot sample results appear to correlate well with those obtained from samples collected over a period of time.

Treatment addresses the **underlying cause** of PLE. **Reduction in dietary fat** intake can aid in decreasing the enteric protein loss.

Suggested Readings

Hardy S, Kleinman RE. Cirrhosis and chronic liver failure. In: Suchy FJ, Sokol RJ, Balistreri WF, eds. *Liver Disease in Children.* 3rd ed. New York: Cambridge University Press; 2007:97–137.

Hyams JS. Ascites. In: Kliegman RM, Behrman RE, Jenson HB, et al., eds. *Nelson Textbook of Pediatrics.* 18th ed. Philadelphia, PA: WB Saunders; 2007:1714.

Nowicki MJ, Bishop PR. Ascites. In: Wyllie R, Hyams JS, Kay M, eds. *Pediatric Gastrointestinal and Liver Disease.* 4th ed. Philadelphia, PA: Elsevier; 2011:187–196.

Proujansky R. Protein-losing enteropathy. In: Walker WA, Goulet O, Kleinman RE, et al., eds. *Pediatric Gastrointestinal Disease.* 4th ed. Philadelphia, PA: BC Decker; 2004:194–202.

Ataxia

INTRODUCTION

Ataxia is a disturbance of coordination or balance that is not caused by a problem of muscle strength. Ataxia is characterized by errors of motor activity with regard to rate, range, direction, timing, duration, and force. The most obvious, and often the initial, manifestation is a wide-based and staggering gait, although more subtle findings such as nystagmus (ocular ataxia), titubation (head bobbing), dysmetria and past pointing (difficulties in fine control of the limbs), and hypotonia may be early signs.

The major causes of acute ataxia differ significantly from those of intermittent or chronic ataxia. However, these can overlap as slowly progressive ataxia may be unrecognized and appear acutely, sometimes in the context of febrile illness or injury. In addition, one may see chronic disability associated with incomplete recovery from intermittent ataxia. Table 17-1 lists the causes of ataxia.

 DIFFERENTIAL DIAGNOSIS LIST

Acute Ataxia
Infectious Causes
- Encephalitis
Postinfectious or Autoimmune Disorders
- Acute cerebellar ataxia
- Guillain–Barré syndrome (GBS)
- Miller–Fisher syndrome
- Acute demyelinating encephalomy-elitis (ADEM)
- Multiple sclerosis
Toxic Causes
- Ethanol
- Anticonvulsants
- Antihistamines
Neoplastic Causes
- Brain stem tumor
- Cerebellar tumor

Paraneoplastic Causes
- Opsoclonus–myoclonus–ataxia syndrome
Psychosocial Causes
- Conversion disorder

Trauma
Miscellaneous Causes
- Migraine headache (benign parox-ysmal vertigo)

Intermittent Ataxia
Metabolic or Genetic Causes
- Dominant recurrent ataxia
- Carnitine acetyltransferase deficiency
- Hartnup disease
- Maple syrup urine disease
- Episodic ataxia type 1 (paroxysmal ataxia and myokymia)

TABLE 17-1	Causes of Ataxia	
Form of Ataxia	**Major Causes**	**Other Causes**
Acute ataxia	Ingestion Acute cerebellar ataxia Guillain–Barré syndrome	Migraine Opsoclonus–myoclonus– ataxia
Acute recurrent ataxia	Migraine Metabolic disease	
Chronic Ataxia	Congenital cerebellar malformations	
Chronic progressive ataxia	Posterior fossa mass Opsoclonus–myoclonus–ataxia	Friedreich ataxia Ataxia–telangiectasia

- Episodic ataxia type 2 (SCA 6, familial hemiplegic migraine)
- Pyruvate decarboxylase deficiency

Miscellaneous Causes
- Migraine headache (benign paroxysmal vertigo)

Chronic or Progressive Ataxia
Neoplastic Causes
- Neuroectodermal tumor
- Posterior fossa tumor
- Glioma
- Astrocytoma
- Ependymoma
- Medulloblastoma

Metabolic or Genetic Causes
- Ataxia–telangiectasia
- Ataxia–oculomotor apraxia
- Friedreich ataxia
- Refsum disease
- Progressive myoclonic epilepsy (Ramsay Hunt syndrome)

Miscellaneous Causes
- Fixed-deficit ataxia—ataxic cerebral palsy, congenital malformations
- Acquired diseases (e.g., systemic lupus erythematosus, hypothyroidism, vitamin E deficiency)

DIFFERENTIAL DIAGNOSIS DISCUSSION
Acute Ataxia
Brain Tumor
Brain stem or cerebellar tumors that **grow rapidly, acutely hemorrhage, or shift** can cause acute decompensation of the brain stem, leading to acute ataxia.

 HINT: Cerebellar hemispheric dysfunction leads to limb ataxia on the same side of the lesion.

Encephalitis
Brain stem encephalitis can be caused by a variety of agents. Common etiologies include Epstein–Barr virus, varicella–zoster virus, enterocytopathogenic human orphan virus, Coxsackievirus, *Mycoplasma,* and borreliosis (Lyme disease). Ataxia occurs, usually in association with other cranial nerve abnormalities, in children

with **diffuse encephalitis;** symptoms typically include altered awareness and seizures. Many children recover completely, although some are left with significant neurologic impairment.

Postinfectious/Autoimmune Disorders

Acute cerebellar ataxia is characterized by the sudden onset of ataxia 2 to 3 weeks after infection. Varicella and Epstein–Barr virus are the most commonly identified triggers, but most often no agent is identified. Children between 1 and 5 years of age are most often affected. Diagnosis often relies on clinical signs because confirmatory laboratory studies are not always present. Cerebrospinal fluid (CSF) may show a mild **pleocytosis** (in about half of cases), and **magnetic resonance imaging (MRI)** may show mildly abnormal signal in the cerebellum (in a minority of patients). Generally, improvement begins within days of presentation, and there is a good outcome within weeks. Corticosteroids are of unproven benefit in the treatment of acute cerebellar ataxia.

Guillain–Barré syndrome (GBS) is a postinfectious demyelinating disease of the peripheral nerves, which can occur in children at any age. It is a postinfectious disorder that usually occurs in otherwise healthy individuals after a nonspecific infection, although certain infections, such as *Campylobacter,* are more often associated. Most affected children will present with progressive, ascending weakness, and areflexia. Up to 15% of patients develop a sensory ataxia before other signs of peripheral demyelination are apparent, and some others, though rare, are dominated by autonomic dysfunction. While GBS is still a potentially serious disorder, even life-threatening, **intravenous immunoglobulin** has dramatically improved the outcome.

Miller–Fisher syndrome is an uncommon variant of GBS, characterized by the sudden onset of ataxia, ophthalmoparesis, and hyporeflexia. Complete recovery within several weeks is the rule.

Acute demyelinating encephalomyelitis (ADEM), like GBS, occurs 1 to 3 weeks following an infection. However, ADEM is a central demyelinating process, affecting the spinal cord and/or brain. Brain stem or cerebellar involvement may cause ataxia. Steroids are the preferred first-line therapy.

Opsoclonus–myoclonus–ataxia syndrome is a paraneoplastic/autoimmune phenomena characterized by the triad of opsoclonus, myoclonus (random, high amplitude, arrhythmic, conjugate eye movements), and ataxia. It is classically seen in patients with neuroblastoma. However, any single symptom or combination of the symptoms may occur in a given patient. When present, the underlying neuroblastoma is often occult. In many cases, there is no underlying tumor, and no trigger for the syndrome is found. The outcome varies widely. Treatment includes long-term steroids or ACTH, but failure to respond to initial approaches may require intravenous immunoglobulin or immune modulation including rituximab.

Trauma

Ataxia may persist for weeks in **post-concussion syndrome**. Trauma can also produce basilar or vertebral artery occlusion accompanied by occipital headache and other cranial nerve dysfunction.

Conversion Disorder

Conversion disorder is characterized by **involuntary alteration or limitation of physical function resulting from psychological conflict**. It must be distinguished from malingering, which implies a willful act (i.e., faking disease). Hysterical abnormalities of gait in children should always be a diagnosis of exclusion. Such disturbances are seen most commonly in older children and adolescents and characterized by findings that do not match expected pathophysiology. For example, some patients will be unable to stand up even though they are able to sit down without difficulty; this is incongruent because sitting requires better balance than standing. Others will stagger and lurch dramatically without ever falling (**astasia–abasia**); this is also incongruent as it takes extra effort and coordination to NOT fall.

Intermittent Ataxia

Postinfectious/Autoimmune Disorders

Multiple sclerosis is a demyelinating disease characterized by recurrent bouts of neurologic symptoms involving different parts of the central nervous system (CNS). Although multiple sclerosis can occur at any age, it is less common in children than in adults. MRI shows numerous white matter "plaques." Acute flares may be treated with **high-dose corticosteroids;** prophylactic therapy to prevent relapses is being studied in children but no immune modulators are approved at present.

Metabolic or Genetic Disorders

Dominant recurrent ataxia is characterized by recurrent bouts of ataxia without a clearly identified metabolic cause. The ataxic symptoms become apparent early in life, usually before 3 years of age. Some affected children demonstrate cerebellar hypoplasia, but this is a variable finding.

Hartnup disease is a rare disorder in which defective amino acid transport in the cells of the proximal renal tubules and the small intestine leads to massive aminoaciduria. These patients are developmentally delayed and have a borderline cognitive impairment. They are photosensitive and develop pellagra-like rashes when exposed to sunlight. Episodic ataxia is frequently reported, sometimes with delirium and emotional lability. The ataxia is triggered by intercurrent infection.

Maple syrup urine disease (intermittent form) is an aminoacidopathy caused by deficiency of a branched-chain decarboxylase leading to bouts of ataxia and encephalopathy. Between attacks of ataxia, the patient's physical examination and IQ are typically normal. During acute exacerbations, the blood and urine exhibit elevated levels of branched-chain amino acids.

Episodic ataxia type 1 (paroxysmal ataxia and myokymia) and **type 2** are autosomal dominant disorders characterized by brief attacks of ataxia that last from minutes to hours. The average age of onset is 5 to 7 years. Patients with this disorder usually respond to **acetazolamide** therapy.

Most patients with **pyruvate decarboxylase deficiency** present with episodic ataxia, dysarthria, and developmental delay. Triggers for attacks of ataxia include infection and a high carbohydrate load. The disorder typically becomes apparent once the child reaches preschool age. Patients have elevated lactate and pyruvate levels during attacks and occasionally following an oral glucose load. Treatment includes a ketogenic diet and the administration of acetazolamide. Prognosis varies and is related to the percentage of preserved enzyme activity.

Chronic or Progressive Ataxia
Congenital Disorders (Ataxia with Fixed Deficit)
Several congenital disorders produce chronic ataxia, including Dandy–Walker malformations, Chiari malformations, and cerebellar hypoplasia. The clinical signs usually appear during infancy or childhood, but these can even be delayed until the patient reaches adulthood. In one recognized variant of cerebral palsy, ataxia is the prominent feature and patients may be hypotonic and hyporeflexic.

Neoplasia
Brain tumors are an important consideration in a child with progressive ataxia, especially those originating in the posterior fossa. Tumors of neuroectodermal origin are the most common solid lesions of the CNS in children, and the second most common childhood malignancy. Posterior fossa tumors are most common in children less than 8 years of age. The most common posterior fossa tumors include **cerebellar astrocytoma, brain stem glioma, and primitive neuroectodermal tumor** or medulloblastoma. More than two-thirds of childhood primary brain tumors are derived from glial elements. Tumors involving the telencephalon are more likely in children <2 years and <8 years of age. CNS tumors arising from the spinal cord are rare at all ages and account for a very small percentage. Cerebellar astrocytoma generally presents with progressive, multiple cranial nerve findings, and ataxia is a late symptom. Ependymoma and medulloblastoma, since they arise in the midline where they can block the CSF movement, more often present with symptoms of increased intracranial pressure. In particular, medulloblastoma may progress especially rapidly.

Metabolic or Genetic Disorders
Ataxia–telangiectasia is a multisystemic disease that most prominently affects the CNS and the immune system. Truncal ataxia usually develops in infancy; drooling and dysarthria are common. The signature vascular lesions involving the conjunctiva and ears are rarely noted before 2 years of age. Complications include sinopulmonary infections (as a result of deficient IgE and IgA) and an increased incidence of neoplasia. Alpha-fetoprotein and carcinoembryonic antigen levels are increased, and immunoglobulin levels are decreased. Treatment usually entails vigorous antibiotic support for infections. There is currently no effective therapy for the neurologic symptoms.

Ataxia–oculomotor apraxia is clinically similar to ataxia–telangiectasia. It is autosomal recessive and has the neurologic features of ataxia–telangiectasia, but symptoms start after 1 year of age, and patients have a normal immunologic status.

Friedreich ataxia is a multisystemic disorder affecting the peripheral nerves, spinal cord, and heart. The ataxia usually begins in childhood with extremity involvement worse than truncal, but ataxia is rarely disabling until young adulthood.

Kyphoscoliosis is common, and there is early loss of position, light touch sensation, and deep tendon reflexes. Diabetes mellitus occurs in 10% to 40% of patients. **Cardiomyopathy** occurs in the majority of patients and is the highest source of mortality.

Refsum disease is an inborn error of phytanic acid metabolism characterized by retinitis pigmentosa, recurrent polyneuropathy, and ataxia. It can be diagnosed by finding elevated serum levels of phytanic acid. Treatment is usually dietary.

Progressive myoclonic epilepsy (Ramsay Hunt disease) is characterized by ataxia, myoclonus, and seizures. Although this disease is usually autosomal recessive, autosomal dominant and mitochondrial cases are also described. Seizures and myoclonus may resolve with appropriate antiepileptic therapy, but the underlying process continues to progress.

Other hereditary disorders that may present with ataxia include Wilson disease, biotinidase deficiency, adrenoleukodystrophy (X-linked), hypobetalipoproteinemia, juvenile sulfatide lipidosis, sea-blue histiocytosis, Leigh disease, and Leber optic neuropathy.

EVALUATION OF ATAXIA

There are two major pitfalls in diagnosing ataxia. The first is confusing ataxia with other gait disturbances. It can be challenging to distinguish ataxia from weakness, dizziness, vertigo, or conversion disorders. Misdiagnosis can be avoided by obtaining a careful history of symptoms, noting evidence of cerebellar dysfunction on neurologic examination, and looking for other features related to ataxia such as dysmetria, intention tremor, and dysdiadochokinesia (difficulty with rapid alternating movements). The second pitfall is misidentification of chronic progressive ataxia as an acute process. The etiology and possible treatments for acute and chronic ataxia are very different, and one would not want to delay appropriate management of a rapidly evolving process.

 HINT: Mild chronic ataxia may be improperly dismissed as clumsiness.

Patient History

After confirming that the symptoms are consistent with ataxia, the next step is to characterize the timing, pattern, and progression of complaints. Unsteadiness can be a nonspecific feature of systemic disease, but ataxia is signaled by coexisting lack of coordination of limb movements or scanning speech. The presence of headache or vomiting may suggest migraine or elevated intracranial pressure as an underlying cause. Other important questions to ask include:

- When were symptoms first noticed, and was there any preceding illness injuries?
- Is there any family history of similar symptoms?
- Is the ataxia acute, intermittent (recurrent), or chronic/progressive?
- Are the symptoms constant, fluctuating, or worsening over time?

- When are the symptoms most notable? For example, difficulty with sitting or head control suggests truncal ataxia correlating with lesions of the cerebellar vermis, while limb ataxia correlates with lesions of the cerebellar hemispheres.
- When did the child have his or her last upper respiratory infection or other viral syndrome?
- Are there any medications in the home the child might have ingested?

Examination

All children should have complete general and neurologic examinations. The following pointers can help clarify the diagnosis of ataxia.

Physical Examination

Ear examination—look for acute or chronic infections, perforations, hemorrhages, or mass lesions. Blowing air into the external ear canal produces vertigo in patients with a fistula of the round or oval window of the labyrinth.

Neurological Examination

Oculovestibular and cranial nerve testing. Careful observation may reveal abnormal movements such as **opsoclonus** (in the opsoclonus–myoclonus–ataxia syndrome), **nystagmus** (suggesting brain stem or cerebellar lesion), or abnormal **saccades** (as in cerebellar lesions). Many normal children have end gaze (physiologic) nystagmus at far lateral gaze in either direction. However, abnormal nystagmus includes spontaneous or induced nystagmus within a normal range of vision. Horizontal nystagmus in only one direction or rotary nystagmus suggests a peripheral cause of vertigo. Vertical, irregular, and variable nystagmus points to a central cause. **Papilledema** suggests increased intracranial pressure, as in intracranial mass lesions or hydrocephalus. Accompanying hearing loss suggests a peripheral cause. If a child can cooperate and march in place, a peripheral lesion of the vestibular system may lead to rotation toward the abnormal side. The presence of **facial weakness, dysarthria, or dysphagia** during the cranial nerve examination is concerning for brain stem or posterior fossa lesion.

Cerebellar testing. Cerebellar testing can help clarify if there is a central component to nystagmus. The **Romberg test** (first standing with feet together, arms outstretched, and eyes open, then with eyes closed) evaluates proprioception that might contribute to a sense of imbalance. If a patient is ataxic and Romberg's test is not positive, it suggests that ataxia is **cerebellar** in nature, that is, depending on localized cerebellar dysfunction instead. A positive Romberg test suggests that the ataxia is sensory in nature.

Others. Although the neurologic examination should focus on vestibular and cerebellar function, a complete examination is necessary to screen for other abnormalities. Evidence of decreased sensation, mild hemiparesis, or other neurologic deficits may indicate an underlying central lesion. Strength testing of isolated muscle groups is essential to clarify the nature of the impairment, particularly when gait abnormality is the presenting complaint. Weakness may also exist in GBS. Impaired joint-position sense or vibration sense suggests a problem in the sensory input that guides our movements in space.

Additional bedside testing that may help clarify the nature of vertigo or syncope include the following:

Orthostatic blood pressure. Blood pressure should be recorded while lying, sitting, and standing to assess for the possibility of orthostatic hypotension.

Valsalva maneuver. The patient should be asked to squat for 30 seconds and then to stand up and strain against a closed glottis. The examiner should note whether this maneuver provokes symptoms suggesting vasovagal syncope or near fainting.

Rapid deep breathing. Reproduction of symptoms by rapid deep breathing within 3 minutes suggests hyperventilation syndrome.

Hallpike maneuver. When the patient is sitting with his legs extended, the examiner rotates the head of the patient approximately 45 degrees and guides the patient's head downward 20 degrees past the edge of the table and allows it to hang 45 degrees to one side. Vertigo with rotational nystagmus indicates benign paroxysmal positional vertigo. In a positive test, the fast phase of nystagmus is seen when the affected ear is turned down closest to the ground.

Laboratory Studies

Laboratory investigations are guided by the presenting signs and symptoms. **Complete serum and urine drug screen** should be performed on all patients presenting with acute ataxia. **Ethanol levels** need to be ordered specifically when ingestion is suspected. If the child takes antiepileptic medication, or such medication is present in the home, **serum levels** may identify toxicity. A complete blood count with differential may identify concomitant infection; **electrolytes** should be checked for metabolic causes of discoordination. **Liver function tests and ammonia** may also be considered. If an infectious or postinfectious illness is suspected, CSF should be sent for cell count, protein, glucose, and culture. Pleocytosis suggests infection or postinfectious illness such as ADEM or acute cerebellar ataxia. Elevated protein may be seen in postinfectious disease, including GBS. If sufficient fluid is collected, it should be sent for specific infectious markers (e.g., **mycoplasma titers**) or markers of demyelination (e.g., **oligoclonal bands**).

Diagnostic Modalities

MRI is the imaging modality of choice when evaluating ataxia. Although computed tomography may be acceptable as an interim screening study while awaiting MRI, it does not adequately assess the posterior fossa, and possible cerebellar and brain stem lesions can be missed. Electroencephalogram is indicated when vertigo is associate with alteration of consciousness.

Hearing testing (audiography) is indicated when there is evidence of hearing loss, ear pain, or tinnitus.

Electronystagmography can allow distinction between central and peripheral causes of vertigo.

Electromyelography and nerve conduction velocity may be useful in assessing for peripheral neuropathy causing sensory ataxia, such as GBS.

Figure 17-1 illustrates the approach to a patient with acute ataxia.

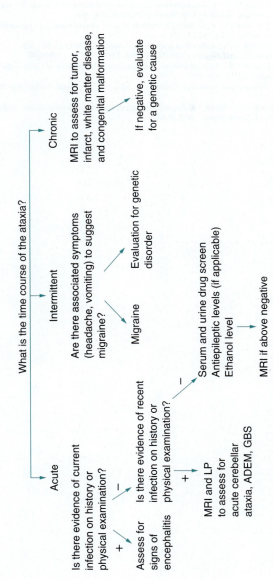

FIGURE 17-1 **Approach to the patient with acute ataxia.** *ADEM,* acute demyelinating encephalomyelitis; *GBS,* Guillain–Barré syndrome; *CSF,* cerebrospinal fluid; *CT,* computed tomography; *EEG,* electroencephalogram; *LP,* lumbar puncture; *MRI,* magnetic resonance imaging.

What is the time course of the ataxia?

Acute

Is there evidence of current infection on history or physical examination?

+
Assess for signs of encephalitis

−
Is there evidence of recent infection on history or physical examination?

+
MRI and LP to assess for acute cerebellar ataxia, ADEM, GBS

−
Serum and urine drug screen
Antiepileptic levels (if applicable)
Ethanol level

MRI if above negative

Intermittent

Are there associated symptoms (headache, vomiting) to suggest migraine?

Migraine

Evaluation for genetic disorder

Chronic

MRI to assess for tumor, infarct, white matter disease, and congenital malformation

If negative, evaluate for a genetic cause

Suggested Readings

Bolduc ME, Limperopoulos C. Neurodevelopmental outcomes in children with cerebellar malformations: a systematic review. *Dev Med Child Neurol.* 2009;51(4):256–267.

Brass SD, Caramano BA, Santos C, et al. Multiple sclerosis vs acute disseminated encephalomyelitis in childhood. *Pediatr Neurol.* 2003;29:227–231.

Casselbrant ML, Mandel EM. Balance disorders in children. *Neurol Clin.* 2005;23:807–829.

Pandolfo M. Freidreich ataxia. *Arch Neurol.* 2008;65(10):1296–1303.

Van Doorn PA, Ruts L, Jacobs BC. Clinical features, pathogenesis and treatment of Guillain-Barre syndrome. *Lancet Neurol.* 2007;7:939–950.

Wells EM, Dalmau J. Paraneoplastic neurologic disorders in children. *Curr Neurol Neurosci Rep.* 2011;11: 187–194.

Young NP, Weinshenker BG, Lucchinetti CF. Acute disseminated encephalomyelitis: current understanding and controversies. *Semin Neurol.* 2008;28:84–94.

Bleeding and Purpura

INTRODUCTION

Purpura, that is, **petechiae and ecchymoses (bruises),** and excessive bleeding are caused by disruptions in one or more of the three stages of normal hemostasis:

- **Vascular phase**—vasoconstriction
- **Primary hemostasis**—platelet plug formation
- **Secondary hemostasis**—fibrin thrombus formation

Disruptions in vascular integrity are characterized by **purpuric lesions;** laboratory tests demonstrate **normal platelet number and function** as well as **normal coagulation**. Disorders of **primary hemostasis** are also characterized by **purpuric lesions,** but **laboratory test results are not normal**. Disorders of **secondary hemostasis** are characterized by **hemarthroses and deep bleeding and abnormal coagulation studies**. Unexplained excessive bruising and bleeding occurring in children with normal hemostasis requires a thorough investigation for nonaccidental trauma.

 DIFFERENTIAL DIAGNOSIS LIST

Thrombocytopenia
Increased Platelet Destruction
Immune-Mediated Thrombocytopenia

- Idiopathic (immune) thrombocytopenic purpura (ITP)
- Evans syndrome
- Autoimmune lymphoproliferative syndrome
- Neonatal, isoimmune, and autoimmune
- Posttransfusion purpura
- Drug related
- HIV infection
- Systemic lupus erythematosus (SLE)

Microangiopathic Process

- Hemolytic uremic syndrome
- Disseminated intravascular coagulation (DIC)
- Thrombotic thrombocytopenic purpura

Decreased Platelet Production

- Congenital amegakaryocytic thrombocytopenia
- Thrombocytopenia with absent radii
- Inherited bone marrow failure syndromes (Fanconi anemia, dyskeratosis congenital, cartilage-hair hypoplasia)
- Aplastic anemia

- Vitamin B_{12} or folate deficiency
- Viral infection—varicella–zoster virus, measles virus, rubella, cytomegalovirus, Epstein–Barr virus
- Drugs

Bone Marrow Infiltration
- Leukemia
- Malignancy metastatic to bone marrow
- Myelofibrosis
- Storage diseases
- Osteopetrosis

Platelet Sequestration
- Splenomegaly
- Large hemangiomas (Kasabach–Merritt syndrome)

Disorders of Platelet Function
- Bernard–Soulier disease
- Glanzmann thrombasthenia
- Wiskott–Aldrich syndrome
- May–Hegglin anomaly
- Platelet granule defects
- Drug-induced abnormalities (e.g., aspirin, ibuprofen)
- Uremia

Disruption in Vascular Integrity
- Trauma (accidental or nonaccidental)
- Henoch–Schönlein purpura (HSP)
- Telangiectasia syndromes
- Drug-induced vasculitis
- Purpura fulminans
- Bacterial (e.g., *Neisseria meningitidis,* streptococcal toxins)
- Viral (e.g., measles, influenza)
- Rickettsial—Rocky Mountain spotted fever
- Parasitic—malaria
- Connective tissue disorders
- Ehlers–Danlos syndrome
- Osteogenesis imperfecta
- Vitamin C deficiency

Clotting Factor Deficiencies
- von Willebrand disease (vWD)
- Hemophilia—factor VIII or IX deficiency
- Other congenital factor deficiencies
- Vitamin K deficiency
- Liver disease
- Disseminated intravascular hemolysis
- Anticoagulants (heparin, warfarin)

DIFFERENTIAL DIAGNOSIS DISCUSSION I: BLEEDING AND PURPURA IN CHILDREN

Idiopathic (Immune) Thrombocytopenic Purpura

ITP, the **most common cause of low platelet counts** in childhood, can be categorized as **newly diagnosed** (thrombocytopenia resolves within 3 months of diagnosis), **persistent** (thrombocytopenia for 3 to 12 months), or **chronic** (thrombocytopenia for >12 months). Although ITP can occur at any age, the **peak incidence** in children is **between** the ages of **2 and 6 years**. The most recent definitions of ITP use a platelet count of less than $100 \times 10^3/\mu L$ ($100 \times 10^9/L$). Primary ITP occurs in situations where the cause of thrombocytopenia is not known and secondary ITP when the cause of thrombocytopenia is known.

Etiology

The exact cause of primary ITP is unknown, but the disorder is thought to be due to **immune-mediated destruction of platelets**. Although the stimulus inciting this immunologic response is often not known, in children, a **viral illness** may precede the signs and symptoms of ITP.

Clinical Features

Children with ITP appear **otherwise well but have rapid onset of purpuric lesions**. They rarely have signs and symptoms of significant bleeding such as intracranial hemorrhage, but **epistaxis** occurs in about a third of patients. Clinical findings of lymphadenopathy and hepatosplenomegaly should alert the physician to a diagnosis other than ITP (e.g., malignancy, metabolic disorder).

Evaluation

A complete blood count (CBC) often demonstrates isolated thrombocytopenia. Hemoglobin values may be low due to significant blood loss or immune-mediated red cell destruction. Additional laboratory studies (depending on the situation) should include a direct antibody test (DAT) and a reticulocyte count. The peripheral blood smear may demonstrate large platelets, but prominent schistocytes or immature lymphocytes should lead the physician to consider other diagnoses such as thrombotic thrombocytopenic purpura or acute leukemia. Other causes of thrombocytopenia (e.g., SLE) should be considered, particularly in adolescent girls. Immunoglobulin levels should be performed when common variable immune deficiency is suspected.

 HINT: Evans syndrome (autoimmune hemolytic anemia with immune-mediated thrombocytopenia) should be suspected in patients with thrombocytopenia and anemia. Patients with Evans syndrome have a positive DAT, evidence of hemolysis, and usually require more intensive intervention than those with ITP alone.

Routine **bone marrow aspiration** to evaluate acute ITP is usually not necessary. **Increased platelet precursors** (megakaryocytes) are often present on histologic examination of bone marrow aspirate in patients with ITP.

Treatment

Many believe that treating patients with newly diagnosed ITP and isolated skin manifestations (petechiae and bruising) is **unnecessary** as the disease process often will resolve over a short period of time without major sequelae. However, if a child experiences **significant bleeding such as prolonged epistaxis, treatment is warranted**. Treatment options include **intravenous immunoglobulin** (IVIG) (800 to 1,000 mg/kg), **steroids** (2 mg/kg/day), and, in Rh-positive children, **anti-D immune globulin** (50 to 75 µg/kg). Rapidity of response and drug side effects should be considered when considering therapeutic options. IVIG or anti-D immune globulin administration may be associated with a more rapid increase in platelet count than steroid therapy. However, aseptic meningitis has been associated with IVIG and significant intravascular hemolysis with anti-D immune globulin. Anti-D administration should be avoided in children with severe anemia, evidence of immune-mediated red cell destruction such as a positive DAT, those who are Rh-negative, and those with a history of splenectomy. The Food and Drug Administration recommends close monitoring for hemolysis in all patients

TABLE 18-1	Causes of Disseminated Intravascular Coagulation (DIC)
Infection	Bacterial, viral, fungal, rickettsial
Cardiovascular disorder	Shock
Toxins	Snake bites
Tumors	Myeloid leukemia
Trauma	Massive generalized or head trauma
Hematologic disorder	Hemolytic transfusion reactions
Miscellaneous causes	Burns, purpura fulminans, severe asphyxia

treated with anti-D immune globulin. If steroids are initiated, they should be tapered as quickly as possible to avoid long-term side effects. In situations where a patient with known ITP requires therapy, it is best to use whatever therapy has been beneficial for that patient in the past.

Intracranial hemorrhage and life-threatening hemorrhage, although rare in patients with ITP, may be fatal. Therefore, **treatment is mandatory** if the ITP patient has **major head trauma, abnormal neurologic examination, or copious blood loss. High-dose steroid therapy with IVIG** administration should be initiated rapidly before more detailed evaluations. In patients with ongoing life-threatening bleeding, **continuous platelet transfusions, emergent splenectomy, or both** may be necessary.

Disseminated Intravascular Coagulation

Etiology
DIC is a **consumptive coagulopathy** characterized by **intravascular coagulation and fibrinolysis** resulting in clotting factor deficiencies and thrombocytopenia in association with an underlying disease (Table 18-1).

> **HINT:** Sepsis should be considered an etiology for any critically ill child until proven otherwise.

Clinical Features
Children with DIC usually **appear ill and bleed from multiple sites**. In neonates, DIC usually manifests as **gastrointestinal bleeding or oozing from skin puncture sites**.

Evaluation
In patients with DIC, laboratory values show a normal or **decreased platelet count, increased prothrombin time (PT) and partial thromboplastin time (PTT), decreased fibrinogen, and increased fibrin split products or D-dimer levels**. A peripheral blood smear is significant for **schistocytes, fragmented red blood cells,** and normal or **decreased platelets**.

Treatment

Treatment is directed toward managing the underlying disorder and **replacing coagulation factors and platelets**.

Henoch–Schönlein Purpura
Etiology

HSP is an **acquired inflammatory small-vessel vasculitis** due to immunoglobulin A subclass 1 (IgA1), C3 and immune complex deposition in blood vessel walls and the renal mesangium. **HSP is most common in early childhood** and often is a self-limited benign illness.

Clinical Features

Diffuse inflammation of the small vessels causes **abdominal pain, joint pain or arthritis, and palpable purpura**. Renal involvement occurs in 50% of patients. Most patients have a **prodromal upper respiratory infection** 1 to 3 weeks before the onset of illness. The **hallmark** of this disorder on physical examination is a **symmetric pattern of purpura,** primarily involving the **buttocks and lower extremities**. In some patients, purpura are also found on the extensor surfaces of the arms but the palms and soles are spared.

Evaluation

Hematuria, proteinuria, and cellular casts on urinalysis confirm nephritis in patients with HSP. The CBC, PT, and PTT are normal unless major gastrointestinal blood loss has occurred, in which case the **patient may be anemic**.

Treatment

HSP, a **self-limited disorder,** usually resolves in 1 to 6 weeks. Treatment primarily involves supportive therapy. **Corticosteroids,** used to manage renal complications, may be helpful to alleviate persistent or severe gastrointestinal and musculoskeletal symptoms but should be used cautiously in patients with suspected renal insufficiency.

Von Willebrand Disease
Etiology

vWD, the **most common inherited bleeding disorder,** is characterized by quantitative or qualitative abnormalities in von Willebrand factor (vWF). Patients with vWD can be classified as having **type 1, type 2, and type 3** vWD, according to the clinical history and laboratory test results. Type 1, occurring in approximately 65% to 80% of vWD patients, is due to a quantitative decrease in vWF and is inherited in an autosomal dominant fashion with variable penetrance. Type 2, occurring in 15% to 20% of patients, is due to a qualitative change in vWF and is inherited in an autosomal dominant or recessive pattern. Type 3 (autosomal recessive) is a rare and more severe bleeding disorder in which vWF levels and factor VIII:coagulant (factor VIII:C) are significantly decreased.

Clinical Features

Children with vWD present with **mucocutaneous bleeding, including epistaxis, gum oozing, menorrhagia, easy bruising, and bleeding after surgery**.

Patients with type 3 (severe) vWD may develop **joint and intramuscular bleeding**.

Evaluation

Screening coagulation studies may demonstrate a **prolonged PTT**, although this may be normal in patients with mild vWD. Specific laboratory studies for vWD include vWF activity (ristocetin cofactor), factor VIII-related antigen (vWF), and factor VIII:C evaluation. Patients with vWD may have decreased factor VIII:C activity, decreased vWF, decreased ristocetin cofactor, or a combination of the three findings (see section on "Etiology").

Treatment

Multiple treatment options are available for patients with vWD, depending on the type of vWD and the reason for treatment. **Desmopressin acetate,** an analog of vasopressin, is often used to treat or prevent bleeding episodes in patients with **type 1** vWD, although its use is controversial in patients with type 2B and platelet-type vWD. **Type 2B and type 3 patients** can receive **factor VIII concentrate** with retained vWF activity, and those with the rare **platelet-type vWD** may need **platelet transfusions,** depending on their past experience with blood products.

Hemophilia A and B (Factor VIII and Factor IX Deficiencies)

Etiology and Incidence

Factor VIII deficiency (hemophilia A) occurs in 1 of every 10,000 live male births, and factor IX deficiency (hemophilia B) occurs in 1 of every 40,000 live male births. Most patients have a **family history of bleeding disorders,** but spontaneous mutations are responsible for about 30% of cases of hemophilia.

Clinical Features

Children with factors VIII and IX deficiencies develop similar clinical features depending on the severity of the factor deficiency. In **infancy,** there can be **excessive bleeding after circumcision, intracranial hemorrhage, or bruising at injection sites**. However, many children with hemophilia do not bleed after circumcision. Later in **childhood,** patients develop **easy bruisability, large hematomas, and hemarthroses or intramuscular hemorrhages** (the hallmarks of hemophilia). Patients with severe factor deficiencies can experience **bleeding episodes spontaneously or following trauma**. Patients with **moderate or mild factor deficiencies** rarely have spontaneous hemorrhages, but are at risk for **post-traumatic bleeding** and bleeding after **surgical procedures**. The **most common cause of morbidity is recurrent hemarthroses**.

Evaluation

Laboratory evaluation should include a **platelet count,** a **PT,** and a **PTT**. In patients with factor VIII or IX deficiency, the PTT is prolonged, but the PT is normal. Therefore, in patients with an isolated prolonged PTT, levels of factors VIII and IX deficiency should be measured. Patients with severe factor VIII or IX deficiency have factor activity levels of <1%. Patients with moderate disease have levels of 1% to 5%, and those with mild disease have levels of 5% to 20%.

Treatment

The most **serious hemorrhages** in patients with hemophilia are **intracranial, retropharyngeal, retroperitoneal,** and those involving the **airway**. The goal of treatment in these circumstances is to achieve a factor activity level of 100% and to offer appropriate supportive therapy.

- **Intracranial hemorrhage.** In patients with severe factor deficiency, intracranial hemorrhage may be spontaneous; therefore, any patient with severe factor deficiency who has a change in mental status or other neurologic findings should be treated for an intracranial hemorrhage until radiologic studies prove negative. Intravenous access and factor replacement should occur before obtaining a head computed tomography scan. Factor VIII and IX deficiencies cause poor secondary clot formation, so that bleeding usually occurs hours after the initial trauma. Therefore, a negative head computed tomography scan does not exclude a slowly developing intracranial hemorrhage. Many clinicians admit children following head trauma, particularly those who have severe factor deficiency, to inpatient wards for observation, with frequent neurologic examinations.
- **Intramuscular bleeding** can be massive, leading to shock. The muscles of the thigh and the iliopsoas muscle in particular can accommodate large volumes of blood. Patients with hemophilia should be admitted to the hospital for close monitoring and bed rest if bleeding occurs in these areas. Extensive intramuscular bleeding can compromise vascular blood flow and cause compartment syndromes. Tingling, numbness, or loss of pulses in an extremity requires immediate factor replacement to 100% and an orthopedic evaluation.
- **Joint bleeds (hemarthroses)** require treatment with factor products and immobilization to avoid chronic complications (e.g., decreased mobility, contractures). The goal of factor replacement for hemarthroses depends on the child's individual bleeding history, but in general, factor replacement should be aimed at obtaining an activity level of 30% to 50% for 1 to 2 days. If recurrent hemarthroses have developed in the affected joint (the so-called target joint), then higher factor activity levels should be obtained. Today, many patients receive factor on a regular or "prophylactic" schedule to prevent recurrent joint bleeds. This approach to hemophilia treatment requires the guidance of a hematologist or a hemophilia specialist.
- **Moderate hemorrhages** involving muscles, hematomas, or lacerations usually require treatment to reach a peak factor activity level of 30%. Oral mucosa bleeding may require factor correction and a-aminocaproic acid or tranexamic acid therapy. These antifibrinolytic therapies decrease mouth bleeding by inhibiting clot breakdown and are contraindicated in patients with hematuria or DIC.
- **Hematuria** can occur spontaneously in patients with severe hemophilia, or after trauma in patients with moderate-to-mild disease. Treatment is directed toward cessation of bleeding while avoiding obstruction, which could lead to an obstructive uropathy. Factor replacement, hydration, and bed rest are recommended.
- **Replacement therapy for dental or surgical procedures.** Patients with factors VIII and IX deficiencies must receive replacement therapy before dental, surgical, or

other general procedures, including laceration repair, suture removal, or spinal tap. The patient's hematologist should be consulted before initiating any procedures.

- **Factor inhibitors.** Of patients with factor VIII deficiency, about 10% to 25% develop factor inhibitors (i.e., antibodies to factor VIII). Patients who do not improve clinically after receiving the appropriate dosage of factor and who have complied with supportive care measures (e.g., splinting, avoidance of weight bearing with hemarthroses) should be evaluated for the presence of a factor inhibitor. Patients with factor inhibitors require alternative treatment options.

Factor XI Deficiency

This is an autosomal disorder primarily affecting persons of **Ashkenazi descent**. This bleeding disorder is **mild,** including **epistaxis, menorrhagia, and postoperative bleeding**. The **PTT is prolonged** in these patients and the diagnosis is confirmed by a factor-specific assay. The factor XI levels do not always predict bleeding risk.

Factor XII Deficiency

This is characterized by a **prolonged PTT** with a **normal PT and bleeding time**. Factor XII-deficient patients are **not at risk for increased bleeding**.

Infection-Related Purpura

An **acute febrile illness** associated with a **petechial rash** may indicate a **benign, self-limited viral process,** or a **severe, life-threatening bacterial illness** (e.g., meningococcal infection). Therefore, ill-appearing **children with fever and petechiae should be considered septic until proven otherwise**.

Infections can cause purpura by a wide variety of mechanisms. Severe bacterial infections are often associated with DIC. Viral illness can be associated with thrombocytopenia from increased platelet destruction (e.g., ITP) or from decreased production. In addition to causing thrombocytopenia, bacterial, fungal, and viral illnesses can cause **platelet dysfunction and vascular abnormalities**.

Drug-Related Purpura

Drug-induced thrombocytopenia in the hospital setting is most often caused by **chemotherapeutic agents** that suppress bone marrow activity. **Heparin, quinidine, digoxin, penicillin, and seizure medications** (e.g., valproic acid) can cause immune-mediated thrombocytopenia, which generally **reverses when the drug is discontinued**. Some drugs, such as **H$_2$ blockers,** are associated with **idiopathic thrombocytopenia**.

Drug-induced platelet dysfunction as a result of cyclooxygenase enzyme inhibition is seen with **aspirin-containing compounds** and to a lesser degree with **nonsteroidal anti-inflammatory drugs** such as ibuprofen. **Penicillins and cephalosporins** can also cause platelet dysfunction, particularly in children with systemic disease. Platelet function should **return to normal** 7 to 10 days after the offending drug is discontinued.

DIFFERENTIAL DIAGNOSIS DISCUSSION II: BLEEDING AND PURPURA IN NEONATES

Bleeding and purpura in the neonate presents a slightly different differential diagnosis than bleeding in the child.

 HINT: Patients whose mothers took aspirin, phenytoin, warfarin, or thiazide diuretics are at increased bleeding risk during the neonatal period.

Vitamin K Deficiency (Hemorrhagic Disease of the Newborn)
Etiology
In the past, vitamin K deficiency was **primarily a disease of breast-fed infants** because cow's milk contains 4 to 10 times the amount of vitamin K found in human breast milk. As a result, vitamin K prophylaxis is recommended for all newborns at birth to prevent hemorrhagic disease in the high-risk breast-fed group.

Clinical Features and Evaluation
Presently, vitamin K deficiency is most common in breast-fed infants who did not receive vitamin K prophylaxis. Affected infants may present with **excessive bleeding at 2 to 5 days of age and have prolongation of the PT and PTT**. However, late bleeding, between 2 and 12 weeks of age, can occur with increased rates of intracranial hemorrhage and mortality.

 HINT: Ill neonates who are transferred from other institutions may not have received vitamin K before transport. Infants of mothers taking phenobarbital are at increased risk for hemorrhagic disease of the newborn.

Treatment
Treatment is the administration of **1 mg vitamin K1 parenterally. Fresh-frozen plasma can be given if there is significant bleeding**.

Neonatal Alloimmune (Isoimmune) Thrombocytopenia
Etiology
Neonatal alloimmune (isoimmune) thrombocytopenia is characterized by **moderate-to-severe isolated thrombocytopenia**. This **antibody-mediated destruction of platelets** is analogous to hemolytic disease of the newborn and occurs when **maternal antibodies** that are directed against paternal antigens found on the patient's platelets cross the placenta, entering the patient's circulation. These antibodies cause increased platelet destruction in the neonate. The most common offending antigen is PLA-1. Thrombocytopenia will persist as long as the maternal antibodies are found in the patient's circulation, usually within **21 days**.

Clinical Features
The infant with neonatal alloimmune (isoimmune) thrombocytopenia is generally well appearing but may have **petechiae, ecchymoses, and mucosal membrane**

bleeding within the **first 48 hours of life,** depending on the platelet count. Petechiae and ecchymoses can be found at **injection sites** as well as at pressure points, such as the **extensor surfaces of the knees** and on the **abdomen** where diapering causes pressure. **Intracranial hemorrhage** is reported in 10% to 15% of patients.

Evaluation

Thrombocytopenia **can be severe,** with a platelet count of <20,000/mm³. The mother's platelet count is normal. **Finding maternal antibodies to paternal platelets** strongly suggests this diagnosis. The diagnosis is confirmed by isolating alloantibodies in the mother's serum, but the results are often negative.

Treatment

In the absence of bleeding, many recommend keeping the platelet count >30,000/mm³ for the first few weeks of life. **If bleeding is severe or** signs of **intracranial hemorrhage** are present, **treatment is critical. Transfusing the infant with the mother's washed, irradiated platelets** increases the platelet count because the mother's platelets are lacking the antigen against which the antibody is aimed. IVIG and corticosteroids can increase the infant's counts, and some clinicians prefer the pharmacological approach to therapy. In **emergent situations, PLA-1(–) platelets or single-donor platelets** can be used if maternal platelets are not available.

Neonatal Autoimmune Thrombocytopenia

Etiology

This type of thrombocytopenia is **secondary to an autoimmune disorder in the mother** (e.g., ITP, SLE, lymphoproliferative disorder, hyperthyroidism). Antibodies are found in maternal and patient platelets of patients with this condition.

Clinical Features and Evaluation

Infants are well appearing and may develop **petechiae within the first 2 days of life**. The diagnosis is made by the clinical presentation of the mother and infant. The infant should have a **low platelet count with a normal PT and PTT**.

Treatment

IVIG should be administered to **patients showing signs of bleeding**. Steroid therapy should be considered in **patients who do not respond to IVIG**. Life-threatening hemorrhage should be treated with **high-dose steroids and continuous platelet transfusion**.

Nonimmune Causes of Thrombocytopenia

Consumptive coagulopathies (e.g., DIC) and coagulopathies associated with **sepsis, asphyxia, respiratory distress, or necrotizing enterocolitis** are the most common nonimmune causes of thrombocytopenia in ill neonates. Thrombocytopenia **secondary to thrombus formation from renal vein thrombosis or catheter-related thrombi** is also a frequent occurrence. Thrombocytopenia after exchange transfusion or extracorporeal membrane oxygenation is a normal finding. Nonimmune causes of thrombocytopenia in the sick neonate also include **congenital viral infections and hyperbilirubinemia treated with phototherapy**.

Kasabach–Merritt syndrome should be considered in neonates with thrombocytopenia and hemangiomata.

> **HINT:** Patients of diabetic mothers are at increased risk of polycythemia and renal vein thrombosis.

> **HINT:** If congenital anomalies are present on physical examination of a neonate with purpura or abnormal bleeding, thrombocytopenia with absent radii, Wiskott–Aldrich syndrome, Fanconi anemia, Chédiak–Higashi syndrome, and trisomy 21 should be considered.

Treatment is directed toward treating the underlying problem, factor replacement with fresh-frozen plasma and cryoprecipitate, and platelet transfusions (if needed).

EVALUATION OF BLEEDING AND PURPURA
Patient History

When evaluating a child with abnormal bleeding, a careful history and physical examination can direct the approach to patient management (Table 18-2). Important questions to ask pertain to the following:

Onset of symptoms. Acute onset of purpura is consistent with an acquired disorder. Recurrent purpura since infancy suggests an inherited abnormality. The physician should ask questions about bleeding or bruising episodes since birth, such as epistaxis, menses, or excessive bleeding after surgical procedures (e.g., circumcision, tonsillectomy, dental extractions). These questions should be made in reference to family members as well as the patient. A child who presents with repeated hemarthroses and a history of requiring a blood transfusion after an uncomplicated surgical procedure most likely has a congenital bleeding disorder, whereas normal hemostasis after major surgical procedures (e.g., a tonsillectomy) makes the diagnosis of an inherited disorder of hemostasis less likely. Of note, for patients with severe hemophilia —50% of those who are circumcised in the newborn period without factor replacement do not have excessive hemorrhage.

> **HINT:** Remember that children may not have been exposed to situations such as surgery that would reveal a disorder of hemostasis.

- **Location.** The location of the bleeding is important. Unilateral epistaxis in a child who frequently traumatizes his nasal mucosa is usually normal. However, prolonged bilateral epistaxis in a child covered with bruises and petechiae is abnormal.
- **Medication history.** Certain drugs, especially aspirin and ibuprofen, are associated with platelet dysfunction. Some drugs can exacerbate bleeding in a patient

TABLE 18-2	Clinical Evaluation of Pediatric Patients with Suspected Bleeding Disorders
Question	**If the Answer Is "Yes," Consider...**
History	
When the child bleeds from an injury, does the bleeding stop and then resume?	Coagulation disorder
Does the patient have a history of fever?	Infection
Does the patient have neurologic manifestations?	Meningococcemia, TTP
Is there a history of a viral prodrome?	HUS, ITP, HSP
Has the patient had repeated episodes of bleeding gums, prolonged bleeding from cuts, or massive bleeding from surgical procedures? Has the patient developed large hematomas at vaccination sites? Did the patient experience prolonged bleeding as a result of circumcision?	Congenital disorder
Do family members have problems with easy bruising or abnormal bleeding?	Congenital disorder
Is the patient currently taking aspirin, ibuprofen, antibiotics, antihistamines, or steroids?	Drug-related purpura
Has the patient received multiple blood or platelet transfusions in the past as well as recently?	Posttransfusion purpura and platelet alloimmunization
Could the child have ingested rat poison?	Warfarin toxicity
Does the patient have a history of delayed wound healing or umbilical stump bleeding?	Factor XIII deficiency
If the patient is a neonate, did the mother take phenytoin? Is the patient an infant who is exclusively breast-fed?	Vitamin K deficiency
Physical examination	
Are predominant findings on examination hemarthroses?	Coagulation disorder, nonaccidental trauma
Are predominant findings on examination-isolated petechiae or ecchymosis?	Platelet disorder, HSP
Are purpura symmetric and predominantly located on the legs and buttocks?	HSP
Are ecchymotic lesions extensive and in various stages of resolution?	Physical abuse
Is there lymphadenopathy with hepatosplenomegaly?	Leukemia, lymphoma, infection, Evans' syndrome, ALPS
Are there palpable purpura with a history of minimal trauma?	Platelet disorder, coagulation disorder, HSP
Is there umbilical stump bleeding?	Factor XIII deficiency
Is there jaundice and bruising?	Hepatic disease (factor deficiency)

ITP, idiopathic (immune) thrombocytopenic purpura; *TTP,* thrombotic thrombocytopenic purpura; *HSP,* Henoch–Schönlein purpura; *HUS,* hemolytic uremic syndrome; *ALPS,* autoimmune lymphoproliferative syndrome.

with an underlying bleeding disorder. Children with vWD may bruise more easily after taking cough preparations or antihistamines.

Physical Examination

The physical examination should include the **skin, mucous membranes,** and **fundi**. The type of lesions, pattern of lesions, and the location, size, and stage of resolution of the lesions should be documented.

Types of Lesions

- **Petechiae** are small (<3 mm in diameter), macular, nonblanching erythematous lesions. They are most common on the face and chest but may involve any skin area.
- **Ecchymotic lesions** are large and can be macular, tender, or raised. Recent injuries are usually purple, fading over time to yellowish brown. Palpable ecchymotic lesions (raised lesions with a central nodule) are rarely a normal finding in children but are found often in boys with hemophilia.
- **Purpura fulminans** (purplish black, well-demarcated, stellate lesions with central necrosis) are usually associated with DIC. They can be extensive and painful.

Findings Suggestive of a Bleeding Disorder

A child who meets any of the following criteria should be screened for a bleeding disorder:

- Excessive purpura involving many sites, particularly areas not normally traumatized (e.g., flexor surfaces of the arms or the axillary and inguinal regions)
- Many purpuric lesions of the same stage
- Palpable ecchymotic lesions
- Observed purpura or bleeding that exceeds what is expected for the child's activity level
- Purpura, excessive bleeding, or both in an ill-appearing child

Laboratory Evaluation

The diagnosis of a bleeding disorder in a child may not be straightforward. Children with abnormal laboratory values may not be at risk for excessive bleeding, whereas those with normal laboratory values may be. Children with **factor XII deficiency or lupus anticoagulants** are **not at risk for increased bleeding,** although their PTT values are prolonged. Conversely, children with **factor XIII deficiency or vasculitic disorders** have normal laboratory values but are at **increased risk for bleeding**.

A laboratory screening evaluation includes the following:

- **CBC with a platelet count.** Thrombocytopenia is a platelet count <150,000/mm^3. Thrombocytopenia determined by automated systems should be confirmed by peripheral blood smear examination.

    PT and PTT. Normal values for PT and PTT vary according to the patient's age and the testing system used in the coagulation laboratory. The PT measures the activity of factors II, V, VII, and X. The PTT measures factors V, VIII, IX, X,

XI, and XII. The PT reflects the extrinsic and common pathways of coagulation, whereas the PTT evaluates the intrinsic and common pathways.

> **HINT:** Blood for PT and PTT analysis must be obtained from a blood vessel large enough to provide free-flowing blood. Blood obtained for PT and PTT via "difficult sticks" may falsely decrease the laboratory values.

- **Peripheral blood smear.** Platelet, red blood cell, and white blood cell morphology can be helpful in narrowing the differential diagnosis. Large platelets are seen in ITP, Bernard–Soulier syndrome, and May–Hegglin anomaly. Small platelets are seen in Wiskott–Aldrich syndrome. Schistocytes accompanying a

TABLE 18-3	Treatment of Common Childhood Bleeding Disorders	
Bleeding Disorder	**Treatment Potential**	**Complications of Therapy**
Idiopathic (immune) thrombocytopenic purpura (ITP)[a]	Intravenous immunoglobulin	Headaches, neutropenia, volume overload, aseptic meningitis, allergic reactions, virus transmission
	Steroids	Partial treatment of leukemia, psychosis, fluid imbalance, hypertension, psychosis
	Anti-D immune globulin	Hemolysis, headaches, allergic reactions
	Continuous platelet transfusion (for life-threatening hemorrhage)	Virus transmission, transfusion reactions
Disseminated intravascular coagulation (DIC)	Fresh-frozen plasma	Virus transmission, allergic reactions
	Platelet and packed red blood cell transfusion	Virus transmission, transfusion reactions
	Cryoprecipitate	Virus transmission
HSP hypertension	Steroids[b]	Fluid imbalance, psychosis
Neonatal isoimmune thrombocytopenia	Transfusion of mother's washed, irradiated, or PLA-1 negative platelets, IVIG, or steroids	—
Platelet function abnormalities	Platelet transfusion (for life-threatening hemorrhage)	Virus transmission, transfusion reactions
von Willebrand disease (vWD)	Desmopressin acetate (DDAVP)	Thrombocytopenia in patients with type 2B or platelet-type vWD
Type 2B and platelet-type vWD	Platelet transfusion or cryoprecipitate administration	—

[a]The necessity of treating acute ITP is controversial.
[b]Considered for patients with gastrointestinal or joint symptoms.

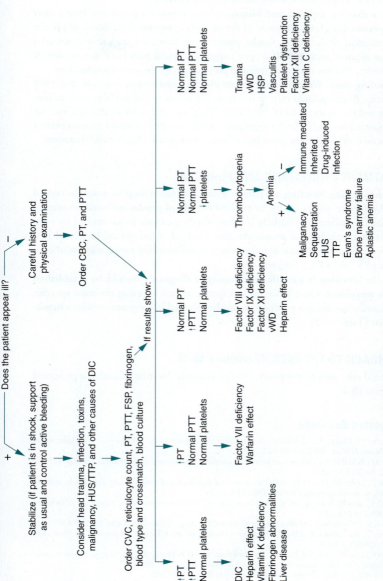

FIGURE 18-1 Evaluation of a pediatric patient with bleeding or purpura. *CBC*, complete blood cell count; *DIC*, disseminated intravascular coagulation; *FSP*, fibrin split products; *HSP*, Henoch–Schönlein purpura; *HUS*, hemolytic uremic syndrome; *PT*, prothrombin time; *PTT*, partial thromboplastin time; *TTP*, thrombotic thrombocytopenic purpura; *vWD*, von Willebrand disease; ↑, increased; ↓, decreased.

decreased platelet count suggest a microangiopathic process. White blood cell blasts on the peripheral blood smear suggest leukemia.

- **Bone marrow aspirate and biopsy.** A bone marrow aspirate and biopsy may be obtained to clarify the cause of the thrombocytopenia (i.e., increased platelet destruction or decreased platelet production). Increased megakaryocytes on a bone marrow aspirate and biopsy suggest increased peripheral destruction of platelets, whereas decreased megakaryocytes suggest decreased production.
- **Bleeding time.** Bleeding times reflect platelet number and function, and vWF activity. Bleeding times vary according to the experience of the laboratory technician and the cooperation of the patient. They are not reliable in children and not performed routinely. Platelet aggregation studies can be performed to assess platelet function, although these must be performed in a special coagulation laboratory.

TREATMENT OF BLEEDING AND PURPURA

Life-threatening bleeding in a patient without a known diagnosis must be treated before a specific diagnosis can be established. **Blood products** should be used to stabilize the patient, particularly if active bleeding cannot be controlled by pressure or other mechanical means. At least 5 mL of blood should be placed in a sodium citrate tube before blood-product transfusion for coagulation studies, a CBC, a PT, and a PTT are performed.

If the **bleeding is not life threatening,** a **diagnosis should be established before treatment**. Once a diagnosis is made, treatment (using the most specific, safest, and cost-effective product) should be initiated in conjunction with a **hematologist** (Table 18-3).

APPROACH TO THE PATIENT (FIGURE 18-1)

A general approach to the patient with a potential bleeding disorder is presented in Figure 18-1.

Suggested Readings

Blanchette VS, Carcao M. Childhood acute immune thrombocytopenic purpura—20 years later. *Semin Thromb Hemost.* 2003;29:605–617.

Geddis AE, Balduini CL. Diagnosis of immune thrombocytopenia purpura in children. *Curr Opin Hematol.* 2007;14:520–525.

Katsanis E, Luike KJ, Hsu Li M, et al. Prevalence and significance of mild bleeding disorders in children with recurrent epistaxis. *J Pediatr.* 1988;113:73–76.

Khair K, Liesner R. Bruising and bleeding in infants and children—a practical approach. *Br J Haematol.* 2006;133:221–231.

Manno CS. Difficult pediatric diagnoses: bruising and bleeding. *Pediatr Clin N Am.* 1991;38:637.

Medeiros D, Buchanan GR. Idiopathic thrombocytopenic purpura: beyond consensus. *Curr Opin Pediatr.* 2000;12(1):4–9.

Neunert C, Lim W, Crowther M, et al. The American Society of Hematology 2011 evidence-based practice guideline for immune thrombocytopenia. *Blood.* 2011;117:4190–4207.

Pramanik AK. Bleeding disorders in neonates. *Pediatr Rev.* 1992;13:163.

Provan D, Stasi R, Newland AC, et al. International consensus report on the investigation and management of primary immune thrombocytopenia. *Blood.* 2010;115:168–186.

Saulsbury FT. Henoch-Schönlein purpura. *Curr Opin Rheumatol.* 2001;13(1):35–40.

CHAPTER 19

Kan N. Hor
Bradley S. Marino

Chest Pain

INTRODUCTION

Chest pain in children and adolescents is common and produces a high level of anxiety in both patients and families because of its perceived association with fatal heart disease in adults. Chest pain may lead to emergency department visits (accounting for 0.5% of all pediatric visits), school absences, and an unnecessary restriction of activities. **Despite the degree of concern it generates, and with the exception of a few uncommon serious conditions, chest pain symptoms in children and adolescents are rarely associated with a cardiac etiology and are usually benign and self-limited.** For these reasons, the workup of chest pain is directed toward ruling out the rare serious causes. A complete, detailed history and physical examination usually can determine the cause and identify patients who require further evaluation or acute intervention. Cardiac conditions are a rare but potentially serious cause of chest pain and should be considered, particularly when a child presents with chest pain associated with syncope or a family history of syncope or sudden cardiac arrest.

 DIFFERENTIAL DIAGNOSIS LIST

Cardiac Causes
Anatomic Lesions
- Severe aortic stenosis (subvalvar, valvar, supravalvar)
- Severe pulmonary stenosis
- Aortic root dissection
- Coronary artery anomalies
- Mitral valve prolapse (MVP)

Acquired Lesions
- Myocarditis
- Pericarditis
- Hypertrophic cardiomyopathy
- Coronary vasospasm (variant angina) and myocardial infarction
- Pulmonary hypertension
- Postpericardiotomy syndrome

Arrhythmia
- Sinus arrhythmia
- Supraventricular arrhythmia
- Premature atrial contractions/supraventricular tachycardia (SVT)
- Ventricular arrhythmia
- Premature ventricular contractions/ventricular tachycardia (VT)

Noncardiac Causes
- Idiopathic
- Costochondritis
- Slipping rib
- Precordial catch syndrome
- Overuse pain
- Trauma

- Pleural effusion
- Pneumonia with or without pleurisy
- Pulmonary embolism
- Reactive airway disease
- Pneumothorax

- Upper or lower respiratory infection resulting in persistent cough
- Gastroesophageal reflux
- Hiatal hernia
- Gastritis
- Peptic ulcer disease

DIFFERENTIAL DIAGNOSIS DISCUSSION

The differential diagnosis of cardiac chest pain in children includes inflammation of the myocardium or pericardium, arrhythmias, and structural abnormalities such as aortic stenosis, subaortic stenosis, coronary artery anomalies, MVP, and rarely, coronary vasospasm and myocardial infarction. A physical examination, electrocardiogram (ECG), and chest radiograph (CXR) can rule out many of these possibilities.

Myocarditis and Pericarditis

In patients referred to a pediatric cardiologist for evaluation of chest pain, the most common serious causes of cardiac chest pain are myocarditis and pericarditis. **Myocarditis usually follows a febrile viral illness.** Patients typically present with symptoms of shortness of breath, nonspecific chest pain, anorexia, or malaise. A physical examination may reveal the presence of an S3 gallop rhythm. The CXR typically reveals cardiomegaly, although early in the illness it may reveal normal heart size. The ECG may reveal ST segment depression and T-wave abnormalities, especially in the inferior or lateral leads (II, III, AVF, V6, and V7). In these patients, the myocardium is inflamed and ventricular dysfunction and congestive heart failure is common. Myocardial inflammation may also affect the conduction system, and patients with myocarditis may present with arrhythmias. These arrhythmias tend to improve when the inflammation resolves. In patients who develop a chronic cardiomyopathy, arrhythmias may persist. **Pericarditis** more frequently presents with acute onset of sharp chest pain, which is lessened by leaning forward. Pericarditis results from inflammation of the pericardium and may result from infections, uremia, neoplasm, trauma, or autoimmune disorders. In patients with a small pericardial fluid collection, the physical examination may reveal a friction rub. In patients with a large pericardial fluid collection around the heart, pericardial tamponade may be present, resulting in distended neck veins, diminished heart sounds, and pulsus paradoxus. In the presence of a large pericardial effusion, the ECG may reveal low-voltage QRS complexes. In patients with pericarditis, the CXR usually demonstrates cardiomegaly. Myocarditis and pericarditis occur after a viral inflammatory process (e.g., coxsackievirus, adenovirus, echovirus, and parvovirus). A viral polymerase chain reaction test on a sample of blood may help determine the specific cause. Since Lyme disease may cause myocarditis, Lyme titers should be obtained for a patient who presents with chest pain and a history of a tick bite in an endemic area. Other inflammatory causes of pericarditis include autoimmune disorders, such as lupus erythematosus.

Aortic and Subaortic Stenosis

A history of chest pain in a child who also has a significant murmur may suggest left ventricular outflow tract obstruction caused by aortic stenosis or subaortic stenosis. In these patients, chest pain may indicate ischemic pain. Pain occurs during exercise because the ability to increase cardiac output is limited by the left ventricular outflow obstruction. The limited cardiac output, coupled with a fall in systemic vascular resistance during exercise, results in coronary hypoperfusion and subsequent myocardial ischemia.

Physical findings in patients with aortic stenosis can include a systolic ejection click, a harsh systolic ejection murmur over the base of the heart that radiates to the carotid arteries, and frequently a palpable thrill in the suprasternal notch. These patients may have a normal ECG or an ECG that suggests left ventricular hypertrophy. A patient with a significant murmur and chest pain should be referred to a cardiologist for an echocardiogram.

Hypertrophic Cardiomyopathy

Another variation of left ventricular outflow tract obstruction is hypertrophic cardiomyopathy. Since hypertrophic cardiomyopathy can occur as an inherited autosomal dominant disorder, a thorough family history is helpful. These patients have a systolic murmur that is enhanced on standing or subjection to the Valsalva maneuver. These maneuvers decrease left ventricular volume and thus increase the degree of outflow obstruction.

Coronary Artery Anomalies

Anomalous left coronary artery is uncommon. Most patients with anomalous left coronary artery from the pulmonary artery present as infants in a shock-like state. The pulmonary artery pressure falls as the pulmonary vascular resistance falls during the neonatal period, resulting in a decreased coronary perfusion pressure into the anomalous left coronary artery. This may result in coronary artery hypoperfusion and myocardial ischemia. In children and adolescents with anomalous left coronary artery from the pulmonary artery, an anomalous insertion of the left coronary artery into the aorta may result in the coronary artery coursing between the great vessels or having an intramural course; this anatomy is associated with myocardial ischemia and sudden death. The key to diagnosis is a thorough history that reveals symptoms at peak exercise. The pathophysiology is related to inadequate coronary perfusion during exercise, by compression between the great vessels, relative ostial stenosis of the anomalous coronary artery, or coronary steal phenomenon from collateral coronary vessels connecting the right coronary and the anomalous left coronary artery attached to the pulmonary artery. When patients with an anomalous left coronary present, their ECG is often abnormal with evidence of left ventricular hypertrophy and abnormal ST segments or inverted T waves in the left precordial leads.

When a child or adolescent presents with chest pain, it is important to inquire about previous Kawasaki disease. Fifteen percent of patients with Kawasaki disease develop coronary artery aneurysms in the subacute phase of the illness about 3 to

6 weeks after diagnosis. Studies have reported up to 2% mortality in patients with Kawasaki disease occurring in the first few months after diagnosis resulting from myocardial infarction or arrhythmia. More than half of all aneurysms resolve spontaneously. Healing of the coronary artery aneurysms following the inflammatory phase may result in areas of stenosis. Similar to any coronary obstruction, myocardial flow reserve and perfusion is decreased during exercise. Therefore, chest pain in children and adolescents with a previous history of Kawasaki disease and coronary artery changes should be considered ischemic until proven otherwise.

Arrhythmia

Patients who present with symptoms of chest pain or chest pain and dizziness with or without syncope may experience arrhythmias. Younger children may perceive palpitations as chest pain, and the additional symptoms of dizziness or syncope suggest an arrhythmia and require evaluation. All patients suspected of having arrhythmias should have an ECG during initial evaluation. In addition to obtaining a rhythm strip to assess for rhythm disturbances, all baseline intervals should be assessed for heart block and for prolonged QTc syndrome. This interval can be prolonged secondary to electrolyte imbalance (hypocalcemia), medications (class I antiarrhythmics such as quinidine and procainamide, antidepressants, and antipsychotics), or due to the long QTc syndrome. Patients with prolonged QTc syndrome are prone to ventricular arrhythmias and should be referred to a cardiologist for further evaluation and therapy.

Sinus Arrhythmia

Arrhythmias can also present as isolated chest pain. In sinus arrhythmia, normal in children, the heart rate slows during inspiration because of increased venous filling of the heart and thus larger volume for cardiac output. Then, the heart rate increases during expiration because of the reduced venous return. School-aged children, who have increased body awareness, may perceive this arrhythmia as abnormal.

Supraventricular Arrhythmia

The most frequent pathologic arrhythmia in infancy and childhood has a supraventricular origin and may be perceived as chest pain in younger children. This includes premature atrial contractions and SVT. Patients who present to the emergency department with chest pain and tachycardia should first have a 12-lead ECG. Supraventricular and ventricular arrhythmia can generally be distinguished on the basis of the QRS and P-wave morphology and the rate of tachycardia. SVT is usually a narrow complex tachycardia with rates of approximately 200 beats per minute, depending on the age of the patient. For treatment strategies for SVT see Chapter 75, "Tachycardia."

Ventricular Arrhythmia

Patients with VT can also present with chest pain. VT generally is noted as a wide QRS tachycardia with a rate of 120 to 240 beats per minute, generally not as rapid as SVT for the same age range. When present, VT is a medical emergency because this rhythm can rapidly deteriorate into ventricular fibrillation. For treatment guidelines for VT see Chapter 75, "Tachycardia."

Mitral Valve Prolapse

MVP may also be associated with chest pain and is a common finding in adults. Its prevalence and clinical significance in pediatrics is controversial. In some studies, up to 15% of a normal population has MVP on echocardiography. In children, the incidence of MVP is ~6%. Although MVP is usually asymptomatic, a history of nonexertional chest pain, palpitation, and, rarely, syncope may be elicited. However, in the pediatric population, chest pain occurs equally in the normal population and in those with MVP.

The diagnosis of MVP is best made on physical examination and confirmed by echocardiography. Physical findings include a mid-to-late systolic click and possibly a short systolic murmur resulting from mild mitral regurgitation. The click is accentuated by standing or with the Valsalva maneuver, which both decrease ventricular filling and move the click from late to midsystole.

Patients suspected of MVP should be referred to a pediatric cardiologist for an echocardiogram to confirm the diagnosis. There is no longer a requirement for bacterial endocarditis prophylaxis in patients with MVP with mitral regurgitation. Because patients with MVP have a small but finite incidence of arrhythmias, patients with chest pain who are found to have MVP should be considered for a workup for an arrhythmia.

Aortic Root Dissection

When evaluating chest pain in patients with known or suspected connective tissue disease, the physician must consider aortic root dissection or rupture. The chest pain is unrelenting and becomes quite severe radiating through the back. Patients with aortic dissection may present with significant cardiorespiratory distress with signs of diminished cardiac output. Careful physical examination may reveal stigmata of Marfan syndrome or other connective tissue diseases.

Postpericardiotomy Syndrome

Postpericardiotomy syndrome, a frequent complication of open-heart surgery, is characterized by fever, chest pain, and pericardial and pleural effusions. These signs may develop 1 to 12 weeks after intracardiac surgery in ~30% of patients. Although the etiology of the syndrome is unknown, evidence points to a viral and/or autoimmune cause. Postpericardiotomy syndrome is diagnosed after excluding other conditions such as endocarditis and pneumonia. In many cases, the syndrome is self-limiting and occurs only once, but in other cases the symptoms may be recurrent. On physical examination, patients often demonstrate tachycardia and a pericardial friction rub. The pericardial rub disappears either with improvement or with further accumulation of pericardial fluid. Systemic fluid retention and hepatomegaly can also occur. Anti-inflammatory agents, such as salicylates and steroids, represent the most commonly used drugs. Although analgesics with codeine or oxycodone are important for the patient's symptomatic relief, early recognition of the syndrome is the key to limiting the discomfort and possible complications associated with this condition.

EVALUATION OF CHEST PAIN
Patient History
In all patients with a chief complaint of chest pain, it is important to elicit a thorough history of events surrounding the onset of chest pain as well as any aggravating and relieving factors. Important general questions define the type, location, duration, sequence of onset of the pain and association with activity, and syncope. Does the pain awaken the child from sleep? Further questions should be directed to separating out the specific organ system most responsible for the symptoms. Pain that worsens with respiration or deep breathing may suggest bronchospastic or pleuritic pain. Patients with an associated history of cough and fever are most likely to have pneumonic or bronchospastic chest pain. A pleural catch is a sharp sudden pain that limits respiration and can be relieved with a deep breath. Musculoskeletal chest pain can be produced with movement, should be well localized, and is reproducible by specific movement or palpation. Costochondritis produces pain on palpation of the costochondral joints. Gastrointestinal pain can be diffuse, is often pre- or postprandial, and may present as a deep or burning pain.

Physical Examination
The physical examination in the child with chest pain should include complete cardiac, respiratory, and upper body musculoskeletal examination. Vital signs should include blood pressure recordings from the right arm and at least one lower extremity. The heart rate and rhythm should be assessed. Is it regular or irregular? Is the respiratory effort normal? With reference to the cardiac examination, findings of a murmur, an irregular heart rate, or additional heart sounds other than S1 and a split S2 would warrant further investigation and may prompt referral to a pediatric cardiologist. Respiratory examination should be directed toward the symmetry of respiratory effort and the presence of abnormal sounds. The musculoskeletal system should be assessed for palpable abnormalities or pain on motion or palpation.

Laboratory Studies
If one is evaluating a child with a chief complaint of chest pain, and a specific diagnosis is not strongly suspected or confirmed by history and physical examination, then a PA and lateral CXR and a 12-lead ECG should be completed. If the history suggests an arrhythmia, then, in addition, a Holter monitor or a transtelephonic event monitor should be used depending on the frequency and duration of the arrhythmia.

APPROACH TO THE PATIENT
Chest pain is a common complaint in the pediatric age group, but the incidence of heart disease in this group is low. The diagnostic approach is to pursue

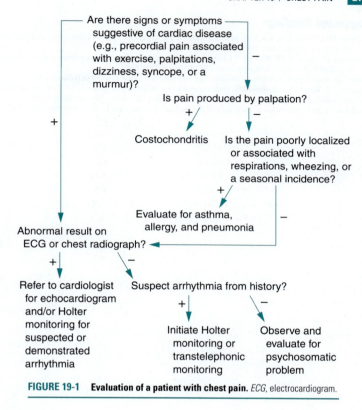

FIGURE 19-1 **Evaluation of a patient with chest pain.** *ECG,* electrocardiogram.

associated signs or symptoms suggestive of cardiac disease (Figure 19-1). These include:

- A history suggestive of myocarditis, such as a recent viral illness, fever, and malaise
- Suspicion of arrhythmia
- Syncope with chest pain
- ECG abnormalities
- Cardiomegaly on CXR
- A significant cardiac murmur

If any of these findings are present with chest pain, further investigation and referral to a pediatric cardiologist are warranted. In patients with respiratory-type chest pain, especially pain brought on by exercise or that limits exercise, referral to a pediatric pulmonologist may be useful to establish a diagnosis of exercise-induced asthma. In the asymptomatic child with a normal ECG and CXR, close observation without referral is appropriate.

Suggested Readings

Drossner DM, Hirsh DA, Sturm JJ, et al. Cardiac disease in pediatric patients presenting to a pediatric ED with chest pain. *Am J Emerg Med.* 2011;29(6):632–638.

Hambrook JT, Kimball TR, Khoury P, Cnota J. Disparities exist in the emergency department evaluation of pediatric chest pain. *Congenit Heart Dis.* 2010;5(3):285–291.

Reddy SR, Singh HR. Chest pain in children and adolescents. *Pediatr Rev.* 2010;31(1):e1–e9.

Sivarajan VB, Vetter VL, Gleason MM. Pediatric evaluation of the cardiac patient. In: VL Vetter, ed. *Pediatric Cardiology: The Requisites in Pediatrics.* Philadelphia, PA: Mosby Elsevier; 2006:1–30.

Thull-Freedman J. Evaluation of chest pain in the pediatric patient. *Clin N Am.* 2010;94(2):327–347.

Child Abuse

INTRODUCTION

Physicians are responsible for **identifying cases of suspected abuse and reporting them** to the proper authorities for investigation. Diagnosing physical abuse can be challenging. The history provided is often misleading, and the injuries may not be pathognomonic. The presentation varies according to the injury sustained. Possible presentations include single or multiple injuries, unusual or unexplained bruising, a change in mental status, an acute life-threatening event (ALTE), respiratory distress, an inability to use an extremity, nonspecific complaints of gastrointestinal disease, and unexpected cardiorespiratory arrest.

 DIFFERENTIAL DIAGNOSIS LIST

Child abuse injuries can result in various physical findings that are also observed in children with physical diseases.

Infectious Diseases
- Meningitis
- Sepsis
- Osteomyelitis
- Congenital syphilis
- Dermatitis herpetiformis
- Impetigo
- Staphylococcal scalded skin syndrome
- Erysipelas
- Purpura fulminans
- Disseminated intravascular coagulation

Metabolic or Genetic Diseases
- Osteogenesis imperfecta
- Ehlers–Danlos syndrome
- Scurvy
- Rickets
- Glutaric aciduria type I
- Copper deficiency
- Menkes disease

Congenital or Vascular Diseases
- Congenital indifference to pain
- Unusual skeletal variants
- Arteriovenous malformation
- Aneurysm
- Arachnoid cyst
- Vasculitis (e.g., Henoch-Schönlein purpura)

Hematologic Diseases and Disorders of Coagulation
- Idiopathic thrombocytopenic purpura
- Leukemia
- Vitamin K deficiency
- Hemophilia
- von Willebrand disease

- Hemophagocytic lymphohistiocytosis
- Liver disease resulting in coagulopathy
- Disseminated intravascular coagulation
- Factor deficiencies

Dermatologic Disorders
- Mongolian spots
- Epidermolysis bullosa
- Erythema multiforme

- Contact dermatitis, including phytophotodermatitis
- Cultural practices—*cao gio* (coining), cupping, and moxibustion

Neoplastic Disorders
- Brain tumor

Miscellaneous Disorders
- Benign external hydrocephalus

COMMON PRESENTATIONS
Bruises
Differential Diagnosis
Abuse should be suspected in a child with a given history of minor trauma who has extensive bruises or bruises on multiple body planes. Bruises that are in different stages of resolution, centrally located, or patterned (e.g., loop marks, finger marks, belt marks) also suggest abuse. Bruises in young infants who are not yet cruising are highly suspicious.

Many conditions can mimic inflicted bruises:

- **Accidental bruises** are usually found over bony prominences and are distally located. They are few to moderate in number.
- **Mongolian spots,** most commonly found in infants with dark complexions, are often located over the buttocks and lower back (but may be found in other locations).
- **Hematologic disorders** (e.g., idiopathic thrombocytopenic purpura, leukemia, vitamin K deficiency, coagulopathies, disseminated intravascular coagulation). Children with coagulopathies can have bruising that varies from mild to severe. The distribution of bruises in children with a bleeding diathesis should not be isolated to unusual locations.
- **Dermatologic disorders** (e.g., erythema multiforme, contact dermatitis, including phytophotodermatitis from lime or lemon juice) can be associated with or resemble bruises.
- **Cultural practices** can also be associated with patterned bruises (e.g., coining). It is useful to be familiar with the cultural practices of subpopulations in the community.
- **Genetic diseases** (e.g., Ehlers–Danlos syndrome, osteogenesis imperfecta) are usually associated with other physical stigmata.
- **Henoch-Schönlein purpura** is associated with lesions that are typically located on the buttocks and legs; in addition, joint, abdominal, renal, or (less commonly) central nervous system (CNS) manifestations are present.

Evaluation
If child abuse is suspected, the **size, location, shape, and color of the bruises** should be **carefully documented.**

When a bleeding diathesis is suspected, a complete blood cell (CBC) count with platelet count, a prothrombin time, a partial thromboplastin time (PTT), and a von Willebrand panel serve as initial screens. Additional testing will vary depending on the clinical scenario. Consultation with a pediatric hematologist is recommended for further evaluation.

Treatment

Most bruises require **no specific treatment** and resolve over days to weeks, depending on their size. Severe beatings, especially over the buttocks or thighs, can result in **myoglobinuria and acute renal failure**. Myoglobinuria is treated with **hydration**.

Burns

Differential Diagnosis

Abusive burns are **most common in infants and toddlers**. Some burn patterns (e.g., immersion burns) are highly specific for inflicted injury. **Immersion burns** are associated with toilet accidents or other behaviors (e.g., vomiting) that require "cleaning" the child. The pattern of burn distribution often identifies the cause—the feet, lower legs, buttocks, and genitals are burned with clear lines of demarcation, but the knees, upper legs, and other parts of the body that were not submerged are spared.

Many conditions can mimic abusive burns:

- **Accidental burns** include burns from hot liquid spills, burns resulting from contact with a clothes iron or curling iron, car-seat buckle burns, chemical burns, and sunburns. Accidental burns are common pediatric injuries, and most pediatric burns are accidental. The history should be compatible with the distribution and severity of the burn.
- **Infection** (e.g., staphylococcal scalded skin syndrome, impetigo, erysipelas) may be associated with fever and an ill appearance. Impetigo can be misidentified as cigarette burns.
- **Cultural rituals** may be associated with burn-like lesions.
- **Ingestions**. Buttocks burns have been described after the ingestion of senna-containing laxatives.

Evaluation

Record areas of **partial and full-thickness burns** on an **anatomic chart and calculate the percentage of body area burned** using age-appropriate estimates (see Chapter 76, "Thermal Injury"). Additional injuries should be sought. Children aged **<2 years** with suspicious burns should have a **skeletal survey** to assess for occult skeletal trauma.

Treatment

Detailed treatment recommendations are provided in Chapter 76, "Thermal Injury."

Fractures

Differential Diagnosis

Although most pediatric fractures are accidental, abuse should be suspected when **unexplained fractures** are identified. Virtually any bone can be injured in cases of child abuse, and no single type of fracture is diagnostic of abuse.

The following are the most commonly seen skeletal injuries:

- **Diaphyseal fractures** are the most common type of fracture in both abusive and accidental trauma cases. This type of fracture should cause more concern for abuse in nonambulatory infants.
- **Spiral fractures** are associated with twisting of the limb. These fractures are often accidental in ambulatory toddlers and children. They should cause more concern for abuse in young infants, especially if the humerus or femur is involved.
- **Metaphyseal fractures** are subtle injuries, most commonly identified by a skeletal survey. These fractures are sometimes associated with abusive head trauma. Although metaphyseal fractures are highly suspicious for abuse, the possibility of healing rickets or congenital syphilis should be considered. These fractures are difficult to date radiographically and usually heal without casting. They are sometimes not visible acutely and may be better identified by a follow-up skeletal survey 2 to 3 weeks after initial presentation.
- **Rib fractures** are common with abusive head trauma and are seen in infants and young children in association with abuse. Only rarely do they result from direct blows to the chest, minor accidental trauma, cardiopulmonary resuscitation, and metabolic bone diseases. Multiple, bilateral, posterior fractures are very specific for child abuse. Rib fractures are difficult to identify acutely, and oblique views of the chest may improve detection of subtle fractures.
- **Skull fractures** may be accidental. In cases of severe abuse, they may be associated with severe CNS injury. Complex, multiple, bilateral fractures are more common in abused children, although none are independently diagnostic of abuse.
- **Other fracture areas** include the clavicle, vertebrae, pelvis, and face (i.e., the mandible, maxilla, or zygoma).

In addition to accidental and inflicted trauma, other causes of fractures must be considered:

- **Birth trauma**. Fractures of the clavicle, humerus, or femur are occasionally seen with difficult or emergency deliveries, large infants, or breech presentations. By 2 weeks of age, birth fractures should show radiographic signs of healing. Rib fractures are rare, but well described in the literature, and they are usually seen in large newborns.
- **Physiologic periosteal changes**. Periosteal new bone formation of the long bones (which is seen with healing fractures) may also represent a physiologic process. Physiologic periosteal changes involve multiple bones, are symmetric, and are typically seen in the first 2 to 3 months of life. They should not be associated with fracture lines.
- **Osteogenesis imperfecta**. Most forms of osteogenesis imperfecta are identifiable on the basis of the patient history, the family history, and the physical examination. Type IV osteogenesis imperfecta is most apt to be confused with abuse. Blue sclerae, hearing impairment, dentinogenesis imperfecta, wormian bones, osteopenia, hypermobility of joints, easy bruising, short stature, a tendency toward bowing and angulation of healed fractures, and progressive scoliosis suggest osteogenesis

imperfecta. Definitive diagnosis is made by biochemical analysis of cultured skin fibroblasts or DNA analysis.

- **Congenital syphilis.** The osteochondritis, epiphysitis, and periostitis of congenital syphilis can mimic the metaphyseal fractures and periosteal new bone formation associated with child abuse. Pseudoparalysis of affected limbs and swelling and tenderness of the ends of involved bones suggest the diagnosis of syphilis. In addition, other manifestations are often present. Syphilis can be diagnosed by serologic testing.
- **Rickets.** Vitamin D deficiency, renal and hepatic disease, certain medications (e.g., antacids, anticonvulsants, furosemide), and some rare diseases cause rickets, which predisposes bones to fractures. The diagnosis of rickets depends on clinical suspicion, laboratory data (i.e., calcium, phosphorus, alkaline phosphatase, PTH and vitamin D levels) and radiographic evaluation.
- **Osteomyelitis** is usually diagnosed on the basis of the patient's history, physical examination, C-reactive protein, erythrocyte sedimentation rate, and results of blood or bone aspirate cultures.

Evaluation

The evaluation for suspected fractures usually involves obtaining **skeletal radiographs**. A **skeletal survey** is used to **detect occult or healing fractures** and is recommended for **all children aged <2 years** who have injuries suspicious for abuse. The skeletal survey is a less sensitive test in children aged 2 to 5 years and is not generally a useful study in children aged >5 years.

Treatment

Most fractures require **casting**. Some (e.g., **rib fractures, metaphyseal fractures**) usually **do not require specific treatment**.

Abdominal Trauma

Abusive abdominal injuries are uncommon, although they are **underrecognized and underreported**. Severe abdominal trauma is the **second leading cause of death as a result of abuse**. Injuries are usually caused by **blunt trauma** and most often affect the liver and small intestine.

Differential Diagnosis

The **history** is almost always **misleading**. Children who have suffered abdominal trauma as a result of abuse may present with **nonspecific complaints** related to the **gastrointestinal tract** (e.g., bilious vomiting, abdominal pain, anorexia), complaints associated with **peritonitis** (e.g., fever, abdominal pain, lethargy), or **unexplained cardiorespiratory arrest** (as a result of blood loss or sepsis). Approximately 50% of victims have no **external soft tissue evidence** of abdominal injury. Children with minor injuries can be **asymptomatic** yet have laboratory evidence of trauma. The following conditions must be ruled out:

- **Accidental trauma.** Victims of accidental abdominal trauma tend to be older with injuries to a single solid organ. These accidental injuries occur more often outside the home.

- **Infection.** Gastroenteritis, peritonitis from a perforated viscus, hepatitis, pancreatitis, and appendicitis must be ruled out.
- **Metabolic/Genetic.** Ehlers–Danlos syndrome can cause spontaneous intestinal perforation.

Evaluation

A simple **hematologic workup** can be used to screen physically abused children for associated abdominal trauma and may reveal abdominal trauma in asymptomatic children. A CBC, liver function tests, amylase and lipase levels, and urinalysis are recommended. **Abdominal imaging** is recommended for children with significantly abnormal laboratory results.

Treatment

Solid organ injuries, unless severe, are **managed conservatively** and usually do not require surgery. **Hollow viscus tears and severe solid organ injuries** require **surgery**. The outcome is generally favorable if the child survives the acute injury.

Head Trauma and Shaking-Impact Syndrome

Head injury, either as a result of blunt trauma, shaking with sudden deceleration forces, or both, is the **leading cause of mortality and morbidity from child physical abuse**. Victims of inflicted head injury are most **often infants and toddlers**. Older children who die of CNS injury more often have signs of blunt impact to the head.

Differential Diagnosis

Children with head trauma as a result of abuse often present with a **change in mental status, respiratory distress, irritability, lethargy, seizures, ALTE,** or an **increasing head circumference**. Variable degrees of **cerebral edema** may be present initially. The following disorders could also account for these findings and need to be ruled out:

- **Accidental trauma** (e.g., motor vehicle accidents, falls out of windows). Common childhood falls (e.g., falls down the stairs or from the couch or changing table) rarely result in life-threatening head injury.
- **Infection.** Sepsis and meningitis can be differentiated on the basis of the history, physical examination findings, and culture results. Bloody cerebrospinal fluid may be caused by lumbar puncture technique or a subarachnoid hemorrhage. In the latter case, the amount of blood in the fluid does not change significantly from the beginning to the end of the procedure.
- **Gastroesophageal reflux disease,** central or obstructive apnea, and **inborn errors of metabolism** can be associated with ALTE but are usually distinguished from abuse by a lack of associated traumatic findings. Some physicians advocate a retinal examination as a screen for head trauma in infants who present with ALTEs.
- **Intracranial vascular anomalies** (e.g., arteriovenous malformation, ruptured aneurysm, arachnoid cysts) are usually identified by magnetic resonance imaging (MRI) scan but may not be evident immediately after they hemorrhage.

- **Glutaric aciduria type I,** a rare inborn error of amino acid metabolism, can present with acute encephalopathy and chronic subdural hematomas in infancy. Skeletal or other injuries should not be found. Retinal hemorrhages can be seen. Diagnosis is made by metabolic screening tests.
- **Coagulopathy.** Some hematologic disorders, including factor deficiencies, can lead to spontaneous intracranial hemorrhage. In addition, liver disease, acquired platelet disorders, and other primary hematologic diseases can result in intracranial bleeding.

Evaluation

External physical injuries can be absent and do not rule out the diagnosis of abusive head trauma. **Subtle bruises** may be of significance and should be documented. A **computed tomography (CT) scan** of the brain shows **subdural hemorrhage**. MRI is recommended for all infants with suspected intracranial injuries from abuse. For infants with suspected abusive head trauma, a **complete ophthalmologic examination and skeletal survey** are essential.

Treatment

Treatment is aimed at **maintaining cerebral perfusion and limiting cerebral edema**. For severely injured children, intubation and intracranial pressure monitoring may be indicated. Despite aggressive therapy, children with severe injuries often have **poor outcomes**.

Munchausen by Proxy Syndrome

In Munchausen by proxy syndrome, the **parent fabricates or causes a child's illness**. The child is repeatedly presented for medical care, and the parent denies knowing the cause of the "disease." Acute symptoms abate when the parent is separated from the child. Common complaints include apnea, ALTE, gastrointestinal bleeding, hematuria, seizures, recurrent fevers, or recurrent infections.

Diagnosing Munchausen by proxy syndrome requires **eliminating** with reasonable accuracy any **diseases** that may account for the reported symptoms. **Delays are almost universal** because the **perpetrator** (usually the mother) commonly **appears devoted and capable**. The perpetrator is usually alone with the child at the onset of symptoms. The **history** of the acute illness is **often much more severe than the findings** on physical examination.

EVALUATION OF CHILD ABUSE
Patient History

Although many victims of child physical abuse are preverbal, older abused children can often provide a history of abuse, and efforts should be made to **interview an older child alone**. Certain factors in the history given by the caregiver raise the suspicion of abuse:

- A history of trauma that does not correlate with the injuries sustained
- A history that specifically denies trauma to a child with obvious injuries
- A history of injury that does not correlate with the child's development (i.e., the child is developmentally incapable of injuring himself in the manner described)

- A history that changes as more injuries are discovered
- An unexpected or unexplained delay in seeking treatment

Physical Examination

Emphasis should be placed on **detecting subtle signs of injury, neglect, or alternative diagnoses**. Some injury constellations are pathognomonic of abuse. In these cases, the diagnosis can be made even in the absence of a history. The following areas should be covered in the physical examination:

- **Growth.** Plot all growth parameters and compare with previous points if possible.
- **Skin.** Describe any bruises, burns, scars, or rashes in detail (i.e., size, location, pattern, color). The precise location of burns should be noted, including small splash marks, lines of demarcation, and identifiable patterns. Photographs are often used to document injuries but should not replace careful documentation because they may not accurately reflect the characteristics of the injuries.
- **Head.** Palpate for areas of swelling or bogginess, for stepoffs or depressions overlying fractures, and for cephalohematomas. Inspect the scalp for avulsed hair and bruises. Scalp bruising is often difficult to see because of the overlying hair.
- **Ears.** Look for bruises on the pinna. Battle sign (caused by a basilar skull fracture) may be noted. Examine the middle ear for blood behind the tympanic membrane.
- **Eyes.** Note edema, scleral hemorrhage, hyphema, and bruises. A funduscopic examination is essential for infants or young toddlers with suspected CNS injury, which requires an examination by an ophthalmologist.
- **Mouth and oropharynx.** Examine for evidence of trauma. Frenulum lacerations are pathognomonic of child abuse in young infants. Examine the teeth for trauma and caries.
- **Chest.** Feel for evidence of healing rib fractures.
- **Heart and lungs.** Assess for tachycardia, which may be a sign of acute blood loss.
- **Abdomen.** Assess for signs of trauma, including bruising, abdominal tenderness, guarding, and rebound tenderness.
- **Back.** Look for bruises and unusual midline masses, which can represent vertebral injuries.
- **Genitalia, anus, and rectum.** Assess for signs of trauma (see Chapter 69, "Sexual Abuse").
- **Extremities.** Assess for soft tissue swelling, point tenderness, and function.
- **Neurologic examination,** including rating of the patient according to the Glasgow coma scale, is especially indicated for children with suspected head trauma.

Laboratory Studies

The following laboratory studies may be appropriate:

- **Hematologic evaluation.** A CBC with platelet count, prothrombin time, and partial thromboplastin time are indicated for children who present with bleeding or bruising. A von Willebrand panel is sometimes included in the screening process. Additional studies may be needed, and consultation with a hematologist is recommended.

- **Toxicology screens** are indicated for infants or children with unexplained neurologic symptoms (e.g., seizures, lethargy, altered mental status, coma). Standard toxicologic screens vary.
- **Aspartate aminotransferase, alanine aminotransferase, amylase, and/or lipase levels** may be elevated with acute liver or pancreatic injury and are recommended for acutely injured young children in whom the abdominal examination may not be a sensitive indicator of injury.
- **Urinalysis** is performed as a screen for renal or bladder trauma, and it can also detect myoglobinuria and hemoglobinuria. Abused children occasionally develop myoglobinuria as a result of severe muscle injury. Urinalysis shows blood by dipstick but no red blood cells microscopically. An elevated creatine phosphokinase level supports the diagnosis of myoglobinuria and muscle injury in these patients.
- **Bone Health Labs.** For children with fractures, calcium, phosphorus, and alkaline phosphatase can screen for underlying bone disease. 25-Hydroxyvitamin D and PTH levels may also be used.

Diagnostic Imaging Studies

The following studies are commonly ordered for children with suspected abuse-related injuries:

- A **roentgenographic skeletal survey** is indicated for all infants and children <2 years who are suspected of being physically abused. Repeated surveys done 2 to 3 weeks after initial presentation often yield additional injuries and is recommended.
- A **radionuclide bone scan** is sensitive for detecting rib fractures that are <7 to 10 days old, subtle diaphyseal fractures, and early periosteal elevation. This test is most often performed when the skeletal survey is negative but the physician still suspects abuse.
- A **CT scan** is the method of choice for diagnosing acute intracranial, pulmonary, and solid abdominal organ injuries in a seriously injured child. Significant elevations of aspartate aminotransferase and alanine aminotransferase should be evaluated with an abdominal CT scan.
- **MRI scan** is required in cases of abusive head trauma, although in most centers, is not the initial imaging study performed. MRI provides a more thorough evaluation of intracranial injury than CT.

TREATMENT OF CHILD ABUSE

Medical treatment is guided by the diagnosed injuries. Hospitalization is required for patients with serious injuries or illnesses from abuse. Occasionally, patients require **hospitalization if a safe environment cannot be guaranteed** at the time of initial diagnosis.

APPROACH TO THE PATIENT

All cases of *suspected* (not proven) **physical abuse** must be **reported to Child Protective Services** (if abuse is committed by a household member or caretaker), **law enforcement officials** (when the injuries are serious or involve a person outside the home), **or both** (Figure 20-1).

The criteria for reporting suspected child physical abuse depends on the history, examination, and laboratory findings. In some cases, the **injuries alone** are so suggestive of abuse that historical and laboratory data are not needed to reach the threshold for reporting. In other cases, the decision to report is reached only after **considering all factors**. Each state has laws that define child physical abuse, and physicians should be **aware of the laws that apply** in their state of practice.

Figure 20-2 provides a basic approach to initiating the civil and criminal investigation of suspected abuse. Individual state and institutional policies vary and may differ from this general approach. Each case must be weighed individually, with the **safety and well-being of the child** always central to the decision to report.

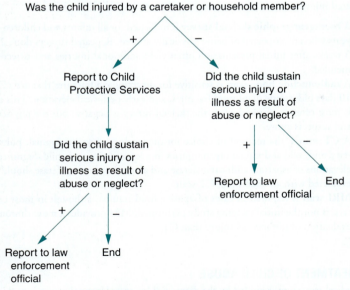

FIGURE 20-1   Reporting child abuse to officials.

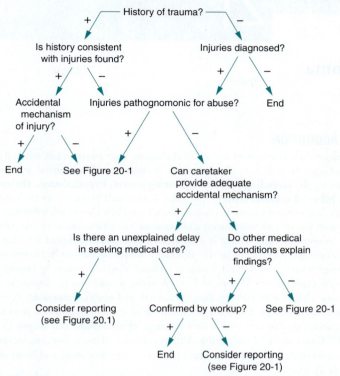

FIGURE 20-2   Approach to initiating the civil and criminal investigation of suspected abuse.

Suggested Readings

American Academy of Pediatrics Committee on Child Abuse and Neglect. Evaluation of suspected child physical abuse. *Pediatrics.* 2007;119:1232–41.

American Academy of Pediatrics Committee on Child Abuse and Neglect. Beyond Munchausen syndrome by proxy: identification and treatment of child abuse in a medical setting. *Pediatrics.* 2007;119:1026–1030.

American Academy of Pediatrics Committee on Child Abuse and Neglect. Abusive head trauma in infant and children. *Pediatrics.* 2009;123:1409–1411.

American Academy of Pediatrics Committee on Child Abuse and Neglect; the Section on Adoption and Foster Care; the American Academy of Child and Adolescent Psychiatry. Understanding the behavioral and emotional consequences of child abuse. *Pediatrics.* 2008;122:667–673.

American Academy of Pediatrics Section on Radiology. Diagnostic imaging of child abuse. *Pediatrics.* 2009;123:1430–1435.

Cooper A, Floyd TF, Barlow B, et al. Major blunt abdominal trauma due to child abuse. *J Trauma.* 1988;28:1483–1486.

Jenny C, Hymel K, Ritzen A, et al. Analysis of missed cases of abusive head trauma. *JAMA.* 1999;281:621–626.

Nimkin K, Kleinman PK. Imaging of child abuse. *Radiol Clin N Am.* 2001;39(4):843–864.

Purdue GF, Hunt JL, Prescott PR. Child abuse by burning—an index of suspicion. *J Trauma.* 1988;28:221–224.

Reece R, Christian CW, eds. *Child Abuse Medical Diagnosis and Management.* 3rd ed. Elk Grove Village, IL: American Academy of Pediatrics; 2008.

21

Nicholas S. Abend

Coma

INTRODUCTION

Consciousness is a state of arousal (wakefulness) with awareness of self and surroundings. Arousal is mediated by the brainstem and subcortical structures, including the **ascending reticular activating system, hypothalamus, thalamus, and bilateral cerebral cortex**. Awareness is mediated primarily by the cerebral cortex, but requires subcortical connections. Coma is a state of altered consciousness with loss of both wakefulness and awareness and characterized by an unarousable unresponsiveness. Coma is a temporary state that is followed by return of consciousness, progression to the minimally conscious state or vegetative state, or progression to brain death. Coma is a clinical diagnosis, made by history and physical examination. History and examination, in addition to diagnostic testing, may elucidate an etiology, direct treatment, and establish prognosis. Between normal consciousness and coma is a spectrum of states of diminished consciousness, subdivided by convention into **lethargy, obtundation, and stupor** (Table 21-1). Coma must be distinguished from delirium, akinetic mutism, locked-in syndrome, minimally conscious state, persistent vegetative state, and brain death (Table 21-2).

> **HINT:** Coma is not a specific disease but is a sign of profound nervous system dysfunction. Depression of consciousness suggests dysfunction of both cerebral hemispheres or that of the reticular activating system of the brainstem.

DIFFERENTIAL DIAGNOSIS LIST

- Traumatic brain injury
- Parenchymal injury (contusions and diffuse axonal injury)
  - Intracranial hemorrhage
  - Epidural hematoma
  - Subdural hematoma
  - Subarachnoid hemorrhage
  - Intracerebral hematoma
- Cerebral edema
- Acute hydrocephalus
- Anoxic ischemic encephalopathy
- Vascular
  - Intracranial hemorrhage
  - Arterial ischemic infract
- Venous sinus thromboses
- Vasculitis

TABLE 21-1	States of Altered Consciousness
Lethargy	Reduced wakefulness, deficits in attention
Obtundation	Blunted alertness, diminished interaction with environment
Stupor	Unresponsiveness with little/no spontaneous movement resembling deep sleep; temporary arousal with vigorous stimulation
Coma	Unarousable unresponsiveness

TABLE 21-2	Coma and Other Disease States of Altered Consciousness
Coma	Arousal and awareness are absent. Sleep/wake cycles are absent. Movements are reflexive and are not purposeful or reproducible. The EEG generally demonstrates diffuse slowing. It is a temporary state that evolves into other states.
Vegetative state	Arousal is present but awareness is absent. Sleep/wake cycles are present. Brainstem and hypothalamic function is sufficiently intact to allow prolonged survival with care. Movements are reflex and are not purposeful or reproducible. The EEG generally demonstrates diffuse slowing. It is considered permanent if it lasts more than 12 mo after traumatic brain injury or 3 mo after nontraumatic brain injury.
Minimally conscious state	Arousal is present and there is partial awareness consisting of minimal but definite behavioral evidence of self or environmental awareness such as following simple commands, making verbalizations, making simple nonreflexive gestures, or reacting appropriately to emotional content of stimuli. A sleep/wake cycle is present. The EEG may contain mild slowing or may be normal. Distinguishing a minimally conscious state from a vegetative state often requires a multidisciplinary team using a responsiveness program.
Akinetic mutism	Both arousal and awareness are present but there is extreme slowing or absence of bodily movement loss and slowed cognition. Sleep/wake cycles are present. The EEG demonstrates diffuse slowing. Caused by damage to bilateral inferior frontal lobes, extensive bihemispheric disease, lesions of the paramedian mesencephalic reticular formation, or posterior diencephalon.
Locked-in syndrome	A state of preserved arousal and awareness, intact sleep/wake cycles, and normal EEG activity with complete paralysis of voluntary muscles. If due to severe neuromuscular disease (e.g., botulism, Guillain–Barre syndrome, neuromuscular blocking medications), then no movement occurs. If due to damage to the corticospinal and corticobulbar pathways below the level of the midbrain, then vertical eye movements may be preserved.
Brain death	Permanent absence of all brain activity, including brainstem function.
Delirium (acute confusional state)	Characterized by impaired attention, fluctuating level of consciousness, disorganization, perceptual disturbances, and increased or decreased psychomotor activity. Recall problems and disorientation are found on examination. It is often associated with acute metabolic, toxic, or endocrine disturbances but may also occur with focal lesions (especially frontal) and seizures.

- Infections/postinfectious/inflammatory
  - Meningitis and encephalitis: bacterial, viral, rickettsial, and fungal
  - Acute demyelinating diseases
    - Acute disseminated encephalomyelitis (ADEM)
    - Multiple sclerosis
    - Acute leukodystrophy
- Inflammatory/autoimmune
  - Sarcoidosis
  - Sjogren syndrome
  - Lupus cerebritis
- Abscess
- Granuloma
- Acute metabolic derangement
  - Hypoglycemia
  - Hyperglycemia (diabetic ketoacidosis and non-ketotic hyperosmolar)
  - Hyponatremia or hypernatremia
  - Hypercalcemia
  - Addison disease
  - Hypothyroidism or panhypopituitarism
  - Uremic coma
  - Hepatic coma
  - Hypercapnia
  - Hyperbilirubinemia

- Cofactors: thiamine, niacin, and pyridoxine
- Inborn errors of metabolism
- Urea cycle disorders
- Amino acidopathies
- Organic acidopathies
- Mitochondrial disorders
- Neoplastic
  - Lymphoma
  - Gliomatosis cerebri
  - Multiple metastases
  - CNS neoplasm causing compression or hydrocephalus or within brain stem
- Toxins
  - Medications: narcotics, sedatives, antiepileptics, antidepressants, analgesics, and aspirin
  - Environmental toxins: organophosphates, heavy metals, cyanide, and mushroom poisoning
  - Illicit substances: alcohol, heroine, amphetamines, and cocaine
- Paroxysmal neurologic disorders
  - Seizures/status epilepticus
  - Acute confusional migraine
- Intussusception
- Psychogenic unresponsiveness

EVALUATION OF COMA

History, physical examination, and diagnostic testing are essential in determining coma etiology so that specific therapies may be instituted. Initial efforts **must identify reversible causes of coma** and normalize vital functions in order to prevent secondary brain injury. An initial approach is listed in Table 21-3. Recent guidelines have also been published online (see "Suggested Readings").

History

History taking should include a detailed description of events leading to the onset of coma, with particular attention to **timing, exposures, and accompanying symptoms**. **Rapidly developing somnolence** suggests a metabolic, toxic, or infectious etiology. **Sudden onset of coma without trauma** suggests spontaneous intracranial hemorrhage or seizure. **Slowly progressive loss of consciousness** suggests hydrocephalus, expanding mass lesion, or indolent infection. **Preceding headache** with positional changes or with Valsalva maneuver suggests increased

TABLE 21-3	**Initial Evaluation of Coma**

- Airway, breathing, and circulation assessment and stabilization.
  - Ensure adequate ventilation and oxygenation.
  - Blood pressure management depends on considerations regarding underlying coma etiology. If hypertensive encephalopathy or intracranial hemorrhage, then lower blood pressure. If perfusion-dependent state such as some strokes or elevated intracranial pressure (ICP), then reducing blood pressure may reduce cerebral perfusion.
  - Identify and treat hypoglycemia (thiamine may be given first in adult patients).
- Draw blood: Consider electrolytes, ammonia, arterial blood gas, liver and renal function tests, complete blood count, lactate, pyruvate, and toxicology screen.
- Neurological assessment.
  - GCS score.
  - Assess for evidence of raised ICP and herniation.
  - Assess for abnormalities suggesting focal neurologic disease.
  - Assess for history or signs of seizures.
- If there is concern for infection and LP must be delayed, then provide broad-spectrum infection coverage (including bacterial, viral, and possibly fungal).
- Give specific antidotes if toxic exposures are known.
  - For opiate overdose administer naloxone.
  - For benzodiazepine overdose consider administering flumazenil.
  - For anticholinergic overdose consider administering physostigmine.
- Identify and treat critical elevations in ICP.
  - Neutral head position, elevated head by 20–30 degrees, sedation.
  - Hyperosmolar therapy with mannitol 0.5–1 g/kg or hypertonic saline.
  - Hyperventilation as temporary measure.
  - Consider intracranial monitoring.
  - Consider neurosurgical intervention.
- Head CT (noncontrast).
- Treat seizures with IV anticonvulsants. Consider prophylactic anticonvulsants.
- Investigate source of fever and use antipyretics and/or cooling devices to reduce cerebral metabolic demands.
- Detailed history and examination.
- Consider: lumbar puncture, EEG or extended long-term EEG monitoring, magnetic resonance imaging, metabolic testing (amino acids, organic acids, acylcarnitine profile), autoimmune testing (ANA panel, anti-thyroid antibodies), thyroid testing (TSH, T3, T4).

intracranial pressure (ICP) from hydrocephalus or mass lesion. **Headache with neck pain** or stiffness suggests meningeal irritation from inflammation, infection, or hemorrhage. **Fever** suggests infection, but its absence does not rule it out, particularly in infants under 3 to 6 months of age or in immunocompromised children. **Recent fevers or illness** suggests an autoimmune process like ADEM. **Abnormal movements** or a fluctuating mental status may suggest nonconvulsive seizures or post-ictal state. Questions about possible toxic ingestions should include a survey of **medications and poisons in the home** and environment, even if not readily accessible to the child. **Travel history** may explain exposure to infections prevalent in certain areas, such as Lyme in the northeastern United States; insect bite history is also helpful but may be misleading. Recent **exposure to kittens** in a comatose child with axillary or inguinal lymphadenopathy may be a clue to infection with *Bartonella henselae* (cat scratch encephalopathy). A history of recurrent abdominal pain may suggest **intussusception**.

Eliciting a **history of trauma,** whether accidental or nonaccidental, is crucial and understanding the mechanism of injury can direct further investigation. Delay of hours between trauma and loss of consciousness can be seen with epidural hematoma. Discordance between the history of trivial trauma and the findings of extensive injury or delay in seeking treatment should raise suspicion of **child abuse**.

The child's **past medical history** may provide valuable information. Prior episodes of unexplained coma suggest intermittent metabolic disease, recurrent toxic ingestions, or **Munchausen by proxy syndrome**. Developmental delay and pre-existing neurological abnormalities may suggest inborn errors of metabolism, but are also independent risk factors for epilepsy, thus raising suspicion of a prolonged post-ictal state. Recent weight changes or other constitutional abnormalities suggest endocrine dysfunction or an oncologic process. In a child with known cardiac disease, circulatory collapse and hypoxic ischemic encephalopathy should be considered.

Examination

The **Glasgow coma scale** (GCS) is a reproducible way to rate any patient with altered consciousness using three areas of response to stimuli, eye opening, verbal response, and motor response, and has been adapted for use in children (Table 21-4). Often, intubation and mechanical ventilation are indicated in a child with deteriorating mental status whose GCS is ≤8.

> **HINT:** Initial evaluation must focus on the usual ABCs of resuscitation since abnormalities may result in secondary brain injury.

General examination should be directed toward uncovering clues to the etiology of coma and to the sequelae of nervous system dysfunction, starting with **vital sign** abnormalities. Hypotension, whether from sepsis, cardiac dysfunction (which may be primary or secondary to severe neurological injury), or toxic ingestion, may lead to poor cerebral perfusion, resulting in diffuse hypoxic ischemic injury. Hypotension may also occur with Addison disease, hypothyroidism, sepsis, or systemic hemorrhage. Hypertension is seen with increased ICP as a physiologic response to maintain cerebral perfusion pressure. Hypertension with bradycardia and a change in respirations (**Cushing's triad**) is a sign of impending brain herniation (see below). Hypertension in the setting of coma may also be the product of a nonspecific sympathetic response or ingestion of stimulants such as amphetamines, cocaine, and hallucinogens. Severe hypertensive encephalopathy (posterior reversible leukoencephalopathy syndrome) can cause visual changes, seizures with prolonged post-ictal state, or coma. Differentiating reactive or compensatory hypertension from a primary hypertensive encephalopathy is essential in guiding blood pressure management. **Respiratory patterns** may be of some localizing value in patients with primary central nervous system abnormalities (Table 21-5).

TABLE 21-4   Glasgow Coma Scale and Modification for Children

Sign	Glasgow Comas Scale	Modification for Children	Score
Eye opening	Spontaneous	Spontaneous	4
	To command	To sound	3
	To pain	To pain	2
	None	None	1
Verbal response	Oriented	Age appropriate verbalization, orients to sound, fixes and follows, and social smile	5
	Confused	Cries, but consolable	4
	Disoriented—inappropriate words	Irritable, uncooperative, aware of environment—irritable, persistent cries, and inconsistently consolable	3
	Incomprehensible sounds	Inconsolable crying, unaware of environment or parents, restless, and agitated	2
	None	None	1
Motor response	Obeys commands	Obeys commands and spontaneous movement	6
	Localizes pain	Localizes pain	5
	Withdraws	Withdraws	4
	Abnormal flexion to pain	Abnormal flexion to pain	3
	Abnormal extension	Abnormal extension	2
	None		1

TABLE 21-5   Respiratory Patterns

Name	Description	Localization
Cheyne-Stokes	Alternating hyperpnea and apnea	Extensive bihemispheric dysfunction or diencephalic dysfunction or metabolic suppression
Kussmaul	Rapid, deep, and regular	Pontomesencephalic or acidosis
Central neurogenic hyperventilation	Rapid and deep hyperpnea	Bihemispheric, midbrain, and pons
Apneustic	Prolonged pause at end of inspiration	Lower pons
Ataxic	Irregular in rate and tidal volume	Medulla
Agonal gasps	Terminal respiratory pattern	Bilateral lower brainstem

Fever may occur with infection and also occur with subarachnoid hemorrhage, pontine hemorrhages, traumatic brain injury, thyrotoxicosis, and drug ingestion (cocaine, amphetamines, anticholinergics, and cyclic antidepressants). **Hyperthermia** should be treated aggressively with anti-pyretic medications or cooling devices to reduce cerebral metabolic demands as outcome in many types of brain injuries is worse with hyperthermia. Patients who have coma secondary to hypoxic ischemic encephalopathy may benefit from therapeutic hypothermia. **Hypothermia** suggests cold exposure, sepsis, hypoglycemia, hypothyroidism, Addison disease, or ingestion (alcohol, barbiturates, opioids, and sedatives). Abnormalities in respiratory rate and pattern may indicate primary pulmonary pathology, acid–base derangement, or nervous system dysfunction.

A focused general examination should follow vital sign evaluation. Resistance to either flexion of the neck (**Brudzinski's sign**) or extension of the knee with the hip flexed (**Kernig's sign**) may indicate meningeal inflammation/irritation. Midface or skull base fractures are suggested by periorbital (raccoon eyes) or retroauricular (Battle sign) **ecchymosis**. Clear fluid leakage from the nose or ears may suggest skull fractures with associated cerebrospinal fluid leak. Skin examination provides information about trauma (bruises and lacerations), infection (e.g., superficial lacerations and lymphadenopathy in cat scratch fever, erythema migrans in Lyme disease, petechiae and purpura in meningococcemia), fat emboli due to long bone fracture (petechiae), and systemic autoimmune disease (butterfly rash of systemic lupus erythematosus). Purpura may occur with meningococcal infection, thrombotic thrombocytopenic purpura, vasculitis, or disseminated intravascular coagulation. Organomegaly raises suspicion of metabolic, hematologic, or hepatic disease. Dry skin suggests anticholinergic agent overdose while sweating suggests organophosphate poisoning, hypoglycemia, thyroid storm, or malignant catatonia.

A detailed **neurologic examination** is directed toward localizing brain dysfunction, identifying coma etiology, and determining early indicators of prognosis. In a comatose child, the neurologic examination focuses on response to stimuli, brainstem function, and motor function. Determining whether a child is unresponsive often involves verbal followed by tactile stimulation. Stimuli may include sternal rubbing, rubbing ribs, pressing supraorbital nerve, pressure on the condyles at temporomandibular joint, or nail-bed pressure. It is critical to determine that the patient is not unresponsive due to a locked-in syndrome or psychogenic unresponsiveness if more noxious tactile stimuli are utilized and to avoid injury or bruising (especially if anticoagulated) in all patients.

> **HINT:** Frequent, standardized, detailed neurological examinations are critically important in detecting expanding lesions or increasing ICP, which require immediate treatment.

A comatose child may be flaccid, or may display **decorticate** (flexion of the arms and extension of the legs—usually due to bihemispheric dysfunction with intact brainstem function) or **decerebrate** posturing (extension and internal rotation of all limbs—usually due to global metabolic derangements or brainstem pathology.

Cranial nerve examination is important in assessing the brainstem. Pupils are examined first by observing the size of both pupils in dim light, and then by assessing reactivity to a bright light shined in each eye. Asymmetric pupil size (**anisocoria**) is caused by unilateral dysfunction of the oculomotor nerve (CN III), which innervates the pupillary constrictors, or of the sympathetic fibers, originating in the midbrain, which innervate the pupillary dilators. Oculomotor nerve palsy causes pupil dilation, ptosis, and ophthalmoparesis in the affected eye and may be due to **uncal herniation**. Impairment of sympathetic fibers (**Horner syndrome**) leads to pupil constriction and a small degree of ptosis in the affected eye. In traumatic coma, Horner syndrome may be an important clue to dissection of the carotid artery. Fixed eye version may suggest an ongoing seizure. Fundoscopic examination may reveal **papilledema** associated with increased ICP (though early in the process papilledema may be absent), **retinal hemorrhages** in shaken baby syndrome, or flame-shaped hemorrhages and **cotton-wool spots** in hypertensive encephalopathy. Abnormalities of eye position and motility may be signs of cortical, midbrain, or pontine dysfunction. Pupil and ocular movement abnormalities seen in coma are summarized in Table 21-6.

TABLE 21-6	Pupil and Eye Movement Abnormalities in Coma	
Etiology/Localization	**Pupil Appearance**	**Eye Movement**
Cerebral hemisphere		Fixed conjugate eye deviation (toward side of injury or away from side of ongoing seizure).
Metabolic	Small and reactive	
Hypothalamic	Small and reactive	
Tectal	Large, fixed, and hippus	
Pontine	Pinpoint	Horizontal gaze palsies.
Midbrain	Mid-position and fixed	Vertical and horizontal gaze palsies. Dorsal compression may result in upgaze paresis (so have tonic down gaze), papillary lightnear dissociation, lid retraction, and nystagmus.
CN III Palsy (uncal herniation)	Ipsilateral pupil dilated and fixed	Depression and abduction of eye (down and out).
CN IV Palsy (often in traumatic brain injury)		Hypertropic eye.
CN VI Palsy (injury or due to elevated intracranial pressure [ICP])		Failure of adduction.
Severe hypoxic ischemic encephalopathy	Bilateral dilated and fixed	
Narcotic, barbiturate overdose	Bilateral small and reactive	

Oculocephalic reflexes are tested by holding the patient's eyelids open and quickly moving the head to one side. In a comatose patient with an intact brainstem, the eyes will move in the direction opposite the head motion (i.e., if the head is moved to the right, the eyes will move conjugately to the left). After several seconds, the eye may return to a neutral position. Oculocephalic reflexes should not be tested if the patient has sustained cervical spine trauma. The oculovestibular reflex (**cold calorics**) is also a test of brainstem function. For testing to be accurate the patient must have an open external auditory canal so initial examination of the ear and canal is essential. With the head of bed at 30 degree, 120 cc of ice water is introduced into the canal with a small catheter. A conscious patient would experience nystagmus with slow deviation toward the irrigated ear and fast correction away from the ear (the mnemonic COWS—*Cold Opposite, Warm Same*—applies to the fast phase of nystagmus). In a comatose patient, the eyes tonically deviate toward the irrigated ear and remain fixed in that position. No movement will be seen if the brainstem vestibular nuclei or their connection to eye movement pathways are impaired. Five minutes should be allowed before the second ear is tested to allow rewarming of the first ear. Other brainstem reflexes are summarized in Table 21-7.

TABLE 21-7	Brainstem Reflexes		
Reflex	**Technique to Examine**	**Normal Response**	**Anatomy**
Pupils	Response to light	Pupillary constriction	Midbrain. Afferent: CN II and chiasm Efferent: CN III and sympathetic fibers
Oculocephalic	Turn head side to side	Eyes move conjugately in direction opposite to head.	Pons Afferent: CN VIII Efferent: CN III and CN VI
Vestibulo-oculocephalic	Cold caloric	Conjugate deviation toward stimulation with fast nystagmoid movements away.	Pons Afferent: CN VIII Efferent: CN III and CN VI
Corneal	Stimulation	Blink	Pons Afferent: CN V Efferent: CN VII
Cough	Stimulation	Cough	Medulla. Afferent and efferent: CN IX and X.
Gag	Stimulation	Gag	Medulla. Afferent and efferent: CN IX and X.

Further Investigation

All children should have an urgent **bedside glucose measurement** upon arrival; laboratory glucose for confirmation should be sent even if normal, since hypoglycemia alone may cause coma, and hypoglycemia in association with other etiologies may worsen outcome. Hypoglycemia must be treated urgently with intravenous dextrose infusion. Hyperglycemia may occur in diabetic ketoacidosis and requires specific management. Further laboratory testing should be guided by the suspected etiology. Arterial **blood gases and electrolytes** should be considered, since abnormalities may cause coma or may occur secondary to intracranial abnormalities. **Liver function tests** should be considered since hepatic encephalopathy may cause coma, and hepatic injury can occur in the setting of systemic hypoxic ischemic injury. A **complete blood count with differential and coagulation profile** is indicated to detect infection, anemia, disseminated intravascular coagulopathy, lead encephalopathy, or sickle cell disease. **Blood and urine cultures** should be obtained when an infectious etiology is suspected. **Toxin screens** should be considered in all children and include acetaminophen, salicylate, and ethanol levels. Specific tests for medications found in the home should be carried out as necessary. Ammonia, lactate, and pyruvate may be performed to screen for **metabolic disorders**. If abnormal or the history is suggestive of metabolic disease, then measurement of organic acids, amino acids, and acylcarnitine profile may be indicated.

Once resuscitation is performed, a **head CT** (without contrast) should be performed in all children with unknown etiology to look for intracranial bleeds, space-occupying lesions (i.e., tumor or abscess), edema, or focal hypodensities (i.e., ADEM, herpes simplex encephalitis, infarction, or hydrocephalus). If trauma is suspected, then cervical spine imaging is required to assess for cervical spine injury or instability. If the child is intubated, then a chest radiograph may be needed to evaluate for tube placement, and may also identify rib fractures, pneumothoraces, or widened mediastinum. If nonaccidental injury is suspected, then a skeletal survey may be required.

Lumbar puncture should be performed if the patient is febrile, infection is suspected, or no other etiology can be determined. It should be deferred and treatment initiated for possible infection (bacterial and viral and sometimes fungal) if there is clinical or radiological evidence for intracranial hypertension. A normal CT does not rule out elevated ICP, so opening pressure should always be measured. Cerebrospinal fluid should be tested for cell count (in the case of a traumatic tap preferably both the first and the last tubes to help differentiate true findings), glucose, protein, gram stain, bacterial culture, viral PCR, additional fungal or tuberculosis cultures when suspected clinically, and lactate (which may be elevated in metabolic/mitochondrial diseases).

An **electroencephalogram** (EEG) can be a helpful adjunctive study. It can detect significant background changes (i.e., triphasic waves suggestive of metabolic encephalopathy or focal slowing with sharp waves associated with herpes simplex encephalitis) and may identify subclinical (nonconvulsive) seizure activity. As described below, a prolonged EEG may be required to detect subclinical seizures.

If the cause of coma remains unknown, additional studies may be directed at uncommon causes of coma in pediatrics such as Hashimoto's encephalitis (**thyroid** function tests and thyroid autoantibodies), cerebral **vasculitis** (erythrocyte sedimentation rate [ESR], antinuclear antibody [ANA] panel, and possibly angiography), or paraneoplastic disorders. Once the patient has been stabilized, and if the etiology of coma remains unclear, a brain magnetic resonance imaging may be performed for diagnostic and prognostic purposes.

Treatment

Recent guidelines including evaluation and management flowcharts are published online (see "Suggested Readings"). Evaluation of the airway, breathing, and circulation must begin the assessment, and continuous cardiopulmonary monitoring and frequent GCS assessment are crucial. Hypoxia, hypotension, hypoglycemia or hyperglycemia, hyperthermia or hypothermia, and anemia worsen the prognosis of coma and must be treated aggressively and quickly. If needed, intubation should be performed using a rapid-sequence intubation and all patients should be assumed to have a full stomach and cervical spine injury. Supplemental oxygen is generally administered. If shock is present, isotonic fluids should be administered since hypotonic fluids may worsen cerebral edema. If elevated ICP is suspected, then neurosurgical consultation regarding an ICP monitor should be considered. Frequent examinations are required to detect any change that may require urgent management. Two issues that often arise as the primary problem is treated include elevated ICP and seizures.

Elevated Intracranial Pressure

Causes of increased ICP in coma include intracranial hemorrhage, other space-occupying lesion, and cerebral edema. Cerebral edema may be vasogenic (leakage of fluid from blood vessels with altered blood–brain barriers into the interstitial space) or cytotoxic (accumulation of intracellular water after failure of energy-dependent sodium potassium pumps). **Herniation** may result in brainstem compression and may compress arteries resulting in secondary infarction. Thus, herniation syndromes often herald impending catastrophic deterioration and death unless ICP is lowered rapidly by medical or surgical means. Other than Cushing's triad, signs of herniation depend on location of herniation syndrome (Table 21-8). Treatment for intracranial hypertension generally begins with ICP >20 mm Hg in patients with ICP monitors. Initial management involves head position (elevating head to 30 degrees) and ensuring adequate sedation, analgesia, and neuromuscular blockade is administered. Additional management includes intravenous **hyperosmolar therapy** (mannitol or 3% normal saline) and **hyperventilation** (to achieve a pCO_2 of 35 mm Hg). Further reduction in pCO_2 may be necessary to achieve rapid but temporary reductions in cerebral blood flow and thus ICP, but excessive or prolonged hyperventilation may lead to vasoconstriction, further compromise cerebral perfusion, and exacerbation of hypoxic ischemic injury. Barbiturate coma or moderate hypothermia may reduce cellular energy requirements and may thus help protect the brain during periods of hypoxia and ischemia. Similarly, providing adequate sedation and paralysis may

TABLE 21-8	Herniation Syndromes	
Herniation Syndrome	**Location**	**Signs**
Subfalcine herniation	Increased pressure in one cerebral hemisphere leads to herniation of cingulated gyrus underneath falx cerebri.	Anterior cerebral artery compression and infarction leads to paraparesis.
Uncal herniation	Uncus of the temporal lobe is displaced medially over the free edge of the tentorium.	Ipsilateral third nerve palsy (initially dilated but reactive to slight and then progressing to pupil fixed and dilated with ophthalmoplegia (eye deviated down and out). Ipsilateral hemiparesis from compression of the contralateral cerebral peduncle (Kernohan's notch). Other signs of brainstem dysfunction from ischemia secondary to compression of posterior cerebral artery.
Cerebellar tonsillar herniation (foramen magnum herniation)	Increased pressure in the posterior fossa leads to brainstem compression.	Loss of consciousness from compression of reticular activating system. Focal lower cranial nerve dysfunction. Respiratory and cardiovascular function can be significantly affected early with relative preservation of upper brain stem function such as pupillary light reflexes and vertical eye movements. Progresses to loss of all brainstem reflexes, flaccid paralysis, and ataxic respirations.
Central herniation	Increased pressure in both cerebral hemispheres causing downward displacement of the diencephalon through the tentorium, causing brainstem compression.	*Diencephalic stage:* Withdraws to noxious stimuli, increased rigidity, or decorticate posturing; small reactive pupils with preserved oculocephalic and oculovestibular reflexes; yawns, sighs, or Cheyne-Stokes breathing. *Midbrain stage:* Decerebrate posturing or no movement; midposition pupils which may become irregular and unreactive; abnormal or absent oculocephalic and oculovestibular reflexes; hyperventilation. *Pons stage:* No spontaneous motor activity; mid-position fixed pupils; absent oculocephalic and oculovestibular reflexes; ataxic respirations. *Medulla stage:* Generalized flaccidity; absent pupillary reflexes and ocular movements; ataxic or slow irregular respirations, death.
Transcalvarial herniation	Increased pressure leads to herniation through a skull defect (traumatic or surgical).	Dysfunction of involved brain.

further reduce energy demand and prevent spikes in ICP. Maintaining a neutral neck position and head of bed elevation at 20 to 30 degrees may improve venous drainage. **Surgical decompression** by removal of mass lesions or craniotomy to provide more space may be life-saving.

 HINT: Herniation syndromes suggest impending catastrophic deterioration and must be recognized and treated rapidly.

Seizures

Subclinical seizures in critically ill patients are an underrecognized phenomenon, so the index of suspicion in a comatose child should be high. Studies of children with altered mental status in the ICU and the emergency room have demonstrated that ~25% have **subclinical seizures**. Only about half can be detected with a 1-hour EEG recording, so often more prolonged EEG monitoring is required. Anti-epileptic medications may successfully terminate these seizures, and consideration should be given to benzodiazepines, phenytoin/fosphenytoin, phenobarbital, levetiracetam, fosphenytoin, and valproic acid.

Suggested Readings

Posner JB, Saper CB, Schiff N. *Plum and Posner's Diagnosis of Stupor and Coma.* 4th ed. New York: Oxford University Press; 2007.

Stevens RD, Bhardwaj A. Approach to the comatose patient. *Crit Care Med.* 2006;34(1):31–41.

The Paediatric Accident and Emergency Research Group. *The Management of a Child (aged 0–18 years) with a Decreased Conscious Level,* 2006. http://www.nottingham.ac.uk/paediatric-guideline/ (Accessed March 2011).

Constipation

INTRODUCTION

Constipation is difficult passage of **hard bowel movements,** usually associated with a decrease in the frequency of bowel movements to **<2 stools per week**. Approximately 3% to 5% of pediatric primary care visits in the United States are for constipation. Estimates of the true prevalence of constipation vary between 1% and 30%. In the majority of reports, the peak prevalence is during pre-school years without gender preference.

Since normal stool frequency varies by age from early in life (Table 22-1), no single definition of constipation neatly fits into pediatric practice. **Breast-fed infants** can defecate as many as 12 times per day, whereas with the introduction of solids or formula, stool frequency decreases and consistency is more solid. There is a decline in stool frequency from >4 stools per day in the first week of life to 1 or 2 stools per day at the age of 4 years. About 97% of 1- to 4-year-old children pass stool three times daily to once every other day. By 4 years of age, 98% of normal children are toilet trained. This developmental process cannot be accelerated by early or high-intensity toilet training. Concerns related to defecation problems are responsible for 25% of outpatient visits to pediatric gastroenterologists.

Infant dyschezia occurs when there is painful defecation with the passage of soft stools. Infants strain, cry, and turn red or purple in the face with defecation effort. It results from failure to coordinate increased abdominal pressure with pelvic floor relaxation. Symptoms persist for 10 to 20 minutes, begin in the first few months of life, and resolve within a few weeks.

Most common complaints are infrequent bowel evacuation, hard small feces, abdominal pain, and painful evacuation of large-caliber stools that may clog the toilet. **Fecal incontinence** (voluntary or involuntary evacuation of stool into the underwear) is often a complaint. Although constipation is common and varies in severity, the complaint should not be ignored. It is important to identify the small percentage of patients with organic causes of constipation. In addition, children with functional constipation will benefit from not only improvement in bowel movements, but also with the psychosocial aspects of constipation if diagnosed and treated early.

TABLE 22-1	Normal Frequency of Bowel Movements	
Age	**Bowel Movements per Week[a]**	**Bowel Movements per Day[b]**
0–3 mo of age		
Breast milk	5–40	2.9
Formula	5–28	2.0
6–12 mo of age	5–28	1.8
1–3 yr of age	4–21	1.4
>3 yr	3–14	1.0

[a]Approximate mean ±2 standard deviations.
[b]Mean.
Reprinted with permission from a medical position statement of the North American Society for Pediatric Gastroenterology and Nutrition, *J Pediatr Gastroenterol Nutr.* 2006;43:e1–13.

 DIFFERENTIAL DIAGNOSIS LIST

Nonorganic Causes
Diet
Excessive cow's milk intake
Insufficient dietary water intake
Introduction to solids
Low fiber intake
Underfeeding/malnutrition
Functional
Irritable Bowel Syndrome
Psychological
Anorexia nervosa
Anxiety disorders
Attention deficit disorder
Situational
Hospitalization
Overzealous toilet training
Resistance to toilet training
Sexual abuse
School bathroom avoidance
Toilet phobia
Voluntary withholding

Organic Causes
Anatomic Causes
Anal stenosis
Anterior displaced anus (ectopic anus)
Imperforate anus
Intestinal bands

Malrotation
Prune belly
Rectal/perirectal abscess
Rectoperitoneal fistula
Sacral teratoma (pelvic mass)

Infectious Causes
Chagas disease
Postviral irritable bowel syndrome
Streptococcal perianal dermatitis
Tetanus

Inflammatory and Autoimmune Disorders
Amyloidosis
Celiac disease
Ehlers–Danlos syndrome
Inflammatory bowel disease
Milk protein allergy
Mixed connective tissue disease
Scleroderma
Systemic lupus erythematosus

Metabolic and Genetic Causes
Adrenal insufficiency
Cystic fibrosis (meconium ileus)
Diabetes insipidus
Diabetes mellitus (neuropathy)
Hypercalcemia

Hyperparathyroidism
Hypokalemia
Hypomagnesemia
Hypothyroidism
Mitochondrial disease
Multiple endocrine neoplasia 2B
Panhypopituitarism
Pheochromocytoma
Renal tubular acidosis

Neurogenic/Neuromuscular Causes

Cerebral palsy
Down syndrome
Familial dysautonomia
Hirschsprung disease
Intestinal pseudoobstruction
Myelomeningocele
Myotonia
Neurofibromatosis
Spinal cord injury
Spinal cord tumor
Spinal muscular atrophy

Static encephalopathy
Tethered cord
Visceral myopathies
Visceral neuropathies

Pharmacological Causes

Antacids with aluminum and calcium
Anticholinergics
Antihistamines
Antidepressants
Antipsychotics
Antispasmodics
Anticonvulsants
Diazoxide
Diuretics
Iron supplements
Narcotics
Ursodiol

Toxic Causes

Botulism
Lead
Vitamin D

DIFFERENTIAL DIAGNOSIS DISCUSSION

Chronic constipation has a broad differential. The major etiologies of constipation can be broadly divided into organic and nonorganic. Functional constipation is a subset of nonorganic constipation. In most cases, the etiology is functional. One must always consider organic causes such as **Hirschsprung disease, neurogenic problems, metabolic disorders, and anatomic defects,** which are often detected in infancy.

Nonorganic Constipation

Chronic constipation is often functional. The pediatrician can usually identify functional constipation by a **thorough history and physical examination**. Onset frequency usually occurs during one of the three periods: in infants transitioning to formula or solids, in toddlers acquiring toilet skills, or at the beginning of school. Children are described as standing on their toes, stiffening their legs, or hiding in a corner. The pain a child experiences is from the normal propagating contractions pushing against a closed external anal sphincter. **Fecal incontinence** occurs when stool seeps out around the distal fecal mass and leaks when the pelvic floor is relaxed (e.g., sleep), with fatigue or attempts at flatus and is occasionally mistaken for diarrhea. Physical examination includes assessing the anal tone and presence of stool in the rectal vault by rectal examination. In patients with functional constipation, the rectal examination causes the child to react with acute fear and negative behaviors.

In such a situation, examination of the perineum is important, and digital examination may be deferred to facilitate a therapeutic alliance with the child.

A number of predisposing factors appear to be associated with the onset of functional constipation. **Painful defecation** is a crucial but often silent clue as a potential trigger for chronic fecal retention and fecal soiling. **Toilet training** is often a potential trigger. To master toilet training, a toddler must develop the interest and ability in retaining a bowel movement until it can be released into the toilet. This behavior often leads to less frequent defecation and, at times, hard painful stools. This problem may be exacerbated if toilet training is vigorously encouraged before the child is developmentally ready. The **American diet** is a potential contributor to chronic constipation. Although a balanced diet of fruits, vegetables, and fiber maybe useful in preventing mild constipation, there is little evidence that fiber alone is effective in the treatment of chronic constipation.

Regardless of the etiology, once constipation is triggered, a **positive feedback-type mechanism** ensues. Retained stool in the distal colon begins to lose water across the intestinal wall. As water is resorbed, fecal motility slows, more water is lost, and the feces harden. A **buildup of desiccated stool** causes **painful defecation** that leads to **ongoing stool retention**. Over time, the rectum and distal colon accommodate the growing fecal mass and, consequently, the **rectosigmoid enlarges.** Under these conditions, a child's **ability to sense rectal fullness diminishes,** and he or she may not appreciate the need to defecate. A classic sign of chronic constipation is the large, infrequent (up to 1 week or more) stool that clogs the toilet. The passage of hard stools frightens the child and results in fearful determination to avoid defecation. Such children respond to the urge to defecate by contracting the anal sphincter and gluteal muscles, attempting to withhold. **Encopresis, or involuntary fecal soiling,** is for all families a source of tremendous stress. It is a complication of severe functional constipation that occurs when watery stool from the proximal colon leaks around the fecal obstruction, passing involuntarily per rectum. Parents or caretakers may misinterpret encopresis as diarrhea. Severe constipation may also lead to rectal prolapse.

Evaluation

The medical evaluation of constipation must differentiate functional from organic- or medication-related causes. The **Rome III criteria** are used for the diagnosis of functional defecation disorders (Tables 22-2). In the **absence of alarm signals** such as weight loss, anorexia, delayed growth, delayed passage of meconium, urinary incontinence, passage of bloody stools (in the absence of anal fissure), fever, vomiting, diarrhea, or other extraintestinal symptoms, functional constipation is the most likely etiology. In most cases of functional constipation, laboratory tests are unnecessary. Any **predisposing factors** (i.e., low fiber intake, difficult toilet training), coupled with **telltale signs** such as infrequent or abnormally large stools or stool-withholding behavior or soiling, strongly suggest the diagnosis. **Social stigma** caused by excess flatulence and the odor of encopresis is

TABLE 22-2	Rome III Criteria for Functional Constipation

Neonate/Toddler	Children/Adolescent
Must include 1 mo of *at least two* of the following in infants up to 4 yr of age:	Must include two or more of the following in a child with developmental age of at least 4 yr with insufficient criteria to meet irritable bowel syndrome:
1. Two or fewer defecations per week 2. At least one episode per week of incontinence after the acquisition of toileting skills 3. History of excessive stool retention 4. History of painful or hard bowel movements 5. Presence of a large fecal mass in the rectum 6. History of large-diameter stools that may obstruct the toilet	1. Two or fewer defecations in the toilet per week 2. At least one episode of fecal incontinence per week 3. History of retentive posturing or excessive volitional stool retention 4. History of painful or hard bowel movements 5. Presence of a large fecal mass in the rectum 6. History of large-diameter stools that may obstruct the toilet.
Accompanying symptoms may include irritability, decreased appetite, and/or early satiety. The accompanying symptoms disappear immediately following passage of a large stool.	Criteria fulfilled at least once per week for at least 2 mo before diagnosis.

Adapted from Hyman P, Mill P, Benninga M, et al. *Gastroenterology.* 2006;130:1519–1526.

not unusual. Physical examination may reveal palpable stool in the abdomen. The anus should be checked for **fissures, hemorrhoids** (rare in childhood), surrounding **dermatitis,** and **abnormal position**. An **anteriorly displaced anus (ectopic anus)** is defined by the anal position index, the ratio of anus-fourchette distance in girls and anus-scrotum distance in boys to the distance between coccyx and fourchette/scrotum. For females, an abnormal ration is >0.45 and for boys, >0.54. Digital rectal examination almost always demonstrates abundant stool in the rectal vault. External sphincter tone and anal wink reflex should be intact. A thorough **neurologic examination,** including inspection of the sacral area for sinuses or tufts of hair, is important.

The clinician must **screen for occult blood** in all constipated infants or any child with abdominal pain, failure to thrive, intermittent diarrhea, or a family history of either colon cancer or polyps. Measurement of **abdominal transit time** with radio-opaque markers by with abdominal radiographs is an option to evaluate for efficacy of clean out and the presence of a megarectum, which is common in functional constipation. In the absence of soiling, a child with normal transit time does not require further evaluation. When there is **soiling with a normal transit time,** treatment relies on **behavioral modification,** sometimes with **psychological evaluation**. Since stool impaction may cause urinary stasis, the need for urinalysis and culture must be weighed.

Treatment

Management of constipation may be as simple as a **dietary change** for simple constipation or as complex as a program of **cleanout, bowel "retraining,"** and **family education** with close follow-up.

Infants with simple constipation often do well with **stool softeners** such as sorbitol-containing juices (prune, apple, pear), karo syrup, lactulose, or barley malt extract. A glycerin suppository usually relieves the acutely constipated infant. Enemas, mineral oil, and stimulant laxatives are contraindicated in infants.

In severely constipated children, **disimpaction** with either oral or rectal medication precedes maintenance therapy. Disimpaction with oral agents has been shown to be effective with the use of **high-dose mineral oil, polyethylene glycol, magnesium citrate, senna, or bisacodyl**. It is recommended that these laxatives be used either alone or in combination. Possible side effects include electrolyte abnormalities. Available rectal agents include **phosphate, saline, or mineral oil enemas** followed by polyethylene glycol for oral lavage. Cleanout is initiated with a mineral oil enema to soften the fecal mass and lubricate the rectal canal. A hypertonic phosphate enema is administered 30 minutes later. Tap water, herbal, and soapsuds enemas should not be used at home because they are associated with water intoxication, bowel perforation, and bowel necrosis. Failure to achieve disimpaction at home may require **hospitalization** for nasogastric lavage with polyethylene glycol or high volume enemas.

Following disimpaction, **maintenance therapy** lasting months and sometimes years is initiated. Children should **decrease cow's milk intake** and consume a **balanced diet** including whole grains, fruits, and vegetables. Osmotic laxatives such as **lactulose and polyethylene glycol** (miralax) are often used as maintenance therapy. Miralax is a safe nonstimulant laxative available to infants over the age of 6 months at a dose of 0.5 to 1.5g/kg, not to exceed 17 g daily. Occasionally, stimulant laxatives such as senna or bisacodyl are used for short-term "rescue" therapy to avoid recurrent impaction. **Mineral oil** is a maintenance lubricant given in doses of 1 to 3 mL/kg/day. Mineral oil should not be used when there is risk for aspiration (infants, swallowing dysfunction) and fat-soluble vitamins in the form of a multivitamin supplement should be taken daily with mineral oil.

Behavioral modification involves unhurried toilet sitting for child's age two to three times a day ~20 minutes after meals. A footstool is often helpful in maximizing Valsalva maneuver. Parents should understand the basic pathophysiology of constipation and be taught to provide consistent positive reinforcement. Praise for successful toileting is essential. A simple **reward system** such as stickers on a calendar can be effective and provides a useful record for the physician at follow-up. Some evidence indicates that biofeedback may be a valid short-term mode of therapy in chronic constipation. **Psychology evaluation** is often important in continued progress.

Organic Causes

Although not as common as functional constipation, there are multiple organic causes of constipation (see "Differential Diagnosis List"). **Cow's milk intolerance** has been associated with various gastrointestinal disturbances including constipation. Rectal inflammation from the allergic response can lead to recurrent anal fissures and ongoing constipation.

Hirschsprung disease (congenital aganglionic megacolon) is the **most common cause of lower intestinal obstruction in newborns**. It is the result of failure of the neural crest cells during 8 though 12 weeks' gestation to migrate completely during colonic development. Neural crest cells normally participate in the formation of submucosal and myenteric parasympathetic ganglia; thus, incomplete migration gives rise to an aganglionic intestine having sustained sympathetic contraction. Consequently, the affected aganglionic segment, which always extends proximally from the internal anal sphincter, blocks the peristaltic wave resulting in a functional bowel obstruction. The incidence is approximately 1 in 5,000 live births and the male-to-female ratio is 4:1. Hirschsprung disease should be considered in children who **fail to pass meconium** within the first 48 hours of life. More than 90% of normal neonates and <10% of children with Hirschsprung disease pass meconium within the first 24 hours of life.

Hirschsprung disease is unusual beyond infancy, but the diagnosis should always be considered in any constipated toddler or school-aged child (Table 22-3). Eighty percent of cases are limited to some portion of the rectosigmoid region. Much less frequently, aganglionosis of the entire colon with or without some small-bowel involvement occurs. The length of bowel involvement correlates with the

TABLE 22-3	Comparison of Functional Constipation and Hirschsprung Disease	
Constipation	**Functional Disease**	**Hirschsprung Disease**
Symptoms as a newborn	Rare	Almost always
Late onset (>3 yr)	Common	Rare
Difficult bowel training	Common	Rare
Stool size	Large	Small, ribbon-like
Urge to defecate	Rare	Common
Obstructive symptoms	Rare	Common
Enterocolitis	Rare	Sometimes
Failure to thrive	Rare	Common
Abdominal distention	Rare	Common
Stool in rectal ampulla	Common	None
Barium enema	Copious stool No transition zone	Delayed evacuation Transition zone
Rectal biopsy	Normal	No ganglion cells Increased anticholinesterase staining
Anorectal manometry	Distention of rectum causes relaxation of the internal anal sphincter	Failure of internal anal sphincter relaxation

timing of diagnosis. Patients with short-segment disease may not be identified until childhood (or rarely, go undetected into adulthood), whereas those with more extensive involvement present in infancy with bilious vomiting, abdominal distension, failure to thrive, and refusal to feed. Fecal soiling is rare except in ultrashort segment Hirschsprung disease. The most feared complication of Hirschsprung disease, **enterocolitis,** may be an initial manifestation. Increased intraluminal pressure from bowel obstruction is thought to mechanically diminish mucosal blood flow and in turn compromising mucosal integrity and allow bacteria and fecal toxins into the bloodstream. Progression is rapid and septic patients are febrile with abrupt onset of foul-smelling bloody diarrhea, abdominal distention, and bilious emesis. The mortality rate in advanced enterocolitis approaches 20% to 30%. In addition to several rare genetic disorders, there is an association with **Trisomy 21, congenital cardiac anomalies** (especially septal defects), and **neuroblastoma**.

Imperforate anus is an anorectal malformation often associated with other gastrointestinal manifestations including tracheoesophageal abnormalities, duodenal atresia or obstruction, and malrotation. Other anorectal malformations to consider include **anteriorly displaced anus (ectopic anus)** defined by the anal position index, greater than a ratio of 0.45 for girls and 0.54 for boys, **anal stenosis, retroperitoneal fistula,** and **sacral teratoma**.

Cystic fibrosis is the most common inherited disease among Caucasian people, affecting approximately 1 in 2,500 live births. **Meconium ileus** is the presenting problem in 10% to 20% of newborns with cystic fibrosis, pathognomonic of the diagnosis. Episodes of bowel obstruction may plague older children and adults, can be termed meconium ileus equivalent or distal intestinal obstructive syndrome. Many patients are hospitalized for hydration and treatment and may require surgical intervention to alleviate the obstruction.

Other organic causes to consider include **infantile botulism,** a neuroparalytic syndrome resulting from the neurotoxin of the microorganism *Clostridium botulinum,* **lead, and Vitamin D intoxication**. Metabolic causes to screen for include **electrolyte abnormalities and hypothyroidism. Intestinal pseudoobstruction,** caused by either nerve or muscle disorders resulting in obstructive symptoms without mechanical obstruction, can either be congenital or acquired. Symptoms include abdominal distention, vomiting, and nausea, among others. **Colonic manometry** is necessary to make the diagnosis. Neurogenic bowel dysfunction occurs in children when diseases such as **myelomeningocele, tethered cord, lipomeningocele, cerebral palsy, or lumbosacral spinal cord tumors** interfere with the normal neurologic control of defecation.

Evaluation

Physical examination findings suggesting an organic etiology include decreased lower extremity tone or strength, lower spine abnormalities, failure to thrive, abdominal distention, a tight, empty rectum in the presence of palpable fecal mass, absent anal wink, absent cremasteric reflex, or patulous anus. In a patient with obstructive symptoms, such as **Hirschsprung disease,** the abdomen is often distended, and the anal sphincter tone is usually increased. The **rectum is typically**

empty, and as the examining digit is withdrawn, there may be a forceful gush of liquid stool. Children with short-segment Hirschsprung disease may have stool in the rectal vault.

Further testing should be pursued if the child fails to respond to conventional therapies including disimpaction, laxatives, and behavioral modification. Testing should be initiated earlier in patients who have evidence of an organic etiology. Several diagnostic methods are available, but they vary in reliability. In children with significant constipation in the neonatal period, and especially in those with delayed passage of meconium, an **unprepped contrast enema** to investigate the possibility of Hirschsprung disease should be considered. A transition zone, or narrowed distal colonic segment that abruptly transitions to a dilated bowel, is characteristic. The contrast enema may also reveal a nondistensible rectum, a classic sign of Hirschsprung disease. Absent rectal air on a prone abdominal radiograph suggests Hirschsprung disease. A **transition zone** may not be apparent in neonates, because of insufficient time to develop colonic dilation, or in infants who have undergone rectal washouts, examinations, or enemas and requires further investigation. Gold standard for diagnosis is a **rectal biopsy**. Consider referral to a pediatric gastroenterologist for possible **anorectal manometry** to assess the internal anal sphincter's response to artificial balloon distention. A normal internal sphincter relaxes with balloon distention, whereas an aganglionic sphincter either remains contracted or increases its tone with distention. When anorectal manometry results are abnormal, rectal biopsy samples can be obtained and interpreted by experienced practitioners to provide a definitive diagnosis.

In patients with evidence of **spinal dysraphism or neurological impairment, magnetic resonance imaging** to investigate tethered cord and spinal cord tumors should be considered. Typical findings include a history of spinal cord trauma, weakness or dysesthesia of the lower extremities, fecal incontinence after successful toilet training, or urinary incontinence. Myelomeningocele-spinal dysraphism in the lumbosacral region can cause constipation and megarectum, but these problems more often manifest as urinary and fecal incontinence. Sacral cysts or fistulae should be identified in the newborn nursery and evaluated by ultrasound.

In children who are refractory to conventional therapies, **laboratory studies** to screen for serum measurements of thyroid-stimulating hormone, thyroxine, electrolytes, calcium, magnesium, lead, and celiac disease should be considered prior to referral to a pediatric gastroenterologist. Referral to a pediatric gastroenterologist should be made for motility testing for patients who have no obvious organic cause for constipation and who fail to respond to aggressive treatment.

Treatment

Organic etiologies for constipation are treatment specific. Anorectal malformations require consultation by a surgeon for **surgical intervention**. Children with imperforate anus usually respond well to surgical intervention with a posterior sagittal anorectoplasty. The treatment of Hirschsprung disease is surgical resection of the aganglionic bowel with temporary placement of a diverting ostomy proximal to the affected segment. More than 90% of patients ultimately have normal bowel function. Before surgery, management of enterocolitis in the intensive care setting includes nasogastric and rectal decompression, antibiotics, and correction of fluid and electrolyte imbalances.

Management of patients with neurogenic bowel dysfunction depends on the type, severity, and location of the lesion. Children with moderate-to-severe impairment benefit from **interdisciplinary collaboration** among physicians, occupational therapists, and behavioral or mental health specialists.

Suggested Readings

Baker SS, Liptak GS, Colletti RB, et al. Evaluation and treatment of constipation in infants and children: evaluation and treatment. Recommendations of the North American Society for Pediatric Gastroenterology, Hepatology and Nutrition. *J Pediatr Gastroenterol Nutr.* 2006;43:e1–e13.

Burgers R, Benninga MA. Functional nonretentive fecal incontinence in children: a frustrating and long-lasting clinical entity. *J Pediatr Gastroenterol Nutr.* 2009;48(Suppl 2):S98–S100.

Di Lorenzo C. Pediatric anorectal disorders. *Gastroenterol Clin N Am.* 2001;30(1):269–287.

Gariepy CE, Mousa H. Clinical management of motility disorders in children. *Semin Pediatr Surg.* 2009;18(4):224–238.

Hyman PE, Di Lorenzo C. *Pediatric Gastrointestinal Motility Disorders.* New York: Academy Professional Information Services; 1994.

Hyman PE, Milla PJ, Benninga MA, et al. Childhood functional gastrointestinal disorders: neonate/toddler. *Gastroenterology.* 2006;130:1519–1526.

Maffei HV, Vicentini AP. Prospective evaluation of dietary treatment in childhood constipation: high dietary fiber and wheat bran intake are associated with constipation amelioration. *Gastroenterology.* 2011;52(1):55–59.

Muller-Lissner S. The pathophysiology, diagnosis, and treatment of constipation. *Dtsch Arztebl Int.* 2009;106(25):424–432.

Pijpers MA, Bongers ME, Benninga MA, et al. Functional constipation in children: a systematic review on prognosis and predictive factors. *J Pediatr Gastroenterol Nutr.* 2010;50(3):256–268.

Taitz LS, Wales KH, Urwin OM, et al. Factors associated with outcome in management of defecation disorders. *Arch Dis Child.* 1986;61:472–477.

Van den Boerg MM, Benninga MA, Di Lorenzo C. Epidemiology of childhood constipation: a systemic review. *Am J Gastroenterol.* 2006;101(10):2401–2409.

Weaver LT. Bowel habit from birth to old age. *J Pediatr Gastroenterol Nutr.* 1988;7(5):637–640.

CHAPTER 23

Richard M. Kravitz

Cough

INTRODUCTION

Cough is one of the most common presenting symptoms in children. The duration of the symptoms determines the level of concern and degree of workup that is warranted. An **acute cough,** lasting <3 weeks, is frequently related to an infectious illness and is often self-limited. This chapter is concerned with **chronic cough,** a cough that persists for ≥3 weeks and suggests a potentially more serious underlying cause. A cough has three components. First, there is an **inspiratory phase,** when the patient takes a deep breath. The inspiratory phase is followed by **closure of the glottis and contraction of the expiratory muscles**. During this phase, intrathoracic pressure increases. Finally, the **glottis opens,** allowing the previously inspired air to be expelled at a high velocity (about 60 to 70 mph). The function of coughing is to shake irritants loose from the airway mucosa and move them proximally (if the irritant is located distally) or expel them (if the irritant is located proximally).

 DIFFERENTIAL DIAGNOSIS LIST

Infectious Causes
Bacterial Infection
- Bacterial pneumonia
- Sinusitis
- Tuberculosis (TB)
- Pertussis
- Chlamydia infection
- Mycoplasma infection

Viral Infection
- Upper respiratory tract infection
- Viral pneumonia
- Bronchiolitis—respiratory syncytial virus infection, parainfluenza infection
- Croup
- Influenza

Fungal Infection
- Aspergillosis
- Allergic bronchopulmonary aspergillosis
- Histoplasmosis
- Coccidioidomycosis

Toxic (Irritant) Causes
- Cigarette smoke
- Industrial pollutants
- Wood-burning stoves
- Cleaning solvents
- Perfumes/colognes

Neoplastic Causes
- Teratoma
- Lymphoma

- Leukemia
- Metastatic malignancy

Congenital Causes
Pulmonary Malformations
- Bronchogenic cysts
- Cystic adenomatoid malformation
- Congenital lobar emphysema
- Pulmonary sequestration

Vascular Malformations
- Aberrant innominate artery
- Double aortic arch
- Airway hemangiomas

Gastrointestinal Malformations
- Esophageal duplications
- Tracheoesophageal fistula

Genetic Causes
- Cystic fibrosis
- Immotile cilia syndrome

Inflammatory Causes
- Asthma
- Allergies
- Sarcoidosis

Psychosocial Causes
- Psychogenic (habitual) cough
- Paradoxical vocal cord dysfunction

Miscellaneous Causes
Pulmonary Disorders
- Bronchopulmonary dysplasia
- Laryngotracheobronchomalacia

- Foreign body in airway
- Bronchiectasis

Ears, Nose, and Throat Disorders
- Foreign body in the nose or ear canal
- Postnasal drip
- Middle ear effusion
- Paralyzed vocal cord
- Swallowing dysfunction with secondary aspiration

Cardiovascular Disorders
- Congestive heart failure
- Pulmonary edema

Gastrointestinal Disorders
- Gastroesophageal reflux disease (GERD) with or without secondary aspiration
- Diaphragmatic or subdiaphragmatic mass
- Foreign body in the esophagus

Immunologic Disorders
- Congenital immunodeficiency with a secondary infection

Medications
- Beta-blockers (e.g., propanolol)
- Angiotensin-converting enzyme (ACE) inhibitors (e.g., captopril, enalapril, lisinopril)

DIFFERENTIAL DIAGNOSIS DISCUSSION
Asthma
Asthma, the **most common chronic illness in children,** affects 5% to 10% of children in the United States.

Etiology
The underlying cause of asthma is unknown, although airway inflammation is known to be a major component. The triad of **airway inflammation, smooth muscle hyperreactivity, and reversible airway obstruction** is characteristic for patients with asthma.

Numerous triggers can precipitate an asthma flare-up, including viral upper respiratory tract infections, sinus infections, exercise, exposure to cold air, weather changes, exposure to allergens (e.g., dust, cockroaches, animal dander, pollen, grass, mold, or certain foods such as shellfish or peanuts), exposure to strong odors (e.g., cigarette smoke, strong chemicals, perfumes), and emotional states (e.g., fear, laughing, crying).

Clinical Features

Asthma symptoms are secondary to airway obstruction brought about by airway inflammation and mucus production and/or increased airway resistance from bronchospasm. **Wheezing** is the classic presentation of asthma, but other symptoms include chronic coughing (often referred to as cough-variant asthma), shortness of breath, and chest pain or tightness.

Evaluation

A detailed history and physical examination are integral to making the diagnosis of asthma. Wheezing, rhonchi, coarse or decreased breath sounds, or a prolonged expiratory phase may be noted on pulmonary examination. Lung sounds can also be entirely normal at the time of examination, even in patients with a significant history.

Spirometry with a bronchodilator response is used to assess for asthma. In patients with asthma, an obstructive pattern with post-bronchodilator improvement in lung function is frequently seen. If spirometry is not available, a handheld peak-flow meter can be substituted.

 HINT: Pulmonary function testing can be normal in many patients with asthma. If asthma is strongly suspected in spite of normal results on pulmonary function testing, then provocational testing (e.g., exercise testing, methacholine challenge) may be indicated to help document airway hyperreactivity. Exercise testing is specific in patients with exercise-induced asthma, whereas the more sensitive methacholine challenge can detect more subtle degrees of airway hyperreactivity.

Treatment

Proper treatment of asthma entails both pharmacologic and nonpharmacologic modalities. For most patients with asthma, ideal therapy includes the use of a daily anti-inflammatory medication along with a rescue bronchodilator given on an as needed basis to treat breakthrough symptoms. Short bursts of oral steroids are often helpful for treating acute flare-ups of asthma, although the side effects of long-term use preclude their use as a chronic maintenance medication (though in severe cases, chronic daily or every other day oral steroids may be needed to adequately control symptoms).

- **Anti-inflammatory medications** include mast cell stabilizers (e.g., cromolyn sodium, nedocromil calcium), inhaled steroids (e.g., beclomethasone, fluticasone, budesonide, ciclesonide, mometasone), and leukotriene inhibitors (e.g., zileuton, zafirlukast, montelukast).

- **Bronchodilators.** β_2-agonists (e.g., albuterol, levalbuterol, terbutaline, pirbuterol) are the most effective and commonly used bronchodilators for rescue therapy. Long acting β_2-agonists (e.g., salmeterol, formoterol) may be used in combination with inhaled steroids (e.g., Advair®-salmeterol+fluticasone; Symbicort®-formoterol+budesonide, Dulera®-formoterol+mometasone) to provide improved symptom control and pulmonary function values when inhaled steroids alone prove insufficient at controlling the patient's asthma (of note, these long acting beta agonists should never be used as monodrug therapy when treating asthma). Methylxanthine derivatives (e.g., theophylline) and parasympathetic antagonists (e.g., atropine, ipratropium) may also be used (although they are not routinely used in children).
- **Nonpharmacologic management** entails patient education (to improve self-management), environmental control and prevention skills (to decrease exposure to asthmatic triggers and the likelihood of developing an asthma attack), and home monitoring with a peak-flow monitor (to objectively assess pulmonary status so that appropriate interventions can be instituted and their effects assessed).

Cystic Fibrosis
Etiology
An autosomal recessive disorder, cystic fibrosis is the **most common genetic disease affecting whites**. The gene is located on chromosome number 7 and codes for a transmembrane protein (cystic fibrosis transmembrane conductance regulator (CFTR)-protein) that functions as a chloride channel. The most common abnormality is an amino acid defect consisting of the deletion of a phenylalanine (the delta F508 mutation). The disease is characterized by **multiorgan involvement**. Chronic sinopulmonary infections (facilitated by excess altered mucus production in the respiratory tract), pancreatic insufficiency, and abnormalities of the exocrine glands and reproductive tract are major manifestations. In the lungs, dry, thickened secretions hinder clearance of pulmonary secretions. Impaired airway clearance, in combination with abnormal colonization with organisms (e.g., *Staphylococcus aureus, Pseudomonas aeruginosa*), leads to the development of bronchiectasis and permanent lung damage.

Clinical Features
Major symptoms include a chronic, productive cough, yellow-green sputum, chest congestion, hemoptysis, steatorrhea, poor weight gain, failure to thrive, and meconium ileus or meconium ileus equivalent (intestinal obstruction).

Evaluation
A detailed family history should be obtained as well as growth patterns and stool characteristics. Cardinal features noted on physical examination may include tachypnea, retractions, bronchial breath sounds, wheezes, crackles, a prolonged expiratory phase, nasal polyps, upper airway congestion, digital clubbing, reduced height and weight, rectal prolapse, and hepatomegaly and splenomegaly.

The following laboratory studies are indicated:

- **Chloride sweat test.** Pilocarpine is used to stimulate sweat collection. The sweat chloride level is considered to be elevated if ≥60 mEq/L.
- **Sputum culture.** *P. aeruginosa* and *S. aureus* are the bacterial pathogens most often responsible for the chronic sinopulmonary infections. Other organisms, such as *Burkholderia cepacia, Stenotrophomonas maltophilia,* and *Alcaligenes xylosoxidans,* are also seen and tend to be more resistant to therapy.
- **Complete blood cell (CBC) count.** A CBC should be obtained to rule out anemia and to assess for leukocytosis. Hypersplenism has also been reported (evidenced by leukopenia and thrombocytopenia).
- **Liver function tests** are ordered to assess for hepatobiliary disease and obstruction.
- **Prothrombin time (PT).** A PT should be obtained to assess vitamin K sufficiency.
- **Vitamin A, E, and D** levels should be measured to assess for possible fat-soluble vitamin deficiency.
- **Fecal fat analysis.** A 72-hour stool collection should be obtained to assess the degree of pancreatic insufficiency. Fecal elastase may also be measured.
- **Oxygen saturation analysis and pulmonary function tests** should be performed to assess the degree of pulmonary involvement (arterial blood gas analysis is not necessary in most cases).
- **Genetic testing** is indicated. More than 70% of patients have the delta F508 mutation.

> **HINT:** All children with recurrent sinopulmonary infections, steatorrhea, growth failure, or poorly controlled asthma which does not respond to appropriate therapy should be tested for cystic fibrosis.

> **HINT:** All siblings of patients with cystic fibrosis should be tested for cystic fibrosis using the chloride sweat test. They should also undergo genetic analysis because they have a two in three chance of being a carrier (this should be after the proband's genetic mutation has been identified).

> **HINT:** Newborn screening is now available in most states. Only the most common CFTR mutations, however, are tested, so it is possible that patients with the less common alleles may be missed. If cystic fibrosis is suspected, a sweat test is still indicated as to not miss diagnosing this serious illness.

Treatment

Therapy is directed toward maintaining optimal pulmonary function and nutritional status:

- **Daily airway clearance** with chest physiotherapy, breathing exercises, and (frequently) inhaled bronchodilators is indicated. The efficacy of mucolytic agents such as Mucomyst® is questioned; however, Pulmozyme® and hypertonic saline have been demonstrated in clinical studies to improve lung function.

- **(Chronic) antibiotic therapy** is frequently used to help suppress the effects of chronic bacterial colonization. Inhaled antibiotics, such as high-dose tobramycin (TOBI®) or the recently approved inhaled aztreonam (Cayston®) given on alternating months, have been found to maintain pulmonary function and decrease hospitalization rates when compared with placebo in prospective studies. Alternatively, oral azithromycin given on a 3 day per week schedule has also proven useful in maintaining good pulmonary health.

- **(Acute) antibiotic therapy** is used to treat acute exacerbations of cystic fibrosis. Symptoms of these exacerbations include increased cough and mucus production, wheezing, shortness of breath, decreased exercise tolerance, decreased appetite, weight loss, and general malaise. Oral antibiotics (in combination with increased airway clearance) can often treat these symptoms when they are mild. In cases with more severe symptoms or when oral antibiotics have not been successful, broad-spectrum intravenous antibiotics are required. These are usually given in the inpatient setting and consist of at least two different antibiotic classes being utilized as to decrease the development of antibiotic resistance and potentially augment each other's efficacy.

- **Pancreatic insufficiency** is treated with the administration of supplemental enteric-coated pancreatic enzymes along with multivitamins (in particular, the fat-soluble vitamins A, D, E, and K). Vitamin K administration is frequently required; especially if the patient chronically takes antibiotics or if the PT is increased (vitamin K should be given intramuscularly if the PT is seriously elevated or if the patient is actively bleeding).

- **Hemoptysis** is a complication usually indicating a severe exacerbation of underlying infection. Treatment is with antibiotics as outlined earlier; however, it may be necessary to withhold chest physiotherapy until the bleeding subsides (12 to 24 hours). Most episodes of hemoptysis manifest as blood streaks and respond to a treatment course of antibiotics. Massive hemoptysis, although rare, is a medical emergency that usually results from erosion of an underlying bronchial vessel into a bronchus. This is frequently treated with bronchial artery embolization.

- **Other major emergencies** in patients with cystic fibrosis include acute intestinal obstruction, massive hemorrhage from esophageal varices, liver failure, pulmonary hypertension, cor pulmonale with cardiac failure, pneumothorax, and chronic hypoxemia.

Sinusitis

Sinusitis, characterized by inflammation and infection of the mucosal lining of the sinuses, is a common cause of chronic cough.

Etiology

In an otherwise healthy host, sinus infections are usually a **complication of upper respiratory tract infections** (i.e., bacterial superinfection following a viral infection).

The usual bacterial pathogens include *Streptococcus pneumoniae, Haemophilus influenzae, and Moraxella catarrhalis.*

Clinical Features

Sinusitis can present in a variety of ways. Common features include persistent symptoms of an upper respiratory tract infection, chronic cough, a mucopurulent nasal discharge, headaches, and malodorous breath.

Evaluation

The diagnosis can be made clinically, based on the history and physical examination. Physical examination findings may include tenderness over the affected sinus and erythema of the nasal mucosa, with or without a mucopurulent nasal discharge. The physical examination, however, may be normal. Radiographic studies that can aid in the diagnosis include **sinus films and computed tomography (CT)** of the sinuses. Opacification of the sinuses, mucosal thickening, or the presence of an air-fluid level are typical findings.

Treatment

The usual treatment for sinusitis is a prolonged course of **antibiotics,** usually lasting 14 to 21 days. Therapy should be directed toward the usual bacterial pathogens. The concomitant use of topical nasal **decongestants** is only recommended for 4 to 7 days. **Surgical drainage** of the sinus is sometimes used in refractory cases.

Bronchiectasis

Bronchiectasis is a condition in which the bronchi are damaged, leading to the development of bronchial dilation with the loss of underlying airway support structures (e.g., cartilage and elastic tissue). Acute or chronic inflammation and recurrent infections are also associated with bronchiectasis. Bronchiectasis is the end result of numerous insults to the lung and can be **reversible** (e.g., cylindrical bronchiectasis) or **permanent** (e.g., saccular bronchiectasis).

Etiology

Some of the more common causes of bronchiectasis include **infection** (e.g., following severe pneumonia caused by *S. aureus, S. pneumoniae,* adenovirus, or influenza virus), **genetic conditions** (e.g., cystic fibrosis, immotile cilia syndrome), **recurrent aspiration events,** or a **retained foreign body**.

Clinical Features

Chronic coughing with excessive sputum production (bronchorrhea) is a cardinal sign of bronchiectasis. In severe cases, hemoptysis and recurrent fevers may also be seen.

Evaluation

- **Physical findings** are related to the extent of the disease. Although the pulmonary examination can be normal early in the course of disease, one is apt to find coarse breath sounds, rhonchi, rales, and expiratory wheezes as the disease progresses. Digital clubbing is also seen in advanced disease.
- **Chest radiographs** typically show thickened bronchial walls in the peripheral lung, although early in the course of disease the films may be normal. Other findings include recurrent atelectasis and localized hyperinflation.

- **Chest CT scans** are more sensitive than radiographs for defining the extent of the disease, especially in patients with milder cases. Typical findings include bronchial wall thickening extending to the periphery, cystic changes in the bronchi, and air-fluid levels in the damaged bronchi.
- **Other studies** may prove useful in the evaluation of the patient with bronchiectasis. These studies depend on the past medical history and can include a sweat test (if cystic fibrosis is to be considered); bronchoscopy (if a foreign body is suspected or if respiratory cultures are desired); an immunologic evaluation (if recurrent pneumonia has occurred); a pH probe or milk scan (if GERD is suspected), or a swallowing evaluation (if aspiration is a concern).

Treatment

Treatment should be directed toward the underlying cause of the bronchiectasis, if one can be identified:

- **Airway clearance.** Maintenance of good pulmonary toilet is important, regardless of the cause of the bronchiectasis. Aiding in the removal of excessive secretions and preventing superinfection can help prevent further bronchial damage. Aerosolized bronchodilators, chest physiotherapy, and postural drainage promote the removal of excess mucus.
- **Antibiotics.** Oral or intravenous antibiotics may be indicated for patients with acute exacerbations of bronchiectasis exacerbated by a bacterial infection. Chronic prophylactic antibiotic use to prevent exacerbations is controversial and should be determined on a case-by-case basis.
- **Surgery.** In certain patients with well-localized bronchiectasis, surgical removal of the affected lung can be curative. Surgery, however, should only be performed when medical management has failed and the likelihood of disease progression after surgery is minimal.

Immotile Cilia Syndrome
Etiology

Immotile cilia syndrome is an autosomal recessive disease characterized by abnormal function of the cilia. Histologic defects in the cilia may include abnormalities in the dynein arms, defects in the radial spokes connecting the microtubules that form the cilia, and defects in the microtubules themselves.

Clinical Features

Patients with immotile cilia syndrome typically present with recurrent episodes of **otitis media, sinusitis, chronic cough, and pulmonary infections**. Physical findings include recurrent otitis media, chronic sinus drainage, nasal polyps, pulmonary findings suggestive of bronchiectasis, and, in more severe cases, digital clubbing (secondary to the bronchiectasis). **Situs inversus** is seen in 50% of cases.

> **HINT:** The triad of sinusitis, bronchiectasis, and situs inversus is referred to as **Kartagener syndrome**.

HINT: Male infertility secondary to abnormally functioning sperm is common.

Evaluation

Frequently, the diagnosis is made by clinical history and by ruling out other causes. It can be difficult to diagnose the condition definitively. Approaches include **electron microscopic evaluation** of the cilia to determine their ultrastructure (tissue is usually obtained via nasal mucosa scrapping or tracheal biopsy), examination of the **ciliary beat frequency or waveform** (under light microscopy), and the **saccharin test** (a drop of saccharin is placed in the nose and the length of time it takes the patient to taste the sweetness is measured).

Radiographic findings (chest radiograph or CT scan) are similar to those of cystic fibrosis and bronchiectasis. Sinus films typically show pansinusitis.

Treatment

Treatment is the **same as for bronchiectasis**. Maintaining adequate pulmonary drainage is the key to minimizing lung damage. Recurrent otitis media is frequently treated with the placement of myringotomy tubes. Chronic use of antibiotics is controversial.

Allergic Rhinitis

Allergic rhinitis is characterized by chronic or recurrent watery nasal discharge and can represent a very common cause of chronic cough.

Etiology

Allergic rhinitis is an IgE-mediated response to agents found in nature. These allergens generate IgE antibodies which bind to mast cells. When a sensitized patient is then re-exposed to this allergen, it binds to the IgE antibody leading to mast cell degranulation. Several chemicals are released from these mast cells, in particular, histamine, which leads to the symptoms described below. Depending on the specific antigen triggering this response, the allergic rhinitis may be seasonal or perennial (throughout the year).

Clinical Features

Allergic rhinitis can present with a variety of symptoms, the more common include rhinorrhea, sneezing, coughing, recurrent throat clearing, allergic shiners, Dennie lines, conjunctivitis, and nasal and ocular itching. Physical examination may reveal pale and boggy nasal turbinates with a watery discharge evident. Cobblestoning of the eyelids and posterior oropharynx along with a postnasal drip are frequently evident.

Evaluation

Although the diagnosis can be made by history, allergy testing can be useful for identifying the specific antigens responsible for these symptoms. Skin testing (simple prick testing) can identify agents to which the patient has been sensitized. A positive skin test correlates well (although not fully) with clinical symptoms.

Radioallergosorbent testing (RAST) measures IgE levels to various antigens. Although highly specific, there is not as much correlation between a positive RAST test and clinical symptoms as is seen with positive skin testing, especially with low-level positive RAST values.

 HINT: Positive RAST and skin testing identify antigens to which the patient has been exposed and to which they have mounted an IgE-medicated response. One must then clinically correlate these positive test results to the actual clinical symptoms. A positive "allergy test" does not tell you what you are allergic to, just what you are sensitized to.

Treatment

Treatment for allergic rhinitis involves both pharmacologic and nonpharmacologic measures.

- **Pharmacologic management.** Antihistamines and nasal steroids are the mainstays of pharmacologic therapy. Antihistamines block the effects of the histamine released by mast cell degranulation. The older first-generation antihistamines (i.e., diphenhydramine, hydroxyzine) tend to be sedating, whereas the newer second-generation antihistamines (i.e., loratadine, cetirizine, fexofenadine) do not cross the blood–brain barrier and are nonsedating.

  As with asthma therapy, anti-inflammatory agents help stop the inflammatory cascade associated with mast cell degranulation and/or prevent the mast cells themselves from degranulating. Nasal steroids (i.e., triamcinolone, fluticasone, budesonide) are the mainstay of therapy to control the symptoms of allergic rhinitis. Other agents found to be effective in controlling allergic rhinitis include the leukotriene inhibitor montelukast and the mast cell stabilizer (nasally inhaled) cromolyn.

  Immunotherapy (commonly referred to as "allergy shots") is also an effective therapy for treating allergies. This is especially useful when antihistamines and nasal steroids are ineffective. It consists of recurrent subcutaneous injections of a particular antigen at increasing concentrations, which desensitizes the body to that particular antigen.

- **Nonpharmacologic management.** Many nonpharmacologic therapies are available to help control allergies. Avoidance of the specific antigen is very effective at diminishing symptoms. Removing pets from the household (or at least minimizing exposures) can be a useful adjunctive therapy. Control of dust mites can be accomplished by maintaining low humidity in the household, washing bedsheets in hot water, encasing pillows and mattresses in plastic sheets, and removing dust-attracting agents (i.e., stuffed animals, window blinds) from the patient's room. Cleaning up loose food and the use of exterminators can decreases cockroach exposures.

Gastroesophageal Reflux Disease (GERD)

Gastroesophageal reflux disease is discussed in Chapter 82, "Vomiting."

TABLE 23-1	Types of Cough
Quality	**Likely Diagnosis**
Staccato	Pertussis or parapertussis infection
Bark-like (seal-like) or brassy	Croup
Throat clearing	Postnasal drip, possibly secondary to sinusitis or allergies
Foghorn-like and occurring only when awake	Pathognomonic for a psychogenic (habitual) cough

EVALUATION OF COUGH
Patient History
Present Illness
The present illness should be defined:

- What is the duration of the cough?
- How frequent is the cough?
- When does the cough occur (e.g., upon awakening, later in the evening)?

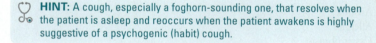

> **HINT:** A cough, especially a foghorn-sounding one, that resolves when the patient is asleep and reoccurs when the patient awakens is highly suggestive of a psychogenic (habit) cough.

- What does the cough sound like (Table 23-1)?
- Is the cough productive or nonproductive for sputum?

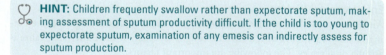

> **HINT:** Children frequently swallow rather than expectorate sputum, making assessment of sputum productivity difficult. If the child is too young to expectorate sputum, examination of any emesis can indirectly assess for sputum production.

- Were there any precipitating events (e.g., infection, choking episode, allergies)?
- Are there any triggers for the cough (Table 23-2)?

TABLE 23-2	Triggers for Coughing
Trigger	**Associations**
Cold air, exercise, or upper respiratory tract infections	Asthma
Supine position	Postnasal drip, GERD
Eating	GERD, tracheoesophageal fistula, aspiration

GERD, gastroesophageal reflux disease.

- Are there accompanying symptoms (e.g., rhinorrhea, watery eyes, headaches, fever, poor weight gain or weight loss, symptoms of food malabsorption, wheezing)?
- How many school days (or work) have been missed?
- Is the cough improving or getting worse?
- What medications is the child currently taking? ACE inhibitors can cause a chronic cough and β_2-antagonists can precipitate bronchospasm in patients with asthma.
- What is the patient's travel history?
- Are other family members ill?

Past Medical History

Important information to be gathered includes the following:

- The patient's birth history
- Information regarding any previous illness or surgery
- Information regarding allergies
- The patient's immunization status

Family History

The patient's parents should be queried about a family history of any of the following disorders:

- Asthma
- Allergies
- Cystic fibrosis
- Emphysema
- Sarcoidosis
- TB

Environmental History

An environmental history can sometimes prove useful in identifying the exacerbating factors in patients with a chronic cough, especially if the underlying cause is asthma or allergies. The following are important factors:

- **Home heating system.** Forced-air heating systems that use a duct network can carry dust through the house. Radiator and baseboard heating are much less likely to cause a problem for children with allergies.
- **Wood-burning stoves.** Older stoves often do not burn wood efficiently. The incompletely burned wood releases hydrocarbons that can be a potent, noxious irritant for patients with asthma.
- **Location of the home.** In rural and suburban settings, patients are exposed to numerous aeroallergens, whereas in urban environments, patients are exposed to industrial irritants, dust mites, and cockroaches.
- **Condition of the home.** Dusty homes can aggravate allergies. If the basement is cool and damp, the possibility of mold exposure exists. Older homes, especially in overcrowded urban areas, can have cockroaches, which are recognized as a potent allergen and can lead to poorly controlled allergies and asthma.

Construction within the home can expose the child to various noxious irritants, ranging from dust to paint and chemical odors. Mold spores can also be released into the air. For patients with severe dust allergies, removing the carpeting, drapes, blinds, and stuffed animals from the patient's room and encasing the mattress and pillow in plastic may help minimize exposure to dust mites.

- **Cigarette exposure.** Smoking in the home can be a potent trigger for coughing, particularly in children with asthma. Children exposed to cigarette smoke have a higher incidence of asthma, recurrent upper respiratory tract infections, and recurrent sinusitis or otitis media. This cigarette smoke effect can be seen even when the parents do not smoke in direct contact with the child.
- **Pets.** Exposure to pets can be a problem for children with allergies and asthma.
- **Child care.** Recurrent exposure to other children increases the likelihood of the child developing recurrent upper respiratory tract infections.

Physical Examination

The following should be noted on physical examination:

- **General appearance**—height and weight and degree of distress
- **Skin**—eczema and rashes
- **Head, ears, eyes, nose, and throat**—watery eyes, cerumen in the ear, sinus tenderness, nasal discharge, pale or boggy nasal turbinates, postnasal drip, and pharyngeal cobblestoning (i.e., a cobblestone-like appearance to the mucosa that is seen in patients with allergic disease)
- **Lungs**—respiratory rate, chest appearance, retractions, and breath sounds (rhonchi, rales, wheezes) and their symmetry
- **Heart**—murmur
- **Extremities**—cyanosis and clubbing

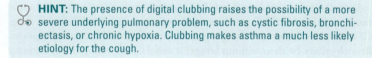

HINT: The presence of digital clubbing raises the possibility of a more severe underlying pulmonary problem, such as cystic fibrosis, bronchiectasis, or chronic hypoxia. Clubbing makes asthma a much less likely etiology for the cough.

Laboratory Studies

Selection of laboratory studies is based on a thorough history and physical examination.

Suspected Asthma

- **Pulmonary function testing** can help confirm the diagnosis of asthma by demonstrating reversible obstructive lung disease or significant airway hyperreactivity. This test can be reliably done in children as young as 5 years old.
- **Pulmonary function provocational testing** can be used to assess for airway hyperreactivity in cases with normal pulmonary function values. A decrease of pulmonary function by 20% during a **methacholine challenge** or 15% during an **exercise challenge** is diagnostic of asthma.

Suspected Allergy

- **Diagnostic skin testing** is the most accurate test for determining atopy; skin testing is best done in patients >2 years.
- **CBC with differential.** Eosinophilia suggests an allergic component.
- **IgE level.** Elevation suggests an allergic component.
- **RAST** is used in the evaluation of allergy but is not as clinically sensitive as skin testing.

Suspected Infection

- **Purified protein derivative (PPD)** is used to rule out TB. Tine testing is no longer recommended as a screening test. The usual dose of PPD for the Mantoux tuberculin skin test is 5 TU given as an intradermal injection.
- **Sputum culture with gram stain** is indicated for patients who have a productive cough. Acid-fast staining should be done if TB is suspected.

Suspected Immunologic Disorder

A CBC with differential; quantitative IgG, IgA, and IgM levels; functional antibody levels (to assess B lymphocyte function); an anergy panel (to assess T lymphocyte function); and an HIV test are indicated.

Other Disorders

- **Sweat chloride test.** A sweat chloride of ≥ 60 mEq/mL is diagnostic of cystic fibrosis.
- **α_1-Antitrypsin (α_1-AT) level.** An α_1-AT level with genetic variants should be obtained in patients with emphysema to rule out α_1-AT deficiency.
- **ACE level.** The ACE level may be elevated in patients with sarcoidosis.

Diagnostic Modalities

- **Radiographic studies.** Radiographs or CT scans of the chest or sinuses may be indicated. A barium swallow should be considered for most infants with chronic cough to rule out GERD, tracheoesophageal fistula, or vascular ring or sling. GERD can also be assessed for by a gastric emptying (milk) scan or a pH probe.
- **Bronchoscopy (with or without lavage)** is useful for inspecting airway anatomy and dynamics, detecting a foreign body, and sampling lung material for culture.

TREATMENT OF COUGH

To treat a chronic cough properly, its underlying cause must be determined. Symptomatic relief, however, should be considered when the cough causes discomfort, interferes with the patient's ability to sleep or perform well in school, and there is otherwise *no specific* therapy available. Symptomatic cough medications fall into three classes: expectorants, antitussives, and mucolytic agents.

- **Expectorants** help moisturize secretions, making it easier for the patient to cough up sputum. The most effective expectorant is water; patients should be advised to drink plenty of fluids. Another effective expectorant is guaifenesin, found in numerous over-the-counter cough and cold preparations.

- **Antitussive agents** fall into two classes: peripherally acting and centrally acting medications. Peripherally acting agents (e.g., diphenhydramine) work by decreasing the sensitivity of the cough receptors in the lung. Centrally acting agents (e.g., codeine, dextromethorphan) act on the cough center located in the medulla. They abate coughing by decreasing the stimulus to cough. Dextromethorphan is as effective as codeine but is not a narcotic and thus not habit forming. Dextromethorphan is available in several over-the-counter cough preparations, usually in combination with antihistamines, expectorants, or both. Codeine is available only with a prescription and can be obtained as a single agent or mixed with other cough and cold preparations. Antitussive agents are not indicated when the child is otherwise well and not bothered by the cough.

- **Mucolytic agents** (e.g., Mucomyst, Pulmozyme) help patients who have thick, tenacious sputum (e.g., patients with cystic fibrosis). These agents help break up the mucus and, with the aid of chest physiotherapy, allow the patient to expectorate sputum more easily. These agents are not indicated in otherwise healthy individuals.

Cochrane meta-analysis reviews of the literature have demonstrated no improvement in cough with over the counter antitussive preparations when compared to placebo. This lack of efficacy, along with their potential for clinically significant side effects, has lead the FDA to advise against their use in children under 2 years of age, with special care being recommended if used in children 2 to 5 years old. Preference should be given to single drug versus multiple medication-containing preparations.

Suggested Readings

Black P. Evaluation of chronic or recurrent cough. In: BC Hillman, ed. *Pediatric Respiratory Disease: Diagnosis and Treatment.* Philadelphia: WB Saunders; 1993:143–154.

Chang AB, Asher MI. A review of cough in children. *J Asthma.* 2001;38(4):299–309.

de Jongste JC, Shields MD. Cough-2: Chronic cough in children. *Thorax.* 2003;58:998–1003.

Food and Drug Administration. Public health advisory: FDA recommends that over-the-counter (OTC) cough and cold products not be used for infants and children under 2 years of age. http://www.fda.gov/Drugs/DrugSafety/PostmarketDrugSafetyInformationforPatientsandProviders/DrugSafetyInformationforHeathcareProfessionals/PublicHealthAdvisories/ucm051137.htm.

Irwin RS, Boulet LP, Cloutier MM, et al. Managing cough as a defense mechanism and as a symptom. A consensus panel report of the American College of Chest Physicians. *Chest.* 1999;114:133S–181S.

Katcher ML. Cold, cough and allergy medications: uses and abuses. *Pediatr Rev.* 1996;17:12–17.

Smith SM, Schroeder K, Fahey T. Over-the-counter medications for acute cough in children and adults in ambulatory settings. *Cochrane Database Syst Rev* 2008;(1):CD001831.

Wilmott RW. Cough. In: MW Schwartz, ed. *Pediatric Primary Care: A Problem-Oriented Approach.* St. Louis: Mosby; 1997:216–224.

CHAPTER 24

Beth Ann Johnson
Bradley S. Marino

Cyanosis

INTRODUCTION

Cyanosis is a physical sign characterized by a bluish discoloration of the mucous membranes, skin, or nail beds. Cyanosis results from hypoxemia (decreased arterial oxygen saturation) or abnormal hemoglobin molecules. Cyanosis does not become clinically apparent until the absolute concentration of deoxygenated hemoglobin is at least 3.0 g/dL and sometimes not until 5 g/dL. The ability to detect cyanosis varies with skin color and total hemoglobin level. Studies have shown that detection of cyanosis by the clinically trained eye is unreliable with significant inter-observer variability. Due to the potential inaccuracy of clinical assessment, providers should exert caution when making judgments about patient's oxygenation based on visual perceptions alone.

The differential diagnosis of cyanosis is broad, encompassing multiple organ systems. Included in this differential are the following abnormalities: intracardiac right-to-left shunting, intrapulmonary ventilation-perfusion mismatch, impairment of oxygen diffusion across the alveolus, alveolar hypoventilation, and diminished affinity of hemoglobin for oxygen. The degree of cyanosis is affected by the total hemoglobin concentration and by any factor that affects the O_2 dissociation curve (pH, P_{CO_2}, temperature, and ratio of adult-to-fetal hemoglobin). Cyanosis will be evident sooner and be more pronounced under the following conditions: high hemoglobin concentration (polycythemic patient), lower pH (acidosis), elevated P_{CO_2}, elevated temperature, and elevated ratio of adult-to-fetal hemoglobin.

Detection of cyanosis and concomitant hypoxemia is important for several reasons. Cyanosis is often one of the first signs of many neonatal diseases including congenital heart disease (CHD). And importantly, cyanosis may be an early sign of cardiorespiratory failure. Early identification of cyanosis and prompt intervention may be life saving.

Central cyanosis refers to discoloration of the trunk, lips, and mucus membranes. Central cyanosis should not be confused with **acrocyanosis** (blueness of the distal extremities only). Acrocyanosis is caused by peripheral vasoconstriction and is a normal finding especially during the first 24 to 48 hours of life. **Differential cyanosis** is present when the oxygen saturation in the right upper extremity is greater than the lower extremities. Fetuses have minimal blood flow through the fluid-filled lungs due to high pulmonary vascular resistance. As a result, blood crosses from the right side of the heart (pulmonary artery) to the left side of the heart (aorta) in utero via the patent ductus arteriosus (PDA). The arteries that supply the right arm arise from the ascending aorta prior to the insertion of the PDA and are considered "pre-ductal;" therefore, the right upper extremity oxygen saturation represents the saturation of the blood leaving the left ventricle. The arterial saturations measured in either lower extremity are considered "post-ductal," as the arterial supply to the lower extremities occurs after the point of ductal insertion in the aortic isthmus. If the ductus arteriosus is patent following delivery, deoxygenated blood may continue to shunt from the pulmonary artery to the descending aorta leading to desaturation in the lower extremities. In the neonatal period, differential cyanosis is observed commonly in patients with persistent pulmonary hypertension of the newborn (PPHN) or CHD lesions with left ventricular outflow tract obstruction (e.g., interrupted aortic arch, coarctation of the aorta, and critical aortic stenosis). Differential cyanosis is an important diagnostic finding in the evaluation of a cyanotic newborn.

In the unusual situation where the pre-ductal saturation is lower than the post-ductal saturation, **reverse differential cyanosis** is present. Reverse differential cyanosis results from transposition of the great arteries (TGA) with PPHN or TGA with concurrent left ventricular outflow obstruction (Table 24-1).

DIFFERENTIAL DIAGNOSIS LIST

Cardiac
Ductal-Independent Mixing Lesions
- Truncus arteriosus
- Total anomalous pulmonary venous return without obstruction
- D-transposition of the great arteries[a]

Lesions with Ductal-Dependent Pulmonary Blood Flow
- Tetralogy of Fallot with pulmonary atresia[b]
- Ebstein anomaly[b]
- Critical pulmonic stenosis
- Tricuspid atresia[b] with normally related great arteries[b]
- Pulmonary atresia with intact ventricular septum

Lesions with Ductal-Dependent Systemic Blood Flow
- Hypoplastic left heart syndrome
- Interrupted aortic arch
- Critical coarctation of the aorta

- Critical aortic stenosis
- Tricuspid atresia with transposition of the great arteries[b]

Pulmonary
Primary Lung Disease
- Respiratory distress syndrome
- Meconium aspiration
- Pneumonia
- Persistent pulmonary hypertension of the newborn
- Pulmonary hypoplasia
- Diffusion impairment
- Ventilation-perfusion mismatch

Airway Obstruction
- Choanal atresia
- Vocal cord paralysis
- Laryngotracheomalacia

Extrinsic Compression of the Lungs
- Pneumothorax
- Chylothorax

[a]A PDA may improve mixing, especially with an intact ventricular septum.
[b]Most forms.

TABLE 24-1　Categories of Cyanosis

	Pre-Ductal Saturations	Post-Ductal Saturations	Diagnostic and Physical Findings	Differential Diagnosis	Work-up or Investigation Indicated	Initial Treatment
Central Cyanosis	Low	Low	Blue discoloration of the trunk, lips, and mucus membranes	Concerning for cardiac, pulmonary, neurologic or metabolic impairment and requires investigation	Yes	Dependent on cause and recommendations of expert consultants
Acrocyanosis	Normal	Normal	Blueness discoloration of the distal extremities only	Normal finding in the first 24 hours of life	No	None
Differential Cyanosis	High	Low	The O_2 saturation in the right upper extremity is greater than the lower extremities	Consistent with the diagnosis of PPHN or CHD lesion with LVOTO	Yes	PGE₁ Infusion and Cardiology Consultation
Reverse Differential Cyanosis	Low	High	The O_2 saturation in right upper extremity is lower than the lower extremities	Consistent with the diagnosis of TGA with PPHN or TGA with LVOTO	Yes	PGE₁ Infusion and Cardiology Consultation

Key: CHD, congenital heart disease; LVOTO, left ventricular outflow tract obstruction; O_2, oxygen; PGE₁, prostaglandin E₁; PPHN, persistent pulmonary hypertension of the newborn; TGA, transposition of the great arteries.

- Hemothorax
- Diaphragmatic hernia
- Pleural Effusion
- Bronchogenic cyst

Neurologic
- Central nervous system dysfunction
- Drug-induced depression of respiratory drive
- Cerebral edema
- Intracranial hemorrhage
- Central apnea

Respiratory Neuromuscular Dysfunction
- Spinal muscular atrophy
- Infant botulism
- Neonatal myasthenia gravis

Hematologic
- Methemoglobinemia
- Polycythemia

Other
- Sepsis
- Hypoglycemia
- Hypoventilation

DIFFERENTIAL DIAGNOSIS DISCUSSION
Methemoglobinemia
Etiology
Methemoglobin is an altered state of hemoglobin in which the ferrous form of iron has been oxidized to the ferric state making the heme moiety unable to carry oxygen. Methemoglobinemia is an increased concentration of methemoglobin in the blood that may lead to serious tissue hypoxia or even death. Methemoglobin may occur because of hereditary abnormalities of hemoglobin as well as exposures to oxidizing toxins. Toxic causes include analgesics (e.g., benzocaine), aniline dyes, some antimicrobials (e.g., dapsone, sulfonamides), azo compounds, and nitrites. Young infancy is a period of increased risk for methemoglobinemia as protective enzyme systems within the red blood cell which normally act to maintain a methemoglobin level <1% have lower activity and fetal hemoglobin is more readily oxidized than adult hemoglobin. Methemoglobinemia has also been described during diarrheal illnesses and is likely secondary to nitrite-forming bacteria in the gut.

Clinical Features
Patients with methemoglobinemia present with cyanosis and abnormal pulse oximetry (often high in comparison to degree of cyanosis) and low measured oxygen saturation by blood gas analysis.

Evaluation
Bedside diagnosis of methemoglobinemia entails placing a drop of the patient's blood on a piece of filter paper. After 30 seconds of exposure to air, normal blood appears red, whereas blood taken from a patient with methemoglobinemia appears chocolate brown. Methemoglobin levels are measured as part of a blood gas by co-oximetry.

Treatment
Methylene blue given intravenously reduces the abnormal ferric hemoglobin molecule back to the ferrous state. Methylene blue therapy is usually reserved

for methemoglobin levels >20% because lower levels typically resolve with supportive care alone. Methylene blue is contraindicated in patients with glucose-6-phosphate dehydrogenase deficiency because it may cause a severe hemolytic anemia.

EVALUATION OF CYANOSIS
Neonates
Patient History
Important information to obtain from the history includes a complete birth history that comprises maternal history; prenatal, perinatal, and postnatal complications; history of labor and delivery; history of maternal infection; and neonatal course should be obtained.

Specific questions to include:

- When did the mother's membranes rupture?
- What medications did the mother receive during labor and how long ago was the last dose?
- Is there a history of birth asphyxia?
- What was the baby's gestational age and birthweight?
- How old was the baby when the first episode of cyanosis occurred?
- What is the severity of desaturation?
- Is differential or reverse differential cyanosis present?
- What part of the body is involved?
- What are the infant's pulse, temperature, and respiratory rate?
- Does the baby have normal or decreased muscle tone?
- Does the baby have a vigorous or weak cry?
- Does the baby exhibit signs of respiratory distress?

Physical Examination
- **General assessment and vital signs.** The initial physical examination should focus on the vital signs and the cardiac and respiratory examinations, assessing for signs of respiratory distress or impending cardiorespiratory failure. If the patient has impending cardiorespiratory failure, quickly address respiratory and cardiac support needs of the patient based on the 2010 Pediatric Advanced Life Support (PALS) Guidelines as further evaluation continues.
- **Skin color.** Blue or dusky mucous membranes are consistent with cyanosis. Skin color has an impact on the diagnosis; in light-skinned patients, cyanosis is usually noted with an arterial oxygen saturation of <88%; in dark-skinned patients, the arterial oxygen saturation must be lower.
- **Respiratory examination.** Evaluate for rales, stridor, grunting, flaring, retractions, and evidence of consolidation and/or effusion. An increased respiratory rate, grunting, nasal flaring, and/or retractions are signs of respiratory distress. Hyperpnea (increased respiratory rate) with cyanosis but without signs of respiratory distress is frequently observed in patients with CHD. Whereas tachypnea with nasal flaring, grunting, and retractions often reflects a pulmonary cause of

cyanosis. Apnea is commonly related to prematurity, intracerebral problems, or medication.

- **Cardiovascular examination.** On cardiovascular examination palpation and auscultation should be performed to assess for abnormal precordial impulse, systolic or diastolic murmurs, S_1 or S_2 splitting abnormalities, and/or the presence of an S_3 or S_4 gallop, ejection click, opening snap, or rub. Absence of a heart murmur does not rule out CHD as several of the most severe cardiac lesions produce only a soft flow murmur in the neonatal period or no murmur at all. Severe cyanosis without a heart murmur suggests transposition of the great arteries. If splitting of S_2 is able to be auscultated confirming the presence of two patent outflow tracts, pulmonary atresia and aortic atresia may be ruled out. Examination of the extremities should focus on the strength and symmetry of the pulses in the upper and lower extremities, evidence of edema, capillary refill time, and cyanosis of the nail beds. Hepatomegaly may be consistent with right ventricular or biventricular heart failure.

Additional Evaluation

The goal of the initial evaluation of the hemodynamically stable but cyanotic neonate is to determine whether the cyanosis is cardiac or noncardiac in origin. Preductal and post-ductal oxygen saturations, as well as four extremity blood pressures should be documented. An electrocardiogram (ECG), chest radiograph, and hyperoxia test should be performed.

Four extremity blood pressure measurements demonstrating a right upper extremity systolic blood pressure at least 10 mm Hg greater than the lower extremity is consistent with arch hypoplasia, coarctation of the aorta, or other lesions with ductal dependent systemic blood flow with a restrictive ductus arteriosus. The **chest radiograph** is obtained to determine the size of the heart and whether the pulmonary vascularity is increased or decreased. The **ECG** evaluates the heart rate, rhythm, axis, intervals, forces (atrial dilation, ventricular hypertrophy), and repolarization (abnormal Q wave pattern, ST/T waves, and corrected QT interval).

The **hyperoxia test** consists of obtaining a baseline right radial (pre-ductal) arterial blood gas measurement with the child breathing room air and then repeating the blood gas measurement after the child has inspired 100% Fio_2 for 10 minutes. **Pulse oximetry measurements are not appropriate for interpretation of the hyperoxia test.** A Pao_2 > 150 mm Hg in 100% oxygen essentially rules out cardiac disease, whereas a Pao_2 < 50 mm Hg in 100% oxygen is highly suspicious for CHD.

Other appropriate laboratory studies may include serum glucose, a complete blood count (CBC) with differential, blood cultures, and urine cultures. If infection is strongly suspected, a lumbar puncture may be indicated. The combined results of the preceding tests should point the clinician in the direction of the cause of the cyanosis. If a cardiac cause is deemed likely, a **cardiology consultation and echocardiogram** should be obtained (Table 24-2).

TABLE 24-2	Initial Assessment of Infants with Central Cyanosis

History
Physical exam
Chest radiograph
ABG/hyperoxia test
CBC/blood cultures/sepsis evaluation
Serum glucose
EKG
Cardiology consultation ± echocardiogram

Treatment

Cyanotic infants require immediate assessment of **airway, breathing, and circulation**. It is crucial to quickly determine if cardiorespiratory failure is present and respond urgently to the patient's needs. Emergent stabilization of the cyanotic infant may include endotracheal intubation, volume resuscitation, and/or inotropic/vasoactive medications. **Prostaglandin E_1** (PGE_1) acts to maintain ductal patency or re-open a restrictive ductus arteriosus. Administration of PGE_1, via continuous intravenous infusion, should be started in any infant with suspected ductal-dependent CHD.

OLDER CHILDREN

Patient History

Important information to obtain from the history includes:

- What are the onset, duration, and frequency of cyanotic episodes?
- Have there been previous episodes of cyanosis?
- Is there associated coughing, wheezing, or stridor?
- Were there any precipitating factors?
- What is the child's medication history?
- Has the child's growth and development been normal?
- Has the child had any contact with anyone with an infectious disease?
- What is the child's family history?

Physical Examination

- **General assessment and vital signs.** As with neonates, the initial physical examination should focus on the vital signs and the cardiac and respiratory examinations, assessing for signs of respiratory distress or impending cardiorespiratory failure. If cardiorespiratory failure is present or pending, quickly address respiratory and cardiac support needs of the patient based on the 2010 PALS Guidelines as further evaluation continues.
- **Respiratory examination.** The child should be assessed for rhinorrhea, otitis media, pharyngitis, and sinusitis. Hoarseness, drooling, stridor, and breath sounds (e.g., rales, wheezing) should be noted. If epiglottitis is suspected, the pharynx should not be examined.

- **Cardiovascular examination.** On cardiovascular examination palpation and auscultation should be performed to assess for abnormal precordial impulse, systolic or diastolic murmurs, S_1 or S_2 splitting abnormalities, and/or the presence of an S_3 or S_4 gallop, ejection click, opening snap, or rub. The pulse rate and blood pressure in all four extremities should be carefully reviewed.

Laboratory Studies and Diagnostic Modalities

Appropriate studies may include:

- A CBC with differential and a blood culture
- Arterial blood gas analysis (if the cyanosis is severe)
- Pulmonary function tests
- A chest radiograph

Treatment

Cyanosis in the older child is almost always respiratory or neurologic in origin. Care is supportive and may require intubation and ventilation for respiratory failure.

Children with Tetralogy of Fallot may have attacks of paroxysmal hyperpnea and cyanosis that occur in association with crying or agitation. These attacks (**"Tet" spells**) occur most commonly in infants 3 to 18 months of age, especially during times of dehydration. Treatment involves delivering 100% oxygen, placing the patient in the knee–chest position, and administering intravenous isotonic fluids or morphine sulfate. Long-term therapy may include propranolol, and phenylephrine is used for severe, refractory cyanosis while awaiting surgical intervention.

Suggested Readings

Dahshan A, Donovan GK. Severe methemoglobinemia complicating topical benzocaine use during endoscopy in a toddler: a case report and review of the literature. *Pediatrics.*2006;117(4):e806–e809.

Driscoll DJ. Evaluation of the cyanotic newborn. *Pediatr Clin North Am.* 1990;37(1):1–23.

Marino BS, Bird GL, Wernovsky G. Diagnosis and management of the newborn with suspected congenital heart disease. *Clin Perinatol.* 2001;28(1):91–136.

O'Donnell CP, Kamlin CO, Davis PG, et al. Clinical assessment of infant colour at delivery. *Arch Dis Child Fetal Neonatal Ed.* 2007;92(6):F465–F467.

Sasidharan P. An approach to diagnosis and management of cyanosis and tachypnea in term infants. *Pediatr Clin North Am.* 2004;51(4):999–1021, ix.

Stevenson DK, Benitz WE. A practical approach to diagnosis and immediate care of the cyanotic neonate. Stabilization and preparation for transfer to level III nursery. *Clin Pediatr (Phila).* 1987;26(7):325–331.

Tingelstad J. Consultation with the specialist: non-respiratory cyanosis. *Pediatr Rev.* 1999;20(10):350–352.

Zorc JJ, Kanic Z. A cyanotic infant: true blue or otherwise? *Pediatr Ann.* 2001;30(10):597–601.

Dehydration

INTRODUCTION

Dehydration is a total body fluid deficit and a cause of hypovolemic shock. It occurs when total fluid loss is greater than fluid intake. It is not a diagnosis in itself but rather a symptom of another process. The most common cause of dehydration brought to medical attention is gastroenteritis. Dehydration can be classified based on the degree of dehydration with 5% representing mild dehydration, 5% to 10% representing moderate dehydration, and 10% representing severe dehydration. If serum electrolytes are assessed, the dehydration can be further classified based on serum sodium. This chapter focuses primarily of dehydration from gastroenteritis.

DIFFERENTIAL DIAGNOSIS LIST

Increased Output
- Gastroenteritis
- Vomiting
- Pyloric stenosis
- Appendicitis
- Pancreatitis
- Small bowel obstruction
- Intussusception
- Lower lobe pneumonia
- Pyelonephritis
- Increased intracranial pressure
- Diarrhea
- Malabsorption
- Inflammatory bowel disease
- Celiac disease

- Cystic fibrosis
- Increased insensible losses (fever, sweating, hyperventilation, etc.)
- Renal losses (diabetic ketoacidosis, diabetes insipidus, Bartter syndrome, etc.)

Decreased Intake
- Voluntary (pharyngitis, stomatitis, respiratory distress, etc.)
- Physical restriction (infant/elderly, coma, child abuse, etc.)

Translocation of Fluids
- Burns
- Hypoproteinemic states (ascites, peripheral edema, etc.)

DIFFERENTIAL DIAGNOSIS DISCUSSION
Gastroenteritis
Physiology
Under normal physiologic conditions, water comprises 70% of lean body mass in children and adults and 75% in infants. Two-thirds of the fluid is intracellular and

one-third is extracellular. Of the extracellular fluid, 75% is interstitial and 25% is intravascular. Fluid that is lost from the body often has an electrolyte composition similar to plasma. Most of the fluid deficit during the early stages of dehydration is from the extracellular space, but with time, the fluid losses equilibrate and fluid leaves the intracellular space. During the recovery phase, fluid administered to the patient is in the extracellular space and will need time to re-equilibrate with the intracellular space.

Etiology

Gastroenteritis can be caused by viral, bacterial, or parasitic pathogens. The predominant cause in developed countries is viral. Rotavirus is known to cause more serious illness than other viral causes. Worldwide, all children have had at least one episode of rotavirus gastroenteritis by 5 years of age.

Clinical Features

Gastroenteritis typically starts with the acute onset of vomiting, which may be persistent and severe. Clinicians should consider other etiologies in a child presenting with vomiting alone, but the subsequent development of diarrhea may clarify a diagnosis of viral gastroenteritis. The overall course of illness typically lasts about 5 to 7 days.

 HINT: The onset of abdominal pain prior to the vomiting should make the clinician consider appendicitis.

Children with dehydration from gastroenteritis may develop electrolyte abnormalities. Approximately one-third of patients who are moderately dehydrated have hypoglycemia. These children appear listless. Less commonly, patients have elevated serum sodium. This hypernatremia represents a free water deficit. The sodium acts osmotically to draw water from the cellular compartment extracellularly. This results in a state of intracellular dehydration. The acute manifestations of hypernatremia include early neurologic irritability (e.g., seizures). The degree of dehydration may be more difficult to assess in these children because most of the clinical findings of dehydration are caused by decreased extracellular fluid; one clue may be the presence of "doughy" skin. Conversely, hyponatremia results in intracellular swelling. These patients also may present with neurologic symptomatology, primarily seizures, lethargy, and coma.

Evaluation

Evaluation of dehydration focuses on a thorough history and physical examination. Historical points to consider include possible exposures to other children who have been sick, timing of the symptoms, number of episodes of vomiting and diarrhea, or presence of blood or bile. Exposure to well water, camping, or recent travel may raise the suspicion for an etiology other than viral gastroenteritis. High fever with bloody diarrhea would be concerning for bacterial dysentery.

A thorough physical examination can aid in confirming the diagnosis. The examiner should assess the overall appearance of the child for the presence of lethargy or listlessness that may be associated with dehydration. Other common examination features include an assessment of the urine output, the presence and quality of tear production, the quality of the mucous membranes (moist, tacky, or dry), the capillary refill (measured at the distal fingertip, considered prolonged if >2 seconds in an warm ambient environment), assessment of the skin turgor, assessment of the heart rate and distal pulses, as well as assessment of the fontanelle in the infant. Research on assessing the degree of dehydration has been helpful in creating a framework within which to evaluate a dehydrated patient. A recent meta-analysis presents data that are helpful (Table 25-1). If a finding is present, it may increase the likelihood of dehydration. For example, the likelihood ratio for the presence of prolonged capillary refill is 4.1 with a 95% confidence interval that ranges from 1.7 to 9.8. We can interpret this to mean that if prolonged capillary refill is present, then the odds of the child having at least 5% dehydration are 4.1 times higher than if prolonged capillary refill was not present. The examination findings in the meta-analysis that significantly increase the likelihood of dehydration include prolonged capillary refill, abnormal skin turgor, and abnormal respiratory pattern. Conversely, some findings if they are absent decrease the likelihood of the patient being 5% dehydrated. For example, the likelihood ratio for the absence of poor overall appearance is 0.46 with a 95% confidence interval that ranges from 0.34 to 0.61. We can interpret this to mean that the odds are less than half as likely for the patient to be at least 5% dehydrated if there is a normal general appearance. The findings that would decrease the likelihood of significant

TABLE 25-1	Signs and Symptoms of the Presence of at Least 5% Dehydration	
Finding	Likelihood Ratio if Present (95% CI)	Likelihood Ratio if Absent (95% CI)
Prolonged capillary refill	**4.1 (1.7–9.8)**	0.57 (0.39–0.82)
Abnormal skin turgor	**2.5 (1.5–4.2)**	0.66 (0.57–0.75)
Abnormal respirations	**2.0 (1.5–2.7)**	0.76 (0.62–0.88)
Sunken eyes	1.7 (1.1–2.5)	**0.49 (0.38–0.63)**
Dry mucous membranes	1.7 (1.1–2.6)	**0.41 (0.21–0.79)**
Cool extremity[a]	1.5, 18.8	0.89, 0.97
Weak pulse[a]	3.1, 7.2	0.66, 0.96
Absent tears	2.3 (0.9–5.8)	0.54 (0.26–1.13)
Increased heart rate	1.3 (0.8–2.0)	0.82 (0.64–1.05)
Sunken fontanelle	0.9 (0.6–1.3)	1.1 (0.82–1.54)
Poor overall appearance	1.9 (0.97–3.8)	**0.46 (0.34–0.61)**

Adapted from Steiner MJ, DeWalt DA, Byerley JS. Is this child dehydrated? *JAMA*. 2004;291(22):2746–2754.
[a]These findings were only evaluated in two studies and a pooled value was not obtained. The range of the point estimates is presented.
The likelihood ratio (LR) is interpreted such that the likelihood of dehydration would increase if the LR if present is >1.0. Clinically useful values have a LR positive value of ≥2 with a 95% confidence interval (CI) that does not cross 1.0. Furthermore, the LR if absent means the likelihood of dehydration would decrease if the sign was absent. Clinically useful values have a LR negative value of <0.5 and have a 95% CI that does not cross 1.0. The values in bold are the clinically helpful values.

TABLE 25-2	Four-Point Dehydration System

Overall poor appearance
Absent tears
Dry mucous membranes
Delayed capillary refill

Adapted from Gorelick MH, Shaw KN, Murphy KO. Validity and reliability of clinical signs in the diagnosis of dehydration in children. *Pediatrics*. 1997;99(5):E6.
The patient is assigned one point for each feature present. A score of zero indicates no dehydration present. A score of 1 indicates mild dehydration (<5%). A score of 2 indicates moderate dehydration (5%–10%). A score of 3 or 4 indicates severe dehydration (>10%).

dehydration if they were absent include dry mucous membranes, sunken eyes, and poor overall appearance.

Although helpful, these summary statistics on physical examination findings are often hard to implement clinically. However, one high-quality study of a 10-point dehydration scoring system took a subset of four symptoms and was able to demonstrate that the subset of four findings had the same diagnostic accuracy as the larger 10-point dehydration score presented. The 4-point dehydration score consists of poor overall appearance, absent tears, dry mucous membranes, and delayed capillary refill (Table 25-2). One point is awarded for each feature present. The interpretation is that a score of 0 out of the 4 features represents no dehydration present, 1 of the 4 represents mild dehydration (<5%), 2 or 3 of the 4 features represents moderate dehydration (5% to 10%), and a score of 4 of the 4 features represents severe dehydration (>10%). This 4-point system is a clinically useful score because most practitioners already assess and can easily remember these four features.

Electrolytes

There is no role for the routine evaluation of electrolytes in dehydrated patients. They should be checked as directed by the clinical evaluation, particularly if an unusual history or examination finding suggests an electrolyte abnormality. Electrolytes do not assist in determining if dehydration is present; they are helpful to determine the degree of acidosis present and if there is a need for specialized treatment because of hypernatremia or hyponatremia. It is important to appreciate that approximately one-third of moderately dehydrated patients are concurrently hypoglycemic.

 HINT: One-third of moderately dehydrated patients are also hypoglycemic.

Treatment
Emergency Treatment

Emergency treatment focuses on identifying and addressing life-threatening issues. The presence of severe dehydration and shock requires aggressive fluid resuscitation. The clinician should place an intravenous line and administer sequential 20 mL/kg boluses of isotonic fluids. Therapy is directed at restoring circulating volume and perfusing vital organs. If there is a need, blood products can be used to restore intravascular volume. After the shock has been addressed, appropriate therapy can be continued.

The fluid deficit can be calculated from the percentage of dehydration present. The fluid lost during gastroenteritis has a specific gravity near one. Hence, the weight loss approximates the fluid deficit. By determining the percent dehydration as discussed previously or if a well and dehydrated weight are known, the fluid deficit can be determined. Five percent of a liter is 50 mL. Hence, 5% dehydration requires 50 mL/kg fluid replacement. Likewise, 10% dehydration is 100 mL/kg.

> **HINT:** Mild (<5%) dehydration requires about 50 mL/kg fluid replacement; moderate (5% to 10%) dehydration requires 100 mL/kg fluid replacement.

> **HINT:** The fluid deficit can be administered over a 4-hour period. Therapy can be initiated under medical supervision. If the patient is performing oral rehydration therapy (ORT) well, they can be discharged to home to continue the fluid replacement.

> **HINT:** Ondansetron is helpful in decreasing emesis associated with gastroenteritis. The oral dissolving tablet can be used prior to starting therapy.

Oral Rehydration Therapy

ORT is recommended as the initial therapy of choice by the American Academy of Pediatrics, the World Health Organization (WHO), and the Centers for Disease Control and Prevention for mildly and moderately dehydrated children and can even be used for severely dehydrated children. ORT is not simply giving the patient Pedialyte or a sports beverage to drink. That would be considered an oral challenge. Rather, ORT is the frequent administration of small volumes of an appropriate oral rehydration solution (ORS) on a regular schedule. Although ORT is effective at rehydrating dehydrated children in an emergency department (ED) setting, its use in the United States has been limited. The most frequent obstacles to successful oral rehydration in the ED are false perceptions that oral rehydration is too slow or not a definitive procedure. Physicians and nurses hold these beliefs as frequently as parents. Generally, 5 minutes spent preparing for and describing ORT to the family reduces or eliminates these obstacles. ORT spares the child the pain of an intravenous (IV) line, promotes more direct parental involvement in the management of the child's dehydration, and teaches the parents a skill that can be used for the ongoing illness and the next time the child becomes dehydrated. After starting ORT, frequent reassessments should be made. If the patient is not tolerating the therapy, then parenteral fluids should be administered.

The administration of ondansetron prior to initiating ORT has improved the success rate of ORT to >80%. If a patient is going to fail with ORT, it generally happens early in the treatment process, typically within 30 minutes.

 HINT: 10 mL of unflavored Pedialyte administered with a syringe over a 5-minute period is one method of ORT. The volume can be increased as tolerated and the interval can be shortened.

Use of an appropriate ORS assists in ensuring success. The physiology of ORT uses the passive absorption of water from the intestines using the sodium–glucose cotransport mechanism. This cotransport is maintained even in the case of severe gastroenteritis when there is significant sloughing of the brush border of the small intestine. The optimal stoichiometric carbohydrate (i.e., glucose) to sodium ratio is 1:1. This ratio is maintained by the WHO in their two ORSs (Table 25-3). The original WHO ORS was developed for cholera and has a higher sodium concentration of 90 mEq/L. The WHO has recently manufactured a second ORS that has a reduced sodium concentration of 75 mEq/L. This second ORS is designed for treatment of dehydration from both viral and bacterial gastroenteritis. Other commercial products are designed for the rehydration phase of ORT, specifically Rehydralyte. The more commonly used Pedialyte is actually a maintenance solution and not technically a rehydration solution; however, it is effective at treating mild to moderate dehydration from gastroenteritis. The commercial products have a higher glucose concentration and therefore deviate from the 1:1 ratio of carbohydrate to sodium. Often, children may refuse the ORS because it has a salty taste. This tends to occur more commonly in older children or children who are minimally dehydrated. As an alternative in mild dehydration, a sports beverage diluted 1:1 with water may be more palatable. Administration of a saltine cracker would increase the sodium administered for this rehydration technique. Table 25-4 lists the fluids that are not appropriate for rehydration solutions for dehydration from gastroenteritis.

 HINT: Syringe administration often helps the child to swallow the ORS despite the salty taste. Children may refuse the ORS when offered in a cup or bottle.

ORT may fail. Typical reasons include patient refusal, parental noncompliance with administration recommendations, persistent emesis, and losses greater than the amount of fluid administered. Additionally, children and parents have a hard time staying awake and performing rehydration during the middle of the night. Patients dehydrated from stomatitis or pharyngitis may refuse oral fluid because of pain. Addressing pain in these patients may assist in avoiding parenteral fluids.

Subcutaneous Fluid Therapy

Subcutaneous fluid administration is a method of administering fluids parentally. The technique utilizes the enzyme hyaluronidase to augment the absorption of

TABLE 25-3 **Appropriate Oral Rehydration Solutions**

Solution	Sodium (mEq/L)	Potassium (mEq/L)	Chloride (mEq/L)	Base (mEq/L)	Carbohydrate % (mmol/L)	Osmolarity (mmol/L)	Carbohydrate-to-Sodium Ratio
WHO solution (1)	90	20	80	10	2% (111)	311	1:1
WHO solution (2)	75	20	65	10	1.4% (75)	245	1:1
Rehydralyte	75	20	65	30	2.5% (139)	329	2:1
Pedialyte	45	20	35	30	2.5% (139)	269	3:1

TABLE 25-4 **Inappropriate Oral Rehydration Solutions**

Solution	Sodium (mEq/L)	Potassium (mEq/L)	Chloride (mEq/L)	Base (mEq/L)	Carbohydrate % (mmol/L)	Osmolarity (mmol/L)	Carbohydrate-to-Sodium Ratio
Gatorade	20	3	17	3	4.6% (58)	330	12:1
Coca-Cola	2	<1		13	12% (112)	>600	—
Apple juice	3	32	2	0	12.4% (120)	730	230:1
Chicken broth	250	8	250	0	0	500	—

TABLE 25-5	Difficult Venous Access Score		
Feature	**0 points**	**1 point**	**2 points**
Vein visible	Yes		No
Vein palpable	Yes		No
Prematurity (<38 wk gestation)	No		Yes
Age	≥3 yr	1–2 yr	<12 mo

Adapted from Yen K, Riegert AM, Gorelick MH. Derivation of the DIVA score: A clinical prediction rule for the identification of children with difficult venous access. *Pediatr Emerg Care.* 2008;24(3):143–147.
A score of 4 or more correlates to 50% first attempt success rate with IV placement.

isotonic fluids administered subcutaneously. This method was common prior to the introduction of intravenous therapy in the 1950s, but fell out of favor due to complications when inappropriate fluids were administered. Isotonic fluids should be utilized to avoid iatrogenic hyponatremia. The development of a human recombinant form of the hyaluronidase enzyme has renewed interest in this technique. Studies are currently underway to further clarify the role of subcutaneously administered fluids for rehydration. It has been shown to rehydrate mild and moderately dehydrated children and could be considered as a "bridge therapy" while intravascular access is obtained in severe dehydration. Consideration for this technique should be given to children who are anticipated to have difficult venous access (Table 25-5).

 HINT: Subcutaneous fluid therapy is a method of administering fluids parentally if there is difficulty in obtaining intravenous access.

Intravenous Fluid Therapy

If administration of ondansetron and an attempt at ORT was unsuccessful or the patient is severely dehydrated, then IV fluid rehydration is warranted. Current recommendations for IV fluid rehydration focus on goal-directed therapy. Replacement of the fluid deficit and maintaining ongoing losses are the primary goals. Sequential fluid boluses may be required with frequent reassessment to assess for improved perfusion, urine output, continued emesis, etc. Boluses should be made with isotonic fluids; frequently normal saline or lactated Ringer's solution is used. The bolus volume is 20 mL/kg. Glucose should not be included in the bolus because the amount of glucose in a 20 mL/kg bolus would be two to four times the amount of glucose required for documented hypoglycemia. After the bolus volume has been administered, glucose-containing IV fluid can be started at 1.5 times maintenance. The child should be encouraged to take enteral feeds. Younger children may require hospitalization until they demonstrate adequate oral intake. Older children can be rehydrated in the ED and discharged to home to continue the therapy unless extenuating circumstances require the continued administration of IV fluids.

Electrolyte Abnormalities

Hypoglycemia is common in dehydrated patients, particularly patients who are moderately dehydrated **(see Chapter 32, "Electrolyte Disturbances")**. ORT addresses the hypoglycemia by providing glucose in the treatment phase. During IV fluid therapy, the practitioner should assess for hypoglycemia as indicated. Treatment for documented hypoglycemia is 0.5 g/kg of glucose. This amount can be easily calculated by using the "rule of 50." Fifty divided by the concentration of dextrose solution to be used (e.g., D5, D10, D25, D50) provides the number of milliliters per kilogram that equal 0.5 g/kg of glucose.

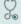 **HINT:** The Rule of 50 can be used to calculate the correct amount of dextrose to give to a hypoglycemic patient. The milliliters per kilogram of dextrose containing fluid multiplied by the dextrose concentration equals 50.

Suggested Readings

Gorelick MH, Shaw KN, Murphy KO. Validity and reliability of clinical signs in the diagnosis of dehydration in children. *Pediatrics.* 1997;99(5):E6.

Harting L, Bellemare S, Wiebe N, et al. Oral versus intravenous rehydration for treating dehydration due to gastroenteritis in children. *Cochrane Database Syst Rev.* 2006;3:CD004390.

Spandorfer PR, Alessandrini EA, Joffe MD, et al. Oral versus intravenous rehydration of moderately dehydrated children: a randomized, controlled trial. *Pediatrics.* 2005;115(2):295–301.

Steiner MJ, DeWalt DA, Byerley JS. Is this child dehydrated? *JAMA.* 2004;291(22):2746–2754.

Yen K, Riegert A, Gorelick MH. Derivation of the DIVA score: a clinical prediction rule for the identification of children with difficult venous access. *Pediatr Emerg Care.* 2008;24(3):143–147.

Diabetes

INTRODUCTION

Diabetes mellitus is a disorder of glucose metabolism characterized by **hyperglycemia** caused by insulin deficiency. Diabetes encompasses several clinical syndromes including, but not limited to, **type 1 diabetes mellitus (T1D),** characterized by rapid onset, a tendency toward ketoacidosis, and absolute insulin deficiency; and **type 2 diabetes (T2D),** associated with obesity, insulin resistance, a lesser likelihood of ketoacidosis, and nonabsolute dependence on insulin for survival. Both types of diabetes are associated with similar long-term complications. T1D affects ~1 in 350 children by the age of 18 and is more common in children of European background. T2D is more commonly seen in African American, Native American, and Latino children, but its prevalence is increasing in all ethnic groups.

DIFFERENTIAL DIAGNOSIS LIST

Infectious Disorders
Urinary tract infection (UTI)
Gastroenteritis
Pneumonia
Sepsis

Toxic Disorders
Salicylate ingestion
Steroid use
Diuretic use

Endocrine and Metabolic Disorders
Hypercalcemia
Diabetes insipidus
Inborn error of metabolism

Miscellaneous Disorders
Renal glucosuria
Stress hyperglycemia

Psychosocial Disorders
Psychogenic polydipsia
Enuresis

EVALUATION OF DIABETES
Patient History
Polyuria, polydipsia, and polyphagia are classic symptoms:

- **Weight loss and poor growth** may go undetected.
- **Nausea, vomiting, and lethargy** occur as the child's illness progresses to diabetic ketoacidosis (DKA).

- **A precipitating event** (intercurrent illness or stress) often prompts medical attention.

Physical Examination

Physical examination is usually normal early in the course of disease. Later findings can include the following:

- **Signs of dehydration** (e.g., tachycardia, poor skin perfusion, hypotension)
- **Hyperpnea (Kussmaul respirations),** a sign of metabolic acidosis
- **Fruity odor to the breath,** a sign of ketosis

Laboratory Studies

The diagnosis of diabetes may be made in one of four ways:

- **Fasting blood glucose** (BG) **level** ≥ 126 mg/dL
- **Random BG level** ≥ 200 mg/dL in the setting of symptoms of diabetes
- **Two-hour BG level** ≥ 200 mg/dL during an oral glucose tolerance test
- **Hemoglobin A1c level** ≥ 6.5%

The presence of glucose in the urine is suggestive but NOT diagnostic for diabetes.

Other biochemical parameters may be normal until the development of DKA, at which time:

- **Serum electrolyte panel** may reveal hyponatremia (sodium level < 136 mEq/L) from hyperglycemia and hypertriglyceridemia; hypokalemia or hyperkalemia (potassium level < 4.0 mEq/L or > 6.0 mEq/L, respectively), or a metabolic acidosis (bicarbonate level < 15 mEq/L).
- **Arterial or venous blood gases** may reveal a metabolic acidosis (pH < 7.3, partial pressure of carbon dioxide [Pco_2] < 35 mm Hg).
- **Complete blood cell count** may reveal elevated white blood cell count even in the absence of infection.

DIFFERENTIAL DIAGNOSIS

UTI and nocturnal enuresis. The early signs of diabetes (i.e., polyuria, nocturia) may be mistaken for UTI or nocturnal enuresis. Urinalysis, however, demonstrates the presence of glucose and ketones and the absence of markers of infection.

Renal glucosuria (a condition in which glucose is excreted in the urine at normal BG levels) may be mistaken for diabetes. Diabetes should never be diagnosed by the presence of glucosuria alone: An elevated BG or hemoglobin A1c level is required for the diagnosis of diabetes.

Other metabolic disorders may present with acidosis and dehydration, but a history of polyuria, polyphagia, and weight loss with an elevated BG is characteristic of diabetes.

Gastroenteritis and surgical abdomen. The abdominal pain and vomiting of DKA may be mistaken for gastroenteritis or a surgical abdomen, but DKA may be differentiated not only from these disorders but also from other metabolic diseases by the distinct history of polyuria, polydipsia, and a characteristic fruity odor to the breath.

Intercurrent febrile illnesses or the **administration of glucocorticoids** for inflammatory conditions may cause an insulin-resistant state and precipitate hyperglycemia, glucosuria, and even small amounts of ketonuria (known as "stress hyperglycemia"). These conditions must be differentiated from true diabetes. In patients who do not have diabetes, resolution of the fever and acute illness or discontinuation of the medications should result in normalization of the blood sugar. It is important to go back and determine whether the typical symptoms of polydipsia and polyuria are present. In the absence of these symptoms, the diagnosis of diabetes is less likely. Occasionally, however, a latent case of true diabetes may be discovered. In these cases, the presence of anti-islet cell antibodies or an elevated hemoglobin A1c value may be useful in establishing the proper diagnosis.

Asthma or pneumonia. The Kussmaul respirations that occur with progressive acidosis may resemble asthma or pneumonia, but auscultation and radiography reveal clear lung fields.

TREATMENT OF DIABETES

Optimal care requires the efforts of the child, the family, and a team of physicians, nurses, dietitians, and counselors specializing in the treatment of children with diabetes. The physician's primary responsibilities are the **prompt recognition of symptoms** leading to a definitive diagnosis, **referral** to a pediatric diabetes center, and **continued supervision** of the child's medical care. Children with diabetes should attend a multidisciplinary pediatric diabetes center at least every 3 months or more frequently if treatment goals are not being met.

Treatment goals are the maintenance of BG and hemoglobin A1c levels as close to normal as possible, avoidance of severe hypoglycemia, and optimization of the child's normal physical and psychosocial growth and development. To accomplish these goals, the child must not only take insulin or oral antidiabetic medications but also monitor the blood sugar several times during the day, exercise, and adhere to the prescribed meal plan. Family members should be trained to monitor blood sugars, give insulin, recognize and treat low blood sugar reactions, and provide support. **Psychosocial factors are critical** in the management of children with diabetes, and potential problems should be addressed by experienced behavioral or family therapists.

Insulin

The goal of diabetes therapy is to maintain the BG levels as close to normal as possible. For the child with T1D, this means reliance on multiple doses of insulin daily. These may be administered either by subcutaneous injections via syringe or via continuous subcutaneous insulin infusion using a portable wearable pump (insulin pump therapy). In both cases, insulin dosages are customized to mimic the body's pattern of basal insulin delivery between meals and overnight, with spikes in insulin release (boluses) for meal-related carbohydrates. Insulin doses

TABLE 26-1	Pharmacokinetics of Common Insulin Preparations		
Insulin	**Onset**	**Peak**	**Duration**
Rapid-acting insulin analogs: Lispro (Humalog) Aspart (NovoLog) Glulisine (Apidra)	10–15 min	1–3 hr	3–5 hr
Short-acting (regular)	0.5–1 hr	2–4 hr	4–8 hr
Intermediate-acting (NPH)	2–4 hr	4–10 hr	10–18 hr
Long-acting analogs: Glargine (Lantus) Detemir (Levemir)	2–3 hr 1 hr	None None	24 hr Up to 24 hr

must be individually titrated, and even in one individual, insulin needs typically change from day to day because of variations in meals, physical activity, illness, and other factors. Table 26-1 shows the most commonly used insulin preparations. Table 26-2 gives recommended insulin adjustments.

Fixed-dose (split mix) insulin regimens are often employed early in the course of diabetes while children and families are still learning to manage the disease. Insulin doses are generally kept constant and given as mixtures of rapid/intermediate-acting or rapid/long-acting to minimize the number of daily injections. Such regimens typically consist of the following:

TABLE 26-2	Adjustments for Fixed-Dose Insulin Regimens[a]	
Blood Glucose	**Time**	**Recommended Action**
High	Pre-breakfast	Increase evening intermediate or long-acting insulin; if this results in nighttime lows, may need to eliminate bedtime snack
Low	Pre-breakfast	Decrease evening intermediate- or long-acting insulin or increase bedtime snack content
High	Pre-lunch	Increase morning rapid-acting insulin first; then intermediate-acting if needed
Low	Pre-lunch	Decrease morning rapid-insulin first; then intermediate-acting if needed
High	Pre-dinner	Increase morning intermediate-acting insulin; if these results in midday lows, extra shot of rapid-acting insulin may be needed after school
Low	Pre-dinner	Decrease morning intermediate-acting insulin
High	Bedtime	Increase evening rapid-insulin
Low	Bedtime	Decrease evening rapid-acting insulin

[a]For basal-bolus regimens, the long-acting insulin analog is titrated to produce a fasting morning BG level in the target range. Meal bolus doses are titrated to yield normal BG levels at the next meal.

Two-thirds total daily dose before breakfast—one-third as rapid-acting, two-thirds as intermediate-acting.

One-third total daily dose before dinner—half as rapid-acting, half as intermediate or long-acting (the intermediate- or long-acting insulin can alternatively be given at bedtime).

Flexible (basal-bolus) regimens require more frequent injections than split-mix regimens but are ultimately more effective in controlling both hyperglycemia and hypoglycemia. In these regimens, a fixed dose of long-acting insulin analog is given once or twice daily to provide the basal insulin requirement, and smaller doses of rapid-acting insulin analogs are given with each meal or snack based on the carbohydrate content of the coming meal and the BG level at the time of the meal, for example:

At breakfast: 0.4 to 0.5 Unit/kg long-acting insulin analog.

Before each meal: 1 Unit rapid-acting insulin analog for every 15 g of carbohydrate in the coming meal *plus* 1 Unit for every 100 mg/dL elevation of the BG level over the target (e.g., 1 extra unit if BG > 200 and target BG = 100).

Insulin pumps have emerged as a preferred means of insulin delivery because of the ability to vary basal and bolus rates easily. Basal rates can be decreased to prevent nighttime or exercise-related hypoglycemia or increased for periods of illness. Bolus doses can be given without the need for a separate injection; and the newer pumps contain software that can determine the proper bolus dose when the current BG level and carbohydrate content of the coming meal are entered. Some newer insulin pumps also work with continuous glucose monitors to provide the glucose levels in real time.

Insulin injection sites should be rotated among the arms, legs, buttocks, and stomach to avoid lipoatrophy or lipohypertrophy. Insulin pump infusion catheters are commonly inserted in the abdomen or buttocks and should be changed every 2 to 3 days.

Oral antidiabetic medications are not indicated in the treatment of T1D in children but play an important role in T2D. The insulin sensitizer **metformin** may be considered the first-line medication if lifestyle interventions such as diet and physical activity are insufficient to normalize BG levels. Metformin may be initiated at a dose of 500 mg daily and increased to a maximum of 1,000 mg twice daily. Common side effects are nausea, anorexia, and gastrointestinal discomfort, which may be lessened if the drug is taken with food and the dose increased gradually. Insulin secretagogues (sulfonylureas, meglitinide analogs) and the other insulin sensitizers (rosiglitazone, pioglitazone) are less commonly used because of the relative scarcity of pediatric data and the side effect of weight gain.

Complications of Insulin Therapy

Hypoglycemia is the most common acute complication of diabetes management. Typical symptoms include hunger, headache, lethargy, dizziness, irritability, confusion, sweating, and tachycardia. Mild symptoms are easily treated with oral glucose (e.g., glucose tablets, orange juice). **Severe hypoglycemia** may lead to seizures and coma. These are treated with glucagon, 1 mg, given intramuscularly. All children with diabetes should carry oral glucose tablets with them at all times and keep glucagon at home. **Recurrent hypoglycemia** should be corrected aggressively.

Intercurrent Illnesses and DKA

Intercurrent illnesses should be managed with more frequent BG and urine ketone monitoring, increased fluid intake, and supplementary insulin if needed for hyperglycemia or ketosis. It should be stressed that children with T1D always needs insulin, even if they are not eating because of illness; in this instance, the short-acting insulin may be withheld and the long-acting insulin reduced to prevent hypoglycemia. Urine ketones should be monitored as an indication to increase insulin dosages. If BG levels cannot be maintained in the normal range, intravenous fluids containing dextrose may be necessary. Table 26-3 describes the management of ketosis and DKA.

Monitoring

The goals of **BG monitoring** are to gauge the effectiveness of the current medication regimen and minimize episodes of hypoglycemia. The availability of accurate,

---

TABLE 26-3   Guidelines to Treatment of Acute Illness

Mild Illness ("Sick Days")

Insulin
Variable; stress of illness masy increase insulin requirements, particularly in presence of fever and ketones; however, smaller more frequent doses may be needed if child is not eating well or vomiting

Fluids
Increase oral fluid intake to prevent dehydration, reduce hyperglycemia, and clear ketones; sugar-containing fluids preferable if glucose levels are low and child requires more insulin to clear ketones

Monitoring
More frequent BG monitoring is important during sick days; every 2 to 3 hr for young children or in setting of vomiting or decreased oral intake

Ketoacidosis (DKA): Glucose ≥ 200 mg/dL, pH < 7.3, or Bicarbonate < 15 mEq/L

Intravenous Fluids
10–20 mL/kg 0.9% saline bolus to restore intravascular volume, then replace deficit slowly over 48 hr using isotonic fluids (0.9% saline)
Nothing by mouth until acidosis corrected (serum HCO_3 >15 mEq/L)

Sodium
Deficit 10 mEq/kg—replace with normal saline in rehydration fluid

Potassium
Deficit 5–10 mEq/L—start after patient urinates
If K ≥ 4.0, add 40 mEq/L
If K < 4.0, add 60 mEq/L
Give potassium as 1:1 potassium chloride:potassium phosphate to help replace phosphate deficit. Monitor serum calcium

Insulin
0.1 Unit/kg per hr (the amount of glucose in the intravenous fluids and the rate of insulin infusion should be titrated to lower the blood sugar 50–100 mg/dL per hr)

easy-to-use home glucose meters has facilitated home monitoring of blood sugars and adjustment of therapy. The BG should be monitored before each meal and before the bedtime snack, with more frequent monitoring when the child is sick, vomiting, or having symptoms of hypoglycemia. Glucose levels 2 to 3 hours after meals may be checked to gauge the effectiveness of meal-dose insulin or in patients not on insulin therapy, to determine whether to initiate insulin. When blood sugar levels are out of the target range, prompt modifications should be made to the insulin regimen (see Table 26-2). **Urine should also be monitored** for ketones during periods of intercurrent illness, fever, vomiting, or when the blood sugar persistently exceeds 240 mg/dL. Continuous glucose monitoring devices are a valuable adjunct to periodic BG testing, by providing up-to-date glucose information in real time as well as alarms for hypo- or hyperglycemia. They have been shown to improve glucose levels in patients who are not meeting glycemic targets and to reduce hypoglycemia in subjects who are already meeting targets. However, they can be uncomfortable and difficult to use.

Diet

Medical nutrition therapy is central to the management of diabetes in children but differs markedly between T1D and T2D. For children with T1D, knowledge of the carbohydrate content of meals and snacks is important for determining insulin doses. Children on fixed insulin regimens should aim for consistency in carbohydrate content (e.g., 60 to 75 g for each meal, 15 to 20 g for snacks) so that the proper amount of insulin is "matched" for the meal. Children on flexible insulin regimens may vary their meal-related insulin dosages depending on the carbohydrate content of their meal (e.g., 1 Unit of rapid-acting insulin for every 15 gm of ingested carbohydrate). For children with T2D, in whom obesity and insulin resistance may be significant factors, adherence to a meal plan designed to promote gradual, sustained weight loss may be more important than the actual carbohydrate content. Low-carbohydrate diets are not recommended in children with T1D; these diets promote weight loss but have not been well studied in children with T2D.

Exercise

A regular exercise program is important for optimal health and blood sugar control in the child with T1D, and it is absolutely necessary for management of the child with T2D. Exercise lowers blood sugar levels and insulin requirements and improves insulin sensitivity. It is also a useful tool to lower the blood sugar level acutely. However, vigorous exercise should be avoided in the presence of ketosis.

Psychosocial Factors

The management of diabetes is particularly stressful for the child and the whole family unit. Children should be screened regularly for signs of depression, anxiety, and stress. Similarly, because the safe management of a child with diabetes requires responsible care on the part of the adult caretakers in the house, the clinician should also assess parenting skills, coping strategies, and adjustment in the parent, along with parent–child interactions. Referral to a behavioral or family therapist is necessary when problems are identified.

Complications and Comorbidities

Proper long-term care of the child with diabetes includes monitoring for chronic complications (nephropathy, neuropathy, retinopathy, and cardiovascular disease) as well as associated medical conditions that occur with greater frequency in children with T1D (autoimmune thyroid disease, celiac disease, and adrenal insufficiency). Routine monitoring of blood pressure, annual laboratory screening of thyroid, and tissue transglutaminase levels and urinary albumin excretion rates, and referral for dilated ophthalmological examinations should be performed in all children of pubertal age or with diabetes duration of >5 years.

Suggested Readings

American Diabetes Association. Standards of medical care in diabetes –2011. *Diabetes Care.* 2011;34(Suppl 1): S11–S61.

Rosenbloom AL, Silverstein JH, Amemiya S, et al. Type 2 diabetes in children and adolescents. *Pediatr Diabetes.* 2009;10(Suppl 12):17–32.

Silverstein J, Klingensmith G, Copeland K, et al. Care of children and adolescents with type 1 diabetes: a statement of the American Diabetes Association. *Diabetes Care.* 2005;28:186–212.

Wolfsdorf J, Glaser N, Sperling MA. Diabetic ketoacidosis in infants, children, and adolescents: a consensus statement from the American Diabetes Association. *Diabetes Care.* 2006;29:1150–1159.

Diarrhea, Acute

INTRODUCTION

Acute diarrhea is defined as stools with **increased water content and frequency** for a period of **<5 to 7 days**. Most cases of acute diarrhea are of infectious (predominantly viral) origin and are self-limited. Approximately 5% of children with acute diarrhea require medical evaluation. Acute diarrhea is occasionally the presenting symptom of a life-threatening condition. The differential diagnostic considerations for acute diarrhea overlap with those for chronic diarrhea (see Chapter 28, "Diarrhea, Chronic").

DIFFERENTIAL DIAGNOSIS LIST

Infectious Causes
Viruses
Rotavirus
Enteric adenoviruses
Caliciviruses (e.g., Norovirus)
Enteroviruses
Astroviruses

Bacteria
Salmonella species
Shigella species
Campylobacter species
Yersinia enterocolitica
Pathogenic *Escherichia coli*
Aeromonas
Clostridium difficile
Vibrio species

Parasites
Giardia species
Cryptosporidium species
Entamoeba histolytica
Blastocystis hominis

Systemic
Otitis media
Urinary tract infection (UTI)

Hepatitis
Sepsis

Toxic Causes
Foodborne illness
Pharmacologic agents—iron, laxatives, and antibiotics
Plant or mushroom toxicity
Household cleaners or soap
Serotonin syndrome
Neonatal drug withdrawal

Metabolic or Genetic Causes
Adrenal insufficiency
Congenital adrenal hyperplasia (CAH)
Disaccharidase deficiency
Hyperthyroidism

Inflammatory Causes
Appendicitis
Inflammatory bowel disease
Eosinophilic gastroenteritis

Anatomic Causes
Intussusception
Partial bowel obstruction

Hirschsprung disease/toxic megacolon

Miscellaneous Causes

Dietary factors—malnutrition, specific food intolerance (e.g., lactose or fructose intolerance), overfeeding, and sorbitol

Other malabsorption—celiac disease and cystic fibrosis

Systemic illness—hemolytic uremic syndrome (HUS), Henoch-Schönlein purpura (HSP) and immunodeficiency

Functional—irritable bowel syndrome

DIFFERENTIAL DIAGNOSIS DISCUSSION

Infectious Diarrhea

Etiology

Infectious diarrhea can be **viral, bacterial, or parasitic** in origin. Transmission is usually by the fecal–oral route. A specific causative agent is not identified in most patients with infectious diarrhea.

Clinical Features

Infectious diarrhea most often affects young children, especially those in child-care. Children commonly present with crampy abdominal pain, vomiting, and 6 to 10 watery bowel movements per day. Associated symptoms (e.g., fever, vomiting, abdominal pain, rash, joint pain) often support an infectious cause. On examination, the abdomen is usually nondistended and soft, with diffuse or no tenderness. Bowel sounds may be hyperactive.

Although the clinical syndrome is rarely specific for a particular pathogen, diagnostic clues do exist (Table 27-1). The history may also provide clues regarding the cause:

- There is a **seasonal predilection** for many pathogens; viral infections are more common during the winter, and bacterial infections occur more frequently in the summer.
- The abrupt onset of diarrhea, with no vomiting prior to the onset of diarrhea, suggests **bacterial enteritis**.
- Bloody diarrhea and fever are seen most commonly in **bacterial enteritis**, although **parasitic** (*Cryptosporidium*) infection should be considered in children with these symptoms who attend daycare.
- A **history of contact** with other ill individuals, **child-care attendance, travel,** or certain exposures may provide clues regarding the specific causative agent. For example, *Giardia lamblia* infection is more common in individuals who drink well water or contaminated water while camping, and *Campylobacter, Salmonella, and G. lamblia* can be transmitted through contact with pets. Infectious organisms common to the child-care setting include rotavirus and other viruses, *Giardia, Cryptosporidium, Campylobacter, and Shigella* species.
- **Swimming** in contaminated water is a common source of exposure to infectious organisms, particularly *Shigella, Giardia, Cryptosporidia, and Entamoeba* species and *E. Coli* 0157:H7. Many waterborne parasites are resistant to chlorination.

TABLE 27-1	**Common Causes of Infectious Diarrhea**				
Causative Agent	**Peak Age**	**Season**	**Incubation Period**	**Fever**	**Character of Stools**
Rotavirus	4 mo–3 yr	Winter	1–3 d	Variable	Watery and foul smelling
Noroviruses	School age	Fall–Winter	12–96 hr	Rare	Loose to watery
Salmonella	1 mo–2 yr	Summer	8–48 hr	Common	Green, slimy, "rotten egg" odor and occasionally bloody
Shigella	1–5 yr	Summer	1–7 d	Common	Watery, bloody, and odorless
Campylobacter	1–5 yr	Summer	1–7 d	Common	Watery; may be bloody
Yersinia	1 mo–2 yr	Winter	1–14 d	Common	Mucoid; may be bloody
G. lamblia	School age	All year	1–4 wk	Rare	Loose, greasy, pale, and of protracted duration
Entamoeba histolytica	All ages	All year	1–4 wk	Variable	May be mucoid and bloody
Cryptosporidia	1–5 yr	Summer	2–14 d	Common	Watery; may be bloody

- *Clostridium difficile* infection occurs predominantly in children who have received **antibiotics** during the preceding 3 weeks.
- **Antacid therapy with H$_2$ blockers or proton pump inhibitors** increases susceptibility to bacterial pathogens.

Evaluation

- **Methylene blue staining of the stool** can be used to screen outpatients who may require a bacterial stool culture and may occasionally identify *G. lamblia*. Although the presence of sheets of polymorphonuclear leukocytes suggests bacterial enteritis and the need for bacterial stool culture, the absence of leukocytes does not eliminate the possibility of a bacterial infection. A jar specimen provides a better yield than does a diaper or swab specimen.
- **Stool culture** is generally recommended for patients who are hospitalized or are in child-care or institutional settings, and those who have underlying chronic conditions, severe or bloody diarrhea, toxic appearance, exposure to bacterial enteritis, or persistent diarrhea on dietary therapy. Some laboratories only test for *Campylobacter, Yersinia,* and pathogenic *E. coli* by special request. *C. difficile* culture and toxin analysis may be helpful in children with antibiotic exposure. (Of note, the asymptomatic carrier rate for *C. difficile* is 30% to 50% in neonates and 3% after 12 months of age.)

- **Antigen tests of stool.** Specific testing for rotavirus, giardia or cryptosporidia is generally unnecessary, but may be considered for selected patients who are hospitalized or have prolonged illness, and for epidemiologic purposes (e.g., during outbreaks).
- **Ova and parasites (O&P).** A stool examination for the presence of O&P should be considered for children who attend child-care or who have traveled outside of the country, particularly if the diarrhea is protracted. Identification of *Cryptosporidium* may require use of a modified auramine acid-fast stain.

Treatment

Antimicrobial agents are not necessary for many patients despite bacterial enteritis. **Antibiotics are contraindicated in some settings.** For example, antibiotic administration may prolong intestinal carriage of *Salmonella* and may increase the risk of HUS in *E. coli* O157:H7 infection. Antibiomicrobial treatment may be indicated to reduce the duration of the illness, or to reduce transmission of the organism. Because of increasing resistance, antimicrobial susceptibility testing should be performed on all isolates of *Salmonella, Shigella, and E. Coli.*

- ***Campylobacter jejuni.*** Erythromycin can be administered orally for 5 to 7 days to reduce fecal shedding, shorten illness, and prevent relapse. Azithromycin is an alternative therapy. For severely ill children, consider intravenous administration of erythromycin, cefotaxime, or an aminoglycoside. Tetracycline is an alternative treatment for children >8 years.
- ***Shigella.*** Most *Shigella* infections do not require treatment. To shorten the duration of illness and reduce contagion, trimethoprim-sulfamethoxazole (TMP-SMX) administered orally or intravenously for 5 days is the treatment of choice. If the organism is sensitive, ampicillin can be used instead. Ceftriaxone and azithromycin are alternatives.
- ***Salmonella.*** Enterocolitis should only be treated in those patients at risk for developing invasive disease, such as infants <3 months, children with hemoglobinopathies (including sickle cell disease), malignancies or immunocompromise (e.g., those with AIDS, those undergoing therapy with immunosuppressive agents, and those with splenic dysfunction), children with cardiac disease at risk for endocarditis, and those with *Salmonella typhi* infection, *Salmonella* bacteremia, or enteric fever. Ampicillin or TMP-SMX may be administered for 7 to 14 days if the organism is sensitive. Alternatives are intravenous ceftriaxone or cefotaxime. Neonates and patients with meningitis may require different doses, and patients with osteomyelitis need extended treatment (e.g., for 4 to 6 weeks).
- ***Clostridium difficile.*** Metronidazole should be administered orally for 7 to 10 days after discontinuing administration of other systemic antimicrobials if possible. Vancomycin can be administered orally for seriously ill patients or for those in whom treatment has failed.
- ***Vibrio cholera.*** Most *Vibrio* infections do not require treatment. Oral doxycycline (single dose) or tetracycline (for 3 days) are the drugs of choice in children >8 years. TMP-SMX, doxycycline, and cefotaxime are alternative therapies.

- **Enterotoxigenic *E. coli*.** Treatment is not typically recommended, but TMP-SMX for 3 days may be administered.
- **Enteroinvasive *E. coli*.** TMP-SMX or ampicillin (if the organism is sensitive) may be used. Azithromycin is an alternative therapy.
- ***Giardia lamblia*.** Metronidazole (5 to 7 days), tinidazole, or nitazoxanide are the drugs of choice. Furazolidone orally for 7 to 10 days is an alternative therapy.
- ***Cryptosporidium*.** Treatment is not generally needed for immunocompetent children. Nitazoxanide is the agent of choice. This drug has limited efficacy in HIV-infected patients.
- ***Entamoeba histolytica*.** Metronidazole orally or intravenously for 10 days or tinidazole for 3 days can be administered to patients with symptomatic colitis or extraintestinal disease. Either method of treatment must be followed by iodoquinol administered orally for 20 days or paromomycin for 7 days. Additional agents may be needed in the case of severe or invasive disease. If the patient is asymptomatic, iodoquinol alone is used for 20 days. Alternative treatments for asymptomatic infection are also available.
- ***Cyclospora*.** TMP-SMX is administered for 7 to 10 days.

Foodborne Illness
Etiology
Foodborne diarrhea may occur secondary to ingestion of an infectious agent or ingestion of a preformed toxin. A number of pathogens may be transmitted in contaminated water or food or via food handlers. Table 27-2 lists the common sources of foodborne diarrhea.

Clinical Features
The **simultaneous, acute onset of gastroenteritis** among individuals who have shared a meal is typical of foodborne illness. These illnesses generally last for **<24 hours**. Vomiting is prominent in most food poisonings and usually has its onset prior to diarrhea. The severe vomiting of *Staphylococcus aureus* toxin illness begins 1 to 6 hours after ingestion of contaminated meat products. Symptoms of *Clostridium perfringens* toxin illness are seen 12 hours after ingestion and typically include secretory diarrhea without vomiting.

 HINT: The onset of symptoms the same day as the ingestion suggests that a preformed toxin is the causative agent. Symptoms that begin 24 hours to several days after ingestion suggest enteric pathogens as the cause.

Evaluation
Food poisoning is mainly a clinical diagnosis. Stool cultures may be obtained for detection of enteric pathogens. *C. perfringens* infection may be confirmed by culture of the contaminated food source.

Treatment
Generally, only supportive care is required. Antimicrobial administration is recommended for some enteric pathogens.

TABLE 27-2	Common Sources of Foodborne Gastroenteritis
Source	**Infectious Agent or Toxin**
Meat	*S. aureus* toxins *C. perfringens* toxin Pathogenic *E. coli* Campylobacter *Salmonella* *Aeromonas*
Pork chitterlings and poultry	*Yersinia enterocolitica, Bacillus cereus* *Salmonella* *Shigella* *C. jejuni*
Eggs and shellfish	*Salmonella* *Salmonella* *V. cholerae* *V. parahaemolyticus* Caliciviruses
Fish	Ciguatera
Raw milk	*Salmonella* *C. jejuni* *Y. enterocolitica*
Fried rice, dried fruit, powdered milk	*Bacillus cereus*
Mushrooms	Mushroom toxin
Produce	*Shigella, Aeromonas, Salmonella, E. coli* 0157:H7
Apple cider	*E. coli* 0157:H7

Intussusception

Intussusception is discussed in Chapter 9, "Abdominal Pain, Acute."

Hemolytic Uremic Syndrome (HUS)

HUS is discussed in Chapter 78, "Urine Output, Decreased."

EVALUATION OF ACUTE DIARRHEA

Patient History

The initial patient history aims both to establish **hydration** status and to uncover the **cause of the diarrhea**. The adequacy and type of fluid and solid intake and the urine output should be carefully assessed. In addition, note the size, frequency, and character of the stools (e.g., watery, mucoid, bloody, or foul smelling) and any associated symptoms. For example, the presence of ear pain or dysuria suggests a diagnosis of a systemic illness causing the diarrhea.

 HINT: *Shigella* emits a neurotoxin, and seizures may precede the gastrointestinal symptoms.

Physical Examination

- Vital signs, level of consciousness, fontanelles, mucous membranes, skin turgor, and capillary refill. Note signs of dehydration (see Chapter 25, "Dehydration," Table 25-1).
- Skin. Note maculopapular rash (seen in viral gastroenteritis, typhoid, and *Shigella* infection), pallor, petechiae, or purpura.
- Abdomen. Auscultate for the presence and quality of bowel sounds; then percuss and palpate for tenderness, organomegaly, or masses. Focal tenderness alerts the examiner to consider alternative diagnoses and potential complications of infection.
- Rectum. Note focal tenderness; stool can be examined and tested for occult blood.

Laboratory Studies

Laboratory studies are unnecessary for most outpatients with acute diarrhea. However, in addition to the stool examinations previously described, the following studies may be indicated:

- **Urine specific gravity** may be helpful if there is a concern about dehydration.
- **Serum electrolyte analysis** should be obtained in children with moderate to severe dehydration (see Chapter 25, "Dehydration," Table 25-3). Results may suggest inadequate fluid replacement (hypernatremic dehydration) or hypotonic fluid replacement (hyponatremic dehydration). Serum electrolytes may be normal despite significant dehydration.
- A **complete blood cell (CBC) count** may show hemoconcentration caused by dehydration or **bandemia** associated with bacterial enteritis.

  Blood cultures should be obtained if there is suspicion of bacteremia or sepsis.

TREATMENT OF ACUTE DIARRHEA

> **HINT:** Children with diarrhea and no dehydration should continue to be fed age-appropriate diets.

Although children who are severely dehydrated require immediate intravenous fluid replacement, **oral rehydration therapy is the first line of treatment** for all children with mild to moderate dehydration (see also Chapter 25, "Dehydration"). Glucose–electrolyte rehydration solutions contain 75 to 90 mEq/L of sodium, and maintenance solutions contain 40 to 60 mEq/L of sodium. Rehydration with oral rehydration solutions should be performed over 4 to 6 hours.

> **HINT:** Vomiting is not a contraindication to oral rehydration in the mild to moderately dehydrated patient.

Oral maintenance fluids can be administered after rehydration, but **age-appropriate foods** should be reintroduced within 24 hours. Restriction of dietary

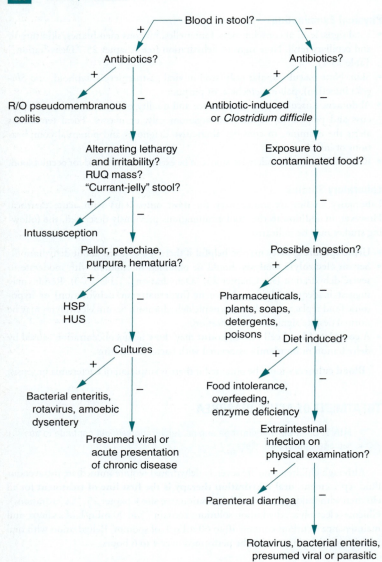

FIGURE 27-1 **Evaluation of a patient with acute diarrhea.** HSP, Henoch-Schönlein purpura; HUS, hemolytic uremic syndrome; R/O 5 rule out; RUQ, right upper quadrant.

intake is associated with greater weight loss than an age-appropriate diet, due to inadequate calorie and protein content. Proper nutrition also helps facilitate mucosal repair after illness. The use of lactose-free formulas and dietary lactose restrictions are not of clear benefit except in the small minority of patients with clinically significant secondary lactase deficiency.

Antidiarrheal medications are not efficacious and are potentially dangerous. They may enhance bacterial proliferation and toxin absorption by promoting reduced gut motility. In addition, they may mask intraluminal fluid loss.

Some studies suggest that bismuth subsalicylate, zinc, and probiotic agents (e.g., *Lactobacillus GG, Saccharomyces boulardii*) may reduce the duration and severity of diarrhea, but these agents are not routinely recommended.

APPROACH TO THE PATIENT (Figure 27-1)

- **Test a stool sample for the presence of gross or microscopic blood.** The presence of blood should be confirmed using a guaiac reagent test, which excludes dyes, medications, and vegetable matter as the source of red stools. Broken skin must also be excluded as a source of blood. Flecks of blood on the surface of the stool are also common in viral illness.
- **Determine whether the child has recently had antibiotic therapy.** Recent antibiotic therapy in a child with bloody diarrhea suggests the presence of pseudomembranous colitis. Recent antibiotic therapy in a child with nonbloody diarrhea suggests the presence of antibiotic-induced gastroenteritis or *C. difficile* infection without colitis.
- **In an afebrile child with bloody diarrhea,** it is particularly important to rule out intussusception (suggested by lethargy, irritability, an abdominal mass, or currant-jelly stools), HUS (suggested by pallor, petechiae, and oliguria), and HSP (suggested by purpura, especially of the buttocks and lower extremities).
- Most patients are diagnosed as having **presumed viral gastroenteritis**.
- Rotavirus gastroenteritis has historically been the most common specific cause of hospitalization for severe diarrhea in infants. Immunization in infancy with an oral, live attenuated rotavirus vaccine is an important preventive measure that is changing the epidemiology of acute diarrheal illness significantly in this age group.

Suggested Readings

American Academy of Pediatrics: *2009 Red Book: Report of the Committee on Infectious Diseases,* 28th ed. Elk Grove Village, Il, American Academy of Pediatrics, 2009.

Amieva MR. Important bacterial gastrointestinal pathogens in children: a pathogenesis perspective. *Pediatr Clin North Am.* 2005;52:749–777.

Atia AN, Buchman AL. Oral rehydration solutions in non-cholera diarrhea: a review. *Am J Gastroenterol.* 2009;104:2596–2604.

Brown KH, Peerson JM, Fontaine O. Use of nonhuman milks in the dietary management of young children with acute diarrhea: a meta-analysis of clinical trials. *Pediatrics.* 1994;93:17–27.

Deenehy PH. Acute diarrheal disease in children: epidemiology, prevention, and treatment. *Infect Dis Clin North Am.* 2005;19:585–602.

Guandalini S. Probiotics for children with diarrhea: an update. *J Clin Gastroenterol.* 2008;42:S53–S57.

Hartling L, Bellemare S, Wiebe N, et al. Oral versus intravenous rehydration for treating dehydration due to gastroenteritis in children. *Cochrane Database Syst Rev.* 2006;3:CD004390.

King CK, Glass R, Bresess JS, et al. Centers for Disease Control and Prevention. Managing acute gastro-enteritis among children: oral rehydration, maintenance and nutritional therapy. *MMWR Recomm Rep.* 2003;52(RR-16):1–16.

Lukacik M, Thomas RL, Aranda JV. A meta-analysis of the effects of oral zinc in the treatment of acute and persistent diarrhea. *Pediatrics.* 2008;121:326–336.

Parashar UD, Alexander JP, Glass RI. Prevention of rotaviral gastroenteritis among infants and children. Recommendations of the Advisory Committee on Immunization Practices (ACIP). *MMWR Recomm Rep.* 2006;55(RR-12):1–13.

Pickering LK. Approach to patients with gastrointestinal tract infections and food poisoning. In: RD Feigin, JD Cherry, GJ Demmler-Harrison, SL Kaplan, eds. *Textbook of Pediatric Infectious Diseases.* 6th ed. Philadelphia: Saunders Elsevier; 2009;621–653.

Sarker SA, Mahalanabis D, Alam NH, et al. Reduced osmolarity oral rehydration solution for persistent diarrhea in infants: A randomized controlled clinical trial. *J Pediatr.* 2001;138:532–538.

Wong CS, Jelacic RL, Habeeb SL, et al. The risk of the hemolytic-uremic syndrome after antibiotic treatment of *E. coli* 0157:H7 infections. *N Engl J Med.* 2000;342:1930–1936.

Diarrhea, Chronic

INTRODUCTION

Stool output of 10 g/kg per day (in infants) or 200 g/kg per day (in children) is defined as diarrhea. Chronic diarrhea is the persistence of loose, frequent stools for 2 to 3 weeks.

Diarrhea can be classified as **secretory, osmotic, inflammatory, or motility related**. Presence of an unabsorbable compound in the lumen of the intestine creates an osmolar load that results in osmotic diarrhea. Secretory diarrhea is caused by an imbalance of water and electrolyte absorption and secretion in the intestine.

 HINT: If diarrhea stops when the patient is given nothing by mouth, this is osmotic diarrhea.

 DIFFERENTIAL DIAGNOSIS LIST

Infectious Causes

Bacterial, parasitic, or viral infection (see Chapter 27, "Diarrhea, Acute")
Small bowel bacterial overgrowth
Postinfectious enteritis
Necrotizing enterocolitis

Toxic Causes

Antibiotics
Laxatives
Mannitol
Motility agents
Chemotherapeutic agents

Neoplastic Causes

Neuroblastoma
VIPoma
Gastrinoma
Lymphoma
Polyposis
Mastocytosis

Metabolic or Genetic Causes

Carbohydrate malabsorption—lactose intolerance, fructose intolerance, glucose–galactose transporter defect, and sucrase–isomaltase deficiency
Fat malabsorption—congenital lipase deficiency, pancreatic disease (cystic fibrosis, chronic pancreatitis, Shwachman syndrome), chronic liver disease, congenital bile salt malabsorption, and Wolman disease
Protein-losing enteropathy (PLE)—intestinal lymphangiectasia or secondary causes
Congenital chloride diarrhea
Congenital sodium diarrhea
Acrodermatitis enteropathica

Hyperthyroidism
Hypoparathyroidism
Congenital adrenal hyperplasia
Diabetes
Lipoprotein disorders

Anatomic Causes
Malrotation
Partial small bowel obstruction
Short bowel syndrome
Blind loop syndrome
Fistula
Pyloroplasty
Hirschsprung disease with
    enterocolitis

Dietary Causes
Overfeeding (food or liquid)
Food allergy
Allergic proctocolitis
Eosinophilic gastroenteritis
Malnutrition
Excessive fructose intake
Fiber
Sorbitol

Inflammatory Causes
Celiac disease
Inflammatory bowel disease
Severe combined
    immunodeficiency
Immunoglobulin A (IgA)
    deficiency
Autoimmune enteropathy
Hemolytic uremic syndrome
    (HUS)

Psychosocial Causes
Munchausen by proxy syndrome

Miscellaneous Causes
Chronic nonspecific diarrhea of
    infancy
Irritable bowel syndrome
Hepatobiliary disorders (hepatitis,
    cholestasis, cholecystectomy)
Encopresis
Radiation enteritis
Neonatal drug withdrawal
    syndrome

DIFFERENTIAL DIAGNOSIS DISCUSSION
Chronic Nonspecific Diarrhea of Infancy
Chronic nonspecific diarrhea of infancy (also known as **toddler's diarrhea**) is the most common cause of diarrhea in children between **6 months and 3 years of age**.

Etiology
The cause is unclear. The disorder may be related to **increased bowel motility or low intake of fat and fiber,** or it may follow a bout of **infectious gastroenteritis**.

Clinical Features
Patients pass **3 to 10 loose stools per day,** usually diminishing in frequency in the evening. The child has a good appetite and appropriate weight gain, although undigested food particles are visible in the stool.

Evaluation
The diagnosis is **by exclusion** of other causes. Workup for infection and malabsorption are negative. Stool testing for occult blood is also negative. Clinically, a history of **excessive intake of juices** and a **diet low in fat and fiber** in a child who is thriving supports the diagnosis.

Treatment

The child's consumption of fruit juice and **excessive fluids should be restricted,** and consumption of **dietary fat and fiber** should be **increased**. Reassure parents that the problem will resolve by the time the child is 2 to 3 years of age.

 HINT: Remember the *four* Fs: *f*ruit juice, *f*luids, *f*at, and *f*iber.

Infectious Enteritis

Infectious enteritis is the **most common cause** of **chronic diarrhea**. Gastrointestinal infections are **usually acute** and resolve in ~**2 weeks,** but sometimes they can persist for as long as **2 months**. Viral gastroenteritis in an infant can be prolonged as a result of the slow healing of the intestinal mucosa. In addition, infections tend to last longer than usual in immunocompromised patients.

Etiology

Common **bacterial causes** of chronic diarrhea include *Salmonella, Shigella, Yersinia enterocolitica, Campylobacter,* enteroadherent *Escherichia coli, Aeromonas, Clostridium difficile, and Plesiomonas.* **Parasitic causes** include *Giardia lamblia, Cryptosporidium, Entamoeba histolytica, and Isospora.* Rotavirus, adenovirus, and norovirus are common **viral causes**.

 HINT: Herpes virus, *Mycobacterium avium-intracellulare, Blastocystis hominis,* Microsporidia, and fungi can cause chronic diarrhea in immunocompromised patients. They usually present with recurrent or prolonged infections.

Clinical Features

***Y. enterocolitica* infection** involves the terminal ileum and can mimic inflammatory bowel disease or appendicitis. It is more common in patients whose normal bowel flora has been changed secondary to antibiotic therapy.

***E. histolytica* infection** can cause colitis. Blood, mucus, or both are seen in the stool, and patients have a fever.

***Giardia lamblia* infection** is usually asymptomatic but may manifest with bloating, abdominal pain, anorexia, chronic diarrhea, and failure to thrive (see Chapter 10, "Abdominal Pain, Chronic").

***C. difficile* infection** most commonly occurs following a course of oral antibiotics, although nonantibiotic associated infections are also common.

Evaluation

A **stool sample** should be obtained for **bacterial and viral culture**. The laboratory should be instructed to culture for all of the most commonly implicated bacteria and viruses. Stool samples for **rotazyme** (an enzyme-linked immunoassay for rotavirus) and assays for *C. difficile* **toxins A and B** should also be obtained.

PCR analysis can be performed for viral infections. **Three stool specimens** should be submitted for **ova and parasites (O&P) analysis**.

Treatment

If the cause is **bacterial,** treatment is with the appropriate **antibiotic** (see Chapter 27, "Diarrhea, Acute"). **Giardiasis** is treated with **furazolidone, metronidazole, or quinacrine** (see Chapter 10, "Abdominal Pain, Chronic"). **Nutritional supplementation** may be required for patients with **viral** diarrhea and **immunocompromised patients**. Probiotics have been shown to be modestly effective for treating acute viral gastroenteritis and preventing antibiotic-associated diarrhea in children.

C. difficile colitis **(pseudomembranous colitis, antibiotic-induced colitis)** is discussed in Chapter 34, "Gastrointestinal Bleeding, Lower."

Parenteral Diarrhea

Etiology

Extraintestinal infection (e.g., upper respiratory tract infection, urinary tract infection [UTI], otitis media, mastoiditis, sinusitis, pneumonia) may be associated with diarrhea. Diarrhea may also be one of the symptoms **associated with other systemic infections** (e.g., toxic shock syndrome, Rocky Mountain spotted fever). The pathogenesis of the diarrhea is unknown.

Clinical Features

The patient may be **otherwise asymptomatic** (e.g., in the case of UTI), or he may have a **range of symptoms** related to the primary illness.

Evaluation

The diagnosis is based on **clinical suspicion**. An appropriate workup for the suspected primary illness should be performed. In an otherwise asymptomatic child, a **urine culture** is necessary.

Treatment

Treatment of the **primary illness** results in resolution of the diarrhea.

Postinfectious Enteritis

Etiology

In **children,** infectious gastroenteritis is usually **uncomplicated;** however, in **infants** (especially those with a borderline nutritional status), **severe mucosal damage** may follow an infectious gastroenteritis. The mucosal damage may result in transient **disaccharidase deficiency** (most commonly lactase deficiency).

Clinical Features

Long after the infectious process has been resolved, the patient experiences **intractable watery diarrhea and nutritional compromise,** manifested as **failure to thrive**. Rarely, evidence of vitamin and mineral deficiency is seen.

Evaluation

The diagnosis is made on the basis of **clinical suspicion**. In some patients, a **lactose breath test** may be appropriate.

Treatment

Temporary **avoidance of dairy products** and introduction of a **lactose-free formula or an elemental formula** are needed to allow the brush borders of the small intestine to heal.

Celiac Disease (Gluten-Sensitive Enteropathy)

Etiology

Gluten-sensitive enteropathy is a hereditary type of malabsorption that is caused by a permanent inability to tolerate gluten, which is present in wheat, barley, and rye. Gliadin, the offending protein, causes severe atrophy of the small intestinal mucosa. This disease is increasingly recognized in all cultures and is thought to affect ~1% of the US population.

Clinical Features

Symptoms usually start ~1 month after gluten is introduced to the diet, but the disease may present at any age. Common manifestations include **apathy and irritability, anorexia, vomiting, chronic diarrhea, steatorrhea, abdominal distension, clubbing of the fingers, and malnutrition** with symptoms and signs related to nutrient deficiency.

Evaluation

The patient should be **screened for IgA antiendomysial antibodies and IgA antitransglutaminase antibodies**. However, IgA deficiency must be excluded. IgA antigliadin antibodies result in a very high false-positive rate, and this screening test is generally not used for celiac disease. Small bowel biopsy remains the gold standard for formally diagnosing celiac disease.

Treatment

Complete removal of gluten from the diet and replacement with corn, rice, or potato starch results in resolution of the symptoms. Complete recovery of the intestinal mucosa is expected in 1 to 2 years.

Encopresis

Etiology

Patients with chronic constipation and impaction may present with what seems like chronic diarrhea as a result of encopresis, or continuous leakage of loose stool around the hard stool. In patients with Hirschsprung disease, diarrhea is usually secondary to enterocolitis (rather than encopresis).

Clinical Features

The patient has a history of constipation. On abdominal examination, hard stool may be palpated, and on rectal examination, the vault is dilated and filled with hard stool.

Evaluation

An **abdominal radiograph** confirms the diagnosis, which is based on clinical suspicion.

Treatment

Treatment entails **evacuation of the bowel,** which can be achieved with oral osmotic agents, stimulant laxative, and/or **multiple enemas. Stool softeners** or an osmotic medication should be prescribed for **several months, and diet and behavioral modification** should take place. Patients with **Hirschsprung disease** require **surgery** for definitive treatment.

Fat Malabsorption
Etiology

Fat digestion and absorption is a complex process. **Lipase** (a pancreatic enzyme), **bile acid secretion** (to help with micellar solubilization), an intact **intestinal brush border** (to facilitate micelle absorption), intact **lipoprotein metabolism,** and an intact **transport mechanism** (to carry the chylomicron to the lymphatics) all play a role. A **defect in any of these steps** may result in fat malabsorption.

Clinical Features

Fat malabsorption is manifested with **diarrhea (bulky, greasy stools), failure to thrive,** and signs and symptoms related to **fat-soluble vitamin deficiency** (e.g., rickets, night blindness, neurologic signs, bleeding tendency).

Evaluation

Fat malabsorption caused by pancreatic insufficiency is suggested by a low concentration of **fecal elastase.** Definitive diagnosis of fat malabsorption requires a **72-hour stool collection** for measurement of fecal fat, which must be compared to dietary fat intake. The workup for the cause of fat malabsorption is extensive, and referral to a **gastroenterologist** is recommended.

Treatment

The **underlying cause** must be identified and treated if possible. All patients with fat malabsorption require **additional calorie intake** to compensate for the excessive fat loss. **Medium-chain triglyceride (MCT)–based formulas** are often preferred. Because MCTs have a smaller molecular weight and higher water solubility than long-chain triglycerides, they are absorbed directly into the portal blood. Patients with fat malabsorption also require **fat-soluble vitamin supplementation.**

Carbohydrate Malabsorption
Etiology

The absorption of carbohydrates involves **amylase** (a pancreatic enzyme); **lactase, isomaltase, and sucrase** (intestinal brush border enzymes); and an intact **transport system.** The most common type of carbohydrate malabsorption is **lactase deficiency** (see Chapter 10, "Abdominal Pain, Chronic"). Congenital carbohydrate malabsorption is rare but has to be considered in the differential diagnosis of diarrhea in a young infant.

Clinical Features

In general, carbohydrate malabsorption syndromes are manifested with **failure to thrive, osmotic diarrhea** (often voluminous and watery), **abdominal cramps, increased flatulence, and borborygmi.**

Evaluation

Detection of reducing substances or a **stool pH 5.0 or less** is indicative of carbohydrate malabsorption. Definitive diagnosis of disaccharidase deficiencies can be made by a specific **hydrogen breath test** or measurement of enzyme activity from **small bowel biopsy**.

Treatment

Symptoms usually resolve with complete **removal of the offending carbohydrate** from the diet. **Supplying the deficient enzyme** may be helpful (e.g., lactase for lactose intolerance).

Protein Malabsorption

Diseases that involve the gastrointestinal mucosa (e.g., Crohn disease, celiac disease) or obstruct lymphatic drainage of the gastrointestinal tract can cause **protein-losing enteropathy (PLE)**. **Primary intestinal lymphangiectasia** is a congenital disorder associated with abnormally dilated lymphatics that results in chronic loss of albumin, immunoglobulins, and other proteins. It is also associated with loss of lymphocytes through the gastrointestinal tract.

Clinical Features

Patients may present with signs and symptoms that reflect the underlying cause, chronic diarrhea, failure to thrive, edema, or recurrent infection.

Evaluation

Patients have hypoalbuminemia, hypoproteinemia, abnormal immunoglobulins, and they may have lymphocytopenia. Hypocalcemia and decreased serum iron and copper levels occur secondary to the loss of binding proteins. Before making the diagnosis of PLE, urinary loss of albumin must be ruled out. Increased stool α_1-antitrypsin (α_1-AT) is the definitive means of diagnosing PLE.

Treatment

The **primary cause** of the PLE should be identified. Patients require a **diet that is rich in protein and MCT oil**.

Allergic Enteropathy

Allergic enteropathy is discussed in Chapter 34, "Gastrointestinal Bleeding, Lower."

Inflammatory Bowel Disease

Inflammatory bowel disease is discussed in Chapter 34, "Gastrointestinal Bleeding, Lower."

EVALUATION OF CHRONIC DIARRHEA

A detailed **history and physical examination** can obviate the need for laboratory evaluation in some cases.

Patient History

- Onset and duration of the diarrhea
- Stool pattern/frequency and aggravating or alleviating factors

- Quality of stool—color; odor; consistency; volume; presence of blood, mucus, or undigested food
- Presence of fever and associated symptoms
- A history of gastroenteritis, constipation, or recurrent pneumonia before the onset of chronic diarrhea
- Dietary history (4 "Fs"—fiber, fluid, fat, fruit juice)
- Recent travel or exposure to infections or treatment with antibiotics
- Medication history
- Pertinent family history

Physical Examination
The following should be noted on examination:

General appearance—hydration status, weight and height, and growth chart
Skin—edema, jaundice, pallor, eczematous rash, bruising, and clubbing
Lungs—wheezing and rales
Abdomen—tenderness, mass (stool, abscess, tumor, or enlarged organs)
Rectum—evidence of perianal disease, rectal prolapse, Hirschsprung disease, and constipation

Laboratory Studies
Initial screening studies may include the following:

- A serum electrolyte panel
- Liver function tests
- Complete blood count with differential
- C-reactive protein and/or erythrocyte sedimentation rate
- Celiac disease panel
- Stool sample for occult blood
- Stool calprotectin is a good screen for evidence of inflammation of the GI tract
- Stool samples for culture, *C. difficile* toxin A and B assay, and O&P
- Urinalysis and urine culture
- Stool electrolytes, anion gap, and osmolarity

    Depending on the suspected diagnosis, additional studies may be indicated:

Carbohydrate malabsorption—stool pH (5.0 or less), reducing substance (positive)
Fat malabsorption—72-hour fecal fat; sweat chloride test; prothrombin time (PT, prolonged); vitamin E and vitamin D levels (may be decreased)
PLE—stool α_1-AT (increased), hypoalbuminemia, lymphopenia, and hypogammaglobulinemia
Small bowel disease—d-xylose test (abnormal)

TREATMENT OF CHRONIC DIARRHEA
The underlying cause of the diarrhea must be identified and treated.

    Consultation with a nutritionist is advisable for patients with disorders such as malabsorption, celiac disease, or allergic enteropathy.

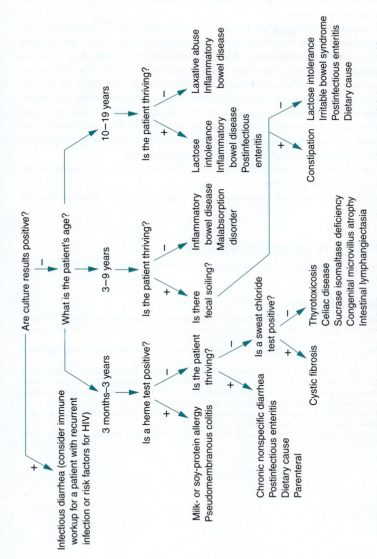

FIGURE 28-1 **Evaluation of a patient with chronic diarrhea.** Most patients are diagnosed as having presumed viral gastroenteritis.

For patients who are not vomiting, an oral glucose electrolyte solution can be given to correct fluid, electrolyte, and acid–base imbalances. Patients may be started on a lactose-free or an elemental formula later, depending on the cause and severity of the diarrhea.

Unstable or malnourished patients should be admitted for stabilization and nutritional rehabilitation. Reinitiation of feeding in a malnourished patient may result in **refeeding syndrome,** which is manifested by an acute drop in serum potassium, phosphate, magnesium, and calcium levels secondary to the sudden intracellular shift of these elements. If these electrolyte abnormalities are not corrected in a timely manner, cardiopulmonary compromise and death may result. All electrolyte imbalances must be corrected before initiation of feeding to prevent refeeding syndrome. A continuous drip of a diluted formula is started, and gradually the rate and concentration are increased while monitoring the patient's electrolytes and calcium, phosphate, and magnesium levels.

Total parenteral nutrition may be required for those with severe malnutrition who cannot tolerate feeding.

Additional nutritional supplementation (e.g., zinc, iron, vitamins) may be required.

APPROACH TO THE PATIENT (Figure 28-1)

A general approach to evaluation of chronic diarrhea is presented in Figure 28-1.

Suggested Readings

Grimwood K, Forbes DA. Acute and persistent diarrhea. *Pediatr Clin North Am.* 2009;56:1343–1361.

Grossman AB, Baldassano RN. Specific considerations in the treatment of pediatric inflammatory bowel disease. *Expert Rev Gastroenterol Hepatol.* 2008;2:105–124.

Heitlinger LA, Lebenthal EB. Disorders of carbohydrate digestion and absorption. *Pediatr Clin North Am.* 1988;35:239–255.

Heyman MB. Lactose intolerance in infants, children, and adolescents. *Pediatrics.* 2006;118:1279–1286.

Hill ID, Dirks MH, Liptak GS, et al. Guideline for the diagnosis and treatment of celiac disease in children: recommendations of the North American Society of Pediatric Gastroenterology, Hepatology, and Nutrition. *J Pediatr Gastroenterol Nutr.* 2005;40:1–19.

Smith MM, Lifshitz F. Excess fruit juice consumption as a contributing factor in nonorganic failure to thrive. *Pediatrics.* 1994;93(3):438–443.

Thomas DW, Greer FR, Bhatia JJS, et al. Probiotics and probiotics in pediatrics. *Pediatrics.* 2010; 126:1217–1231.

Drowning

INTRODUCTION

Terminology

Historically, the terminology used to describe drowning events has been somewhat confusing. The World Congress on Drowning has suggested that the **term *drowning* be uniformly applied** to describe any process in which there is respiratory impairment from submersion in a liquid medium, **regardless of outcome**. Inconsistent terms such as "near drowning," "wet drowning," and "dry drowning" should be abandoned. Similarly, there is no need to distinguish freshwater or saltwater drownings, because it makes little difference in the management of the patient. Water temperature at the time of drowning is significant because children who drown in **very cold water (≤5°C)** may have a **better prognosis**. Drowning usually results in either **severe permanent brain damage or prompt complete recovery**.

Epidemiology

Nationally, drowning is **second only to motor vehicle accidents** as the most common cause of death caused by nonintentional injury in children <19 years. For every drowning death, several children are hospitalized and countless others have submersion events with no morbidity. **Males of all ages** drown at higher rates than females. The **highest rate** of drowning is seen in **children 1 to 4 years** of age. In California, Arizona, and Florida, drowning is the leading cause of death in this age group. The vast majority of deaths in this age group occur in **residential swimming pools**. **Infants** are most likely to drown in **bathtubs,** and these drownings are sometimes the result of **abuse or neglect**. A second peak in drowning deaths occurs in the **teen and young adult** age groups in bodies of **fresh water,** with the highest rate in black males. These deaths are often associated with drug and alcohol use and other risk-taking behaviors.

Most drownings are **preventable**. Passage of legislation that requires proper pool fencing, limits alcohol access at public pools and beaches, and demands pool owners to be proficient in cardiopulmonary resuscitation (CPR) could significantly reduce morbidity and mortality rates. Preventive counseling for parents and swimming lessons for young children may also be helpful.

Pathophysiology

Drowning begins with a period of panic, during which the normal breathing pattern is lost and fluid enters the hypopharynx, triggering laryngospasm. The victim then swallows large volumes of water, which is often aspirated into the lungs once the laryngospasm abates. This cascade results in poor surfactant function, increased capillary permeability, ventilation/perfusion mismatch, and poor lung compliance, all of which leads to acute respiratory distress syndrome (ARDS). **The severe hypoxia that results from this pulmonary injury leads to multisystem organ failure, with cerebral hypoxia causing the majority of morbidity and mortality.** Global anoxic-ischemic injury in turn causes cerebral edema and increased intracranial pressure. Hypothermia may protect the brain by causing a decrease in metabolic demand, but this is true only if the hypothermia occurred at the time of the drowning in extremely cold water.

APPROACH TO THE PATIENT

History

The age of the patient, duration of submersion, temperature of the water, presence of cyanosis or apnea at the scene, performance of CPR at the recovery scene, and amount of time that elapsed until CPR was initiated are all important historical points that influence prognosis and management (Table 29-1). One should also inquire about the possibility of a diving injury, alcohol use, or a past history of a seizure disorder or underlying cardiac dysrhythmia.

Physical Examination

During the physical examination, particular attention should be paid to **assessment of vital signs** (including the temperature) and to the neurologic and respiratory examinations. Frequent reassessment of the patient's **neurologic and respiratory status** is an extremely important component of managing drowning victims.

TABLE 29-1	Prognostic Indicators of Poor Neurologic Outcome in Drowning Victims[a]

At the Scene
Age <3
Submersion time >10 min
Resuscitation delay >10 min
Prolonged resuscitation (>25 min)

In the Emergency Department
Necessity for CPR
Fixed, dilated pupils
Initial ABG pH <7.1
GCS <5

After Initial Resuscitation
Persistent GCS <5
Persistent apnea
Persistent lack of spontaneous, purposeful movements within 24 hr

[a]Applies to victims of warm water near-drownings only. Hypothermic victims of cold water drownings may have a better prognosis.
ABG, arterial blood gas; CPR, cardiopulmonary resuscitation; GCS, Glasgow coma score.

Pupillary response and the **Glasgow coma score (GCS)** (see Chapter 21, "Coma," Table 21-4) should be **assessed serially** to determine the **extent of anoxic-ischemic injury** and the **patient's response to resuscitation** attempts. The child who presents in asystole with fixed, dilated pupils and a **GCS of <5 generally has a poor prognosis** unless he responds fairly rapidly to resuscitation efforts or he has a core temperature of <32°C, following a very-cold-water drowning. In children with a **GCS of >5** at presentation, the **outcome is generally good**. Unfortunately, **neurologic damage** as a result of drowning **cannot be reversed**. The **gag reflex** should be assessed to determine whether the child can protect his or her own airway. The **cervical spine** should be examined for any signs of injury, and if there is any history of diving, a cervical collar should be placed immediately.

Careful attention is paid to the respiratory examination, even in an alert, active child without obvious respiratory distress. **Close monitoring for signs of respiratory involvement** (in the form of serial examinations) **is crucial, even for the initially asymptomatic child**. **Signs of lower respiratory involvement** (e.g., the use of accessory muscles, tachypnea, cough, wheezing, rales, nasal flaring) **may be delayed** for minutes to hours, and the **injury is usually progressive**.

Laboratory and Radiographic Evaluation

Serial pulse oximetry should be used to detect early signs of pulmonary involvement that are not clinically detectable (e.g., oxygen desaturation of <95%).

The following laboratory and imaging studies can also be considered in drowning victims:

- **Electrolyte values** are rarely abnormal. Respiratory or metabolic acidosis may be present and should be corrected.
- **Anticonvulsant levels** in victims with seizure disorders.
- **Cardiac monitoring** is indicated for the severely affected patient or for a patient in whom a cardiac electrophysiologic conduction delay (e.g., a prolonged QT interval) may have precipitated unconsciousness, leading to the drowning episode.
- **Toxicology screens,** including an ethyl alcohol level measurement, may be indicated.
- **Chest radiography** is indicated following intubation or if there are signs of lower airway involvement, but is not required in all submersion victims.
- **Cervical spine films** are indicated for victims of high-impact events.
- **Head CT** if concern for anoxic injury and cerebral edema.

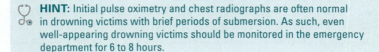

HINT: Initial pulse oximetry and chest radiographs are often normal in drowning victims with brief periods of submersion. As such, even well-appearing drowning victims should be monitored in the emergency department for 6 to 8 hours.

TREATMENT

The **prognosis** of drowning victims is directly related to the duration of the **hypoxic-ischemic injury** and the **adequacy of the initial resuscitation**. Therefore, the **prehospital care** is of paramount importance. **Prompt water rescue** and **bystander CPR** are the best predictors of a good outcome. As soon as possible, the **airway** should be **suctioned** and properly positioned to ensure air entry. See Figure 29-1 for how to manage the airway and breathing of drowning victims. Quality CPR should be initiated for all pulseless patients.

> **HINT:** The Heimlich maneuver is not indicated in drownings and should not delay resuscitation. It should never be considered in the patient who could have a c-spine injury.

Upon arrival to the ED, a **brief, well-executed resuscitation effort** with initiation of **advanced cardiopulmonary life support** measures, if necessary, should be made as information is gathered regarding the accident, the patient's core temperature, and the response to therapy. Resuscitation should be initiated **in all apneic and pulseless victims,** but it should only be **continued for prolonged periods in victims of a cold-water drowning** and then only until the **patient's core temperature exceeds 32°C.** The goal of therapy is to **prevent further anoxic-ischemic injury**.

Respiratory Care

Even children who required no resuscitation and are **asymptomatic** upon arrival at the ED should be **observed and monitored** for any **signs of respiratory impairment** for a minimum of **6 to 8 hours** before discharge. Children who show signs of any **lower respiratory involvement** should be **admitted** and closely **monitored** for the development of **progressive respiratory failure**.

Assisted ventilation (e.g., bag-valve-mask ventilation) is initiated if necessary, and hypoxemic patients may require **continuous positive airway pressure (CPAP),** which helps improve ventilation-perfusion matching in the lungs. **Intubation** is required if the child is apneic, in severe respiratory distress, difficult to oxygenate, or too obtunded to protect her airway. The **stomach** should be **emptied of water** by means of a nasogastric tube once the airway is protected. **Antibiotics** should be reserved for patients with evidence of pulmonary infection or in cases involving grossly contaminated water.

Circulation

The victim should be assessed for **adequacy of circulation**. Drowning patients may be hypotensive due to a "cold diuresis" or due to hypoxic injury to the heart. Therefore, an intravenous line should be started and **normal saline** given in 20 mL/kg aliquots if there are signs of poor perfusion. Poor perfusion usually occurs only in children with severe ischemic injury or pulmonary edema and in those who require mechanical ventilation. Severe drowning victims require

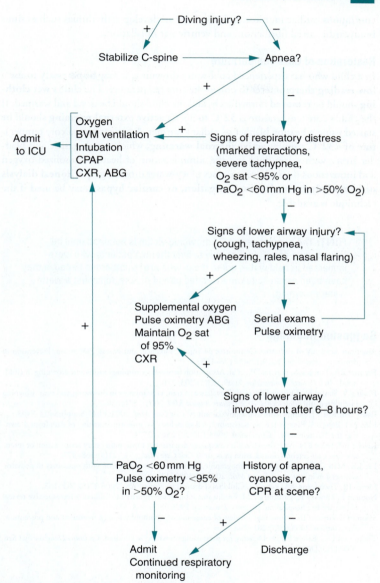

FIGURE 29-1 **Management of the airway and breathing in a drowning victim.** ABG, arterial blood gases; BVM, bag-valve-mask; CPAP, continuous positive airway pressure; CPR, cardiopulmonary resuscitation; C-spine, cervical spine; CXR, chest radiograph; ICU, intensive care unit; O_2 sat, oxygen saturation; Pao_2, arterial oxygen tension.

continuous cardiac monitoring since they can develop arrhythmias such as sinus bradycardia, atrial fibrillation, and ventricular fibrillation.

Restoration of Core Temperature

In a child who has experienced cold-water drowning, it may be necessary to use a **low-reading thermometer** to obtain the core temperature. The child's **wet clothing** should be **removed** immediately, and the child should be dried and warmed. If the child's core temperature is **32°C to 35°C, active external warming** should be started using a heating blanket or radiant warmer. A patient with a core temperature of **<32°C** requires **active internal warming,** which entails gastric and bladder lavage with warm fluid and the administration of heated aerosolized oxygen and intravenous fluids. In severe cases of icy-water drownings, **peritoneal dialysis or hemodialysis, mediastinal irrigation, or cardiac bypass** may be used if the technique is available.

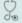 **HINT:** The popular saying "A drowning victim is not dead until he is warm and dead" applies only to hypothermia patients who were immersed in cold water, not to those who are hypothermic because they have been asystolic for an extended period of time, following a warm-water drowning.

Suggested Readings

American Academy of Pediatrics Committee on Injury, Violence, and Poison Prevention. Prevention of drowning. *Pediatrics.* 2010;126(1):178–185.

Brenner RA, Taneja GS, Haynie DL, et al. Association between swimming lessons and drowning in childhood. *Arch Pediatr Adolesc Med.* 2009;163(3):203–210.

Hwang V, Shofer FS, Durbin DR, et al. Prevalence of traumatic injuries in drowning and near drowning in children and adolescents. *Arch Pediatr Adolesc Med.* 2003;157(1):50–53.

Ibsen LM, Koch T. Submersion and asphyxial injury. *Crit Care Med.* 2002;30(11 Suppl):S402–S408.

Idris AH, Berg RA, Bierens J, et al. Recommended guidelines for uniform reporting of data from drowning: the "Utstein style." *Circulation.* 2003;108(20):2565–2574.

Lavelle JM, Shaw KN. Near drowning: is emergency department cardiopulmonary resuscitation or intensive care unit cerebral resuscitation indicated? *Crit Care Med.* 1993;21(3):368–373.

Lee LK, Mao C, Thompson KM. Demographic factors and their association with outcomes in pediatric submersion injury. *Acad Emerg Med.* 2006;13:308–313.

Meyer RJ, Theodorou AA, Berg RA. Childhood drowning. *Pediatr Rev.* 2006;27(5):163–168.

Noonan L, Howrey R, Ginsburg CM. Freshwater submersion injuries in children: a retrospective review of seventy-five hospitalized patients. *Pediatrics.* 1996;98(3):368–371.

Salomez F, Vincent JL. Drowning: a review of epidemiology, pathophysiology, treatment and prevention. *Resuscitation.* 2004;63(3):261–268.

Thompson DC, Rivara FP. Pool fencing for preventing drowning in children. *Cochrane Database Syst Rev.* 2000;(2):CD001047.

Ear, Painful

INTRODUCTION

Diseases that produce ear pain are common maladies of childhood. Many cases of otalgia are caused by **acute otitis media**. **Otitis externa** is also commonly seen, especially during the summer months.

 DIFFERENTIAL DIAGNOSIS LIST

External Ear Pain
Infection
Otitis externa (swimmer's ear)
Auricular cellulitis
External canal abscess
Infected preauricular sinus
Herpes simplex virus infection
Herpes zoster

Neoplasm
Neoplasms of the external auditory
canal

Trauma
Lacerations
Hematoma or seroma
Frostbite and burns

Miscellany
Foreign body and cerumen
impaction

Middle and Inner Ear Pain
Infection
Acute otitis media
Myringitis
Mastoiditis

Neoplasm
Rhabdomyosarcoma and
lymphoma
Histiocytosis X

Trauma
Traumatic perforation
Barotrauma

Inflammation
Otitis media with effusion

Miscellany
Eustachian tube dysfunction
Cholesteatoma

Referred Pain
Infection
Dental abscess
Pharyngitis or tonsillitis
Stomatitis
Sinusitis
Cervical lymphadenitis
Retropharyngeal abscess
Peritonsillar abscess
Infected branchial cyst
Parotitis
Meningitis

Neoplasm

Neoplasms of the jaw, oropharynx, nasopharynx, larynx, facial nerve, or central nervous system

Trauma

Oral cavity, pharyngeal, laryngeal, or esophageal trauma or foreign body

Miscellany

Erupting teeth
Impacted teeth
Migraine
Temporomandibular joint dysfunction or arthritis
Bell palsy

DIFFERENTIAL DIAGNOSIS DISCUSSION
Acute Otitis Media
Etiology

Acute otitis media is an infection of the middle ear space that occurs when the **eustachian tube obstructs** and a build-up of fluid in the middle ear (**effusion**) gets **infected by nasopharyngeal secretions**. Obstruction can result from **infection, allergy, enlarged adenoids, decreased eustachian tube stiffness, or inefficient tube opening**. The most common pathogens are (in order of frequency) *Streptococcus pneumoniae,* nontypeable *Haemophilus influenzae, and Moraxella catarrhalis.* With the advent of the heptavalent pneumococcal conjugated vaccine, the incidence of otitis media from *S. pneumoniae* is decreasing; however, the long-term impact of the vaccine has yet to be established. Table 30-1 lists risk factors associated with acute otitis media.

Clinical Features

Symptoms of acute otitis media may include **otalgia, fever, irritability (from the pain), vomiting, diarrhea, hearing loss, anorexia, and otorrhea**. It is common for the patient to have a preceding upper respiratory infection.

 HINT: Parents commonly state that they are concerned about an ear infection because their child is, "pulling on their ears." While many children with otitis media will rub or pull at their ears, this is not a specific sign of the disease.

TABLE 30-1	Risk Factors for Acute Otitis Media
Day care attendance	
Passive cigarette smoke exposure	
Bottle propping	
Formula-fed (as opposed to breastfed)	
Male	
Winter season	
First episode of acute otitis media before 6 mo of age	
Siblings in the home	
Sibling with recurrent acute otitis media	

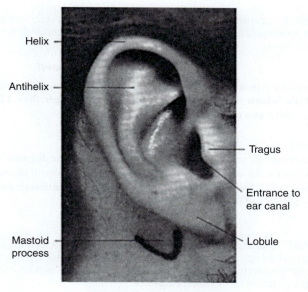

FIGURE 30-1   Anatomy of the ear.

Evaluation

To facilitate examination of the tympanic membrane, the clinician should **properly position the child** in his/her parent's arms, lap, or on the examining table **as well as manipulate the ear** (i.e., pull the pinna posteriorly and superiorly and push the tragus forward by applying traction to the skin in front of the ear). See Figure 30-1 for ear anatomy. If necessary, **remove cerumen** with a curette or by irrigation with water. (However, **irrigation is contraindicated** when a **perforated tympanic membrane** is suspected.)

In acute otitis media, the tympanic membrane is **opaque or cloudy, bulging, red,** and has **decreased mobility**.

> **HINT:** Tympanic membrane erythema alone is not a reliable indicator of acute otitis media. A red tympanic membrane can also be caused by a viral upper respiratory tract infection, by crying, or by efforts to remove cerumen.

Tympanic membrane mobility should be **assessed** using **tympanometry** or **pneumatic otoscopy**—which involves applying positive and negative pressure to the tympanic membrane with a rubber bulb connected by a tube to the otoscope.

HINT: To perform pneumatic otoscopy, use the largest speculum that will fit comfortably in the auditory meatus and fit the speculum tightly to the ear canal.

Laboratory evaluation is usually not necessary. Some clinicians do recommend that **febrile infants** with acute otitis media who are **younger than 12 weeks** undergo a full **sepsis evaluation**.

Treatment
Many patients who have physical findings consistent with the diagnosis of otitis media recover without treatment, and antibiotics afford only small improvement in symptom relief. **Some experts recommend withholding antibiotic treatment** for 48–72 hours and focusing on treatment of pain.

 HINT: In addition to diagnosing the cause of the ear pain, it is important to treat the pain. Acetaminophen or ibuprofen provides adequate pain control for most patients. Anesthetic otic drops are also useful, but should be avoided if a perforation is suspected.

Initially withholding antibiotics helps curtail the emergence of resistant organisms, and **has not been shown to increase incidence of complications** such as mastoiditis or meningitis. However, some studies suggest using antibiotics in **children less than 2 years of age,** and in those with **bilateral otitis media,** shows more significant **benefit in relief of symptoms**. A wait-and-see approach can still be used, but more judiciously in these circumstances. Clinical studies have also shown that **selective use of antibiotics** in patients who **meet stringent criteria** for acute otitis media have **less clinical failure** when treated with antibiotics compared to placebo.

First-line Therapy
- **High dose amoxicillin** (80–90 mg/kg/day divided two or three times a day for a total of 10 days) should be used as first-line therapy in most children. **Twice-a-day dosing improves adherence** over three-times-a-day treatment. Increased dose of amoxicillin is used to overcome moderately **resistant strains of *S. pneumoniae*.** The following increases the risk of resistant organisms:
  - Children less than 2 years of age
  - Recent beta-lactam use
  - Exposure to day care
  - Communities with a high incidence of resistant organisms
- **Amoxicillin** (45 mg/kg/day) can be used in limited circumstances. Most communities have high incidence of resistant *S. pneumoniae;* however, local bacteriologic data should be used to tailor initial antibiotic choice.

- A **5–7 day course** may be sufficient for children over 2 years of age.
  - **Cephalosporins or azithromycin** may be used in patients who are allergic to penicillin, with azithromycin being recommended for those with a history of urticaria or anaphylaxis. Azithromycin should otherwise not be used as a first-line agent.

With appropriate antimicrobial therapy, most children experience **symptomatic improvement within 48–72 hours**. If a patient does not respond fully to amoxicillin, the cause of the otitis may be viral or there may be bacterial resistance.

Second-line Therapy

The choice of a second-line antibiotic depends on the suspected mechanism of resistance. *H. influenzae and M. catarrhalis* produce beta lactamase, therefore **amoxicillin-clavulanate** or a **second-generation cephalosporin** may be used. *S. pneumoniae* alters penicillin binding-proteins; therefore, **high dose amoxicillin** (80–90 mg/kg/day) is recommended if not done initially or a second or third generation cephalosporin. Amoxicillin-clavulanate and cephalosporins including **intramuscular ceftriaxone** may be effective against resistant strains. **Intramuscular ceftriaxone** is not recommended for routine treatment of otitis media. It may be considered **when oral therapy is impossible** or when appropriate **first- and second-line therapy** for *S. pneumoniae* **has already failed**. When used for treatment of resistant organisms, ceftriaxone 50 mg/kg once a day should be given for a total of one to three doses.

> **HINT:** The tympanic membrane does not return to normal appearance for 6–12 weeks. Many times when the ear is examined shortly after an episode of otitis media, the tympanic membrane may appear dull and pink when it is in the healing phase and is not infected.

Infants younger than 4 weeks who present with fever and/or irritability and acute otitis media should be **hospitalized** for **intravenous antibiotic administration,** pending cultures of the blood, urine, and cerebrospinal fluid. **Well-appearing, afebrile infants younger than 4 weeks** may be treated **cautiously as outpatient**s with **careful follow-up**.

Prevention

There is some **controversy** surrounding the administration of **preventive antibiotics** because of the risk of accelerated bacterial resistance and the marginal benefit of prophylaxis found in some clinical trials.

Children who have **repeated cases of otitis media** may need **evaluation for myringotomy**. However, the short- and long-term benefits must be weighed since there is question as to the value of tympanostomy tube placement.

Otitis Media with Effusion
Etiology

Otitis media with effusion (i.e., a **middle ear effusion without** the **clinical manifestations** of acute otitis media) is usually either an **extension** of an **upper respiratory tract infection** or a **sequela** to an episode of acute otitis media.

HINT: When otitis media with effusion follows properly treated acute otitis media, it usually represents the beginning of resolution of the infection (as opposed to persistent infection).

Clinical Features

Most children are **asymptomatic,** although some complain of fullness in the ear, hearing loss and, less commonly, tinnitus and vertigo.

Evaluation

Otoscopy often reveals a retracted tympanic membrane with **decreased mobility**. Laboratory evaluation is not necessary.

Treatment

Most cases of otitis media with effusion **clear spontaneously** without active treatment. The management of otitis media with effusion is undergoing reevaluation. Studies from Europe and the United States show little long-term effect from **insertion of ventilation tubes**. Likewise, treatment with **antibiotics** may have some short-term beneficial effects but the effect does not last when compared with patients not treated with antibiotics. Each case has to be individualized, but the main strategy continues to be **patient observation** for infection and speech difficulties.

 HINT: Decongestants and antihistamines have not been proven effective in the treatment of acute otitis media or otitis media with effusion.

Otitis Externa (Swimmer's Ear)
Etiology

Otitis externa, **an infection of the ear canal and external surface of the tympanic membrane,** results from **chronic irritation** as a result of **excessive moisture** in the ear canal. **Trauma or foreign bodies** in the ear canal can also precipitate otitis externa.

Diffuse otitis externa is most commonly caused by *Pseudomonas aeruginosa and Staphylococcus aureus* (which can also cause **abscesses** in the ear canal). Less commonly, *Enterobacter aerogenes, Proteus mirabilis, Klebsiella pneumoniae,* streptococci, and *Staphylococcus epidermidis* can be implicated and, rarely, fungi and herpes virus causes acute otitis externa.

Clinical Features

The initial symptom of otitis externa is **pruritus** of the auditory canal leading to **ear pain**. The pain **worsens with touching or movement** of the ear and **during chewing**.

HINT: Recent history of swimming is common risk factor for the development of otitis externa. Also, water with higher bacteriologic counts will cause otitis externa more often.

Evaluation

Patients may report **purulent drainage and otorrhea** is often noted in the ear canal on examination. The canal appears **erythematous and edematous,** and the ear is **tender** to palpation or manipulation.

Treatment

Initial management consists of **removing the debris** from the affected ear—wiping the ear canal with a dry cotton swab will usually suffice, but occasionally gentle suction is needed. An **antibiotic otic suspension** or combination **antibiotic–corticosteroid otic** preparation should be instilled in the affected ear three to four times daily for up to 10 days. If a perforated tympanic membrane is suspected, corticosteroids are contraindicated. If the canal is particularly edematous, a wick of cotton or gauze should be inserted into the canal to facilitate medication entry. Patients should be advised that **swimming is to be avoided** during treatment. Failure to respond to **two courses of treatment** or the presence of **severe inflammation** should prompt referral to an **otolaryngologist**.

Prevention

In susceptible patients, prevention of otitis externa entails abstaining from swimming or placing 2% acetic acid solution in each ear canal after swimming or bathing.

Foreign Bodies
Etiology

Foreign bodies rank **second to inflammatory and infectious disorders** of the ear as causes of otalgia. Solid, nonorganic objects are most commonly seen, although live insects can also enter the ear canal.

Treatment

Most foreign bodies can be **gently removed** with an ear curette or otologic forceps. **Insects should be killed** before attempting removal (e.g., with mineral oil, microscope immersion oil, or alcohol). If the object cannot be removed with an ear curette or otologic forceps, **irrigation** of the ear canal with **water at body temperature** is often effective. The stream of water should be directed toward the edge of the foreign body in an attempt to push it toward the external meatus. **Inability to remove the foreign body** necessitates referral to an **otolaryngologist** for removal.

 HINT: If the foreign body is vegetable matter, irrigation should not be attempted because the vegetable matter can swell and occlude the ear canal.

Acute Mastoiditis
Etiology

Acute mastoiditis is one of the **most serious complications of acute otitis media**. Infection of the mastoid air cells in the temporal bone poses a risk because it is contiguous with the posterior and middle cranial fossae, the sigmoid and lateral sinuses, the facial nerve, and the semicircular canals. Although all cases of acute otitis media are characterized by concomitant inflammation of the mucosal lining of the mastoid air cells, clinically significant mastoiditis occurs when the **passageway from the middle ear to the mastoid becomes obstructed**. Acute mastoiditis is most commonly caused by *S. pneumoniae, H. influenzae, M. catarrhalis,* but *Streptococcus pyogenes, S. aureus, P. aeruginosa,* and anaerobic organisms may also be involved.

Clinical Features

Patients with acute mastoiditis present with **persistent otalgia and fever**. **Otoscopy** usually reveals a **bulging, red, and poorly mobile tympanic membrane; purulent drainage** (through a perforation in the membrane) may be visible. **Edema and erythema** can be seen **over the mastoid bone,** obliterating the postauricular crease and **causing the characteristic downward and forward displacement of the pinna**. The **mastoid region** is **tender to palpation**.

Evaluation

A **computed tomography (CT) scan** of the temporal bone reveals **inflammation and destruction of the mastoid**. If the tympanic membrane is perforated, the canal should be cleaned of debris and fresh pus should be obtained for culture.

Treatment

Broad-spectrum **IV antibiotic therapy** covering the most common organisms should be initiated and later narrowed according to culture results when available. A third generation cephalosporin can be initiated as first-line therapy; however, if cephalosporin-resistant *S. pneumoniae,* anaerobes, or methicillin-resistant *S. aureus* are considered potential pathogens then antibiotics should be tailored accordingly. An **otolaryngologist** should be consulted, as **mastoidectomy** may be necessary if there **is poor response to IV antibiotics**. Placement of **ventilating tubes** may be appropriate to ensure continued drainage.

Trauma
Etiology

- **External ear injuries** can be caused by athletic injuries, falls, direct blows to the ear, earrings that tear through the lobe, burns, or frostbite.
- **Middle and inner ear injuries.** The ear canal can be injured by objects used to scratch the ear or to remove cerumen. Traumatic perforation of the tympanic membrane is most commonly caused by poking an object into the ear canal, but trauma to the head and barotrauma can also cause tympanic membrane perforation. Barotrauma occurs when the eustachian tube is obstructed and changes in ambient pressure cannot be transmitted to the middle ear cavity. The increased ambient pressure is transmitted to the vessels of the middle ear mucosa, creating mucosal edema. The pressure differential between the mucosa and the middle ear cavity causes rupture of the mucosal vessels, bleeding into the middle ear, and possibly perforation.

Evaluation

A history of ear trauma may be elicited. The **external ear** should be **examined for hematomas or seromas,** which appear as smooth, blue masses on the lateral auricle and obscure its natural contour. **Microscopic examination** of the tympanic membrane is necessary in patients with suspected traumatic tympanic membrane perforations to ensure that the edges of the perforation do not enter the middle ear cavity. Cholesteatoma formation can occur as a complication if the edges of the ruptured tympanic membrane protrude into the middle ear.

Treatment

- **External ear injuries.** Immediate evacuation of hematomas and seromas of the auricle is necessary to prevent cartilage damage. Use of epinephrine should be avoided when lacerations of the pinna are sutured, because epinephrine causes vasoconstriction and may lead to tissue necrosis.
- **Perforated tympanic membrane.** Clean perforations of the tympanic membrane (i.e., those in which the edges do not enter the middle ear cavity) usually heal spontaneously within 2–3 weeks. The perforation should be kept clean and dry. A patient with a traumatic perforation that does not heal in 3 weeks, or one who experiences vertigo, sensorineural hearing loss, or facial nerve paralysis must be referred to an otolaryngologist.
- **Barotrauma** should be treated with antibiotics to prevent infection of the middle ear hemorrhagic effusion. Patients with barotrauma and acute sensorineural hearing loss or vertigo and those with barotrauma injuries that do not heal require prompt referral to an otolaryngologist.

Suggested Readings

American Academy of Pediatrics and American Academy of Family Physicians Subcommittee on Management of Acute Otitis Media. Clinical practice guideline: diagnosis and management of acute otitis media. *Pediatrics.* 2004;113(5):1451–1465.

American Academy of Family Physicians, American Academy of Otolaryngology—Head and Neck Surgery, American Academy of Pediatrics Subcommittee on Otitis Media With Effusion. Clinical practice guideline: Otitis media with effusion. *Pediatrics.* 2004;113(5):1412–1429.

Bhetwal N, McConaghy JR. The evaluation and treatment of children with acute otitis media. *Prim Care: Clin Office Pract.* 2007;34:59–70.

Spiro DM, Tay KY, Arnold DH, Dziura JD, Baker MD, Shapiro ED. Wait-and-see prescription for the treatment of acute otitis media: a randomized controlled trial. *JAMA.* 2006;296(10):1235–1241.

Edema

INTRODUCTION

Edema refers to the clinical condition in which an excessive amount of fluid accumulates in the **extravascular interstitial space** of the body. The balance of competing Starling forces (hydrostatic and oncotic pressure) between plasma and the interstitium normally favors a small net movement of fluid from the capillary lumen into the interstitial space. This fluid is then collected by the lymphatic system and returned to the venous system via the thoracic duct. Edema occurs when these different forces become unbalanced either from **alterations to capillary hemodynamics** (change in hydrostatic or oncotic pressure gradients across the capillary wall), an **increase in capillary wall permeability, or impaired lymphatic function**. Edema may be **localized or generalized**. Localized edema is found in diseases of the lymphatic system, with venous obstruction, and in conditions associated with increased permeability of the capillary wall (e.g., infection, burns, trauma, and allergic reactions). **Allergic reaction** is the most common cause of localized edema in childhood. Generalized edema usually develops secondary to **hypoalbuminemia** (the main source of plasma oncotic pressure) or **increased hydrostatic pressure** from sodium and water retention. **Minimal-change nephrotic syndrome** (MCNS), although uncommon in and of itself with an annual incidence of 2–7 cases per 100,000 children, accounts for most cases of generalized edema. Severe generalized edema is referred to as **anasarca**. Additionally, localized edema may be seen in the abdomen (ascites) or chest (pulmonary edema or pleural effusions), but are typically associated with generalized edema.

DIFFERENTIAL DIAGNOSIS LIST

A variety of diseases may cause localized or generalized edema, with some contributing to both. They may be classified according to the pathophysiologic mechanism, although for localized edema the location of the edema may be more helpful as an approach to the diagnosis.

Localized Edema (Represent Distinctive Areas of Involvement)
Increased Capillary Permeability

Allergic reaction (insect bites, contact dermatitis, drug or food allergy)

Local trauma
Cellulitis
Angioedema (hereditary, ACE inhibitor induced)

Vasculitis (Henoch–
Schönlein purpura – *scalp,*
Dermatomyositis – *eyelids,*
Kawasaki disease – *hands or
feet*)

Hypothyroidism (pre-tibial
myxedema, periorbital)

Epstein–Barr virus (*bilateral upper
eyelids,* i.e., Hoagland's sign)

Increased Plasma Hydrostatic Pressure

Venous thrombosis

Dactylitis of sickle cell anemia
(*hands or feet*)

Extrinsic venous compression
(tumor, lymphadenopathy)

Cirrhosis (ascites, bilateral lower
extremities)

Impaired Lymphatic Drainage

Regional lymph node trauma or
lymphadenitis

Lymphedema Praecox (*lower
extremities* – 4 times more likely
than upper extremities)

Turner or Noonan syndrome
(*neck, dorsal hands, or feet*)

Filariasis

Milroy's disease

Autoimmune involvement
of lymphatics (sarcoidosis,
Juvenile Rheumatoid Arthritis,
Crohn's)

Generalized Edema
Increased Capillary Permeability

Sepsis

Burns

Serum Sickness

Systemic Inflammatory Response
Syndrome

Hypothyroidism (myxedema)

Other infections (Scarlet Fever,
Rocky Mountain Spotted Fever,
Roseola)

Decreased Plasma Oncotic Pressure (Hypoproteinemia)

Nephrotic syndrome

Hepatic failure (hepatitis,
congenital fibrosis, cystic
fibrosis, metabolic disorders)

Protein-losing enteropathy
(milk protein allergy, Celiac
disease, Menetrier's disease,
inflammatory bowel disease,
Fontan physiology)

Protein-calorie malnutrition
(kwashiorkor)

Severe anemia (hemolytic anemia)

Beriberi

Increased Hydrostatic Pressure

Congestive heart failure

Cirrhosis

Renal failure

Glomerulonephritis
(Postinfectious, hereditary,
IgA Nephropathy,
Henoch–Schönlein,
Membranoproliferative)

Medications (vasodilators,
corticosteroids)

Excessive iatrogenic intravenous
fluid

APPROACH TO THE PATIENT WITH EDEMA

The general approach to children with edema is to first determine the character of the edema, **localized versus generalized,** as their subsequent etiologies are usually quite different. Localized edema can be unilateral or even fixed (not extending further) in distribution, whereas generalized edema would not. Generalized edema often is **dependent** in nature, involving those areas affected by gravity most. This is typically the lower legs and feet in ambulatory children but may include the sacral area in nonambulating children. Generalized edema may also involve tissues that are easily distensible such as the eyelids, but also areas less easily examined like the scrotum or labia. However, localized edema may also be dependent, especially if it involves the lower extremity or scalp, or involve distensible tissues.

> **HINT:** Unilateral swelling of one side of the body after waking up from sleep may still be dependent edema, if the child had slept with that side down.

As both localized and generalized edema can be associated with life-threatening conditions, the immediate evaluation should always be to insure that the patient is stable from a cardiorespiratory standpoint before proceeding. Localized facial edema could concurrently involve the airway while patients with generalized edema could have pulmonary edema and/or cardiac compromise, all potential medical emergencies. An initial inquiry into how the patient is breathing while assessing their respiratory effort (tachypnea, retractions), breath sounds (stridor, wheezing, rales), and heart rate (tachycardia) and heart sounds (S3 or S4 gallop) should be completed before proceeding with any extended work-up.

Localized Edema (Figure 31-1)

As allergic reactions, infection, and trauma are the most common causes of localized edema, symptom history and associated findings should first focus on these possibilities. Edema is often **acute in onset** in these cases with a history of antecedent trauma, either direct to the soft tissue (trauma), causing a break in skin integrity (cellulitis), or from an insect bite. **Pruritis** is often associated with allergic reactions while **erythema or fever** may be seen with cellulitis. The age of onset may also be helpful, as congenital causes of localized edema are fairly limited in scope (birth trauma, Milroy's disease, Turner, or Noonan syndrome) while **lymphedema praecox and hereditary angioedema** tend to develop or worsen closer to puberty. A history of **recurrent swelling episodes,** even if they include different areas of localization, is suggestive of hereditary angioedema, especially if accompanied by recurrent abdominal pain episodes.

Past medical history should inquire into possible risk factors for venous thrombosis, including sickle cell disease, congenital heart disease, venous catheters, or malignancies. A complete medication history should include any new medicines, especially **angiotensin converting enzyme (ACE) inhibitors or oral contraceptives**. A family history of recurrent edema would lend toward hereditary angioedema, as it is an **autosomal dominant** disorder.

The physical exam should focus first on the localization of the edema, as this is often helpful in distinguishing some of the different possibilities. Some disorders have distinctive areas of involvement (see Differential Diagnosis List). Venous and lymphatic obstructions are more common in certain regions and cause edema distal to

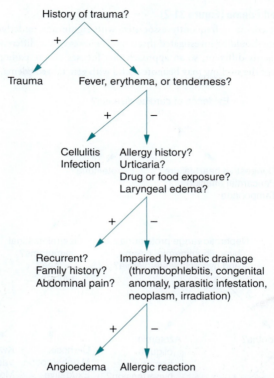

History of trauma?

+ → **Trauma**

− → **Fever, erythema, or tenderness?**

+ → **Cellulitis Infection**

− → **Allergy history? Urticaria? Drug or food exposure? Laryngeal edema?**

+ → **Recurrent? Family history? Abdominal pain?**

− → **Impaired lymphatic drainage (thrombophlebitis, congenital anomaly, parasitic infestation, neoplasm, irradiation)**

+ → **Angioedema**

− → **Allergic reaction**

FIGURE 31-1   Algorithm for diagnosis in a patient with localized edema (not congenital).

the site of obstruction. This may occur peripherally with unilateral extremity swelling or more centrally, as in cirrhosis (portal hypertension with resultant ascites and lower extremity edema) or superior vena cava syndrome (head, neck, and arm swelling). If the edema is **nonpitting,** lymphedema or myxedema should be considered. Other skin findings may include urticaria (allergic reaction, angioedema), erythema (cellulitis), petechiae (vasculitis), or a palpable cord (venous thrombosis). Local lymph nodes should also be palpated for the possibility of obstructed lymphatic return or infection.

The lab and radiologic evaluation for localized edema is rather limited, as most diagnoses should be made by history and physical exam. In a child suspected of having a venous thrombosis, an elevated D-dimer or thrombocytopenia may be suggestive of this possibility, but **Doppler ultrasonography** assessing venous flow (or lack of) proximal to the site of edema would be diagnostic. Once this diagnosis is made, additional coagulation and additional thrombophilic studies (antithrombin III, Protein S, Protein C, and Factor V Leiden) are indicated. With suspected hereditary angioedema, low complement components (C2, C4, C1 inhibitors) may be found.

Generalized Edema (Figure 31-2)

Generalized edema is frequently associated with significant underlying disease and therefore should be investigated thoroughly. However, the different etiologies can be distinctly different, so an approach that focuses on the pathophysiologic mechanism of the swelling may be more useful with generalized edema. Decreased

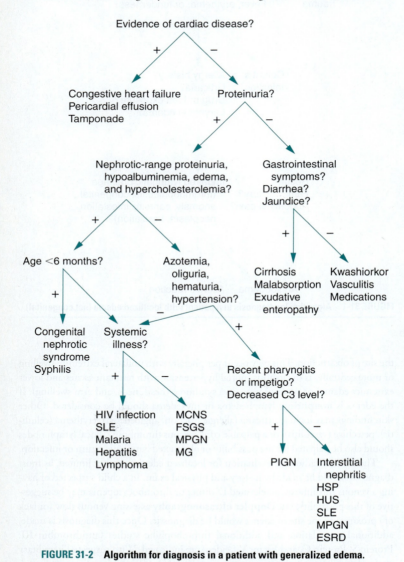

FIGURE 31-2 Algorithm for diagnosis in a patient with generalized edema.

plasma oncotic pressure in most cases will be secondary to a **low serum albumin** (<2.5 gm/dL to cause edema). Increased hydrostatic pressure may be associated with elevated blood pressure or, with congestive heart failure, pulmonary edema and gallop rhythm. Causes of increased capillary permeability are often associated with serious infections, inflammatory responses, or burns which may have a history of either exposure or fever.

The patient history may help in disclosing if there any other **associated symptoms** that may aid in the diagnosis. A decrease in urine output, gross hematuria, or flank pain may be seen in renal failure or glomerulonephritis. Respiratory symptoms such as cough and dyspnea on exertion may be suggestive of congestive heart failure. Diarrhea, abdominal pain, mouth ulcers, jaundice, or blood in stool is suggestive of liver disease or protein-losing enteropathies. Distinctive rashes and joint complaints may be seen with Rocky Mountain Spotted Fever, serum sickness, and some vasculitides.

A recent **exposure history** should include dietary changes, risk of tick bite exposure, and Strep throat or cellulitis, which often occurs 1–4 weeks prior to post-streptococcal glomerulonephritis. **Medication history** should inquire specifically about any corticosteroid or vasodilator (calcium channel blockers, minoxidil) use. **Family history** ought to focus upon any renal diseases, autoimmune disorders, liver diseases, and cystic fibrosis. Lastly, a **social history** should screen for any risk of malnutrition or prenatal exposures (Hepatitis B, HIV), which are less typically seen in developing nations.

The physical exam should include careful attention to the heart, lungs, and abdomen. **Elevated blood pressure** is often seen with volume overload from renal disease. Tachycardia, tachypnea, crackles, murmur, and/or gallop may be seen in patients with congestive heart failure.

> **HINT:** Left ventricular failure may present with pulmonary but not peripheral edema, while right ventricular failure may present with hepatomegaly and peripheral edema. Therefore, edema is not typically seen in children until they are moderately decompensated, and infants more typically present with irritability, feeding difficulties, diaphoresis, and labored breathing.

Decreased breath sounds and dullness to percussion are found with pleural effusion, which is not pathognomonic for a particular etiology but indicative of the degree of edema involvement. **Abdominal distention** and fluid wave may be seen with ascites, while the presence of splenomegaly would be suggestive of portal hypertension. **Oral ulcers and uveitis** may be seen in Crohn's disease. **Skin findings** may include burns, jaundice, dermatitis (kwashiorkor), purpura (Henoch–Schonlein, serum sickness), erythema nodosum (inflammatory bowel disease), sandpaper-like rash (Scarlet Fever), or palm and sole involvement (Rocky Mountain Spotted Fever [RMSF]). **Poor growth** may be seen in chronic kidney or liver disease, malnutrition, and heart failure.

The following studies may be indicated for the evaluation of **generalized edema:** serum albumin; urinalysis including microscopic examination; serum electrolytes, blood urea nitrogen, and creatinine; chest X-ray; echocardiogram; stool α-1-antitrypsin; liver function tests including coagulation studies; complete blood count; and other specific serologic tests.

A pathophysiologic approach to generalized edema may start with first determining if the patient is hypoalbuminemic and, if so, then determining if the low albumin is from renal losses, gastrointestinal losses, or lack of production. Massive proteinuria (4+ on dipstick urinalysis or urine protein-creatinine ratio >2), hypoalbuminemia, and edema characterize nephrotic syndrome (along with hypercholesterolemia), which can be seen in a variety of clinical entities. The most common cause of nephrotic syndrome is **Minimal Change Disease,** accounting for 75% of all cases. It typically presents in children between 2 and 7 years of age, with cases presenting younger often requiring special consideration. Blood pressure is rarely elevated and hematuria, present in a minority of patients, is usually microscopic. However, nephrotic syndrome is not a mutually exclusive diagnosis and may be seen with other disorders, including other glomerulonephritides, or secondary to systemic disorders (malaria, Hodgkin's disease, Hepatitis B or C, congenital syphilis).

> **HINT:** Remember that, although these children do not appear dehydrated, their intravascular volume may be decreased, and they are at increased risk for hypovolemic shock in the setting of vomiting or diarrhea.

If the urinalysis is negative for protein in a hypoalbuminemic patient, then **gastrointestinal etiologies** should be investigated. Patients with diarrhea should be suspected of having a **protein-losing enteropathy,** which can be confirmed by an elevated **stool α-1-antitrypsin** level. This is nonspecific for the cause of enteropathy and more specific investigations may be needed, such as endomyseal antibodies (Celiac disease) or endoscopy. If protein loss in the stool is minimal, then **decreased albumin synthesis** may be the cause of hypoalbuminemia. Screening of liver function tests, including measures of synthetic function like coagulation factors, is indicated. If there is evidence of **hepatitis or cirrhosis,** then further diagnostic testing may be indicated, including viral hepatitis studies, ceruloplasmin levels, serum α-1-antitrypsin levels, and Doppler ultrasonography of the liver. If there is no evidence of protein losses (urine or stool) or impaired liver function in the hypoalbuminemic patient, then focus should, by default, shift **to impaired protein intake** and investigation of other nutritional losses.

If hypoalbuminemia is not present and there are no other overt symptoms to the etiology, then dysfunction of the heart or kidneys should next be evaluated. A chest X-ray showing an enlarged cardiac silhouette and pulmonary edema would be especially suspicious of **congestive heart failure,** especially in the setting of normal or low blood pressure. Brain natriuretic peptide also may be elevated. However, an echocardiogram showing impaired cardiac function is diagnostic of heart failure and may also aid in giving a more specific structural etiology to the failure. **Renal failure** can be diagnosed easily by an elevated serum creatinine; however, this does not indicate if the failure is acute or chronic. Acute kidney injury can be caused by different etiologies including hypovolemia, acute vesicoureteral obstruction, nephrotoxic medications, systemic inflammatory response associated with cardiopulmonary bypass, hemolytic-uremic syndrome, interstitial, or glomerulonephritis. Chronic kidney disease is from congenital abnormalities of the urinary tract (renal dysplasia, obstructive uropathy, reflux nephropathy) in a majority of children, but may also be secondary to acquired disorders or genetic disorders with later presentations. A urinalysis with microscopic examination and renal ultrasound would both be indicated to evaluate the causes of renal failure.

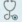 **HINT:** In chronic kidney disease, the sequelae of ongoing impairment of other renal functions may be seen such as significant anemia, hypocalcemia, and secondary hyperparathyroidism, which may also need to be addressed.

As mentioned, **glomerulonephritis** (GN) may present in a variety of ways, including with or without nephrotic syndrome or renal failure. It should be considered if there is both significant blood and protein on urinalysis; however, the presence of red blood cell casts on urine microscopy is pathognomonic. Postinfectious GN is the most common pediatric cause of GN, but other possible causes include IgA nephropathy, Alport syndrome, membranoproliferative GN, and systemic vasculitides (lupus, Henoch–Schonlein purpura). A **serum C3 level** is helpful in determining the cause of GN, while other tests to be considered include **C4 level, antinuclear antibody** (ANA), and **antineutrophil cytoplasmic antibody** (ANCA).

Nonspecific laboratory abnormalities may be seen with possible infectious and inflammatory diagnoses, such as leukopenia or leukocytosis, bandemia, eosinophilia (serum sickness and scarlet fever), thrombocytopenia, hyponatremia (Rocky Mountain spotted fever), acidosis, and elevated transaminases. When other diagnostics have been negative or nonspecific, other tests to consider include blood cultures, thyroid function screening (free T4, thyroid stimulating hormone) and those for specific infectious processes (rapid strep, rickettsial ELISA).

TREATMENT OF EDEMA

In patients with generalized edema, treatment of the primary disease usually results in resolution of the edema. However, because there is a vast array of disorders causing edema, with different pathogenic mechanisms, no single treatment is universal for all edema. Fortunately, it is often not necessary to treat the edema before establishing the diagnosis. One mainstay of edema therapy is **salt restriction,** as it helps to minimize the edema and would not worsen any of the etiologies.

Diuretic administration may be considered, especially with severe edema. Loop diuretics, such as **furosemide,** may be especially effective in addressing issues of increased hydrostatic pressure as seen in congestive heart failure, renal failure, and glomerulonephritis. However, they should be used with caution in patients who may have intravascular depletion, such as in nephrotic syndrome, or at risk for worsening electrolyte imbalance, like cirrhosis. **Spironolactone,** with its sparing of renal potassium losses, is sometimes considered in cirrhosis. Also, diuretics are of little benefit to localized edema caused by obstruction (venous or lymphatic).

Albumin (25 g/dL, 25%) infusions or intermittent dosing may be considered in patients with decreased intravascular oncotic pressure, but **should be used with caution**. This intervention is typically used when there is respiratory compromise (from ascites or pleural effusion), acute kidney injury from intravascular depletion, or risk of skin breakdown from the edema. Its possible complications are **hypertension and pulmonary edema,** so it should not be used in instances when intravascular overload is present such as with glomerulonephritis and cardiac failure.

Other interventions to consider in specific clinical conditions include corticosteroids in minimal change disease, inotropic medications in congestive heart failure, and dietary modifications in malabsorptive disorders or malnutrition.

Suggested Readings

Andreucci M, Federico S, Andreucci VE. Edema and acute renal failure. *Semin Nephrol.* 2001;21(3): 251–256.

Cho S, Atwood JE. Peripheral edema. *Am J Med.* 2002;113:580–586.

Eddy AA, Symons JM. Nephrotic syndrome in childhood. *Lancet.* 2003;362(9384):629–639.

Fenton M, Burch M. Understanding chronic heart failure. *Arch Dis Child.* 2007;92(9):812–816.

Hisano S, Hahn S, Kuemmerle NB, et al. Edema in childhood. *Kidney Int Suppl.* 1997;59:S100–S104.

Kaplan BS, Meyers KEC. *Pediatric Nephrology and Urology: The Requisites in Pediatrics.* Philadelphia: Elsevier Mosby; 2004.

Martin P-Y, Schrier RW. Renal sodium excretion and edematous disorders. *Endocrinol Metab Clin North Am.* 1995;24:459–479.

Rosen FS. Urticaria, angioedema, anaphylaxis. *Pediatr Rev.* 1992;13:387–390.

Electrolyte Disturbances

 DIFFERENTIAL DIAGNOSIS LIST*

Sodium imbalance

Potassium imbalance

Calcium imbalance

Magnesium imbalance

Phosphate imbalance

Metabolic acidosis

Metabolic alkalosis

*Normal pediatric laboratory parameters vary according to age (Table 32-1)

DIFFERENTIAL DIAGNOSIS DISCUSSION

Hypernatremia

Etiology

Definition: Serum sodium >150 mEq/L.

- **Water loss**
  - Unreplaced loss of solute-free water raises the serum sodium concentration and is the most common cause of hypernatremia. Concurrent sodium loss may occur, but with water loss in excess of sodium loss.
  - Major causes:
    - Gastrointestinal (diarrhea, vomiting, or both with inadequate fluid intake)
    - Insensible water loss (fevers, exposure to heat, exercise, infants with poor feeding)
    - Urinary water loss (central or nephrogenic diabetes insipidus, renal disease with urinary concentrating defect, therapy with loop diuretics)
    - Impaired thirst/hypodipsia (hypothalamic lesions, holoprosencephaly, osmoreceptor injury leading to **essential hypernatremia**)
    - Osmotic diuresis (glucose, urea, mannitol) in which urine is hypotonic to plasma due to nonreabsorbed osmotically active solute
- **Excess sodium**
  - Exogenous sodium intake
    - Commonly iatrogenic (oral or intravenous sodium chloride or sodium bicarbonate)
    - Salt poisoning in infants and toddlers
  - Sodium retention
    - Mineralocorticoid excess can result in mild hypernatremia with reset osmostat

TABLE 32-1	Normal Serum Pediatric Laboratory Values (found at http://www.pediatriccareonline.org)
Sodium (Na⁺)	**136–145 mEq/L**
Potassium (K⁺)	**Newborns** 4.5–7.2 mEq/L **2 d–3 mo** 4.0–6.2 mEq/L **3 mo–1 yr** 3.7–5.6 mEq/L **1–16 yr** 3.5–5.0 mEq/L
Bicarbonate (HCO₃⁻)	**Newborns** 17.2–23.6 mEq/L **2 mo–2 yr** 19–24 mEq/L **Children** 18–25 mEq/L
Calcium (Ca⁺⁺)	**Newborns** 7.0–12.0 mg/dL **0–2 yr** 8.8–11.2 mg/dL **>2 yr** 9.0–11.0 mg/dL
Magnesium (Mg⁺)	1.5–2.5 mEq/L
Phosphorus (P)	**Newborns** 4.2–9.0 mg/dL **6 wk–19 mo** 3.8–6.7 mg/dL **19 mo–3 yr** 2.9–5.9 mg/dL **3–15 yr** 3.6–5.6 mg/dL **>15 yr** 2.5–5.0 mg/dL

- **Intracellular water movement**
  - Occurs during seizures or exercise due to transient intracellular increase in osmotically active molecules (lactic acid)

Clinical Features
- Variable and nonspecific
- Depend on the magnitude of hypernatremia and the rate of change
- Irritability, lethargy, weakness, MS changes, increased deep tendon reflexes, seizures, and cramping
- Water loss can be accompanied by dehydration, volume depletion, and weight loss
- Sodium excess can have weight gain, mild volume expansion, and edema

Evaluation
Hypernatremia associated with water loss can cause osmotic fluid shift from the intracellular to the extracellular space, with relative sparing of the extracellular fluid (ECF) volume.

Physical examination:

- Assess weight change if possible. Weight loss may occur even in the absence of ECF volume depletion
- Assess **adequacy of ECF compartments**
  - Intravascular compartment: peripheral pulses, perfusion, temperature, and capillary refill time
  - Interstitial compartment: skin turgor, tears, and mucous membrane appearance

Laboratory Studies
- Basic metabolic panel
- Urinalysis and urine osmolality, sodium, and creatinine

TABLE 32-2	Assessment of Hypernatremia			
Underlying Cause	**ECF Volume**	**Urine Output**	**Urine Sodium**	**Specific Gravity**
Sodium excess	Increased	Normal or increased	Increased	High
Water loss (DI)	Decreased*	Increased	Decreased	Low
Sodium and water loss (water more than sodium)	Decreased	Decreased	Increased	High

*In states of water loss alone, resulting hypernatremia results in intracellular to extracellular fluid shift, which may initially have relative sparing of ECF volume loss.
DI, diabetes insipidus; ECF, extracellular fluid.

Table 32-2 summarizes the findings suggestive of the various underlying mechanisms of hypernatremia.

Treatment
Inadequate effective circulating volume (ECV) should be **treated promptly** and independently of the serum sodium.

- Normal saline to restore ECV. Initial bolus of 20 mL/kg over about 30 minutes in children without known underlying cardiac or renal disease.
- Close monitoring and reassessment is critical.

After Restoration of ECV
- **Reduce the serum sodium level slowly** (approximately 0.5 mEq/L/hour and no greater than 15 mEq/L in a 24-hour period).
- Assessment of the solute-free water deficit, maintenance needs, and ongoing losses of water ± sodium should be performed. The free water deficit is calculated as follows:
  - **4 mL/kg of free water decreases serum Na^+ by 1 mEq/L**
  - **The free water deficit (L) = 4 mL/kg × wt(kg) × (observed Na^+ − desired Na^+)**
- Hypotonic intravenous fluids at a concentration and rate determined by careful calculation and given over 48 hours is recommended.
- Avoid rapid administration of very hypotonic fluids, which can lead to intracellular water shift, cell swelling, and cerebral edema.
- Monitor serum sodium, fluid balance, and weight closely with any intravenous fluid therapy.
- Patients with **severe total body sodium excess require** judicious use of fluids, with or without furosemide administration, dialysis, or both (under the guidance of a nephrologist).

Hyponatremia
Etiology
Definition: Serum sodium ≤130 mEq/L. All causes of hyponatremia can be considered to be dilutional, depletional, or both (Table 32-3).

- **Dilutional hyponatremia.** The total body water is generally expanded and is increased relative to total body sodium.

TABLE 32-3	**Causes of Hyponatremia**

Dilutional Hyponatremia
Water intoxication (excess ingestion or iatrogenic administration)
Edema-associated states
Congestive heart failure
Nephrotic syndrome
Renal failure
Hepatic failure
Neuromuscular blockade (e.g., pancuronium-induced)
Excess antidiuretic hormone (ADH)* (nonedematous state)
Exogenous administration
Syndrome of inappropriate antidiuretic hormone (SIADH)
Hypothyroidism
Reset osmostat
Hyperglycemia

Depletional Hyponatremia
Renal sodium wasting (e.g., Fanconi syndrome, states of aldosterone resistance)
Adrenal sodium wasting (e.g., adrenal insufficiency)
CAH (21-hydroxylase deficiency)
Diuretic therapy
Osmotic diuresis (e.g., glucosuria)
Gastrointestinal fluid losses with hypotonic replacement
Excessive perspiration associated with large sodium loss (e.g., cystic fibrosis)

*Conditions associated with increased ADH or an ADH-like effect and hyponatremia include pain, vomiting, central nervous system disorders (e.g., trauma, infection, neoplasia), intrathoracic conditions (e.g., infection, mechanical ventilation), and some drugs (e.g., narcotics, barbiturates, carbamazepine, nonsteroidal anti-inflammatory agents [NSAIDs], cyclophosphamide, vincristine).
CAH, congenital adrenal hyperplasia.

- **Depletional hyponatremia.** There is a decreased (or normal) amount of total body water and a deficit of sodium in excess of water.
- **Pseudohyponatremia.** Sodium is not distributed throughout the serum and its concentration is artificially lowered. Causes of pseudohyponatremia include hyperlipidemia and hyperproteinemia. Na^+ decrease = $0.002 \times$ lipid concentration in mg/dL (hyperlipidemia) and $0.25 \times$ (protein in g/dL -8) (hyperproteinemia).
- **Severe hyperglycemia.** Hyponatremia may occur from osmotic movement of water out of cells. Na^+ decreases by 1.6 mEq/L per 100 mg/dL rise in glucose.

Clinical Features
- Variable and nonspecific
- Depend on the magnitude of hyponatremia and the rate of change
- Lethargy, weakness, encephalopathy, and seizures

Evaluation
Physical examination:

- Assess weight change and status of ECF volume as with hypernatremia.

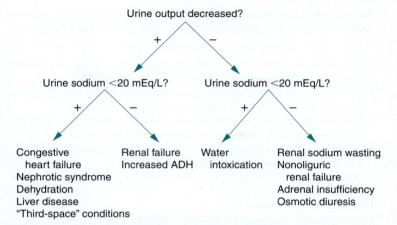

FIGURE 32-1 **Narrowing the differential diagnosis for the underlying cause of hyponatremia.** ADH, antidiuretic hormone.

Laboratory Studies
- Basic metabolic panel
- Serum osmolality: Estimated by doubling the serum sodium level (mEq/L) and adding 10 or the following equation:

$$\text{Serum osm} = 2 \times \text{Na}^+ \text{ (mEq/L)} + \text{Glucose}/118 + \text{BUN}/2.8$$

- Urine osmolality
- Urine sodium
- Serum and urine uric acid (helpful in SIADH)
- Calculation of the fractional excretion of sodium (FE_{Na}) can be useful when the urine sodium concentration is borderline (e.g., 19 to 21 mEq/L):

$$FE_{Na} = (U_{Na} \times P_{Cr})/(U_{Cr} \times P_{Na}) \times 100\%$$

Figure 32-1 demonstrates how the differential for the specific cause of the hyponatremia can be narrowed on the basis of urine output and urine sodium excretion.

Therapy
In all cases of hyponatremia, therapy should aim to treat the underlying etiology. Management of fluid and sodium balance varies according to the category of hyponatremia.

 Depletional hyponatremia: Associated with a water shift to the intracellular fluid (ICF) compartment. Therefore, careful assessment and prompt restoration of the **ECF and intravascular volume** are critical.

- **Compromised ECV.** Restore promptly with the administration of isotonic saline, initially with an intravenous bolus of 20 mL/kg, given rapidly over about 30 minutes. Additional isotonic fluid boluses may be indicated after patient reassessment.

- **Sodium deficit.** The sodium deficit should be calculated and measures taken to restore the sodium level. The sodium deficit can be calculated as follows:

  $$Na^+ \text{ deficit (mEq)} = 0.6 \times wt \text{ (kg)} \times (\text{desired } Na^+ - \text{observed } Na^+)$$

- Rapid increase in serum sodium with 3% saline is required in symptomatic patients (e.g., hyponatremia-induced seizures) 0.5 mEq/mL.
  - Volume of 3% (mEq) = (target Na^+ − observed Na^+) × wt (kg) × f_D (f_D − distribution factor, for Na^+ 0.6–0.7 L/kg body weight).
  - In acute hyponatremia, the sodium level should be corrected to 125 mEq/L or to a level slightly higher than that associated with symptoms.
  - In chronic hyponatremia, rapid correction can lead to osmotic demyelinization syndrome or central pontine myelinolysis.
  - Target rate of Na^+ rise in asymptomatic patients: 0.5–1 mEq/L/hour or 10–20 mEq/24 hour.

  Dilutional hyponatremia:
- General principle of treatment is restriction of fluid.
- Exceptions include edematous states with hypoalbuminemia, where there is risk of intravascular volume depletion.
  - Restrict sodium, as it may contribute to worsening of associated edema.
- SIADH: Treatment approach
  - Uncommon in pediatrics, usually transient. See Table 32-3 for medications causing SIADH.
  - ADH is fixed regardless of variation in intake, ECF volume, or serum osmolality.
  - Fluid restriction to approximately 2/3 of maintenance.

 HINT: Serum sodium concentration is maintained within a narrow range by adjustments in water intake and excretion in response to ADH secretion and thirst. Abnormalities in serum sodium are therefore predominantly a result of abnormalities in water balance, with or without a significant contribution from sodium itself; however, sodium may be a predominant factor in certain specific sodium derangements.

Hyperkalemia
Etiology
- **Transcellular potassium shifts** are the most common cause of hyperkalemia in childhood. Potassium shifts from the ICF to the ECF in the following conditions:
  - Metabolic acidosis
  - Beta-adrenergic blockade
  - Strenuous exercise
  - Insulin deficiency, hyperglycemia, and hyperosmolality
  - Hyperkalemic periodic paralysis

HINT: The presence of acidosis does not always account for the hyperkalemia and may lead to failure to recognize and treat another cause.

TABLE 32-4	Drugs Associated with Hyperkalemia

Potassium-sparing diuretics (spironolactone, triamterene, amiloride)
Potassium supplements (e.g., potassium chloride)
Potassium-containing penicillins
Stored blood
Calcineurin inhibitors (cyclosporine, tacrolimus)
Nonsteroidal anti-inflammatory drugs (NSAIDs)
Heparin
Angiotensin-converting enzyme (ACE) inhibitors
Beta-adrenergic blockers
Chemotherapeutic agents

- **Increased potassium intake**
  - Potassium supplements, drugs containing potassium (e.g., potassium penicillins), salt substitute use, and blood transfusions (stored blood). Hyperkalemia usually occurs in the context of impaired renal potassium excretion.
- **Decreased renal excretion of potassium**
  - Renal failure
  - Medications (Table 32-4)
  - Renal tubular acidosis (RTA) – Type IV or voltage-dependent distal (Type I) RTA
  - Mineralocorticoid deficiency (adrenal insufficiency, congenital adrenal hyperplasia (CAH), hyporeninemic hypoaldosteronism, and primary mineralocorticoid deficiency).
  - Mineralocorticoid resistance (transient condition in newborn, associated with renal injury, or due to pseudohypoaldosteronism).
- Increased endogenous cellular release of potassium is associated with hypoxic or toxic cell death, burns, intravascular hemolysis, rhabdomyolysis, and acute tumor lysis syndrome.
- Pseudohyperkalemia – Movement of potassium out of cells during or after specimen collection.
  - Hemolysis
  - Leukocytosis or thrombocytosis
  - Familial pseudohyperkalemia (temperature-dependent leakage of potassium out of cells)

Clinical Features
Symptoms of hyperkalemia are neither predictably present nor specific. They include muscle weakness, decreased deep tendon reflexes, ileus, anorexia, tingling of the mouth and extremities, malaise, and tetany.

Evaluation
Laboratory Studies
- Serum electrolyte panel; serum calcium, magnesium, and glucose
- Urinalysis, urine potassium, and creatinine (to calculate the transtubular potassium gradient or TTKG)

- Other tests (e.g., imaging, endocrine, or genetic studies) based upon clinical suspicion
- ECG
- Peaked T waves (especially in precordial leads) and prolonged PR intervals or a widened, prolonged QRS complex
- Late life-threatening ECG changes include flattened P or T waves (or both) with ST segment depression, a sine wave pattern, and tachyarrhythmias or bradyarrhythmias

Treatment

If the ***verified*** potassium level is high or there are hyperkalemic signs and symptoms, emergency measures should be initiated. Table 32-5 summarizes the options for the management of hyperkalemia. Indications for urgent or emergent treatment include the following:

- A potassium value above 7.0 mEq/L
- A rapidly increasing potassium concentration
- A clinical state in which the potassium level is expected to continue to increase (e.g., rhabdomyolysis)
- Renal failure
- Symptoms of hyperkalemia

> **HINT:** Avoidance of hyperkalemia is critical in patients with kidney disease and reduced glomerular filtration rate (GFR). These patients require frequent lab monitoring. Some may require restriction of potassium intake, avoidance of certain medications (e.g., renin-angiotensin system blockade), and use of potassium-free solutions for intravenous fluid therapy. All patients receiving intravenous fluids with potassium should have renal function assessed prior to administration.

Hypokalemia

Etiology

- **Severely limited nutrition** (e.g., anorexia nervosa, renal excretion can adjust to more moderate limitations in potassium intake)
- **Increased gastrointestinal losses** (e.g., vomiting, diarrhea, cathartic abuse)
- **Increased skin losses** (e.g., excessive sweating, burns)
- **Increased renal losses**—Fanconi syndrome, RTA, Bartter syndrome, diuretic therapy, osmotic diuresis (e.g., glucosuria), hyperaldosteronism, CAH, 11-*b*-hydroxysteroid dehydrogenase deficiency (or inhibition with natural licorice ingestion), Liddle syndrome, Gitelman syndrome (magnesium-losing tubulopathy), salt-wasting nephropathies, excess adrenocorticotropic hormone (ACTH), drugs (Table 32-6), magnesium depletion, chloride depletion, loss of gastric secretions, and polyuria
- **Transcellular potassium shifts**—alkalosis (metabolic and respiratory), excess insulin, beta-adrenergic activity, hypokalemic periodic paralysis, and certain drugs (Table 32-6)

TABLE 32-5	Treatment of Hyperkalemia			
Agent	**Indication**	**Mechanism of Action**	**Dose**	**Side Effects/ Potential Problems**
10% calcium gluconate	ECG changes	Stabilizes membranes	1 mg/kg IV over 5–10 min	Hypercalcemia
Sodium bicarbonate*	ECG changes or very high K^+ level	Shifts K^+ to intracellular compartment	1 mg/kg IV over 5–10 min	Sodium load
Glucose plus insulin	ECG changes or very high K^+ level	Shifts K^+ to intracellular compartment	0.25–0.5 g/kg glucose plus 0.3 U insulin/g glucose over 30–60 min	Hyper- or hypo-glycemia
Albuterol (Beta-agonist)	ECG changes or very high K^+ level	Shifts K^+ to intracellular compartment	1.25–2.5 mg by nebulizer	Tachycardia
Kayexalate resin	To remove K^+ from body	K^+ binds to resin in gut	1 g/kg PO or PR in 50%–70% sorbitol	Constipation
Furosemide	Symptomatic hyperkale-mia	Enhances urinary K^+ excretion	1–2 mg/kg IV	May not be enough renal func-tion to be effective
Hemodialysis or perito-neal dialysis	Decreased renal func-tion	Removes K^+ in dialysate	—	Risks associ-ated with dialysis
Exchange transfusion	ECG changes or very high K^+ level	Donor blood must be washed and have had most K^+ removed	Double volume	Risks associ-ated with exchange transfusion

*Sodium bicarbonate and calcium salts are incompatible in intravenous solutions.
ECG, electrocardiogram; IV, intravenous; K^+, potassium; PO, oral; PR, rectal.

 HINT: The administration of intravenous glucose, especially in high concentrations, may worsen hypokalemia by stimulating insulin release, which increases cellular uptake of potassium.

Clinical Features

Signs and symptoms: variable and nonspecific.

- **Neuromuscular signs** include weakness, paralysis, tetany, ileus, ureteral aperistalsis, lethargy, confusion, autonomically mediated hypotension, and rhabdomyolysis.

TABLE 32-6	**Drugs Associated with Hypokalemia**

Drugs Associated With Increased Renal Loss

Aminoglycoside toxicity
Amphotericin B
Cisplatin
Penicillins in high doses
Corticosteroids
Diuretics (except for potassium-sparing ones)

Drugs Associated With Increased Cellular Uptake of Potassium

Terbutaline
Epinephrine
Beta-adrenergic agents (e.g., albuterol)
Theophylline toxicity
Barium toxicity
Insulin

- **Cardiovascular signs** may include elevated blood pressure, bradyarrhythmias, and tachyarrhythmias.
- **Renal and metabolic abnormalities** include impaired renal concentrating capacity and polyuria, chronic nephrotoxicity (hypokalemic nephropathy), and impaired insulin secretion (glucose intolerance).

Evaluation

Laboratory Studies

- Serum electrolyte panel; serum calcium, magnesium, and glucose
- Urinalysis, urine potassium, and creatinine (to calculate the transtubular potassium gradient or TTKG).
- ECG changes with severe potassium deficit (<2.5 mEq/L)
  - T-wave flattening, U waves, which give the appearance of a long corrected QT interval (QTc), ST segment depression, and prolonged PR intervals (Figure 32-2)
  - Hypokalemia increases susceptibility to digitalis toxicity
- Other tests (e.g., endocrine or genetic studies) based upon clinical suspicion

Therapy

Potassium deficits frequently occur with other abnormalities (e.g., calcium, magnesium, and chloride depletion) and cannot be completely corrected until the accompanying deficits are repaired.

- **Potassium replacement**
  - Oral route preferred when possible.
  - Oral potassium supplements may cause gastric irritation, vomiting, or may be nonpalatable to a young child.
  - A normal diet usually provides potassium in excess of daily maintenance requirements (2 to 3 mEq/kg). Foods rich in potassium include dried fruits,

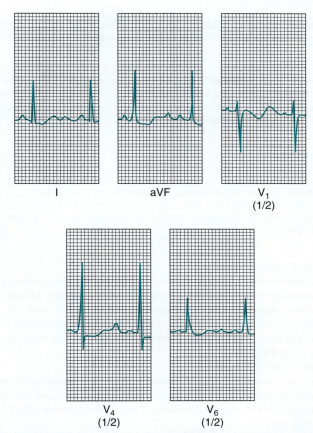

FIGURE 32-2 **Characteristic electrocardiogram (ECG) pattern in a patient with hypo-kalemia.** These tracings are from a 4-year-old with nephrotic syndrome. Note the prominent U waves in all leads with ST segment depression and T wave inversion in leads I, aVF, V$_4$, and V$_6$. (Reprinted with permission from Garson A, Jr. Electrocardiography. In: Garson A, Jr, Bricker JT, Fisher D, et al., eds. *The Science and Practice of Pediatric Cardiology.* 2nd ed. Baltimore, Williams & Wilkins; 1998:772.)

bananas (1.5 mEq/inch), tomatoes, and most other fruits. Prune juice and orange juice provide 16 mEq and 12 mEq of potassium per 8 ounces, respectively.

- Severe or symptomatic hypokalemia: IV potassium, dose not to exceed 0.3 to 0.5 mEq/kg/hour. Because most of the body's potassium is not in the ECF, the serum potassium concentration may not reflect (and does not permit calculation of) the total potassium deficit.
- Ensure intact urine output prior to administration of intravenous potassium. Close monitoring is critical.

> **HINT:** Intravenous potassium at concentrations of ≥40 mEq/L are irritating to small peripheral veins and often result in pain or loss of access site.

> **HINT:** In acute metabolic acidosis, the serum potassium level may be increased owing to extracellular shift while the total body potassium level is diminished. A rule of thumb is that a 0.1 decrease in pH acutely results in an increase in potassium level of 0.7 mEq/L.

Hypercalcemia
Etiology

> **HINT:** Hypercalcemia reduces renal blood flow and, as a result, decreases the GFR; increases sodium, potassium, and magnesium excretion; decreases renal concentrating capacity; and leads to metabolic acidosis.

- Increased calcium absorption
  - Hypervitaminosis D: excess vitamin D administration, increased endogenous vitamin D sensitivity or activity (such as occurs in idiopathic infantile hypercalcemia, sarcoidosis, certain malignancies, and neonatal fat necrosis)
  - High calcium intake—Milk-alkali syndrome, excessive intravenous calcium administration, chronic kidney disease treated with calcium-based phosphate binders and Vitamin D therapy
- Increased bone resorption
  - Hyperparathyroidism, immobilization hypercalcemia, hypophosphatasia, vitamin A intoxication, thyrotoxicosis, skeletal dysplasias, metastatic bone disease, malignancies with associated secretion of parathyroid hormone (PTH)-related peptide (PTHrP)
- **Renal disorders**—Familial hypocalciuric hypercalcemia, thiazide diuretic therapy, and rhabdomyolysis with acute myoglobinuric renal failure
- **Miscellaneous causes**—Lithium therapy, adrenal insufficiency, severe hypophosphatemia, blue diaper syndrome (tryptophan transport defect), theophylline toxicity, and infants with congenital lactase deficiency

Clinical Features

- Variable, more severe at higher serum calcium levels
- Symptoms uncommon at serum levels <12 mg/dL.
- Levels of >16 mg/dL are life threatening and should be treated as an emergency.

> **HINT:** A common mnemonic aid for clinical features of hypercalcemia is "stones, bones, groans, and psychiatric overtones."

- Nephrolithiasis and nephrocalcinosis (stones)
- Myalgias, arthralgias, bone pain, and hypotonia (bones)
- Abdominal pain, nausea, vomiting, constipation, anorexia, xerostomia, and symptoms of pancreatitis (groans)
- Anxiety, depression, fatigue, lethargy, and weakness (psychiatric overtones)
- Other features
  - Renal—Polyuria and polydipsia; decrease in GFR, acute renal insufficiency
  - Cardiovascular—Hypertension, short QT interval, arrhythmia, and heart block

Evaluation
Laboratory Studies
- Total and ionized calcium levels
- Basic metabolic panel; serum phosphorus, alkaline phosphatase, magnesium and serum albumin
- Intact or aminoterminal assay for PTH
- Vitamin D levels (25 OH vitamin D and 1, 25 dihydroxy vitamin D) based on clinical suspicion
- Calcium excretion
  - 24-hour urine collection (normal <4 mg/kg/day)
  - Calcium-to-creatinine ratio from a random sample. (Normal is <0.2 for children >6 years. Normal newborn values are up to 0.86).

Therapy
- **Dehydration** should be corrected, **hydration status** should be closely monitored, and **intravascular volume** should be maintained.
- The underlying cause of the hypercalcemia should be identified and removed.
- Calcium excretion should be maximized via saline diuresis and the use of loop diuretics.
- Other therapies as guided by etiology, symptoms, and severity are as follows:
  - Glucocorticoids
  - Calcitonin (rapid onset, short duration of action)
  - Osteoclast inhibition (slower onset, longer duration of action)
    - Bisphosphonates
    - Gallium nitrate
  - Calcimimetics (Ca-sensing receptor agonists)
  - Dialysis

Hypocalcemia
Etiology
- Binding of circulating calcium (Hyperphosphatemia, alkalosis, citrated blood products, high lactate, pancreatitis)
- Hypovitaminosis D:
  - Dietary ± insufficient sunlight exposure
  - Hepatic disease

TABLE 32-7	**Causes of Hypoparathyroidism**

Decreased Secretion
Genetic
Autosomal dominant
HDR syndrome (hypoparathyroidism, sensorineural deafness, renal dysplasia)
Abnormal processing of preproPTH
Calcium-sensing receptor defect (Autosomal dominant hypocalcemia)
Autosomal recessive
Abnormal processing of preproPTH
Sanjad–Sakati syndrome
Autosomal recessive form of Kenny–Caffey syndrome
Mitochondrial disorders
DiGeorge syndrome – Aplasia/hypoplasia of thyroid gland
Autoimmune
Autoimmune polyglandular syndrome type I
Other
Surgery, infection, and iron overload

End-Organ Resistance
Pseudohypoparathyroidism (types 1 and 2)

- Renal disease
  - Renal failure
  - Vitamin D-dependent rickets
  - Vitamin D resistant rickets
- Hypocalcemia of the newborn
  - Early (within 72 hours of birth)
  - Late (5 to 7 days after birth)
- Hypoparathyroidism/Pseudohypoparathyroidism (Table 32-7)
- Hypomagnesemia (via PTH resistance or decreased secretion in severe cases)
- Medications
  - Those used in treatment of hypercalcemia
  - Those that increase Vitamin D catabolism (i.e., anticonvulsants, isoniazid, theophylline, rifampin)

Hypoalbuminemia results in ↓ total calcium with normal ionized calcium.
Correction factor:

$$Ca = \text{serum } Ca + 0.8 \times (\text{normal albumin} - \text{patient albumin})$$

Clinical Features
- Muscle weakness, fasciculations, or both
- Parasthesia
- Cramping
- Hyperreflexia

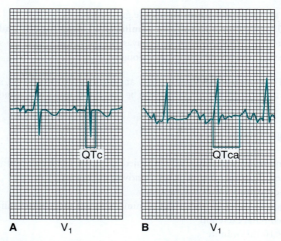

FIGURE 32-3 **(A)** Corrected QT (*QTc*) interval in a healthy newborn. **(B)** Prolonged QTc interval in a patient with hypocalcemia. (Reprinted with permission from Garson A, Jr. Electrocardiography. In: Garson A, Jr, Bricker JT, Fisher D, et al., eds. *The Science and Practice of Pediatric Cardiology.* 2nd ed. Baltimore, Williams & Wilkins; 1998:746.)

- Tetany
  - Chvostek sign (ipsilateral facial muscle spasm with facial nerve stimulation)
  - Trousseau sign (carpopedal spasm with brief ischemia, i.e., blood pressure cuff inflation)
- Seizures
- Psychiatric: Emotional lability, and rarely, confusion, or psychosis
- Cardiovascular
  - Hypotension
  - ECG changes – Prolonged QT interval most common (Figure 32-3)

Evaluation

Laboratory studies include those recommended for evaluation of hypercalcemia. Electrocardiogram should be performed if there is severe hypocalcemia.

Treatment

Based on the symptoms, severity, and etiology.

- **Oral therapy** – Only for correction of **chronic and mildly symptomatic states**.
  - Maintenance need not be precisely known but considered to be 20 to 50 mg/kg/day of elemental calcium.
  - Treatment of hyperphosphatemia – Calcium-based phosphate binders
  - Vitamin D therapy increases absorption of calcium from the gastrointestinal tract and renal reabsorption. Active vitamin D therapy (calcitriol, paricalcitol) is used for secondary hyperparathyroidism associated with chronic renal failure.

Severe symptomatic hypocalcemia (e.g., seizures)
- 10 to 20 mg/kg elemental **calcium administered intravenously and slowly**.
  - Monitor for bradyarrhythmias, extravasation of calcium into the subcutaneous tissues (may cause serious skin sloughs).

> **HINT:** Hypomagnesemia frequently accompanies hypocalcemia, so the magnesium level should always be measured, and if low, should be corrected.

Hypermagnesemia
Etiology
- Excess intake (almost always accompanied by significant renal insufficiency)
  - Magnesium-containing antacids, laxatives, or enemas
  - High-dose intravenous magnesium
  - Newborns–Maternal prepartum administration of magnesium sulfate
- Decreased renal excretion
  - GFR <10 mL/minute
  - Hypothyroidism
  - Familial hypocalciuric hypercalcemia
- Other
  - Lithium
  - Tumor lysis syndrome
  - Diabetic ketoacidosis (DKA)

Clinical Features
Signs and symptoms, including decreased deep tendon reflexes, weakness, confusion, lethargy, and hypotension, relate to adverse effects on neuromuscular transmission and usually appear when the magnesium level exceeds 7 mEq/L.

Evaluation
It is important to assess the GFR and the calcium concentration because hypocalcemia worsens the signs and symptoms of hypermagnesemia.

Therapy
- Identify underlying cause.
- **Continuous heart rate and blood pressure monitoring** are indicated for patients with magnesium levels >5 mEq/L.
- If symptomatic, or if the magnesium level exceeds 7 mEq/L, **intravenous administration of calcium** is indicated to decrease the serum magnesium level temporarily. In patients with severe renal insufficiency, **peritoneal dialysis or hemodialysis** may be required.

Hypomagnesemia
Etiology
- Frequently seen in association with hypocalcemia and hypokalemia
- May also be seen with hypercalcemia (see below)
- Common causes include increased gastrointestinal losses, increased renal excretion, and redistribution (Table 32-8).

TABLE 32-8	Causes of Hypomagnesemia

Increased Gastrointestinal Losses
Small bowel disease or inflammation
Fat malabsorption (including cystic fibrosis)
Laxative abuse
Protein-calorie malnutrition
Gluten sensitivity
Gastroenteritis or chronic diarrhea

Increased Renal Losses
Primary renal tubular magnesium wasting
Gitelman syndrome
Familial hypomagnesemia with hypercalciuria/nephrocalcinosis
Rare mutations (Na-K ATPase, voltage-gated K^+ channel, HNF-1beta)
Postobstructive diuresis
Recovery phase of acute renal failure
Diuretic therapy (thiazides, loop diuretics)
Hypercalcemia
Hypokalemia
Hyperaldosteronism
Drugs (aminoglycosides, amphotericin, cyclosporine)
Hypoparathyroidism or hyperparathyroidism
Renal tubular acidosis
Hyperthyroidism

Redistribution
Refeeding, total parenteral nutrition
Pancreatitis
"Hungry bone" syndrome

 HINT: The association of hypomagnesemia with hypocalcemia and hypokalemia is common but confusing. In some situations, a cause and effect relationship may be in place. For example, hypomagnesemia leads to hypocalcemia as a result of diminished PTH secretion or decreased responsiveness of bone to PTH. Likewise, hypomagnesemia increases renal potassium loss. In other situations, a shared cause (e.g., aminoglycoside toxicity) accounts for the overlap. Attempts to treat one of these deficiencies without recognizing the presence of another will not be successful. It is also important that hypercalcemia can in turn lead to renal loss of magnesium due to competition for transport occurring at the thick ascending limb of the loop of Henle.

Clinical Features

- Difficult to separate from those associated with concomitant electrolyte disturbances.
- Clinical features include weakness, tremors, anorexia, lassitude, and rarely, seizures.

Evaluation

- Laboratory studies: Serum electrolyte panel and serum calcium, phosphorus, alkaline phosphatase, and PTH levels

- ECG
  - Tachycardia (sinus or nodal)
  - Premature beats (supraventricular or ventricular)
  - Changes similar to those seen in hypokalemia (i.e., flat, broad T waves; prolonged PR and QT intervals). Patients with hypomagnesemia also have increased susceptibility to digitalis toxicity
- Urine studies: Fractional excretion of magnesium can help differentiate renal losses versus other causes
  - $FE_{Mg} = U_{Mg} \times P_{Cr}/(P_{Mg} \times 0.7) \times U_{Cr} \times 100$
  - $FE_{Mg} > 2\%$ indicates renal magnesium wasting (assumes normal GFR)

Treatment
- Symptomatic hypomagnesemia
  - **Magnesium sulfate** (25 to 50 mg/kg intravenously via a slow drip or every 4 to 6 hours intramuscularly). Monitor for hypotension.
- Prevention
  - Ensure adequate magnesium in the diet or in parenteral fluids.
  - Normal requirements ~ 4 mg/kg/day (0.3 mEq/kg/day)
  - Note: Oral magnesium supplements can cause diarrhea and should be used with caution in children with renal insufficiency.

Hyperphosphatemia
Etiology
- **Renal failure** (usually associated with a GFR below 50 mL/minute)
- **Increased renal tubular reabsorption (TRP)**
  - Hypoparathyroidism
  - Pseudohypoparathyroidism
  - Hypervitaminosis D
  - Familial tumoral calcinosis (autosomal recessive, increased proximal tubular phosphate transport)
  - Therapy with bisphosphonates
- **Increased phosphate intake**—cow's milk in infants and phosphate-containing enemas
- **Increased endogenous phosphate release**—tumor lysis syndrome and rhabdomyolysis
- **Most hypocalcemic states**

Clinical Features
Hyperphosphatemia is almost always accompanied by hypocalcemia, and signs and symptoms are related to the latter.

> **HINT:** A serious complication of hyperphosphatemia is metastatic or ectopic calcification in vessel walls and tissues. The risk is greatly increased when the calcium X phosphorus product exceeds 70.

Evaluation

- Appropriate laboratory studies include those for the assessment of calcium disorders.
- Assessment of the urine creatinine and phosphate level allows determination of fractional excretion of phosphate ($FEPO_4$): $FEPO_4 = (U_{Phos} \times P_{Cr})/(P_{Phos} \times U_{Cr}) \times 100$.
- The $FEPO_4$ should be between 5 and 20% under normal circumstances. The inverse of this value is called the TRP, and as such is normally $\geq 80\%$. Appropriate variations in these values may occur in states of hyper- or hypophosphatemia if tubular phosphate transport is intact.

Treatment

- **Restrict phosphate intake**
- Oral phosphate binders
  - Calcium carbonate and calcium acetate
  - Sevelamer
  - Lanthanum
  - Aluminum salts should never be used chronically because of the neurotoxicity of aluminum accumulation.
- Phosphate excretion should be maximized by **saline diuresis** if renal function is normal.
- In chronic kidney disease, **peritoneal dialysis or hemodialysis** may be effective.
- Hypocalcemia, if present, should be corrected.

Hypophosphatemia

Etiology

- Redistribution
  - Stimulation of glycolysis (insulin secretion with refeeding syndrome, respiratory alkalosis)
  - Hungry bone syndrome
- Gastrointestinal
  - Decreased absorption (chronic diarrhea, Mg and aluminum antacids that bind intestinal phosphate)
  - Decreased intake (rare)
- Renal losses
  - Hyperparathyroidism
  - Vitamin D deficiency/resistance
  - Primary renal phosphate wasting: X-linked hypophosphatemic rickets, other genetic forms affecting tubular phosphate transport, McCune–Albright syndrome
  - Fanconi syndrome
  - Diuretics with proximal tubule targets (acetazolamide or metolazone)
  - Postrenal transplantation
  - Calcimimetic therapy
  - Acute volume expansion

Clinical Features

Symptoms and signs generally do not occur until the phosphorus level is less than 1.5 mg/dL. Clinical features include muscle weakness, rhabdomyolysis, bone pain, arthralgias, hemolytic anemia, anorexia, nausea, and vomiting.

Evaluation

See evaluation of hyperphosphatemia.

Treatment

- Treat underlying condition.
- Treat **accompanying hypercalcemia**. Often, treatment of the hypercalcemia resolves the hypophosphatemia.
- **Phosphate** administration to increase the serum phosphorus level to 2.0 mg/dL.
  - Given at a rate of 15 to 20 mg/kg/day, either orally or intravenously.
  - Ensure normal renal function prior to treatment.
  - Intravenous phosphate is **contraindicated in the presence of hypercalcemia** because it may lead to the development of metastatic calcifications.

Metabolic Acidosis

Etiology

- Metabolic acidosis may be accompanied by either a normal anion gap (hyperchloremic metabolic acidosis) or a wide anion gap. Table 32-9 summarizes the causes of metabolic acidosis.
- **Renal tubular acidosis (RTA)** is a group of disorders in which hyperchloremic metabolic acidosis occurs because of excess renal tubular loss of bicarbonate, failure to excrete dietary net acid, or both. The many causes of RTA (Table 32-10) can be categorized according to the type: **type 1** (distal or classic)

TABLE 32-9	**Causes of Metabolic Acidosis**

Normal Anion Gap
Gastrointestinal loss of bicarbonate
Diarrhea
Drainage of intestinal fluid (e.g., ileostomy, nasojejunal tube drainage)
Administration of acid
Total parenteral nutrition (e.g., amino acids)
Acute ECF expansion (e.g., following the rapid administration of intravenous fluids)
Renal loss of bicarbonate or failure to secrete net acid
Renal tubular acidosis
Therapy with carbonic anhydrase inhibitors (e.g., acetazolamide)

Wide Anion Gap
Renal failure
Ketoacidosis
Diabetes mellitus
Starvation
Lactic acidosis
Other organic acidosis (e.g., methylmalonic acidemia)
Intoxications (e.g., methanol, salicylates, ethylene glycol)

TABLE 32-10 **Selected Causes of Renal Tubular Acidosis**

Type 1 (Distal or Classic) RTA
Idiopathic
Sporadic
Inherited (autosomal dominant or recessive)
Associated with renal disease
Obstructive nephropathy
Reflux nephropathy
Postrenal transplant
Associated with disorders causing nephrocalcinosis
Medullary sponge kidney
Hyperparathyroidism
Hypervitaminosis D
Associated with systemic disease
Sickle cell disease
Marfan syndrome
Ehlers–Danlos syndrome
Hereditary elliptocytosis
Wilson disease
Associated with autoimmune disorders
SLE
Sjögren syndrome
Polyarteritis nodosa
Hypergammaglobulinemia
Associated with drug toxicity
Amphotericin B
Lithium

Type 2 (Proximal) RTA
Idiopathic or isolated
Sporadic
Inherited (autosomal dominant)
Associated with Fanconi syndrome*
Associated with systemic disease
Cystinosis
Lowe (oculocerebrorenal) syndrome
Galactosemia
Glycogen storage disease
Hereditary fructose intolerance
Tyrosinemia
SLE and other autoimmune disorders
Associated with toxins
Drugs (e.g., aminoglycosides, chemotherapeutic agents)
Heavy metals
Associated with renal disorders
Nephrotic syndrome
Medullary cystic disease
Renal venous thrombosis
Renal transplant rejection
Associated with carbonic anhydrase deficiency
Congenital (sporadic or familial)
Drug-induced (acetazolamide)

(continued)

TABLE 32-10 Selected Causes of Renal Tubular Acidosis (*Cont.*)

Type 4 (Hyperkalemic) RTA
Associated with renal disease
Diabetic nephropathy
Obstructive nephropathy
Hyporeninemic hypoaldosteronism[†]
Associated with aldosterone deficiency
Addison disease
Chronic adrenal suppression
Congenital adrenal hyperplasia (21-hydroxylase defect)
Associated with aldosterone resistance
Pseudohypoaldosteronism
Transient resistance (in newborns)
Associated with drugs
Spironolactone
Triamterene
Amiloride
Chloride shunt (excess reabsorption of chloride)

*Fanconi syndrome is characterized by generalized proximal tubular dysfunction.
[†]Type 4 RTA may be found with any chronic tubulointerstitial nephritis.
RTA, renal tubular acidosis; SLE, systemic lupus erythematosus.

RTA, **type 2** (proximal) RTA, or **type 4** (hyperkalemic) RTA. Table 32-11 summarizes the characteristics of each of these types of RTA.

Clinical Features
- Nonspecific and variable.
- Occasionally overshadowed by the illness or disorder leading to the acidosis.

TABLE 32-11 Characteristics of Renal Tubular Acidosis

	Type 1	Type 2	Type 4
Renal function?	Normal	Normal	Normal or decreased
Failure to thrive?	Yes	Yes	Yes
Polyuria or polydipsia?	Yes	Yes	No
Potassium level?	Normal or low	Normal or low	Elevated
Bicarbonate leak?	Usually	Significant	Small
Urine maximally acid?	No (pH > 6)	Yes (below serum threshold)	Yes
Nephrocalcinosis or nephrolithiasis?	Yes	No	No
Fanconi syndrome?	No	Often	No
Osteomalacia or rickets?	Rarely	If Fanconi syndrome is present	No

- Isolated metabolic acidosis (e.g., RTA) occasionally associated with anorexia and vomiting. Hyperventilation, an almost immediate compensatory response to metabolic acidosis, is often, but not always apparent.
- Chronic acidosis (e.g., RTA) may lead to growth failure due to use of skeleton as a buffer.

Evaluation

The serum bicarbonate concentration is virtually equivalent to the total carbon dioxide value reported with serum electrolytes. The first step in the evaluation of a low bicarbonate level is to **calculate the anion gap:**

$$\text{Anion gap} = (Na^+) - [(Cl^-) + (HCO_3^-)]$$

The normal gap is 12, with a range of 8 to 16.

- If **normal anion gap,** a history of diarrhea or other gastrointestinal losses should be sought. If there is none, an accurate (meter) pH determination using a freshly voided urine sample transported in an airtight container should be obtained, and evaluation for RTA should be undertaken.
- If **anion gap is above 16,** the source of the unexplained anion should be sought. For example, the possibility of lactic acidosis or DKA must be excluded. Although the history is helpful, several laboratory studies may be useful as well. A blood gas analysis should be obtained to assess the pH and arterial carbon dioxide tension ($PaCO_2$) to determine the degree of compensation or the presence of a mixed acid–base disturbance. A blood ammonia level and evaluation of urine for organic acids may be helpful.

> **HINT:** Not all low serum bicarbonate levels indicate metabolic acidosis. Fingerstick carbon dioxide levels are often spuriously low because of prolonged exposure of the blood to air. Decreased bicarbonate concentrations may occur as compensation for chronic respiratory alkalosis.

> **HINT:** Metabolic acidosis may occur with a normal bicarbonate value in children with mixed metabolic acid–base disturbances. For example, an infant with bronchopulmonary dysplasia who is receiving furosemide chronically (metabolic alkalosis) may develop severe diarrhea (metabolic acidosis) and have a normal bicarbonate concentration. Mixed disturbances involving metabolic acidosis may be detected by the "delta-delta," i.e., the difference between the delta anion gap (observed minus normal) and the delta of the serum bicarbonate. Delta-deltas more than and less than zero usually indicate mixed disorders.

> **HINT:** A change in the bicarbonate concentration of 10 mmol/L is expected to lead to a change in pH of 0.15 in the same direction.

Therapy

- Correct/remove the cause (e.g., insulin administration in a patient with DKA). Because the lungs permit the removal of volatile acid as carbon dioxide, it is important to ensure **adequate ventilation**.
- Alkali therapy is not always indicated in the treatment of acute acidosis.
- In chronic acidosis, **alkali therapy** may help prevent growth failure.
- **Bicarbonate therapy** – start at 2 mEq/kg/day and increase as needed.
- In patients with renal bicarbonate loss, up to 20 mEq/kg per day of bicarbonate may be required. Commonly used oral alkalinizing agents in children include the following:
  - **Polycitra syrup** (provides 2 mEq/mL of bicarbonate, 1 mEq/mL of sodium, and 1 mEq/mL of potassium)
  - **Bicitra** (1 mEq/mL of bicarbonate and 1 mEq/mL of sodium)
  - **Sodium bicarbonate tablets,** which supply 650 mg of bicarbonate (8 mEq/tablet)

Metabolic Alkalosis

Etiology

Metabolic alkalosis is often divided into two categories: **chloride sensitive or chloride resistant** (Table 32-12). Chloride-sensitive metabolic alkalosis is associated with a decreased ECF volume, and the urinary chloride level is <10 mEq/L. Chloride-resistant metabolic alkalosis is associated with a urinary chloride level >20 mEq/L.

Clinical Features

As with metabolic acidosis, signs and symptoms are generally those of the underlying disorder. Sudden, **severe** metabolic alkalosis may result in **diminished ionized calcium** levels, leading to hypocalcemic cramps or tetany.

TABLE 32-12	Causes of Metabolic Alkalosis

Chloride Sensitive
Vomiting or nasogastric suction
Chronic diuretic therapy
Chloride-deficient diet
Cystic fibrosis (increased skin loss of chloride)
Congenital chloride diarrhea (autosomal recessive)

Chloride Resistant
Alkali administration (e.g., antacid therapy)
Acute diuretic therapy
Hypokalemic state
Mineralocorticoid excess
Compensation for respiratory acidosis
Bartter syndrome
Liddle syndrome

Evaluation

- The physical examination should focus on assessment of the ECF volume status.
- Laboratory studies
  - Basic metabolic panel
  - Urine electrolyte levels, including chloride
  - In some children, a sweat chloride determination is indicated

> **HINT:** There may be mixed metabolic acidosis and alkalosis occurring together, and the measured bicarbonate concentration may be normal.

> **HINT:** Metabolic alkalosis and frank alkalemia may occur if long-standing respiratory acidosis is corrected suddenly (e.g., with mechanical ventilation). This condition is called "posthypercapnic alkalosis."

Treatment

- Correct volume contraction with normal saline.
- If present, **hypokalemia** should be corrected.
- Diuretic therapy should be decreased or discontinued.
- If applicable, stop alkali therapy.

Suggested Readings

Adrogue HJ, Modios NE. Hypernatremia. *New Engl J Med.* 2000;342(20):1493–1499.

Chon JC, Scheinmann JI, Roth KS. Renal tubular acidosis. *Pediatr Rev.* 2001;22(8):277–286.

Evans KJ, Greenberg A. Hyperkalemia: a review. *J Intensive Care Med.* 2005;20(5):272–290.

Kraut JA, Madias NE. Serum anion gap: its uses and limitations in clinical medicine. *Clin J Am Soc Nephrol.* 2007;2(1):162–174.

Marks KH, Kilav R, Naveh-Many T, et al. Calcium, phosphate, vitamin D, and the parathyroid. *Pediatr Nephrol.* 1996;10(3):364–367.

Moritz ML, Ayus JC. Preventing neurological complications from dysnatremias in children. *Pediatr Nephrol.* 2005;20(12):1687–1700.

Ruth JL, Wassner SJ. Body composition: salt and water. *Pediatr Rev.* 2006;27(5):181–187.

Schwaderer AL, Schwartz GJ. Back to basics: acidosis and alkalosis. *Pediatr Rev.* 2004;25(10):350–357.

CHAPTER **33**

Fran Balamuth
Elizabeth R. Alpern

Fever

INTRODUCTION

Fever is the abnormal elevation of body temperature. It is a **nonspecific sign** of disease. The significance of fever lies in its indication of disease processes. Fever is defined as a core body temperature ≥38.0°C (100.4°F). However, the clinically relevant defined cutoff point of an abnormally elevated temperature is based on a particular child's risk for infection. Fever in neonates or in immunocompromised patients is defined as ≥38.0°C (100.4°F) and in older children as ≥38.5°C (101°F) to 39.0°C (102°F).

Body temperature is usually measured by **rectal thermometry** in infants and young children and by **sublingual thermometry** in older children and adolescents. Because temperature may vary in different areas of the body, tympanic, temporal artery, and pacifier thermometers may not correlate with rectal measurements in young children.

Because fever is an indication of disease, the most important management and therapeutic measures are to determine the underlying cause of the fever (e.g., infection, inflammation, neoplasm). When the underlying disease is treated appropriately, the fever can be managed with antipyretics as needed to make the child comfortable.

 DIFFERENTIAL DIAGNOSIS LIST

Infectious Causes
Systemic
Sepsis
Occult bacteremia
Viral syndrome
Tick-borne infections (Lyme disease, Rocky Mountain spotted fever)

CNS
Meningitis
Encephalitis

Respiratory Tract
Upper respiratory tract infection
Pharyngitis/tonsillitis
Retropharyngeal abscess
Otitis media
Croup
Sinusitis
Pneumonia
Bronchiolitis

Abdominal/Pelvic
Gastroenteritis
Appendicitis

Genitourinary
Urinary tract disease
Pelvic inflammatory disease
Tubo-ovarian abscess

Musculoskeletal
Osteomyelitis
Septic arthritis

Cutaneous
Cellulitis
Abscess

Miscellaneous
Adenitis
Orbital cellulitis
Fever of unknown origin

Toxicologic Causes
Salicylates
Cocaine
Amphetamine
Anticholinergics
Malignant hyperthermia

Neoplastic Causes
Leukemia
Lymphoma

Inflammatory Causes
Acute rheumatic fever
Systemic lupus erythematosus
Juvenile rheumatoid arthritis
Kawasaki disease
Inflammatory bowel disease
Serum sickness
Drug and immunization
reactions

Miscellaneous Causes
Heat stroke
Thyrotoxicosis
Dehydration
Prolonged seizures
Factitious

EVALUATION OF COMMON PRESENTATIONS
Infants Less Than 2 Months of Age
Well-appearing infants (0 to 60 days of age) with a fever (≥38.0°C [100.4°F]) but without an identifiable source of infection are at risk for **occult serious bacterial infections**. These young infants may have only vague or nonspecific signs and symptoms of illness that do not indicate the severity of potential infection.

History
- High risk—prematurity, perinatal complication, pre- and perinatal maternal infection, immunocompromised state (sickle cell disease, HIV), exposure to recent antibiotics, steroids, surgery
- Low risk—full-term gestation, uncomplicated prenatal course

Physical Examination
Physical examination should concentrate on identifying infections that are more common in neonates, such as meningitis, herpes simplex virus encephalitis, omphalitis, pneumonia, bronchiolitis and pyelonephritis.

Screening Tests
Table 33-1 presents the low-risk criteria for three published screening protocols.

TABLE 33-1	Low-Risk Screening Criteria		
	Philadelphia Protocol	**Boston Protocol**	**Rochester Criteria**
History/physical examination	Normal	Normal	Normal
WBC count	5,000–15,000/mm³	<20,000/mm³	5,000–15,000/mm³
Differential	Band-to-neutrophil ratio <0.2		Absolute band count ≤1,500/mm³
Urinalysis	<10 WBC/hpf	<10 WBC/hpf	<10 WBC/hpf
CSF	<8 WBC/hpf	<10 WBC/hpf	
CXR	Normal	Normal	
Stool	If symptoms: negative blood and few WBC on smear		If symptoms: <5 WBC/hpf
Social	Readily available transportation and phone	Readily available transportation and phone	Readily available transportation and phone
Negative predictive value (for SBI) of screen	100%	94.6%	98.9%
Treatment option if low risk	Home without antibiotics and follow-up in 24 hr	Home with Ceftriaxone IM and follow-up in 24 hr	Home without antibiotics and follow-up in 24 hr

CSF, cerebrospinal fluid; CXR, chest X-ray; hpf, high-power field; IM, intramuscular; SBI, serious bacterial infection; WBC, white blood cell.

Management

The management of febrile infants is determined by age, history, and screening tests. Figure 33-1 presents the management options.

Children from 2 to 24 Months of Age

Occult bacteremia is the presence of pathogenic bacteria in the blood of a well-appearing febrile child (usually defined as ≥39.0°C [102°F]) who lacks a focal bacterial source of infection. The current risk of occult bacteremia in an immunized child is less than 1%. This risk increases with increasing temperature or a white blood cell (WBC) count. Occult bacteremia carries a risk of **progression to focal infection, meningitis, or sepsis**. However, in a population immunized with the *Haemophilus influenzae* B vaccine and the conjugate pneumococcal vaccine, the prevalence of occult bacteremia has become so low that routine screening with blood culture for this condition in a well appearing child is no longer recommended. In this population, the most common bacterial isolate causing

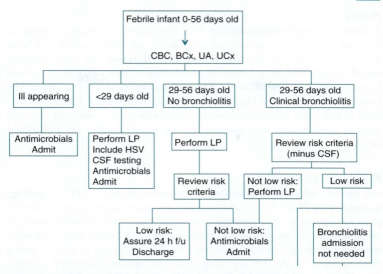

FIGURE 33-1   Management of febrile infants less than 2 months of age. BCx, blood culture; CBC, complete blood cell count; CSF, cerebrospinal fluid; LP, lumbar puncture; UA, urinalysis; UCx, urine culture; HSV, herpes simplex virus; f/u, follow-up.

occult bacteremia is still *Streptococcus pneumoniae,* which usually resolves spontaneously.

Occult urinary tract infections (UTIs) occur frequently in the 2 to 24 month age group. Risk factors for UTI in this age group in girls include temperature >39.0°C [102°F]), non-African American race, age <1 year, and lack of other focal source of infection and fever ≥2 days. It is recommended to consider screening female patients with at least two risk factors. UTI should also be considered in boys, particularly if they are uncircumcised and/or less than 6 months old. See Table 33-2 for risk factors.

TABLE 33-2	Risk Factors for Urinary Tract Infections	
Girls	**Boys**
Temperature ≥39°C (102°F)	Age ≤6 mo
Fever ≥2 d	Uncircumcised penis
Non African American	Lack of other focal source of infection
Age ≤1 yr	
Lack of other focal source of infection	

History

An **immunocompromised state** (e.g., long-term steroid use, oncologic processes, acquired or inborn immunodeficiencies, sickle cell anemia, congenital heart disease) or the presence of an **indwelling medical device** (e.g., ventriculoperitoneal shunts, indwelling catheters) puts a child at increased risk of invasive bacterial infection. The child's **immunization history** is also important. The pneumococcal conjugate vaccine has significantly decreased the risk of bacteremia and other invasive pneumococcal diseases. Prior antibiotic use may mask presenting signs or symptoms of focal bacterial infections and should be noted.

Physical Examination

Any sign of focal **bacterial infection** (e.g., pneumonia, abscess, UTI) or **pathognomonic viral illness** (e.g., varicella, stomatitis) guides diagnosis and treatment plans appropriate for that particular infection. Otitis media is very common in young children and may result from bacterial, viral, or mixed etiology. Viral respiratory infections and gastroenteritis are also common causes of fever in young children. However, the well-appearing child without identifiable focal infection should be evaluated for occult infections such as occult UTI or occult pneumonia. Occult bacteremia should be considered, although in the current vaccination climate, this condition is becoming increasingly rare.

Screening Tests

Blood culture is the gold standard for diagnosing occult bacteremia. However, because of the low incidence of occult bacteremia, this screening test has significant limitations, and broad screening is not currently recommended. Nevertheless, if there is heightened clinical concern for occult bacteremia, screening can be appropriate. In these circumstances, some authorities advocate the WBC count for use as a risk stratification measure when considering expectant antibiotic therapy for the child at risk for occult bacteremia.

Chest radiographs are indicated in children with significant respiratory symptoms or persistent tachypnea.

Urinalysis and culture are helpful for those children with dysuria, foul-smelling urine, prior history of UTI, urinary tract abnormality, or other risk factors for occult UTIs. See Table 33-2 for risk factors associated with occult UTIs in young children.

Management

Patients should be treated with antimicrobial therapy only if a focal of bacterial infection is identified. Antipyretics may be used for comfort. Supportive care including good oral hydration, pain control as needed, and nasal saline/suction or treatment of respiratory symptoms may be helpful. **Close medical follow up in all children with fever is imperative.**

Suggested Readings

Alpern ER, Alessandrini EA, Bell LM, et al. Occult bacteremia from a pediatric emergency department: current prevalence, time to detection, and outcome. *Pediatrics.* 2000;106:505–511.

Alpern ER, Henretig FM. Fever. In: GR Fleisher, S Ludwig, eds. *Textbook of Pediatric Emergency Medicine.* 6th ed. Philadelphia: Lippincott Williams and Wilkins; 2010;266–275.

Bulloch B, Craig WR, Klassen TP. The use of antibiotics to prevent serious sequelae in children at risk for occult bacteremia: a meta-analysis. *Acad Emerg Med.* 1997;4:679–683.

Carstairs K, Tasnen D, Johnson AS, et al. Pneumococcal bacteremia in febrile infants presenting to the emergency department before and after the introduction of the heptavalent pneumococcal vaccine. *Ann Emerg Med.* 2007;49:772–777.

Gorelick MH, Shaw KN. Clinical decision rule to identify febrile young girls at risk for urinary tract infection. *Arch Pediatr Adolesc Med.* 2000;154:386–390.

Jaskiewicz JA, McCarthy CA, Richardson AC, et al. Febrile infants at low risk for serious bacterial infection—an appraisal of the Rochester criteria and implications for management. *Pediatrics.* 1994;94:390–396.

Joffe MD, Alpern ER. Occult pneumococcal bacteremia: a review. *Pediatr Emerg Care.* 2010; 26(6):448–454.

Kaplan SL, Mason EO Jr, Wald ER, et al. Decrease of invasive pneumococcal infections in children among 8 children's hospitals in the United States after the introduction of the 7-valent pneumococcal conjugate vaccine. *Pediatrics.* 2004;113:443–449.

Lee GM, Harper MB. Risk of bacteremia for febrile young children in the post-*Haemophilus influenzae* type B era. *Arch Pediatr Adolesc Med.* 1998;152(5):624–628.

Rothrock SG, Harper MB, Green SM, et al. Do oral antibiotics prevent meningitis and serious bacterial infections in children with *Streptococcus pneumoniae* occult bacteremia? A meta-analysis. *Pediatrics.* 1997;99(3):438–444.

Shaikh N, Morone NE, Lopez J, et al. Does this child have a urinary tract infection? *JAMA.* 2007;298(24):2895–2904.

Shaw KN, Gorelick MH. Urinary tract infection in the pediatric patient. *Pediatr Clin North Am.* 1999;46(6):1111–1124.

Whitney CG, Farley MM, Hadler J, et al. Decline in invasive pneumococcal disease after the introduction of protein-polysaccharide conjugate vaccine. *N Engl J Med.* 2003;348:1737–1746.

Wilkinson M, Bulloch B, Smith M. Prevalence of occult bacteremia in children aged 3–36 months presenting to the emergency department with fever in the postpneumococcal conjugate vaccine era. *Acad Emerg Med.* 2009;16:220–225.

Gastrointestinal Bleeding, Lower

INTRODUCTION

The presence of **blood in the gastrointestinal tract is always abnormal**. Blood in the stool can occur in several forms: **hematochezia** (bright red blood on the stool), **"currant-jelly" stools** (thickened brick-red blood on the stool), **melena** (dark or black stools), or **occult bleeding** (normal-appearing stools that test positive by Hemoccult or guaiac testing).

Blood acts as a cathartic that decreases intestinal transit time. Therefore, hematochezia usually signifies colonic disease (i.e., bleeding from a site between the distal colon and the terminal ileum), but it may be the result of profuse proximal gastrointestinal tract bleeding. Melena usually signifies profuse upper intestinal bleeding (above the ligament of Treitz), whereas currant-jelly stools commonly occur when there is shedding of the intestinal mucosa as a result of an active Meckel diverticulum or intussusception. Normal-appearing stools that test positive for blood suggest slow gastrointestinal tract bleeding. Table 34-1 lists causes of bloody stools by site.

> **HINT:** Rapid upper gastrointestinal tract bleeding should always be considered in any child with first-time bloody stools, and a nasogastric tube should be passed for gastric lavage.

 DIFFERENTIAL DIAGNOSIS LIST

The following are common causes of hematochezia and melena:

Infectious Causes
Bacterial Infection
Salmonella
Shigella
Campylobacter
Yersinia
Enterohemorrhagic *Escherichia coli*
Aeromonas

Plesiomonas
Clostridium difficile

Parasitic Infection
Entamoeba histolytica
Balantidium coli
Necator americanus (hookworm)
Strongyloides stercoralis
Ascaris lumbricoides

TABLE 34-1	Causes of Bloody Stools by Site
Site	**Cause**
Nasopharynx	Epistaxis, gum disease, oral or nasal trauma, tonsillectomy, adenoidectomy
Esophagus	Esophageal stricture, esophagitis, ulcer, varices, eosinophilic enteritis, graft-versus-host disease (GVHD)
Stomach	Gastritis, ulcer, foreign body, vascular anomaly, tumor, duplication, polyp, infection
Duodenum	Ulcer, celiac disease, malrotation, vascular anomaly, post-viral enteritis, parasitic infection
Small bowel	Inflammatory bowel disease, celiac disease, volvulus, malrotation, necrotizing enterocolitis, infection, Henoch-Schönlein purpura, duplication, Meckel diverticulum, vascular anomaly, tumor, eosinophilic enteritis
Colon	Polyp, inflammatory bowel disease, infection, Hirschsprung disease, trauma, sexual abuse, hemorrhoid, tumor, hemolytic uremic syndrome, Henoch-Schönlein purpura, milk-protein or soy-protein allergy, rectal varices, intussusception, volvulus, fissure, solitary rectal ulcer, foreign body, vascular anomaly, GVHD

Viral Infection
Adenovirus
Rotavirus
Cytomegalovirus
HIV

Neoplastic Causes
Leiomyoma
Lymphoma
Adenocarcinoma
Carcinoid

Traumatic Causes
Anal fissure
Foreign body
Sexual abuse

Congenital or Vascular Causes
Meckel diverticulum
Enteric duplication
Arteriovenous malformation (AVM)
Hemangioma
Hemorrhoids
Rectal varices
Esophageal varices (rapid flow)
Hirschsprung enterocolitis

Inflammatory Causes
Juvenile polyps
Polyposis syndromes
Inflammatory bowel disease
Lymphonodular hyperplasia
Necrotizing enterocolitis
Milk- or soy-protein allergy
Eosinophilic gastroenteritis
Graft-versus-host disease
Vasculitis (systemic lupus erythematosus)

Miscellaneous Causes
Rapid upper gastrointestinal bleeding
Intussusception
Volvulus
Solitary rectal ulcer
Coagulopathy
Thrombocytopenia
Anticoagulant drug therapy
Henoch-Schönlein purpura
Hemolytic uremic syndrome

TABLE 34-2	Foods and Drugs Mimicking Blood in the Stool

False Hematochezia	False Melena	False Heme-Positive Stools
Foods that contain red dye	Spinach	Red meat
Juice	Blueberries	Cherries
Candy	Licorice	Tomato skin
Kool-Aid	Purple grapes	Iron supplements
Jell-O	Chocolate	
Tomatoes	Grape juice	
Beets	Bismuth subsalicylate	
Cranberries	Iron supplements	
Cefdinir		

HINT: Certain foods, drugs, and occurrences (e.g., menstrual bleeding, hematuria, swallowed maternal blood) can mimic blood in the stool and must be ruled out (Table 34-2).

DIFFERENTIAL DIAGNOSIS DISCUSSION

HINT: Lower gastrointestinal tract bleeding in children is most often caused by constipation or infection. Bacterial infections often present with acute abdominal pain, fever, and bloody diarrhea.

C. Difficile Colitis (Pseudomembranous Colitis, Antibiotic-Induced Colitis)
Etiology

The toxins produced by *C. difficile* have **cytotoxic effects** on the colonic mucosa. Although *C. difficile* colitis is usually associated with an imbalance of the gastrointestinal flora **following the administration of broad-spectrum antibiotics** (e.g., clindamycin, amoxicillin, cephalosporin), it can develop in patients with **underlying intestinal disorders** (e.g., inflammatory bowel disease) and those who have undergone **recent abdominal surgery, institutionalized patients** (as a result of cross-infection), and, sporadically, in otherwise healthy patients. **Although *C. difficile* can also cause disease in young infants, this age group can have *C. difficile* carriage in the stool without symptoms. After 2 years of age, *C. difficile* toxin-positive stools are pathologic.**

HINT: Antibiotic-induced colitis commonly occurs within 2 weeks of introducing the drug.

Clinical Features

C. difficile is associated with a **wide variety of clinical symptoms**. Patients may be **asymptomatic,** or they may experience **frequent, painful, bloody diarrhea, a sign of severe, life-threatening colitis**. Typically, children present with abdominal pain and frequent bloody, mucus-streaked, foul-smelling, watery stools. Some patients may be **dehydrated**.

Evaluation

Fresh stool specimens (transported on ice or frozen) should be collected and evaluated for the presence of *C. difficile* toxins A and B. In patients with persistent bloody diarrhea and a negative microbiologic evaluation, **colonoscopy** should be performed. Colonoscopy often reveals the classic mucosal pseudomembrane formation (raised yellow plaques).

Treatment

Treatment includes **discontinuation of the inciting antibiotic** and therapy with **oral metronidazole** (see Chapter 27, "Diarrhea, Acute"). Typically, oral metronidazole is the first-line therapy, and can be used for a second course if the symptoms recur. Vancomycin is an alternative antibiotic that is used when patients do not respond to metronidazole. Use of vancomycin as first-line therapy is discouraged because there is potential for creating vancomycin-resistant organisms. Symptoms usually resolve within 3 to 5 days. Recurrent episodes may occur following cessation of therapy; in this situation, repeat treatment and further evaluation for other underlying systemic disorders (e.g., inflammatory bowel disease) are indicated. Good hand-washing with water and soap should be encouraged because the *C. difficile* spores are resistant to regular alcoholic hand rubs. Dehydrated patients require **intravenous fluids** and the short-term introduction of clear liquids.

Meckel Diverticulum

Etiology

Meckel diverticulum is rare overall, but it is the **most common** of all **congenital gastrointestinal anomalies** occurring in 1% to 3% of all infants. The diverticulum is derived from a congenital remnant of the embryonic yolk sac that originates from the antimesenteric border of the intestine. This abnormality is typically located within 2 ft (60 cm) of the ileocecal valve. The diverticulum commonly contains ectopic gastric tissue, which can cause **peptic ulceration** (manifested as painless bright red or currant-jelly rectal bleeding).

 HINT: Enteric duplications (intestinal cysts) originate from the mesenteric border of the bowel and, like Meckel diverticulum, can also contain ectopic gastric tissue and manifest with hematochezia or currant-jelly bleeding.

Clinical Features

Intermittent, painless rectal bleeding in the first decade of life (average 2.5 years) is the most common presentation. A small percentage of patients may present with massive life-threatening rectal bleeding.

Less commonly, bowel obstruction can lead to abdominal pain and bilious vomiting. This is because the diverticulum acts as a lead point to intussusceptions, or internal herniation.

Evaluation

The diagnosis is made either by a **Meckel scan,** a specific nuclear medicine test that uses a radioisotope (technetium-99m pertechnetate) to identify the ectopic gastric mucosa, or by a **nonspecific tagged red blood cell scan** that identifies sites of rapid gastrointestinal bleeding. Routine abdominal radiographs and contrast studies are almost never useful for making the diagnosis of a Meckel diverticulum. Typically, giving H_2 blocker half hour prior to the Meckel scan will enhance radioisotope retention and increase the sensitivity to 85% and specificity to 95%.

Treatment

Surgical excision is performed in all cases of documented Meckel diverticulum.

Colonic Polyps

Etiology

Most juvenile polyps are **inflammatory** in origin. **Polyposis syndromes,** which may involve a few polyps or hundreds of polyps, are typically **genetic** in origin and include inflammatory, hamartomatous, and adenomatous changes. The presence of **five or more polyps** usually carries an **increased risk of cancer**.

Clinical Features

Painless hematochezia in a child aged between 2 and 10 years is the typical presentation. Other common symptoms include **tenesmus, mucus-streaked stools, and rectal (or polyp) prolapse** through the rectum. Rarely, intussusception occurs secondary to a polyp acting as a lead point. Juvenile polyps are usually palpable on rectal examination. As many as 30% of children may develop an **iron-deficiency anemia**.

Evaluation

In the past, barium enemas were used to diagnose colonic polyps. However, there was a high false-negative rate due to stool retention. The present treatment of choice is polypectomy; **colonoscopy** is now the preferred diagnostic tool. In addition to allowing visualization of the entire colon (thus identifying the exact cause and all possible polyps), colonoscopy allows the endoscopist to treat the problem by performing a polypectomy.

Treatment

In the past, conservative therapy consisted of observation with the hope that the polyp would auto-amputate. However, currently, **colonoscopy with polypectomy** is recommended to eliminate the source of bleeding, to identify the presence of other polyps, and to identify the type of polyp so that future management of the patient can be determined. Patients with suspected polyposis syndromes should undergo genetic evaluation to determine cancer risk and recommendations for screening of family members.

Inflammatory Bowel Disease
Etiology
Inflammatory bowel disease is an idiopathic, autoimmune, multifactorial inflammatory condition of the alimentary tract.

Crohn disease may occur in both the upper and the lower gastrointestinal tract and results in chronic intestinal inflammation associated with severe mucosal damage, **transmural wall thickening,** serosal induration, **granuloma formation,** fistula and abscess formation, intestinal strictures, and perforation. The terminal ileum is the most common site of involvement, although the disease may "skip" to noncontiguous areas.

Ulcerative colitis is confined to the colon and rectum and typically causes severe mucosal destruction **without transmural involvement**. Unlike Crohn disease, ulcerative colitis is continuous along the lower gastrointestinal tract, although the rectum may be spared.

 HINT: Toxic megacolon, which presents with fever, ill appearance along with diarrhea, abdominal pain, rectal bleeding, and tenesmus, is a potential complication of ulcerative colitis. This is a true surgical emergency and should be ruled out promptly.

Clinical Features
Children with inflammatory bowel disease usually present with **fever, bloody diarrhea, weight loss, and crampy abdominal pain**. Associated systemic abnormalities in inflammatory bowel disease include growth failure, arthralgias, arthritis, skin lesions (pyoderma gangrenosum, erythema nodosum), perianal disease (rectal abscess, skin tags, or fistula formation), ophthalmologic abnormalities (episcleritis and uveitis), mouth sores, and hepatobiliary disease. Many children with Crohn disease develop an **iron-deficiency anemia** and a **secondary lactase deficiency**.

 HINT: Profuse rectal bleeding, hypogastric pain, and tenesmus usually suggest ulcerative colitis, whereas right lower quadrant pain, weight loss, failure to thrive, and perianal disease typify Crohn disease.

Evaluation
The **physical examination** may reveal abdominal tenderness that is usually focal in the lower quadrants and signs of systemic involvement (e.g., mouth sores, joint involvement, erythema nodosum, pyoderma gangrenosum, perianal disease).

Laboratory studies such as a complete blood count, erythrocyte sedimentation rate, chemistry panel, and C-reactive protein are useful for determining the biochemical abnormalities associated with inflammatory bowel disease. Patients with inflammatory bowel disease often have an elevated erythrocyte sedimentation rate and C-reactive protein, hypoalbuminemia, anemia, and an elevated white blood cell count.

Colonoscopy with biopsy is the test of choice for diagnosing ulcerative colitis and Crohn disease. The diagnosis may be made by visual inspection of the intestinal mucosa (aphthous ulcers and mucosal damage) or by biopsy (granulomas, crypt abscesses, and mucosal inflammation). Upper endoscopy should also be performed to assess for upper tract disease. Video capsule endoscopy can be a useful method to visualize small-bowel lesions in Crohn disease.

Upper gastrointestinal small-bowel follow-through contrast studies are useful for assessing small-bowel (terminal ileal) disease. Magnetic resonance imaging enterography also provides high definition studies to localize sites of involvement.

Treatment

The prognosis depends on aggressive treatment of exacerbations, but aggressive intervention with nutritional support is equally important.

Corticosteroids are the first-line therapy for patients with moderate to severe disease. The recommended dosage (1 to 2 mg/kg/day, with a maximum of 40 mg) is tapered over 4 to 8 weeks, depending on the clinical response.

Immunosuppressive agents (e.g., 6-mercaptopurine, azathioprine, methotrexate) are used in children who have an increased risk for complications from steroid treatment, who require prolonged steroid use, or who are refractory to other treatment regimens. They are also used as maintenance medications after a steroid course. New, more effective medications emerging are the biologic treatments like Remicade, Humira, and Cimzia, which are given as IV infusions or subcutaneous injections.

Oral salicylate derivatives, which help heal the intestinal mucosa, are a mainstay of treatment in patients with mild disease. In the past, sulfasalazine (50 to 100 mg/kg/day) was used for patients with mild to moderate exacerbations. 5-Aminosalicylic acid (5-ASA), the active component, is minimally absorbed and thus acts directly on the mucosa as an anti-inflammatory agent. Recently, mesalamine, which does not require coliform bacteria to metabolize itself to 5-aminosalicylic acid, has been used. The dose is 50 to 100 mg/kg/day.

Antibiotics are effective for patients with perianal disease and mucosal inflammation. Metronidazole, used when there is evidence of bacterial overgrowth, fistulae, or perianal disease, has been effective against anaerobes but also has anti-inflammatory properties.

Surgical intervention, such as resection with colectomy and eventual endorectal pull-through, is useful in patients with ulcerative colitis. Surgery should be avoided, however, in children with Crohn disease unless abscess, fistula, toxic megacolon, perforation, acute obstruction, or uncontrolled bleeding exist.

Nutritional support is paramount to achieve optimal growth. In some cases, enteral nutrition replacing the majority of the patient's calories may induce remission in Crohn's patients. Special issues such as deficiencies in trace elements (e.g., zinc, magnesium, and calcium), protein-losing enteropathy (PLE), and fat malabsorption resulting in vitamin A, D, E, and K deficiency must be addressed. An oral elemental diet, total parenteral nutrition, or both are the primary modes of nutritional support for these patients. The goal is to provide at least 125% to 140% of the recommended daily allowance for calories and protein.

Psychological support is vital because of the chronicity of the disease. It is important to teach adaptive responses to the illness, rather than enabling maladaptive responses to progress.

Hirschsprung Enterocolitis

Etiology

Hirschsprung disease is caused by a **congenital absence of ganglion cells** that normally relax the colon and rectum to allow defecation (see Chapter 22, "Constipation"). An associated enterocolitis occurs secondary to poor colonic motility, stagnation of fecal material in the rectum, dilation of normal bowel, poor circulation due to edema, and ultimately necrosis and breakdown of the mucosal barrier.

Clinical Features

Although Hirschsprung enterocolitis is uncommon, the possibility should be considered in any infant with rectal bleeding who has abdominal distention, foul-smelling diarrhea, a history of delayed meconium passage, constipation, fever, and sepsis. There may also be evidence of intestinal obstruction.

Evaluation

A **barium enema** (unprepped—to prevent dilation of the colonic transition zone) may suggest the diagnosis. Often, a submucosal or full-thickness **rectal biopsy** (demonstrating absence of ganglion cells and hypertrophied nerve bundles) is required to confirm the diagnosis.

Treatment

Infants with suspected Hirschsprung enterocolitis should be placed on **nothing by mouth** and administered **fluids and broad-spectrum antibiotics intravenously**. A **nasogastric tube** should be inserted to decompress the proximal bowel. **Surgical correction** is required to remove the aganglionic bowel segment and to relieve the intestinal obstruction.

Milk-Protein or Soy-Protein Allergy

Etiology

Milk-protein or soy-protein allergy is the **most common immunologic cause of gastrointestinal bleeding** in infants. The most common explanation for milk-protein allergy is that it is caused by an antigen-induced, IgE-mediated reaction with subsequent mast cell activation and eosinophilic infiltration of the intestinal mucosa. Food protein-induced enterocolitis syndrome is another form of intolerance that causes vomiting, bloody stools, irritability, and dehydration. This is usually due to intolerance to cow or soy proteins, but has also been associated with other foods including rice. Food protein-induced proctocolitis also causes blood-streaked stools, and can occasionally cause anemia. Soy and milk proteins are also the common causes of this condition. These two conditions are cell-mediated resulting from activation of T cells and secretion of cytokines.

Clinical Features

Many children have a history of atopic illnesses such as rhinitis, bronchospasm, eczema, and coughing. There are several clinical manifestations, including an

immediate hypersensitivity reaction, a **delayed systemic reaction** (characterized by a rash and headache), and a **gastrointestinal reaction** that occurs several days later. Infants most commonly present with bloody, mucus-streaked **diarrhea, abdominal pain, weight loss, and vomiting**. Patients may also have signs of **anaphylaxis** (e.g., urticaria, bronchospasm, hypotension).

 HINT: Approximately 20% of infants with milk-protein allergy are also allergic to soy, and 1% may also be allergic to most simple foods. Therefore, it is key to eliminate both from the diet.

Evaluation

The diagnosis is usually made on the basis of the **clinical history**. Although a strict placebo-controlled **food challenge test** is the only way to make a definitive diagnosis, food elimination can often strongly suggest the offending agent. Helpful diagnostic tests include a **Wright stain of the stool** (to reveal stool eosinophils) **or endoscopy,** which may demonstrate eosinophilic infiltration of the intestinal mucosa. Peripheral eosinophilia is often present. It is important to note that it may take up to 1 month for the stool guaiac to become negative.

Treatment

Treatment consists of **removing the offending antigen** from the diet. Most children outgrow this condition by 2 years of age, when these foods can be reintroduced in the diet under close observation. Older children who develop food allergies often require a lifetime of avoidance.

Eosinophilic Enteritis
Etiology

Idiopathic eosinophilic gastroenteritis is a rare disorder caused by eosinophilic tissue infiltration and mast cell activation without known antigenic stimulation. Three forms exist: **mucosal infiltration** (vomiting, diarrhea, PLE), **muscular infiltration** (gastric outlet obstruction), and **serosal infiltration** (ascites without other intestinal symptoms). Common sites of involvement include the gastric antrum, esophagus, and colon. Eosinophilic enteritis can produce **severe esophagitis, gastritis, duodenitis, or all three**.

Clinical Features

Patients present with **nausea, vomiting, abdominal pain, and upper or lower gastrointestinal bleeding**. **Hematemesis** results from mucosal infiltration, which promotes an inflammatory response. Other clinical findings include **diarrhea, weight loss, failure to thrive, ascites, and peripheral edema**.

Laboratory findings include peripheral eosinophilia, iron-deficiency anemia, elevated serum IgE levels, and hypoalbuminemia (secondary to PLE).

Evaluation

Initial evaluation includes searching for evidence of mucosal malabsorption using the D-**xylose absorption test** and performing **radiographic contrast studies,** which may show small-bowel edema and ulceration. Definitive diagnosis can be made by **endoscopy with biopsy**.

Treatment

Treatment involves **supportive care, dietary manipulation,** and the administration of **corticosteroids** (in severe cases) and **oral cromolyn sodium**. Long-term care should be coordinated by a pediatric gastroenterologist.

Intussusception

Intussusception is discussed in Chapter 9, "Abdominal Pain, Acute."

EVALUATION OF LOWER GASTROINTESTINAL BLEEDING
Patient History

Travel history. The travel history may suggest an infectious cause.

Events suggesting upper gastrointestinal tract trauma. A recent history of epistaxis, nasogastric, or gastrostomy tube placement, retching (suggestive of a Mallory-Weiss tear), surgery (e.g., tonsillectomy, adenoidectomy), or caustic ingestion may explain melena or heme-positive stools.

Medication history. Melanotic stools can be caused by drug-induced gastritis, for example, from nonsteroidal anti-inflammatory agents or salicylates. In addition, certain drugs can mimic blood in the stool (see Table 34-2). For example, Omnicef (Cefdinir) which is a white liquid can cause red stools. This is due to iron in the child's diet binding to Cefdinir, and resulting in a pigment that appears bright red in the stools.

Physical Examination

Perianal and digital rectal examinations should always be performed in children with hematochezia to look for anal fissure, hemorrhoids, rectal trauma, foreign bodies in the rectum, and signs of sexual abuse (e.g., cutaneous bruising, anal tears, labial or penile irritation).

Abdominal palpation may reveal hepatosplenomegaly, which suggests portal hypertension and possible varices.

Cutaneous examination may reveal hemangiomas (suggestive of an alimentary arteriovenous malformation), purpura on the buttocks and lower extremities (consistent with Henoch-Schönlein purpura), or erythema nodosum and pyoderma gangrenosum (seen in children with inflammatory bowel disease).

Laboratory Studies

Stool culture and **testing for white blood cells** is always indicated for a child who presents with bloody diarrhea.

Diagnostic Modalities

Upper gastrointestinal endoscopy and colonoscopy are the most important tests for the diagnosis of gastrointestinal bleeding and may be therapeutic. Table 34-3 summarizes other diagnostic modalities and their indications.

TABLE 34-3	Useful Diagnostic Tests for Evaluation of Gastrointestinal Bleeding
Test	**Indication**
Meckel scan	Identification of a Meckel diverticulum or intestinal duplication
Tagged red blood cell scan	Identification of a site of rapid intestinal bleeding
Colonoscopy	Evaluation of hematochezia or colonic disease
Upper endoscopy	Evaluation of causes of upper gastrointestinal bleeding proximal to the ligament of Treitz
Angiography	Identification of vascular causes of gastrointestinal bleeding
Barium enema	Identification of anatomic abnormalities of the colon (Hirschsprung disease, intussusception, stricture, and mass)
Upper gastrointestinal series	Identification of anatomic and inflammatory abnormalities of the esophagus, stomach, and small intestine
Enteroclysis	Used when enhancement of the mucosal detail of the small intestine is required
Abdominal radiograph	Identification of foreign body, intestinal obstruction, and mucosal edema (thumbprinting)
Video capsule endoscopy	Identification of bleeding sources in the small bowel

TREATMENT OF LOWER GASTROINTESTINAL BLEEDING

Lower gastrointestinal bleeding can be life threatening. Patients with persistent, rapid bleeding or associated dizziness, fatigue, or severe abdominal pain require immediate evaluation and stabilization:

- Orthostatic vital signs and a complete blood count should be obtained as soon as possible.
- Patients with hypotension or anemia should receive intravenous fluids and blood products (when necessary).
- A plain abdominal radiograph is useful for revealing intestinal obstruction or perforation.
- In patients with significant lower gastrointestinal bleeding, a nasogastric tube should be placed to decompress the bowel and to determine the severity and origin of the bleeding (e.g., from the stomach or esophagus).
- The patient should be admitted under the care of a pediatric gastroenterologist.

Suggested Readings

American Academy of Pediatrics. Clostridium difficile. In: Pickering LK, Baker CJ, Kimberlin DW, Long SS, eds. *Red Book: 2009 Report of the Committee on Infectious Diseases.* 28th ed. Elk Grove Village, IL: American Academy of Pediatrics; 2009, 263–265.

Boyle JT. Gastrointestinal bleeding in infants and children. *Pediatr Rev.* 2008;29(2):39–52.

Brown RL, Azizkhan RG. Gastrointestinal bleeding in infants and children: Meckel's diverticulum and intestinal duplication. *Semin Pediatr Surg.* 1999;8(4):202–209.

El-Matary W. Wireless capsule endoscopy: indications, limitations and future challenges. *J Pediatr Gastroenterol Nutr.* 2008;46(1):4–12.

Feldman M, Friedman LS, Brandy LJ. *Sleisenger and Fordtran's Gastrointestinal and Liver Disease: Pathophysiology, Diagnosis, Management.* Philadelphia, PA: WB Saunders; 2006.

Fox VL. Gastrointestinal bleeding in infancy and childhood. *Gastroenterol Clin North Am.* 2000;29(1):37–66.

Friedlander J, Mamula P. Gastrointestinal hemorrhage. In: Wyllie R, Hyams JS, Kay M, eds. *Pediatric Gastrointestinal and Liver Disease.* Philadelphia, PA: Elsevier Saunders; 2011.

Hoffenberg EJ, Sauaia A, Maltzman T, et al. Symptomatic colonic polyps in childhood: not so benign. *J Pediatr Gastroenterol Nutr.* 1999;28(2):175–181.

Kliegman RM. Adverse reactions to foods. In: Kliegman RM, Behrman RE, Jenson HB, Stanton BF, eds. *Nelson Textbook of Pediatrics.* 18th ed. Philadelphia, PA: Elsevier; 2007, Chapter 150.

Kliegman RM. Intestinal duplications, Meckel diverticulum and other remnants of the omphalomesenteric duct. In: Behrman LE, Kliegman RM, Jenson HB, eds. *Nelson Textbook of Pediatrics.* 18th ed. Philadelphia, PA: Saunders Elsevier; 2007, Chapter 328.

Lee KH, Yeung CK, Tam YH, et al. Laparoscopy for definitive diagnosis and treatment of gastrointestinal bleeding of obscure origin in children. *J Pediatr Surg.* 2000;35(9):1291–1293.

Lowers J, Jaffe A, Zenel J, et al. Visual diagnosis: four infants who have red, bloody stools. *Pediatr Rev.* 2009;30:146–149.

Walker WA, Goulet O, Kleinman RE, et al. *Pediatric Gastrointestinal Disease.* 4th ed. Hamilton, ON: BC Decker; 2004.

Gastrointestinal Bleeding, Upper

INTRODUCTION

The presence of hematemesis usually suggests that the site of bleeding is proximal to the ligament of Treitz. Common sites of upper gastrointestinal (GI) tract bleeding are summarized in Table 35-1.

DIFFERENTIAL DIANGOSIS LIST

Infectious Causes
- Bacterial gastritis—*Helicobacter pylori* infection
- Viral infection—Cytomegalovirus, varicella, herpesvirus, adenovirus
- Fungal esophagitis or gastritis

Toxic Causes
- Drugs—nonsteroidal anti-inflammatory drugs (NSAIDs), aspirin, steroids
- Caustic substances
- Alcohol gastritis

Neoplastic Causes
- Zollinger–Ellison syndrome
- Leiomyoma
- Leiomyosarcoma
- Lymphoma
- Upper GI tract polyps

Traumatic Causes
- Mallory-Weiss tear
- Epistaxis
- Oropharyngeal trauma (e.g., postsurgical trauma)
- Nasogastric or gastric tube trauma
- Foreign body

Congenital or Vascular Causes
- Enteric duplication
- Ulcer with Dieulafoy lesion
- Arteriovenous malformation
- Esophageal or gastric varices

Inflammatory Causes
- Gastric or duodenal ulcer
- Esophagitis (reflux or chemical)
- Gastritis (caustic or chemical)
- Duodenitis
- Eosinophilic gastritis

Miscellaneous Causes
- Hemobilia
- Graft-versus-host disease
- Swallowed maternal blood
- Pulmonary disease (hemoptysis)
- Factitious bleeding (Munchausen by proxy syndrome)

TABLE 35-1	Causes of Hematemesis by Site
Site	**Cause**
Oropharynx	Epistaxis
	Mouth-/nose-/throat-surgery trauma
	Foreign body
Esophagus	Esophagitis
	Esophageal stricture
	Mallory-Weiss tear
	Infection
	Foreign body
	Esophageal varices
Stomach	Ulcer
	Gastritis (drug, infection, caustic ingestion)
	Eosinophilic enteritis
	Graft-versus-host disease
	Vascular abnormality
	Gastric varices
	Duplication
	Tumor
	Gastric polyps
Duodenum	Ulcer
	Eosinophilic enteritis
	Hemobilia

DIFFERENTIAL DIAGNOSIS DISCUSSION

Mallory-Weiss Tear

Etiology

A Mallory-Weiss tear is a **linear mucosal tear of the distal esophagus** that occurs as a result of **forceful vomiting or retching**.

Clinical Features

Bloody streaks are seen in the vomitus.

Evaluation

Mallory-Weiss tears are not visible on radiographs, and definitive diagnosis is via **upper endoscopy**. Initially, the tear appears as a **vertical, linear red streak;** after healing, it is seen as a **white streak** with surrounding erythema. Most times, it is suspected from clinical history and tests are not needed. In any case of hematemesis or coffee ground emesis, nasogastric tube should be placed and normal saline gastric lavage should be performed.

Treatment

Most patients can be managed in the outpatient setting because Mallory-Weiss tears usually **resolve spontaneously**. In severe cases, hospital observation is indicated. Rarely, blood transfusion, vasopressin therapy, or balloon tamponade may be necessary.

Esophagitis

Etiology

Esophagitis **(inflammation of the esophageal mucosa)** can be caused by acid or bile reflux, infection, inflammation, allergy, or caustic ingestions. Esophagitis may result from disorders that promote delayed gastric emptying secondary to vomiting acidic stomach contents.

Clinical Features

Typically, patients complain of **heartburn, chest pain, water brash** (sour taste in the mouth), dysphagia, halitosis, **vomiting, and/or regurgitation**. **Blood-streaked emesis** occurs in patients with severe or untreated esophagitis.

In infants with severe reflux esophagitis, parents may notice pooled bloody secretions on the infant's bedding. In older children with esophagitis, bloody emesis is usually associated with epigastric or chest pain and a history of frequent regurgitation and a "sour taste" in the mouth.

Evaluation

Upper endoscopy is the preferred test because it allows for inspection of the esophageal mucosa. Biopsies of the esophagus can be taken to determine the cause of the inflammation and the degree of histologic involvement.

Upper GI tract radiography is often useful for determining the anatomic configuration of the upper GI tract. This study is most valuable for ruling out other causes of upper GI bleeding (e.g., gastric or duodenal ulcer disease, esophageal strictures).

Treatment

The treatment of esophagitis depends on its cause.

- **Acid reflux esophagitis** is treated with gastric acid blockers (H_2 blockers, or proton pump inhibitors) as first-line therapy. Prokinetic agents may be used in refractory cases.
- **Inflammatory esophagitis** is treated with protective agents, such as sucralfate, gastric acid blockers, and treatment of the underlying inflammatory process (e.g., corticosteroids for Crohn disease and food elimination for allergic eosinophilic esophagitis).
- **Strictures** necessitate dilation, usually accomplished via endoscopy.
- **Infectious esophagitis** is treated with antimicrobials or antifungals.

Gastritis

Etiology

Gastritis **(inflammation of the gastric mucosa)** can be classified as primary or secondary:

- **Primary gastritis** results when acid or bile causes direct mucosal damage.
- **Secondary gastritis** is either a complication of another disease process (e.g., severe burns, systemic illness, Henoch-Schönlein purpura) or is caused by an offending agent (e.g., ingested drugs or corrosives, infections).

Clinical Features

Epigastric pain and vomiting are the most common symptoms of gastritis in children. The pain often occurs during, or just after, meals, and the patient often complains of **nausea and early satiety**. Small amounts of **fresh blood or "coffee ground" material** may be seen **in the vomitus**.

Evaluation

In children, radiographic contrast studies often do not have the sensitivity necessary to show gastritis. **Upper endoscopy** is a more valuable tool; the gastric mucosa can be directly visualized and biopsies can be obtained to determine the cause of the gastritis.

Treatment

Initially, **acid-blocking medications** (e.g., antacids, H_2 blockers) are first-line medications used to protect the stomach lining by raising the gastric pH above 4.0. **Exacerbating drugs** (e.g., aspirin, NSAIDs) **should be eliminated**. Patients with major hemorrhage require **fluid resuscitation and transfusion. Specific causes of gastritis should be identified with endoscopy to better tailor the therapy.**

Gastric or Duodenal Ulcer
Etiology

Ulcers in children are either primary or secondary. Primary ulcers are usually chronic, in the duodenum, commonly caused by *H. pylori*. Secondary ulcers are found in acute illnesses, typically in the stomach, and are caused by NSAIDs, hypersecretory states (Zollinger–Ellison Syndrome), short bowel syndrome, systemic mastocytosis, systemic illnesses, stress from sepsis or shock, intracranial lesions (Cushing ulcer), or severe burn (Curling ulcer). The development of ulcers is also associated with several **systemic diseases,** including sickle cell disease, cystic fibrosis, and asthma.

 HINT: Gastric ulcers are more common in children around 6 years and found in the lesser curvature, whereas duodenal ulcers occur more frequently in older children and are typically found in the duodenal bulb.

Clinical Features

Major symptoms include **upper GI bleeding, abdominal pain, vomiting, anorexia, syncope or dizziness** (secondary to anemia), **weight loss or failure to thrive, and heartburn**. The pain can awaken the child at night or in the early morning. Occasionally, patients will present with melena or bright red blood per rectum due to rapid upper GI bleeding. Symptoms of ulcer disease have often been present for as long as 2 years prior to diagnosis.

Evaluation

Although an upper GI contrast study can confirm the diagnosis in up to 50% of patients, **upper endoscopy** remains the most efficacious test. Upper endoscopy allows identification of the ulcer, determination of the cause (via a biopsy), and, in some cases, treatment (e.g., cauterization in the case of acute bleeding).

 HINT: When the ulcers are multiple or recurrent, rare disorders such as Zollinger–Ellison syndrome or antral G-cell hyperplasia should be considered.

Treatment

Routine medical therapy consists of **gastric acid suppression** (with antacids, H_2 blockers, and proton pump inhibitors) and **mucosal protection** (with sucralfate). **Infectious causes and systemic diseases should be treated** to prevent recurrences. Current treatment of *H. pylori* infection is 7- to 14-day treatment with two antimicrobials (clarithromycin and amoxicillin or metronidazole) and a proton pump inhibitor. Profuse bleeding may require endoscopy with **electrocautery; surgery** is indicated in the rare case of intractable bleeding or perforation.

Esophageal or Gastric Varices

Etiology

Varices occur **secondary to portal hypertension caused by chronic liver disease, vascular obstruction** (Budd–Chiari syndrome), **or portal vein obstruction** (cavernous transformation, thrombosis). The portal hypertension and subsequent vascular shunting cause the development of varices (esophageal, gastric, and rectal) and abdominal caput medusae. Increased vascular pressure results in elevated wall tension, thinning of the blood vessel wall, and, eventually, vascular rupture.

Clinical Features

Painless, profuse vomiting of bright-red blood is often the first sign of bleeding varices. Patients may also present with melena or with bright red blood per rectum. Approximately 25% of children with varices have had no prior diagnosis and present with hematemesis. Patients may have **signs of liver disease** (e.g., jaundice, palmar erythema, spider angiomas). Almost all patients with varices have palpable **splenomegaly**.

Evaluation

A good physical and **abdominal examination is part of the initial evaluation**. There may be **laboratory evidence of liver disease** (e.g., elevated transaminases, low albumin, or abnormal PT/INR). Although radiographic studies may provide some additional information—for example, a contrast study can show the outline of the varices, or an abdominal ultrasound can detect associated liver disease and the direction of blood flow in the portal system—**upper GI endoscopy** is the most accurate method of diagnosing varices.

Treatment

Bleeding varices are an **absolute medical emergency**. The patient must be admitted to a **pediatric intensive care facility** and placed in the care of a **pediatric gastroenterologist**. Upper GI endoscopy is indicated for diagnosis and treatment **(sclerotherapy or variceal banding)**.

EVALUATION OF UPPER GASTROINTESTINAL BLEEDING
Patient History
- Is there a history of prolonged retching or recent stress?
- Could the child be swallowing blood as a result of epistaxis, tonsillectomy or adenoidectomy, trauma to the teeth or gums, or trauma from foreign objects or nasogastric tube insertion?
- Has the child eaten any food that may resemble blood in the vomitus?
- Does the child's medication history include NSAIDs or aspirin (which can cause gastritis) or steroids (which can cause gastric ulcers)?

Physical Examination
- The **nares, mouth, and throat** of any child who presents with hematemesis should be carefully examined.
- The child's **fingernails** should be inspected for evidence of dried blood because digital manipulation of the nose is the most common cause of nosebleeds in children. A negative rectal examination for occult blood should alert the physician to the possibility that epistaxis is responsible for the blood in the vomitus.
- **Hepatosplenomegaly or isolated splenomegaly** almost always occurs in conjunction with portal hypertension and varices. However, splenomegaly may not be present immediately after an acute variceal bleed.
- **Freckles over the lips and under the axilla** may suggest Peutz–Jeghers syndrome with gastric polyps.

Diagnostic Modalities
Upper GI endoscopy and contrast studies are useful for discovering the cause of hematemesis. Although an upper GI contrast study occasionally shows pathognomonic esophageal findings, **upper endoscopy with biopsy** is the study of choice. For children who have recurrent bleeding episodes and for whom endoscopy or contrast studies have been negative, **nuclear medicine bleeding scans** may be useful. The patient must be actively bleeding at the time of the test. Recently, video capsule endoscopy has become available in many centers, and may be useful in identifying a source of obscure GI bleeding.

TREATMENT OF UPPER GASTROINTESTINAL BLEEDING
The first step in the management of a patient with upper GI tract bleeding is to provide supportive care:

- Obtain vital signs and manage the airway, breathing, and circulation.
- Place two large-bore intravenous lines.
- Obtain a complete blood cell count, type and cross-match, serum electrolyte panel, and blood urea nitrogen and creatinine levels.
- Administer crystalloid (normal saline) or a blood transfusion (if necessary).
- Place a nasogastric tube to irrigate the stomach with normal saline.
- Place a central venous catheter for central venous pressure measurement (if indicated).

- Obtain the patient's history and evaluate for prior bleeding episodes or chronic disease.
- Consult a pediatric gastroenterologist.

In addition to supportive care, acute medical management may entail the **intravenous administration of vasopressin or octreotide** to promote vasoconstriction of bleeding blood vessels. These medications are extremely useful in children with active esophageal or gastric varices and ulcers. Patients given vasopressin or octreotide should be monitored in an **intensive care setting** and should be in the care of a **pediatric gastroenterologist**.

Other medical treatments include **endoscopy with sclerotherapy, band ligation or electrocautery and balloon tamponade**. **Surgery** is indicated for patients with uncontrolled bleeding in whom medical treatment has failed.

APPROACH TO THE PATIENT

The **first episode** of upper GI tract bleeding in children should always be **treated as a medical emergency**. Once the patient is stabilized, a careful history and physical examination should be performed to determine the cause of the bleeding.

Suggested Readings

American Academy of Pediatrics. Helicobacter pylori infections. In: Pickering LK, Baker CJ, Kimberlin DW, Long SS, eds. *Red Book: 2009 Report of the Committee on Infectious Diseases.* 28th ed. Elk Grove Village, IL: American Academy of Pediatrics; 2009:321–324.

Boyle JT. Gastrointestinal bleeding in infants and children. *Pediatr Rev.* 2008;29(2):39–52.

Chawla S, Seth D, Mahajan P, et al. Upper gastrointestinal bleeding in children. *Clin Pediatr.* 2007;46(1):16–21.

Feldman M, Friedman LS, Brandy LJ. *Sleisenger and Fordtran's Gastrointestinal and Liver Disease: Pathophysiology, Diagnosis, Management.* Philadelphia, PA: WB Saunders; 2006.

Friedlander J, Mamula P. Gastrointestinal hemorrhage. In: Wyllie R, Hyams JS, Kay M, eds. *Pediatric Gastrointestinal Disease: Pathophysiology, Diagnosis, Management.* 4th ed. Philadelphia, PA: Elsevier Saunders; 2011.

Mileti E, Rosenthal P. Management of portal hypertension in children. *Curr Gastroenterol Rep.* 2011; 13(1):10–16.

Molleston JP. Variceal bleeding in children. *J Pediatr Gastroenterol Nutr.* 2003;37(5):538–545.

Polin RA, Ditmar MF. *Pediatric Secrets.* 4th ed. Philadelphia, PA: Hanley & Belfus; 2005.

Walker WA, Goulet O, Kleinman RE, et al. *Pediatric Gastrointestinal Disease.* 4th ed. Hamilton, ON: BC Decker; 2004.

CHAPTER 36

Craig A. Alter
Wilma C. Rossi
Andrew J. Bauer

Goiter

INTRODUCTION

Goiter (enlargement of the thyroid gland) arises under a variety of clinical circumstances. Morbidity from an enlarged thyroid ranges from simple cosmetic appearance to that associated with carcinoma. The majority of children who present with a goiter have **normal thyroid hormone** levels.

DIFFERENTIAL DIAGNOSIS LIST

Congenital Causes
- Unilateral agenesis
- Dyshormonogenesis (including Pendred syndrome)
- Thyroxine (T_4) resistance
- Thyroid-stimulating hormone (TSH) receptor and Gα protein receptor mutations

Autoimmune Causes
- Chronic lymphocytic thyroiditis (CLT, Hashimoto thyroiditis)
- Graves disease (acquired and neonatal)

Infectious Causes
- Acute suppurative thyroiditis
- Subacute thyroiditis

Toxic Causes
- Lithium carbonate
- Amiodarone
- Iodide-containing drugs

Neoplastic Causes
- Thyroid adenoma
- Papillary thyroid carcinoma
- Follicular thyroid carcinoma
- Medullary thyroid carcinoma
- TSH-secreting adenoma
- Nonthyroid carcinomas—lymphoma, teratoma, hygroma

Metabolic or Environmental Causes
- Iodine deficiency
- Environmental and dietary goitrogens

Miscellaneous Causes
- Sporadic, nontoxic goiter
- Multinodular colloid goiter
- Thyroglossal duct cyst (may simulate a goiter)

DIFFERENTIAL DIAGNOSIS DISCUSSION
Chronic Lymphocytic Thyroiditis (Hashimoto Thyroiditis)
Etiology
Chronic lymphocytic thyroiditis (CLT), an autoimmune condition, is the most common cause of goiter in the pediatric population. Its incidence is highest in adolescent girls, with a **female-to-male ratio of 2:1**.

TABLE 36-1	Signs and Symptoms of Hypothyroidism and Hyperthyroidism
Hypothyroidism	**Hyperthyroidism**
Goiter	Goiter, bruit over thyroid
Lethargy, slow speech	Nervousness, restless sleep
Cold skin, decreased sweating	Sweating, heat intolerance
Bradycardia	Palpitation, tachycardia
Weakness	Fatigue, weakness
Anorexia	Increased appetite
Weight gain	Weight loss
Constipation	Increased stool frequency
Stiff, aching muscles	Tremor of hands and tongue
Edema of face and eyelids	Exophthalmos, lid lag
Dry, coarse skin	Increased skin pigmentation
Hair loss with increased coarseness	Fine hair
Poor growth	Accelerated growth
Delayed puberty and tooth eruption	Poor school performance
Precocious puberty	Moodiness or irritability
Changes in menstrual cycle (menorrhagia)	Changes in menstrual cycle (sporadic to amenorrhea, light flow)

Clinical Features

Some patients with CLT present for medical examination with symptoms of hypothyroidism (Table 36-1). Most have enlargement of the gland without systemic complaints. Rarely, patients with CLT present with symptoms of hyperthyroidism (**Hashitoxicosis**). These children usually progress toward hypothyroidism over a period of months. The thyroid gland itself is diffusely enlarged (although possibly with asymmetry), mobile, nontender, firm, or rubbery. It usually has a granular or pebbly texture but can be smooth. However, in the most severe cases of hypothyroidism and CLT, the thyroid is often so degenerated that it is not easily palpable. Enlargement of the thyroid in CLT may be caused by lymphocytic infiltration or stimulation by the increased TSH. A goiter due to increased TSH stimulation typically decreases with treatment.

There is a family history of thyroid disease in 30% to 40% of patients with CLT. Histologic findings include infiltration of the gland with plasma cells and lymphocytes, parenchymal atrophy, and eosinophilic degeneration of thyroid follicles.

Evaluation

Laboratory studies should include assessment of T_4 and/or free T_4, TSH, and antithyroglobulin and antithyroperoxidase antibodies. In children with CLT, thyroid function tests indicate either a **euthyroid** state (no abnormalities), **compensated hypothyroidism** (normal level of T_4 with increased TSH), or **hypothyroidism** (low level of T_4 with increased TSH). One or both of the antithyroid antibodies are present in 90% to 95% of patients with CLT. These antibodies represent the immunologic response to the presence of elements of thyroid tissue in the bloodstream and are not the cause of the thyroiditis. In general, routine ultrasound (US) imaging of the thyroid is unnecessary. However, patients with Hashimoto disease are at an increased risk of developing thyroid nodules. If the patient presents with an asymmetric gland, or an easily palpated nodule, **US imaging** should be pursued. US imaging will typically reveal thyroid gland enlargement with heterogeneous echotexture. "Pseudonodules" are commonly found, and are distinguished from true nodules by confirming their presence in more than one imaging plane (sagittal and transverse). If a nodule is found, fine needle aspiration biopsy should be performed (see below).

Treatment

If the child is euthyroid at presentation and again at 6 months, yearly monitoring of T_4 and TSH is reasonable, more frequently depending on age, growth, and any other complicating factors. **Thyroid hormone replacement** is indicated for the treatment of overt hypothyroidism and occasionally for compensated hypothyroidism accompanied by a significantly enlarged gland. Initial doses of sodium L-thyroxine at 100 $\mu g/m^2$ of body surface area or 2 to 5 $\mu g/kg$ per day should be adjusted after 6 to 8 weeks of therapy to keep TSH levels in the normal or low normal range and T_4 in the mid to upper range. Shrinkage of the goiter may not occur if the inflammation is long standing and the fibrosis is extensive. Once an appropriate dose of sodium L-thyroxine is established, biannual follow-up is necessary to ensure compliance and appropriate adjustment in dose is made based on normal growth and development. Some may require more frequent laboratory studies.

Spontaneous remission occurs in up to 30% of adolescents. In children where remission seems possible, it is acceptable to discontinue hormone replacement therapy when growth is completed to ascertain whether spontaneous remission has occurred. If this is done, follow-up TSH and free T_4 or total T_4 should be repeated 6 to 8 weeks after stopping levothyroxine.

 HINT: Hypothyroidism can cause either pubertal delay or precocity. If it causes precocious puberty, the growth rate will be slow rather than rapid in contrast to what is seen with other etiologies of precocious puberty.

Sporadic Nontoxic Goiter

Etiology

Sporadic nontoxic goiter is the second most common cause of nontoxic thyroid enlargement in the pediatric population. Its cause is uncertain, although an autoimmune cause is a possibility. There is often a family history of goiter and/or hypothyroidism.

Clinical Features

There is diffuse enlargement of the thyroid gland in asymptomatic adolescents. The gland is enlarged and usually softer and more homogeneous than in CLT.

Nodularity may develop after several years, even in those patients in whom regression has occurred.

Evaluation

There are usually **no antithyroid antibodies,** and the T_4 and TSH levels are normal. Patients should be followed with repeat physical examination and serial thyroid function testing (TSH and T_4) every 6 to 12 months to ensure that thyroid gland dysfunction does not develop. Ultrasound is not indicated unless there is a suspicion of a thyroid nodule.

Treatment

• Treatment with sodium L-thyroxine is not required. In many cases, the goiter resolves with time.

Graves Disease

Etiology

Graves disease, a multisystem autoimmune disorder, is the most common cause of hyperthyroidism in the pediatric population. The incidence in males and females is equal in infancy and early childhood, with a **female predominance occurring in adolescence**. In Graves disease, elaboration of an immunoglobulin G1 antibody stimulates the TSH receptor, resulting in hyperfunctioning follicular cells with increased production and release of thyroid hormone. The predominant antibody acts to stimulate the TSH receptor causing both hyperthyroidism and a goiter. Mild **exophthalmos** is common in pediatric patients with Graves disease; however, it is usually less severe than what is seen in adults with exophthalmos.

Clinical Features

Graves disease presents with signs of hyperthyroidism and thyromegaly. Exophthalmos is occasionally present, and dermopathy (redness and swelling of the skin on the shins and feet) is rare. Children with hyperthyroidism caused by Graves disease often are brought to medical attention because of worsening school performance and a change in behavior (emotional lability and irritability). The majority of symptoms of hyperthyroidism (see Table 36-1) are caused by stimulation of the sympathetic nervous system resulting from increased levels of thyroid hormones.

Evaluation

On physical examination, the thyroid gland is typically symmetrically enlarged, smooth, and nontender. The texture is soft to firm, and the size is variable. The severity of the hyperthyroidism correlates with the size of the gland. Graves disease is rare in a child without a goiter. The child is usually tachycardic with a widened pulse pressure and an active precordium. A vascular bruit may be heard over the gland. Proptosis with stare and upper lid lag is noted in many cases; however, the eye disease in children rarely reaches the severity seen in adults. **Dermopathy,** caused by an accumulation of mucopolysaccharide in the skin and subcutaneous tissue, is uncommon in children.

TABLE 36-2	Laboratory Findings in Graves Disease
Parameter	**Finding Suggestive of Graves Disease**
Total T_4	Levels increased
Free T_4	Levels increased
T_3	Levels increased
TSH	Significantly suppressed and often undetectable
TSI	Elevated
Thyroid antibodies	
Antithyroglobulin and antithyroperoxidase antibodies	May be detected, but not useful in distinguishing Graves disease from Hashitoxicosis
^{123}I uptake study	Increased uptake of the isotope at 6 and 24 hr post-administration is supportive of Graves disease (decreased or patchy uptake is seen in CLT and subacute thyroiditis) A focal area of increased iodine uptake implies a hot nodule

CLT, chronic lymphocytic thyroiditis; ^{123}I, iodine-123; T_3, triiodothyronine; T_4, thyroxine; TSH, thyroid-stimulating hormone; TSI, thyroid-stimulating immunoglobulin.

Table 36-2 shows the laboratory and radiologic studies that support the diagnosis of Graves disease and help distinguish it from other causes of hyperthyroidism.

Treatment

There are three main approaches to the management of Graves disease: antithyroid medications, iodine-131 (^{131}I) ablation therapy, and near-total thyroidectomy. In general, medical management with medications should be the first intervention, followed by either ablation with ^{131}I or surgery. The mainstay of long-term medical treatment in children is the thionamide derivative methimazole. Propylthiouracil (**PTU**) is no longer recommended since fatal liver failure secondary to the drug has been reported. **Methimazole** inhibits the organification of iodide, thus blocking the synthesis (but not the release) of thyroid hormone. Side effects of the medication include skin rash, pruritus, liver toxicity and, rarely, agranulocytosis. If a child on methimazole presents with a severe sore throat, a complete blood cell count should be obtained. Liver enzymes should be monitored and the drug should be discontinued at the first sign of liver toxicity. β-**Blocking agents** are used as adjuvant treatment to control symptoms when long-term therapy is initially introduced; they may be discontinued when the thyroid disease is well controlled. **Remission** is unlikely in children who are severely hyperthyroid, have large goiters, do not respond quickly to treatment with antithyroid drugs, and are under 5 years of age. If a child has a significant reaction to methimazole, then the treatment options include radioiodine ablation or surgery. PTU may be considered, but cross-reactivity occurs in more than 50% of patients, and with the recent black-box warning of PTU-induced fatal hepatitis, this option should be discouraged.

Thyroid Storm (Thyroid Crisis)
Etiology
Thyroid storm is a medical emergency. It is a very rare condition and typically occurs in individuals who have preexisting hyperthyroidism and who are undertreated or noncompliant. Infection, trauma, and surgical procedures are the most common precipitating events. Pneumococcal sepsis is occasionally found. The release of large amounts of thyroid hormone leads to a hypermetabolic state with excessive thermogenesis and significant fluid losses. Increase in temperature can be extreme and life threatening.

Clinical Features
Children with thyroid storm present with fever, tachycardia, tremor, nausea and vomiting, diarrhea, dehydration, and delirium or coma. Occasionally, patients have a true toxic psychosis. The markedly increased cardiac workload can lead to congestive heart failure.

Treatment
Treatment of thyroid storm includes the immediate administration of **short acting β-blocking agents** to suppress the activity of the sympathetic nervous system. Next, **hydration** must be achieved, and appropriate measures must be taken to lower the body temperature slowly. **Methimazole** (0.4 mg/kg, divided, every 8 hours) is administered orally. Thyroid storm remains one of the rare exceptions where **PTU** may be theoretically more efficacious than methimazole due to its ability to block peripheral T_4 to T_3 conversion. Concentrated iodide solution treatment will rapidly terminate the release of thyroxine. It may be administered in the form of Lugol's solution, 5 drops every 8 hours; SSKI, 3 to 5 drops every 8 hours; or sodium iodide, 125 to 250 mg/day intravenously over 24 hours. **Glucocorticoids** which decrease peripheral conversion of T_4 to T_3 may also be helpful. It is critical to treat the underlying condition that precipitated the thyroid storm such as sepsis. Pneumococcal sepsis has been observed in some children who presented thyroid storm.

Thyroid Nodule
Etiology
Up to 2% of children and 13% of adolescents have a thyroid nodule. While nodules are less commonly found in children compared to adults, nodules diagnosed during childhood have increased malignant potential with 25% ultimately diagnosed as malignant compared to 5% to 10% of adults. Several risk factors are associated with development of nodules, to include iodine deficiency, prior exposure to radiation (environment or medical), and previous history of thyroid disease. Up to a radiation dose of approximately 20 Gy, gender, age at exposure, and time since exposure are the most significant modifiers of risk for the development of thyroid nodules and thyroid cancer. In patients without a history of radiation exposure, female gender and increasing age are associated with an increased incidence of nodular disease.

Clinical Features
The majority of nodules are found incidentally during routine physical exam, by a caregiver, or during radiologic evaluation of an unrelated medical condition.

Most children and adolescents are euthyroid at the time of discovery, although there are some data to suggest that patients with hypothyroidism may have an increased risk of developing nodules. On rare occasion, there may be acute discomfort associated with spontaneous bleeding into a large, mixed solid-cystic or purely cystic nodule.

Evaluation

Ultrasound is the most clinically useful tool for determining the morphologic features of the nodule and to determine the location and the number of nodules. The features that should be assessed during US include size, location, composition, echogenicity, outline, and vascular flow (Doppler). Decreased echogenicity, irregular nodule outline, subcapsular location, increased intranodular vascularity, and microcalcifications are associated with increased risk of malignancy. Purely cystic lesions under 1 cm in size are almost universally benign.

For the majority of solid nodules >0.5 cm in size, **fine-needle aspiration biopsy** (FNAB) should be performed. Factors that increase the yield of adequate samples include regular performance of FNAB, US guidance, and immediate, bed-side cytological evaluation. The use of sedation in both children and adolescents is strongly encouraged.

Scintigraphy (thyroid uptake and scan) should be limited to investigating patients with a nodule and suppressed TSH. If investigation is consistent with an autonomously functioning or hot nodule, FNAB may not be necessary as malignant tissue have notoriously poor ability to synthesize thyroid hormone. Treatment for these patients includes either surgical resection or radioiodine therapy.

Treatment

Treatment is dependent on the cytologic results of the FNAB. Inadequate samples should undergo repeat FNAB. Benign nodules should be followed with serial physical examinations and US. Repeat FNAB should be considered based on change in size and/or US features (listed above). Patients with malignant nodules should have preoperative staging to determine regional (cervical) or distal (pulmonary) metastasis. Near total **thyroidectomy** is the surgery of choice for the majority of patients. Consideration for the location and extent of neck dissection is based on preoperative staging. The risk of surgical complications is markedly reduced if the surgery is performed in a hospital with regular medical and surgical experience in the evaluation and treatment of pediatric patients with thyroid nodules and thyroid cancer. For patients with indeterminate cytology and unilateral disease, surgical resection should be considered.

Acute Suppurative Thyroiditis
Etiology

A **fistula tract** may have formed between the left pyriform sinus of the pharynx and the left lobe of the thyroid gland. Because of high endogenous levels of iodine, the thyroid gland is inherently resistant to bacterial infection. However, infections do occur and must be treated promptly to prevent abscess formation.

Clinical Features

Patients present with the **rapid onset of anterior neck pain** associated with dysphagia, pharyngitis, mandibular pain, and a hoarse voice; fever; and signs of systemic toxicity. The thyroid itself is exquisitely tender and nonmobile and an US may show areas of fluid collection. The pain increases with neck extension.

Evaluation

Organisms identified by means of needle biopsy include *Streptococcus pyogenes, Staphylococcus aureus, Streptococcus pneumoniae,* anaerobes, fungi, and parasitic organisms. Marked leukocytosis and an increased sedimentation rate are the most consistent laboratory findings. Thyroid function tests usually are normal, but a transient increase in T_4 levels can occur. Nuclear medicine scanning with iodine-123 (^{123}I) demonstrates decreased uptake of the isotope.

Treatment

Antibiotic treatment should be tailored to the suspected organism. Areas of abscess may require surgical drainage. β-**Blocking drugs** can be used if signs of transient thyrotoxicosis develop. Recovery without residual thyroid disease is the natural course.

Subacute Thyroiditis

Etiology

Subacute thyroiditis is a self-limited inflammation of the thyroid gland that most often is associated with, or follows, a viral illness. Viral agents implicated include mumps virus, adenovirus, coxsackievirus, influenza virus, Epstein–Barr virus, and enteric cytopathic human orphan virus. The incidence is the same in boys and girls.

Clinical Features

It can be difficult to distinguish between subacute and acute suppurative thyroiditis. Patients present for treatment with fever and anterior neck pain. The area over the thyroid may be warm and erythematous. The thyroid is usually tender and enlarged. Signs and symptoms of hyperthyroidism develop because of the release of stored hormone from the inflamed gland. These symptoms can persist for 1 to 4 weeks and can be followed by a 2- to 9-month period of hypothyroidism.

Evaluation

Free and total T_4 and triiodothyronine (T_3) levels are increased in the majority of patients with subacute thyroiditis for a period of several weeks. Most patients do not develop antithyroid antibodies. As in acute suppurative thyroiditis, an ^{123}I scan demonstrates decreased uptake of isotope.

Treatment

Treatment includes the administration of **nonsteroidal anti-inflammatory drugs** and a β-**blocker**. In severe cases, the use of corticosteroids may be indicated. Typically, full recovery of thyroid function occurs. If hypothyroidism develops, it is usually transient, but it should be treated.

Congenital Goiter
Etiology
Most cases of newborn goiter are caused by inborn defects of thyroid hormone metabolism (thyroid dyshormonogenesis). Most defects occur sporadically. Inherited forms occur as either an autosomal recessive or dominant traits. These defects include the following:

- Abnormal iodide trapping or organification
- Iodotyrosine deiodinase defect
- Defects in thyroglobulin synthesis, transport, or processing

A second cause of congenital goiter is the maternal ingestion of **goitrogenic agents** during pregnancy, leading to a transient congenital hypothyroidism in the infant. Pregnant women who have Graves disease are currently treated with either PTU or methimazole. Such treatment usually does not cause congenital hypothyroidism unless very high doses are used.

Evaluation
In dyshormonogenesis, free and total T_4 levels may be normal or low while the TSH is elevated. ^{123}I uptake and scan may reveal a normal or enlarged gland with decreased isotope uptake.

Treatment
As with other causes of congenital hypothyroidism, infants with dyshormonogenesis need treatment with **sodium L-thyroxine** (10 to 15 mcg/kg per day) to ensure adequate T_4 levels are available for normal central nervous system development.

Infants with presumed transient hypothyroidism can be followed closely without treatment for 2 weeks. If the T_4 level remains low and the TSH level is elevated, then treatment should be started. Treatment should be continued for the first 2 to 3 years of life while the brain thyroid-dependent myelinization occurs before one considers a trial off of medication.

EVALUATION OF GOITER
Patient History
The major goals during the initial history are to determine if a child has signs or symptoms of hypothyroidism or hyperthyroidism (see Table 36-1). The rapidity of enlargement of the gland may allow one to focus on an acute process (e.g., suppurative thyroiditis) as opposed to a chronic problem (e.g., CLT). In the case of a solitary nodule or unilateral enlargement, exposure to radiation either for treatment of a medical condition or accidental exposure should be determined. A family history of thyroid disease and/or autoimmune tendency should be elicited.

 HINT: Review of systems at each visit should include whether the child has polyuria and polydipsia to screen for early diabetes mellitus. Fatigue in a child with thyroid disease can be caused not only by inadequately treated hypothyroidism but also by new-onset diabetes mellitus.

Physical Examination

- **Vital signs.** Heart rate and blood pressure findings are important in both hypothyroid and hyperthyroid states.
- **Growth.** Poor linear growth may be the first sign of hypothyroidism associated with CLT. Obesity with normal linear growth argues against hypothyroidism as the cause of increased weight. Accelerated linear growth is common in hyperthyroidism.
- **Neurologic examination.** Restlessness, tremor, and hyperreflexia are common features of hyperthyroidism. In contrast, decreased energy and delayed relaxation phase of deep tendon reflexes are common findings in hypothyroidism.
- **Eye examination.** Exophthalmos, lid lag, eyelid edema, and conjunctival injection are common features of Graves disease.
- **Thyroid examination.** Careful palpation and measurement of the gland is performed with the examiner standing behind a seated or standing patient. The size and texture of the gland, symmetry of enlargement, associated lymphadenopathy, and any tenderness should be noted.

Laboratory Studies

Laboratory studies are guided by the history and physical examination findings. They commonly include evaluation of **T_4 and/or free T_4, TSH, and thyroid antibodies** (antithyroglobulin and antithyroperoxidase). In cases of suspected hyperthyroidism, **T_3** must also be measured because children occasionally manifest predominant T_3 toxicosis with normal or near-normal T_4. Thyroid-stimulating immunoglobulin and/or thyroid-binding inhibitory immunoglobulin antibody levels can also be measured in patients with suspected Graves disease. Elevations in total T_4 are seen in states of **increased binding** such as in pregnancy and use of oral birth control pills with an associated increase in thyroid-binding globulin. Free T_4 assays may be affected by certain medications such as **antiseizure** therapies. Free T_4 by equilibrium dialysis would be an appropriate alternative if one is suspicious of an interfering antibody (heterophile antibody).

Treatment

If an individual with goiter is found to be hypothyroid or hyperthyroid, appropriate treatment with sodium L-thyroxine or antithyroid medications as outlined previously should be initiated. The case of a euthyroid patient is less clear; for example, the presence of antibodies with normal T_4 and TSH does not require thyroid hormone replacement. Instead, close monitoring of thyroid function every 6 to 12 months is an acceptable alternative.

Suggested Readings

American Academy of Pediatrics, Rose SR; Section on Endocrinology and Committee on Genetics, American Thyroid Association, Brown RS; Public Health Committee, Lawson Wilkins Pediatric Endocrine Society, Foley T, Kaplowitz PB, et al. Update of newborn screening and therapy for congenital hypothyroidism. *Pediatrics.* 2006;117(6):2290–2303.

American Thyroid Association (ATA) Guidelines Taskforce on Thyroid Nodules and Differentiated Thyroid Cancer, Cooper DS, Doherty GM, et al. Revised American Thyroid Association management guidelines for patients with thyroid nodules and differentiated thyroid cancer. *Thyroid.* 2009;19(11):1167–1214.

Foley TP. Hypothyroidism. *Pediatr Rev.* 2004;25(3):94–100.

Jaruratanasirikul S, Leethanaporn K, Khuntigij P, et al. The clinical course of Hashimoto's thyroiditis in children and adolescents: 6 years longitudinal follow-up. *J Pediatr Endocrinol Metab.* 2001;14: 177–184.

Jaruratanasirikul S, Leethanaporn K, Suchat K. The natural clinical course of children with an initial diagnosis of simple goiter: a 5-year longitudinal follow-up. *J Pediatr Endocrinol Metab.* 2000;13: 1109–1113.

LaFranchi SH, Austin J. How should we be treating children with congenital hypothyroidism? *J Pediatr Endocrinol Metab.* 2007;20(5):559–578.

Niedziela M. Pathogenesis, diagnosis and management of thyroid nodules in children. *Endocr Relat Cancer.* 2006;13(2):427–453.

Reiners C, Demidchik YE. Differentiated thyroid cancer in childhood: pathology, diagnosis and therapy. *Pediatr Endocrinol Rev.* 2003;1(Suppl 2):230–236.

Rivkees SA, Mattison DR. Ending propylthiouracil-induced liver failure in children. *N Engl J Med.* 2009;360:1574–1575.

Rivkees SA. The treatment of Graves' disease in children. *J Pediatr Endocrinol Metab.* 2006;19(9): 1095–1111.

Thyroid Internet Textbook. Available at: http://www.thyroidmanager.org/thyroidbook.htm. Accessed July 12, 2004.

Waguespack SG, Francis G. Initial management and follow-up of differentiated thyroid cancer in children. *J Natl Compr Canc Netw.* 2010;8(11):1289–1300.

CHAPTER 37

Oluwakemi B. Badaki-Makun
Joel A. Fein

Head Trauma

INTRODUCTION

Head injury in children accounts for up to 650,000 emergency department visits, 95,000 hospitalizations, and 7,400 deaths per year. It is the most significant cause of morbidity and mortality in pediatric trauma patients. The highest injury rates are found in children <4 years. Brain injuries can be subdivided into primary and secondary injuries. Primary injuries occur as a result of a mechanical damage at the time of insult and can be from direct trauma to the brain or shear forces experienced by the neuronal axons as a result of acceleration–deceleration injury. These injuries are usually irreversible. Fatal or irreversible injury is usually a sequela of neuronal cell death and vascular disruption during the first few milliseconds of impact. Secondary brain injuries result from subsequent pathophysiologic changes such as hypoperfusion, hypoxia, edema, and metabolic derangements. **The only injuries that are reversible with therapy are those with secondary effects on the brain and blood vessels, such as cerebral edema and impaired glucose and oxygen delivery to the neurons.**

 DIFFERENTIAL DIAGNOSIS LIST

Focal Injuries
- Scalp lacerations
- Hematoma (subgaleal, subdural, epidural)
- Cerebral contusion
- Fractures

Diffuse Injuries
- Concussion syndrome
- Diffuse axonal injury
- Increased intracranial pressure (ICP)

DIFFERENTIAL DIAGNOSIS DISCUSSION
Scalp Lacerations

Scalp lacerations are common findings in patients with head injuries. Blood loss can be extensive, especially in infants and young children, given the high vascularity of the scalp. The physician should apply direct pressure to stop local bleeding, carefully assess the **depth of the wound,** and evaluate it for **retained foreign bodies**. In addition, the **integrity of the galea aponeurotica** (a tendinous sheath located just above the periosteum) should be evaluated; attention to careful reapproximation of this layer often results in better hemostasis and easier closure of the laceration. Finally, the physician should search for **skull fractures or "step-offs" (dents)**.

Hematomas

Hematoma caused by head injury may exist outside of the confines of the skull (e.g., cephalohematoma, subgaleal hematoma) or inside the skull (e.g., epidural or subdural hematoma). **Intracranial lesions** may require **neurosurgical intervention,** whereas **extracranial lesions** rarely require any treatment other than **supportive care**.

Cephalohematoma

Newborn infants commonly incur a cephalohematoma, in which blood collects between the periosteum and the table of the skull and is therefore prevented from spreading past the midline. This type of injury is common in traumatic deliveries.

Subgaleal Hematoma

A posttraumatic, well-circumscribed "lump" on an older child's head usually represents a subgaleal hematoma.

Epidural and Subdural Hematomas

Epidural hematomas are less often associated with underlying brain injury than are subdural hematomas (Table 37-1).

Subarachnoid Hemorrhage

Common in more severely injured patients, subarachnoid hemorrhage (SAH) results from shearing of small vessels in the pia mater. It is usually associated with other intracranial injuries. Due to the location of the bleed, SAH causes meningeal irritation and the clinical symptoms can mimic meningitis.

Cerebral Contusions and Lacerations

Cerebral contusions are bruises of the cortex and can occur as a **coup injury** (at the contact location) or as a **contre-coup injury** (rebounding, on the opposite side). Late intraparenchymal hematomas may occur.

Cerebral lacerations usually result from **penetrating injury** to the brain or from a **depressed skull fracture**. The clinical manifestations are more often a result of the associated concussion and the underlying brain injury than of the focal lesions themselves.

Skull Fractures

A significant proportion of children seen in emergency departments with head injury have skull fractures. Infants and children with trauma to the parietal area are at higher risk.

Linear Skull Fractures

Linear skull fractures comprise 75% to 90% of all skull fractures. **Usually no treatment is necessary.** However, if the fracture is located over a vascular structure (e.g., the middle meningeal artery), there is an increased incidence of epidural

TABLE 37-1	**Epidural Versus Acute Subdural Hematoma**	
	Epidural Hematoma	**Subdural Hematoma**
Common mechanism	Blunt direct trauma, frequently to parietal or temporal regions, lower forces	Acceleration–deceleration injury, direct trauma, higher forces
Etiology	Arterial or venous (bleed between skull and dura)	Venous (bridging veins between dura and arachnoid membranes)
Incidence	Uncommon	Common
Peak age	Usually >2 yr	Usually <1 yr, peak at 6 mo
Location	Unilateral, commonly parietal	75% Bilateral, diffuse, over cerebral hemispheres
Skull fracture	Common	Uncommon
Associated seizures	Uncommon	Common
Retinal hemorrhages	Rare	Common
Decreased level of consciousness	Common	Almost always (50% present in coma)
Mortality	Rare	Uncommon
Morbidity in survivors	Low	High, due to associated underlying brain injury
Other clinical findings	Dilated ipsilateral pupil, contralateral hemiparesis Period of lucidity prior to acute decompensation and rapid progression to herniation (only 20%)	Decreased level of consciousness Headaches, irritability, emesis
Onset	Acute	Acute (within 24 hr), subacute (within 1 d to 2 wk), or chronic (after 2 wk)
Findings on computed tomography	Lentiform "lens-shaped," usually not crossing suture lines	Lunar "crescent shaped," often not crossing midline (due to falx cerebri)

hemorrhage. **Diastatic ("growing") fractures can develop when meninges get caught between the bone edges** and continue to separate them.

Basilar Skull Fractures

Basilar skull fractures typically occur in the **petrous portion of the temporal bone**. Potential findings on physical examination of a patient with a basilar skull fracture include the following:

- "Raccoon" eyes (ecchymosis below the eyes)
- Battle sign (ecchymosis at the mastoid)
- Hemotympanum (blood behind the eardrum)
- Cerebrospinal fluid (CSF) otorrhea or rhinorrhea
- Cranial nerve dysfunction, especially involving the seventh and eighth cranial nerves

Depressed Skull Fractures

Depressed skull fractures can sometimes be diagnosed clinically, by palpation of the depression of the skull underneath a hematoma, or radiographically, using tangential views of the skull or a computed tomography (CT) scan. **Surgical elevation** may be necessary **if the fracture extends past the inner table of the skull**.

Concussion Syndromes

Concussion syndromes are diagnosed when blunt head injury results in a transient impairment in awareness and responsiveness. According to the American Academy of Neurology, concussions are trauma-induced alterations in mental status that may or may not be associated with loss of consciousness. CT scans are usually normal. Loss of consciousness and amnesia may be important indicators of more severe injury. The **symptoms can last from a few seconds to several hours but in most cases resolve within 7 to 10 days**. Some patients complain of persistent headaches, dizziness, and subtle differences in memory, anxiety level, and/or sleep patterns lasting months after head injury. Pediatric patients are also at higher risk of **second impact syndrome,** which occurs when an athlete sustains a second head injury prior to resolution of symptoms from an earlier concussion. This can lead to severe neurologic sequelae including cerebral vascular congestion, diffuse brain swelling, and death.

Diffuse Axonal Injury

Diffuse axonal injury occurs when nerve fibers are sheared on initial impact. Patients exhibit **persistent functional neurologic deficits** (e.g., a prolonged comatose state) with sometimes absent radiographic abnormalities. Diffuse axonal injury is associated with high morbidity and mortality rates. It is **most frequently associated with child abuse or motor vehicle crashes**.

Increased Intracranial Pressure

Increased intracranial pressure (ICP) **affects the delivery of oxygen and substrate to the brain tissue**. An increase in one component of the intracranial contents (i.e., blood, CSF, or tissue) necessitates a decrease in another component because, under normal conditions, the sum of these compartments in the cranial vault remains constant. Therefore, if the ICP increases to more than the normal limit (15 mm Hg), small changes in the volume of the intracranial contents result in large changes in ICP. The **brain tissue and blood vessels** become **increasingly compressed,** disrupting cerebral blood flow or causing herniation of brain tissue through the dural reflections.

APPROACH TO THE PATIENT

Stabilization

Initial priorities for any severely injured child are **protection of the airway, maintenance of adequate tissue perfusion, and rapid assessment of neurologic status**.

Although the primary injury to the brain is irreversible, the secondary injury may be minimized in the acute care setting.

Airway

Upper airway obstruction is initially managed with proper **adjustment of the head, neck, and mandible** to clear the soft tissues and tongue away from the airway. Stabilization of the cervical spine is considered as a part of the airway evaluation. Before undertaking radiographic and clinical examination of the cervical spine, a **cervical collar** should be used with side immobilization, or manual immobilization should be provided.

Breathing

The head trauma victim with a clear upper airway but decreased breath sounds may have one of many injuries:

- Pneumothorax
- Pulmonary contusion
- Flail chest
- Central nervous system depression

Circulation

Lack of brain perfusion can lead to irreversible neuronal cell damage. **The cerebral perfusion pressure equals the mean arterial pressure minus the ICP.** Therefore, the goal of management is to normalize the mean arterial pressure while minimizing ICP.

Shock should be dealt with aggressively in the trauma patient, regardless of concern about increased ICP. Shock must be addressed as if it were a hypovolemic shock, until proven otherwise; it cannot be presumed to be secondary to spinal cord injury (neurogenic shock). The administration of crystalloid (e.g., normal saline or lactated Ringer's solution) or colloid (e.g., whole blood) should be based on the patient's heart rate, skin perfusion, and urinary output.

Assessment of Neurologic Disability

The **Glasgow coma scale (GCS) score** should be obtained (see Chapter 21, "Coma," Table 21-4), and the **pupils and gag reflex** should be evaluated relatively early to determine the presence of brain herniation as well as the need for endotracheal intubation. The GCS score is a prognostic tool for patients with head trauma (Table 37-2).

TABLE 37-2	Factors Associated with a Poor Outcome in Children with Head Injury

Age <2 yr

Glasgow coma scale (GCS) score <5

Subdural hematoma

Decerebrate or flaccid posture

Coma >24 hr

Management of Increased ICP

- **Hyperventilation** reduces the "blood" portion of the cerebral vault by constricting the cerebral vessels; however, this leads to decreased cerebral perfusion and may result in iatrogenic ischemia in an already traumatized brain. For the latter reason, prophylactic hyperventilation after traumatic brain injury is no longer recommended. The arterial carbon dioxide tension ($PaCO_2$) should be maintained at, or slightly above, approximately 35 mm Hg. Mild hyperventilation ($PaCO_2$ 30 to 35 mm Hg) is an option in patients with persistently increased ICP refractory to sedation, analgesia, CSF drainage, or hyperosmolar therapy.

- **Hyperosmolar therapy** is thought to reduce the "tissue" portion of the intracranial vault by drawing water out of the brain. Hypertonic saline (3% saline, 0.1 to 1 mL/kg per hour as a continuous infusion) may be given for this purpose; Mannitol (0.5 to 1 g/kg intravenously as a single bolus) may also be used for this purpose but may actually increase ICP with continuous use. The presence of hypotension or hypovolemia is a relative contraindication to the use of hyperosmolar agents.

- **Maintenance of normal intracranial pressure** is also facilitated by elevating the head to 30°, correcting systemic hypotension with fluid resuscitation, and taking measures to stop seizure activity, if present.

Further Evaluation

Patient History

A brief history of the **events before, during, and after the traumatic episode** should be obtained, focusing on the timing and mechanism of injury, duration of unconsciousness, presence of amnesia, neurologic assessment at the scene, and any preexisting medical conditions.

Physical Examination

A **secondary survey** should follow soon after the primary survey and include a close inspection of the head, torso, abdomen, genitalia, and extremities. It is important to examine the head for lacerations, depressions, contusions, or signs of basilar skull fracture.

In the comatose patient, a **normal oculovestibular response** implies that the cranial nerve pathways, most proximal to the brainstem (i.e., the third, sixth, and eighth cranial nerves), are intact and that, by association, the neighboring brainstem is functional. Performance of this test can be delayed until after the secondary survey is completed.

The **oculocephalic ("doll's eye") reflex** should not be performed in patients who might have a cervical spine injury.

Diagnostic Modalities

Patients with a GCS >14 and who have none of the symptoms listed in Table 37-3 are highly unlikely to have clinically important traumatic brain injury and do not routinely require a head CT.

Management of Complications

Posttraumatic seizures develop in a small percentage of patients who have experienced head trauma and are classified as immediate (within 24 hours of injury),

TABLE 37-3	Possible Predictors of Clinically Important Traumatic Brain Injury	
	Age <2 yr	Age >2 yr
Loss of consciousness ≥5 sec	√	√
Altered mental status	√	√
Severe mechanism of injury	√	√
Palpable or suspected skull fracture	√	√
Not acting normally per parent report	√	
Occipital or parietal scalp hematoma	√	
Severe headache		√
History of vomiting		√

From: Kuppermann N, Holmes JF, Dayan PS, et al. Pediatric Emergency Care Applied Research Network (PECARN). Identification of children at very low risk of clinically-important brain injuries after head trauma: a prospective cohort study. *Lancet.* 2009;374(9696):1160–1170.

early (within 1 week of injury), and late (occurring >1week after the initial injury). Owing to its rapid onset of action, a **benzodiazepine** should be administered to an acutely seizing patient. **Phenytoin** should be used as a second antiepileptic agent in this setting. Prophylactic antiepileptics may be useful in preventing seizures after traumatic brain injury (TBI) within the first 7 days but have not been shown to be effective in preventing seizures in these patients beyond that point.

TREATMENT OF HEAD TRAUMA
Severe Head Trauma
Treatment consists of **head CT scan and management of intracranial pressure** as needed. Patients with severe head trauma include those with the following characteristics:

- Abnormal neurologic examination
- Persistent seizures
- Persistently altered level of consciousness (GCS score <14)
- Depressed or basilar skull fracture

Moderate Head Trauma
Treatment consists of **12 to 24 hours of observation**. CT of the head may be considered. Patients with "moderate" head trauma include those with a history of amnesia or a brief loss of consciousness but a normal neurologic examination. Patients with persistent or worsening headache, vomiting, or reported seizure activity are also considered to have moderate head injury.

Mild Head Trauma
For the head trauma to be considered **mild,** the patient must have a normal neurologic examination and no reported amnesia. Such patients can be **observed at**

home by a reliable caretaker. The caretaker should bring the patient back to the emergency department if any of the following conditions develop:

- A headache that worsens or is unrelieved by acetaminophen
- Frequent vomiting or vomiting beyond 8 hours post injury
- Change in behavior or gait
- Vision problems
- Fever or stiff neck
- Evidence of clear or bloody fluid draining from the nose or ear
- Difficulty in awakening from sleep
- Seizures
- Bleeding that is unrelieved by the application of pressure for 5 minutes

Concussions

Stepwise return to activity is recommended:

1. Physical and mental rest until asymptomatic
2. Light aerobic exercise
3. Sport-specific exercise
4. Noncontact training drills
5. Full-contact training
6. Return to competition

Each step should last at least 24 hours. A patient cannot return to competitive activity until at least 5 days after the concussion and should **never return to play if persistently symptomatic at rest or with exertion**. Medical clearance is recommended prior to return to full contact training or competitive play.

Suggested Readings

Adelson PD, Bratton SL, Carney NL, et al. Guidelines for the acute medical management of severe traumatic brain injury in infants, children and adolescents. *Pediatr Crit Care Med.* 2003;4:S1–S71.

Halstead ME, Walter KD, Council on Sports Medicine and Fitness. American Academy of Pediatrics. Clinical report–sport-related concussion in children and adolescents. *Pediatrics.* 2010;126(3): 597–615.

Kaye AJ, Gallagher R, Callahan JM, et al. Mild traumatic brain injury in the pediatric population: the role of the pediatrician in routine follow-up. *J Trauma.* 2010;68(6):1396–1400.

Kuppermann N, Holmes JF, Dayan PS, et al. Pediatric Emergency Care Applied Research Network (PECARN). Identification of children at very low risk of clinically-important brain injuries after head trauma: a prospective cohort study. *Lancet.* 2009;374(9696):1160–1170.

CHAPTER 38

Nicholas S. Abend
Donald Younkin

Headache

INTRODUCTION

Headaches are common in children and adolescents. The incidence increases from early childhood to adolescence. Headaches may be classified as primary or secondary (Table 38-1). **Primary** headaches are diagnosed based on groupings of symptoms and signs, and include migraine, tension-type, and cluster headaches. **Secondary** headaches are symptomatic of an underlying intracranial or medical condition. Headaches may also be classified in terms of time course (Figure 38-1). In acute headache, there is a single episode of headache without prior headaches. In acute recurrent headache, there are stereotyped headaches separated by headache-free periods. In chronic progressive headache, there is a gradual increase in headache intensity. In chronic nonprogressive headache, there is a constant steady headache.

DIFFERENTIAL DIAGNOSIS LIST

Acute Headache

Intracranial hemorrhage—subarachnoid, intraparenchymal, subdural, epidural
Meningitis/encephalitis
Infections: Sinusitis, pharyngitis, otitis media
First migraine, tension-type, or cluster headache
Febrile illness-related headache (often related to upper respiratory tract infection)
Dental or Temporo-Mandibular Joint dysfunction
Hydrocephalus
Vasculitis
Intracranial hypertension—primary (pseudotumor) or secondary
Intracranial hypotension
Arterial ischemic stroke
Neoplasm
Hypertension
Ventriculo-peritoneal shunt malfunction
Toxins (carbon monoxide, lead)

Acute Recurrent Headache

Migraine or tension-type headaches
Episodic intracranial hypertension (i.e., ventricular tumor)

TABLE 38-1 | **Simplified International Classification of Headache Disorders**

Primary headache

Migraine

Migraine without aura

Migraine with aura

Hemiplegic migraine (familial or sporadic)

Basilar-type migraine

Childhood periodic syndromes that are commonly precursors of migraine

    Cyclic vomiting, abdominal migraine, benign paroxysmal vertigo of childhood

Retinal migraine

Complications of migraine

    Chronic migraine, status migrainosus, migrainous infarction

Tension headache

    Episodic or chronic

Trigeminal autonomic cephalalgias

    Cluster Headache

    Paroxysmal hemicrania (episodic of chronic)

    Short-lasting unilateral neuralgiform headache attacks with conjunctival injection
       and tearing

Chronic headaches

    New daily persistent headache

    Medication overuse headache

    Transformed migraine or tension headache

    Hemicrania continua

Others

    Exertional, cough, stabbing, hypnic, primary thunderclap

Secondary headache

Acute and chronic posttraumatic headache

Headache attributed to intracranial hematoma (traumatic or nontraumatic)

Headache attributed to head or neck trauma.

Headache attributed to cranial or cervical vascular disorders

Acute ischemic cerebrovascular disorder

Unruptured vascular malformation

Headache due to arteritis

Cerebral venous thrombosis

High CSF pressure

Low CSF pressure

Noninfectious inflammatory disorder

Headache attributed to neoplasm

Epileptic seizures

Headache due to Chiari type I malformation

Headache associated with substance abuse or withdrawal

Intracranial infection

Systemic infection

Hypoxia and or hypercapnia

Dialysis headache

Hypertension

Hypothyroidism

Fasting

Headache or facial pain associated with disorder of cranium, neck, eyes, ears, nose sinuses,
    teeth, and mouth

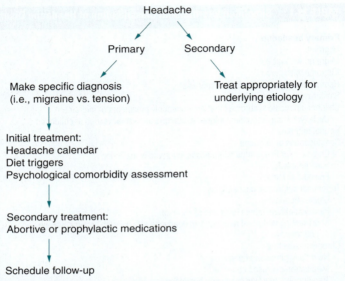

FIGURE 38-1   Temporal patterns of headache. (Adapted from Rothner AD. The evaluation of headaches in children and adolescents. *Semin Pediatr Neurol.* 1995;2:109–118).

Chronic Progressive Headache

Neoplasm
Intracranial hypertension
  (primary or secondary)
Neoplasm
Abscess
Epidural or Subdural Hemorrhage
Vascular Malformation
Toxins (carbon monoxide, lead)

Chronic Nonprogressive Headache

Chronic daily headache
Medication overuse
  headache
New daily persistent
  headache
Psychosomatic
Post-concussion syndrome

DIFFERENTIAL DIAGNOSIS DISCUSSION

> **HINT:** An acute onset severe headache requires urgent evaluation since specific and rapid therapy may be required. A chronic progressive headache is suggestive of an enlarging intracranial lesion and requires neuroimaging evaluation.

Acute Onset (Thunderclap) Headache

Thunderclap headache (or sudden severe headache onset) is uncommon, but recognition and accurate diagnosis of this headache are important because there is often a serious underlying brain disorder that requires specific and urgent therapy.

These include subarachnoid hemorrhage, parenchymal hemorrhage, sinovenous thrombosis, intracranial infection, arterial dissection, pituitary apoplexy, intracranial hypotension, and intermittent hydrocephalus. After a history and physical examination, diagnostic testing often begins with a noncontrast head computed tomography (CT) in which acute blood will be bright. If subarachnoid hemorrhage is suspected and the head CT is nondiagnostic, then lumbar puncture should be performed with two tubes sent for cell count (to differentiate between subarachnoid blood in which the red blood cell count will remain constant and a traumatic tap in which the red blood cell count will decrease from tube 1 to tube 4). If arterial dissection, sinovenous thrombosis, or tumor is suspected, then MRI with and without gadolinium is indicated and may require specific sequences to visualize the neck vasculature or venous sinuses. If intracranial hypertension or hypotension is suspected, then a lumbar puncture with opening pressure is indicated. Generally, neuroimaging is indicated prior to lumbar puncture since mass lesions may pose the risk of herniation with lumbar puncture. Only after appropriate evaluation can more benign etiologies be diagnosed including first or severe migraine or tension headache, cluster headache, or exertion/coital headache.

Migraine Headache

Migraine is the most common primary headache disorder in children. Migraine is defined as five or more attacks of headache that lasts for 1 to 72 hours (shorter than required in adult criteria), with a throbbing or pulsatile quality, moderate to severe intensity, bilateral or unilateral in the frontal or temporal regions, exacerbation or causing avoidance of routine physical activity, associated with nausea and/or emesis, light and sound sensitivity (which may be inferred from behavior), and often a need to sleep. A family history of migraine is often present. Migraine without aura is most common. Migraine with **aura** refers to fully reversible visual, sensory, or language symptoms that generally develop over 5 minutes and last from 5 to 60 minutes. The diagnosis is made clinically, but if there are atypical features or with the first aura, especially without a typical migraine headache associated, neuroimaging is indicated to evaluate for other acute etiologies such as stroke.

Patients may be instructed to keep a headache diary and to ensure adequate sleep, nutrition, and exercise. An attempt to identify dietary triggers (chocolate, cheese, nitrite-containing foods such as processed meats, monosodium gulatamate) may be useful. Eliminating caffeine intake and avoiding medication overuse, both of which may result in chronic headache, may be the useful initial steps. Several neutraceuticals including coenzyme Q10, riboflavin, and magnesium oxide may be useful.

If headaches are infrequent and the child can accurately identify the headache onset, then abortive medications may be indicated. These include ibuprofen, acetaminophen, naproxen sodium, metoclopramide, promethazine, prochlorperazine, dihydroergotamine, and the triptan medications. The triptan medications are thought to act on serotonin receptors of the nerve endings and blood vessels, impacting release of multiple neuropeptides. Triptans are contraindicated if there is history suggestive of cerebral ischemia (complicated migraine), cardiac disease, hypertension, or recent use of ergot medications. Only almotriptan tablets and zolmitriptan nasal spray are FDA approved for use in 12- to 17-year-olds, although all triptans are used in clinical practice. For an individual patient, one triptan may be more effective than others, so failure of one or several triptans does not preclude trying other triptan medications. All are taken at the onset of migraine and may be repeated 2 hours later if the headache persists. These medications may be more effective if used quickly upon headache onset, so a note to allow medication administration at school is often useful. Sumatriptan is available as tablets, injection, or nasal spray. Proper instruction is required for the nasal spray since it is used differently than typical nasal sprays (don't tilt head back and don't inhale). Zolmitriptan is available as a tablet and as a nasal spray. Rizatriptan is available as a standard tablet, disintegrating tablet (useful in pediatric population) or nasal spray. Naratriptan, almotriptan, frovatriptan, and eletriptan are available as tablets. Frovatriptan is longer acting than the other triptans and may be useful for hormonally induced migraines in women. One combination of triptan medication available is sumatriptan–naproxen.

If the headache is frequent (>2 to 3 per week), chronic, has an unclear onset, or abortive medications are inadequate, then prophylactic medications may be indicated. Treatment is titrated up as needed and the goal is to reduce headache frequency over several weeks to months. Cyproheptadine is an antihistamine medication useful for migraine prevention, but often sedating. Antidepressants include the tricyclics amitriptyline and nortriptyline and the serotonin–norepinephrine reuptake inhibitors venlafaxine and duloxetine. Few studies of these medications are available, but amitriptyline is a common first choice. Anticonvulsants including topiramate, valproic acid, levetiracetam, and gabapentin may be useful and are commonly used in the pediatric population for epilepsy management. Valproic acid may cause weight gain, requires blood testing, and has a high teratogenicity risk. The β-blocker proranolol and the calcium channel blocker verapamil may be useful, though the former is contraindicated with asthma. Psychological intervention and biobehavioral feedback may also be beneficial.

For **status migrainosus,** there are a few studies to guide treatment but there is clinical experience with intravenous dihydroergotamine protocols (generally with metoclopramide to reduce nausea), intravenous metoclopramide or prochlorperazine, intravenous valproic acid, or steroids.

 HINT: Triptans are contraindicated in the setting of focal neurological signs.

Tension Headache

Tension headaches last 5 minutes to 7 days (shorter than required in adults), are bilateral, have a pressing/tightening quality of pain, are mild to moderate in severity, are not aggravated by routine physical activity (as vs. migraine), and are not associated with other migrainous features. They may be episodic or chronic (if more than 15 per month). There have been a few studies of treatment in children, but antidepressants (amitriptyline), relaxation training, and biofeedback may be useful.

Trigeminal Autonomic Cephalgias

Cluster headache and the trigeminal autonomic cephalgias consist of repetitive attacks of intense headache that is often excruciating, unilateral, and boring in character accompanied by prominent cranial parasympathetic signs and symptoms such as conjunctival injection and tearing, eyelid edema, nasal congestion and rhinorrhea, facial sweating, and miosis ipsilateral to the headache. Migrainous features such as nausea and photophobia may occur. Attack frequency and duration vary in different syndromes. Cluster headache attacks generally last 15 to 180 minutes, occur every other day to 8 times per day, and often occur in clusters separated by attack-free periods. Attacks lasting 5 seconds to 4 minutes and occurring 5 to 200 times per day occur in short-lasting unilateral neuralgiform headache attacks with conjunctival injection and tearing. Attacks lasting 2 to 30 minutes and occurring up to 5 times per day constitute **paroxysmal hemicrania**. Although rare, accurate diagnosis is important since specific treatments are available. Indomethacin relieves attacks in paroxysmal hemicrania (and hemicrania continua described below). Oxygen and triptans may relieve cluster headache, and prophylactic medications may include verapamil, lithium, valproic acid, and topiramate.

Chronic Daily Headache

In some children, headaches are present for more than 15 days per month. Most of these children had episodic headaches that increased in frequency and eventually became chronic, although in some children headaches may be chronic from the onset (new daily persistent headache). Suggested risk factors for transformation include headaches more than 1 to 3 times per month, obesity, and medication overuse. Medication overuse headache is defined by frequent medication use (>10 to 15 times per month) and may occur with over-the-counter medications, triptans, ergots, and opiods. Medications may be changed to longer acting formulations to help reduce the symptoms of withdrawal, but treatment requires withdrawal of medications and detoxification. Associated psychiatric conditions including anxiety, mood disorders, and somatoform disorders are common and must be treated in conjunction with tapering of the overused medication. **Hemicrania continua** may result in chronic headache with mild associated parasympathetic signs and is relieved with indomethacin.

Pseudotumor Cerebri

Elevated intracranial pressure may result in headache and may be due to a secondary etiology or may be idiopathic (pseudotumor cerebri). Initially, the headache is often position dependent, worsening when lying supine or when waking in the morning and improving when upright. However, this position dependence may be less prominent with more long-standing headache. Many patients develop papilledema due to pressure-related axoplasmic stasis in the optic nerves. Other symptoms include transient visual obscurations and horizontal diplopia (due to abducens nerve palsy with elevated intracranial pressure). Diagnosis is by lumbar puncture. Often, the headache improves after removal of cerebrospinal fluid (CSF), but this improvement is temporary as CSF is reformed several times per day. The diagnosis of idiopathic intracranial hypertension requires **ruling out secondary etiologies** such as sinovenous thrombosis that raise intracranial pressure (most children should undergo magnetic resonance imaging including venography), medication exposure (tetracycline and related compounds including retinoic acid and vitamin A, growth hormone, steroid hormone withdrawal), and endocrine disease (recent weight gain, hypoparathyroidism, Addison disease). **Secondary causes** are common in children and the most common etiologies are otitis media, viral infections, and predisposing medications. Initial measurement and tracking of visual fields is important since permanent vision loss may occur and rapidly progressive vision deterioration may be an indication for optic nerve sheath fenestration to reduce pressure. Secondary etiologies must be treated appropriately. Weight loss is important if there has been recent weight gain. If headache is present but papilledema is absent or mild, then a low salt diet and weight loss may be sufficient. If papilledema is moderate or headache is worsening, then diuretic medications including acetazolamide or furosemide may be provided. If papilledema is severe and visual loss progresses, then optic nerve sheath fenestration may be indicated. If headache is severe or progressive, then lumbar drainage may be indicated.

 HINT: Visual fields must be followed carefully in patients with pseudo-tumor cerebri since there is a risk of permanent visual loss and definitive treatment is available with optic nerve sheath fenestration.

Psychological Comorbidities
Many of the primary headaches including migraine and tension-type headaches, and especially chronic headaches, are associated with psychological comorbidity including depression and anxiety, and the treatment plan must address these issues. Treatment may involve medication, psychological counseling, biofeedback, or relaxation training.

EVALUATION OF THE PATIENT
- Useful questions to help evaluate the type of headache as well as the time course are listed in Table 38-2.
- Physical examination is important since focal signs suggest a secondary etiology of headache.
  - Medical examination
    - Vital signs (blood pressure, heart rate, respirations, temperature)
    - Cervical spine evaluation
    - Meningeal sign evaluation: Kernig, Brudzinski, nuchal rigidity
    - Skull: palpation and bruit assessment
    - Temporomandibular: Joint palpation and range of motion
    - Dental examination
    - Ear and tympanic membrane evaluation

TABLE 38-2	Useful Headache Questions

When did your headache start?

Did it start in a split second or start slowly?

Is there a history of head trauma?

What were you doing when your headache started?

Was this a sudden first headache?

Have you had headaches like this before?

How often do you get headaches?

Are your headaches getting worse or more frequent than they used to be?

Do you have the same kind of headaches all the time or do you have different types of headaches?

How long do your headaches last?

What do your headaches feel like?

How intense are your headaches?

Are there any signs that a headache is going to start?

Do you experience nausea, vomiting, dizziness, numbness, or weakness with the headache?

Do you get eye or nasal tearing with the headache?

What makes your headache better or worse?

Do you have to stop your activity when you have a headache?

Is there a trigger that causes you to get a headache?

Are you taking any medicines for your headache and how often do you take these medications?

Do you have any other health problems?

Does anyone else in your family get headaches?

- Sinus palpation
- Carotid artery bruit assessment
- Skin examination for neurocutaneous signs
- Neurologic examination
  - Head circumference
  - Cranial nerve II (optic nerve): papilledema, visual fields
  - Extraocular movements (CN3, 4, and 6)
  - Pupil size and reactivity
  - Motor: weakness, asymmetry, pronator drift
  - Deep tendon reflexes
  - Sensory examination
  - Coordination: dysmetria, tremor, and uncoordinated or slow rapid alternating movements
  - Gait: including tandem gait
- Indications for neuroimaging are listed in Table 38-3.

APPROACH TO THE PATIENT

See Figure 38-2.

TABLE 38-3 Neuroimaging Indications

Historical features and symptoms
Age younger than 3 yr or inability to provide clear history
Acute onset headache
Worst headache of life
Thunderclap headache
Chronic-progressive pattern
Headache or emesis on awakening or that wakes child from sleep
Headache associated with Valsalva or straining
Unvarying headache location
Occurring in context of psychiatric or cognitive changes
Immunocompromised

Signs
Hypertension
Macrocephaly
Meningeal signs
Focal neurologic symptoms or signs
Papilledema
Neurocutaneous signs

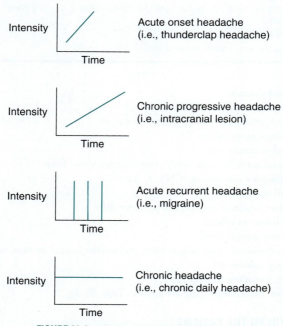

FIGURE 38-2 **Management of pediatric headache.**

Treatment

Appropriate treatment is dependent on the underlying etiology or headache or the specific primary headache diagnosis.

Suggested Readings

Abend NS, Younkin D, Lewis DW. Secondary headaches in children and adolescents. *Semin Pediatr Neurol.* 2010;17(2):123–133.

Gladstein J, Rothner AD. Chronic daily headache in children and adolescents. *Semin Pediatr Neurol.* 2010;17(2):88–92.

Hershey AD. Current approaches to the diagnosis and management of pediatric migraine. *Lancet Neurol.* 2010;9:190–204.

Kabbouche MA, Cleves C. Evaluation and management of mhildren and mdolescents presenting with an acute aetting. *Semin Pediatr Neurol.* 2010;17(2):105–108.

Lewis DW. Pediatric migraine. *Pediatr Rev.* 2007;28(2):43–53.

Lewis DW, Gozzo YF, Avner MT. The "other" primary headaches in children and adolescents. *Pediatr Neurol* 2005;33:303–313.

Lewis K. Pediatric headache. *Semin Pediatr Neurol.* 2010;17(4):224–229.

Ramadan NM, Olesen J. Classification of headache disorders. *Semin Neurol.* 2006;26(2):157–162.

Winner P, Lewis D, Rothner AD, eds. *Headache in Children and Adolescents.* 2nd ed. Hamilton, ON: BC Decker; 2008.

CHAPTER 39

Rebecca Ruebner
Madhura Pradhan

Hematuria

INTRODUCTION

Hematuria, the medical term for the presence of blood in the urine, is a common pediatric problem. Gross hematuria is the visible presence of blood in the urine, whereas microscopic hematuria is usually detected during a routine urinalysis. The incidence of gross hematuria among children presenting to an emergency department is 1.3 in 1,000, whereas 1% to 2% of school-aged children have microscopic hematuria in two or more urine samples. The American Academy of Pediatrics no longer recommends routine screening urinalysis for school-aged children and adolescents.

Hematuria can originate from the glomerulus or the lower urinary tract. Brown, tea-colored, or cola-colored urine is suggestive of glomerular bleeding, whereas bright red urine or presence of visible blood clots is suggestive of bleeding from the urinary tract. Hematuria is first detected by urine dipstick; however, the dipstick will also be positive in the setting of myoglobinuria or hemoglobinuria. Hematuria is confirmed by the presence of red blood cells (RBCs) on microscopic examination of a spun sediment of urine. Microscopic hematuria is defined by the presence of five or more RBCs per high-power field on at least three occasions over a 3-week period in a spun urine sample (see Table 39-1).

DIFFERENTIAL DIAGNOSIS LIST

Macroscopic Hematuria
Glomerular Disease
Acute postinfectious glomerulonephritis (GN)

Immunoglobulin A (IgA) nephropathy—*recurrent, gross hematuria*

Alport syndrome

Thin basement membrane disease

Systemic lupus erythematosus

Membranoproliferative glomerulonephritis (MPGN)

Henoch–Schönlein purpura

Membranous nephropathy

Vasculitis

Infections
Bacterial urinary tract infection (UTI), viral (adenovirus), tuberculosis

Structural Abnormalities
Congenital anomalies

Polycystic kidneys

Trauma

TABLE 39-1	Causes of Discolored Urine
Dark yellow or orange urine	Concentrated urine Rifampin, Pyridium, Macrodantin
Brown or black urine	Bile pigment Methemoglobinemia Homogentisic acid, thymol, melanin, tyrosinosis, alkaptonuria Alanine, cascara, resorcinol
Red or pink urine	Red blood cells, hemoglobin/myoglobin Benzene, chloroquine, deferoxamine, phenazo-pyridine, phenolphthalein Beets, blackberries, red dye Urates

Vascular anomalies—angiomyolipomas, arteriovenous malformations

Tumors

Hematologic
Sickle cell trait/disease
Coagulopathies—hemophilia
Renal vein thrombosis

Hypercalciuria and Nephrolithiasis
Exercise
Medications
Penicillins, polymyxin, sulfa-containing agents, anticonvulsants, warfarin, aspirin, colchicine, cyclophosphamide, indomethacin, gold salts

Others
Dyes (Table 39-1)
Loin pain-hematuria syndrome
Urethrorrhagia

Asymptomatic Microscopic Hematuria
Idiopathic
Thin basement membrane disease
Hypercalciuria
IgA nephropathy
Sickle cell trait or disease

DIFFERENTIAL DIAGNOSIS DISCUSSION
Glomerular Disease
GN (Table 39-2) usually presents with some combination of gross hematuria (often tea- or cola-colored), proteinuria, hypertension, RBC casts, acute kidney injury, and oligoanuria. GN can be categorized according to serum complement (C3) levels at presentation. Causes of hypocomplementemic GN include acute postinfectious GN, membranoproliferative GN, and systemic lupus erythematosus nephritis. The remainder of etiologies is associated with normal complement levels. The most common forms of nephritis are **acute poststreptococcal glomerulonephritis (APSGN) and IgA nephropathy**.

APSGN typically presents 10 to 14 days after an upper respiratory infection with beta-hemolytic streptococci or, in some cases, an episode of impetigo. IgA nephropathy often presents with recurrent hematuria and is commonly associated with a viral prodrome 1 to 3 days before the development of grossly bloody urine.

TABLE 39-2	Distinguishing Features of Glomerular and Nonglomerular Hematuria	
Feature	**Glomerular**	**Nonglomerular**
History		
Burning on micturition	No	Urethritis, cystitis
Systemic complaints	Edema, fever, pharyngitis, rash, arthralgias	Fever with UTI; pain with calculi
Family history	Deafness in Alport syndrome, renal failure	Usually negative, except with calculi
Physical Examination		
Hypertension	Often	Unlikely
Edema	Sometimes present	No
Abdominal mass	No	Wilms tumor, polycystic kidneys
Rash, arthritis	SLE, HSP	No
Urine Analysis		
Color	Brown: tea- or cola-colored	Bright red or pink
Proteinuria	Often	No
Dysmorphic RBCs	Yes	No
RBC casts	Yes	No
Crystals	No	May be informative

HSP, Henoch–Schönlein purpura; *RBC,* red blood cells; *SLE,* systemic lupus erythematosus; *UTI,* urinary tract infection.

All patients with suspected GN should have microscopic urinalysis, blood chemistries including serum creatinine, complete blood count, antistreptolysin O (ASO) titer and/or streptozyme, C3, and antinuclear antibody (ANA) when clinically indicated. The presence of **RBC casts in the urine is diagnostic of a GN**. Renal biopsy may be indicated in some instances, particularly if there is rapidly progressive GN characterized by rapid decline in kidney function.

 HINT: C3 levels should return to normal within 6 to 8 weeks after presentation of APSGN; a persistently low C3 level is suggestive of membranoproliferative glomerulonephritis.

The treatment of acute poststreptococcal nephritis is largely **supportive**. Careful attention to **fluid and electrolyte balance** is essential. **Urine output** should be optimized and diuretics may be needed. **Blood pressure should be carefully monitored and treated aggressively**. Patients with fluid overload need sodium and fluid restriction. Diuretics are first-line therapy for treatment of hypertension.

Alport syndrome is a **hereditary nephritis** associated with **sensorineural hearing loss**. Eighty percent of cases are transmitted as an X-linked dominant trait. The primary genetic defect involves the gene for collagen 4A5.

Alport syndrome presents with intermittent or persistent **microscopic hematuria or episodic gross hematuria**. Hearing deficit typically occurs in late childhood and deafness ultimately develops in 80% of males with X-linked Alport syndrome.

Alport is strongly suggested by a family history of chronic kidney disease associated with hearing loss. Diagnosis is confirmed by renal biopsy or genetic testing.

Urinary Tract Infection

Children with bacterial infections often present with dysuria, fever, burning on micturition, and increased urinary frequency or urgency. Adenoviral cystitis presents with painful gross hematuria. Urine analysis by dipstick is typically positive for nitrites (gram-negative organisms) and leukocyte esterase and reveals white blood cells on microscopic examination. Bacterial UTI is confirmed by >100,000 colony-forming units of a single organism on a clean-catch urine specimen or >50,000 colony-forming units from a catheterized specimen.

Trauma

Traumatic injury to the urogenital tract is frequently seen with blunt force trauma and may be **life threatening,** depending on the severity of injury.

 HINT: The presence of hematuria with minimal traumatic injury is highly suggestive of anatomic abnormalities of the kidney such as polycystic kidney disease.

Hematuria associated with renal trauma requires evaluation by computed tomography (CT) scan, renal ultrasound, or intravenous pyelography.

 HINT: When traumatic injury to the lower urinary tract is suspected, any imaging study involving placement of urethral or bladder catheters should be ordered only after urologic consultation.

Treatment is directed on the basis of severity of injury. Most renal contusions or lacerations can be managed **conservatively;** however, significant lacerations of the kidney or injury to the collecting system or lower urinary tract may require **emergent surgical intervention**.

Malignancy

Wilms tumor accounts for 90% of childhood malignancies that arise from the urogenital tract. Other tumors include renal cell carcinoma, mesoblastic nephroma, rhabdomyosarcoma, hemangioma, and sarcomas. Wilms tumor typically presents as an **abdominal mass with or without associated abdominal pain**. Microscopic hematuria is found in about 50% of patients at presentation, but gross hematuria is unusual. Hematuria as a sole presenting feature of Wilms tumor is exceedingly rare.

Up to 80% of patients with **tuberous sclerosis** may develop hematuria associated with hemorrhage from renal angiolipomas. Renal medullary carcinoma should be considered in patients with sickle cell trait.

Hematologic Causes

Hematuria is a common manifestation of sickle cell hemoglobinopathy and is thought to be caused by sickling and sludging of RBCs in the renal medulla. It can occur in patients with sickle cell disease or trait, is commonly painless, and may be microscopic or gross. Hematuria typically occurs in adolescent males and can be precipitated by trauma, exercise, dehydration, or infection. Papillary necrosis is also seen with severe dehydration and renal infarction.

> **HINT:** Hematuria, both gross and microscopic, is a common complication in patients with sickle cell trait.

Hematuria is rarely the sole finding in a patient with a coagulopathy. However, coagulopathies should be investigated in patients without another source for painless, gross hematuria and a history of bruising/bleeding or a family history of a bleeding diathesis.

Hypercalciuria

Hypercalciuria occurs in states of both **hypercalcemia and normocalcemia**. In normocalcemic patients, the most common cause is idiopathic; other causes include immobilization, Cushing syndrome, distal renal tubular acidosis, and Bartter syndrome. Disorders associated with hypercalcemia include hyperparathyroidism, vitamin D intoxication, hypophosphatasia, tumors, and immobilization bone resorption.

Idiopathic hypercalciuria typically presents with **asymptomatic microscopic hematuria**. As with secondary forms of hypercalciuria, these patients can also present with gross hematuria, renal colic, and dysuria.

The initial screening test for hypercalciuria is a **urine calcium-to-creatinine** (Ca:Cr) **ratio** on a spot urine sample. A ratio of >0.2 in older children and adults is highly suggestive of hypercalciuria. Normal values are higher in infants and young children. Confirmation should be obtained by **24-hour urine collection** with an excretion of >4 mg/kg/24 hours. **Serum chemistries,** including bicarbonate, potassium, calcium, phosphorus, magnesium, creatinine, and urine pH, should also be obtained. A detailed **family history** for stone disease, diet history, and evaluation of medications and nutritional supplements should be sought.

> **HINT:** Hypercalciuria is the most common metabolic abnormality found in patients with renal calculi.

Urolithiasis

Stone disease typically presents with **grossly bloody urine and renal colic**. Presentation with microscopic hematuria, penile pain, and passage of the stone or gravel may also be seen.

A family history of stone disease is frequently noted, particularly in older patients. **Renal ultrasound or CT scan** should be considered. If a stone is suspected, **blood chemistries** including calcium, phosphorus, magnesium, uric acid, and creatinine should be performed. **Urine pH and 24-hour urine collections** for calcium, cystine, oxalate, phosphorus, citrate, and uric excretion should be obtained. However, in young children, this is difficult. Attempts should be made to **recover the stone** or gravel for analysis of mineral content.

 HINT: Simple radiographs can detect kidney stones if the stone is radio-opaque (calcium, oxalate, cystine, or struvite). Uric acid stones and some cystine stones are radiolucent and not seen by plain film.

Management of these patients is twofold. First, acute management includes fluid administration and pain control. Surgical intervention or lithotripsy is indicated in cases of urinary obstruction or recurrent stones with superimposed UTIs. Second, once the cause has been determined, therapy to **prevent stone recurrence** can be implemented, which includes increased fluid intake to ensure dilute hypotonic urine, dietary manipulation, and drug therapy in some cases.

Medications

Microscopic hematuria related to drug exposure is not uncommon. Although some of these medications are commonly used in pediatrics, most are not (see section on "Differential Diagnosis List"). **Cyclophosphamide** is frequently associated with gross hematuria that can be severe in some cases.

Urethrorrhagia

Urethrorrhagia typically presents with **terminal hematuria** or bloody spots in the underwear in boys between **4 and 17 years of age**. The mean age of presentation is 10 years. Dysuria is present in nearly 30% of patients. It can be recurrent, but resolution usually occurs in nearly 92% with an average time course of 10 months (2 weeks to 3 years). Other causes of gross hematuria should be ruled out. Treatment is restricted to **watchful waiting**. Urethral stricture can be caused by cystoscopy; therefore, such procedures should be avoided.

Thin Basement Membrane Disease

This is often referred to as benign familial hematuria. It is transmitted in an autosomal dominant fashion. Diagnosis can be made based on clinical and pedigree data. Criteria for a clinical diagnosis include isolated hematuria, normal kidney function, urine protein excretion and blood pressure, positive family history of hematuria consistent with autosomal dominant transmission, and negative family history of kidney failure. Evaluation of parents' urine may be necessary to consider this diagnosis, which can be confirmed by **renal biopsy** that shows thin basement membranes.

EVALUATION OF HEMATURIA

 HINT: Gross hematuria should be evaluated as soon as possible. In addition, if proteinuria and/or red cell casts are absent, a renal ultrasound should be performed to exclude a malignancy.

Patient History

A **complete and thorough history** is essential for guiding the diagnostic evaluation of hematuria. The following information should be obtained (Figures 39-1 through 39-3):

- Previous episodes of gross hematuria or UTI
- Pattern of hematuria (initial, terminal)

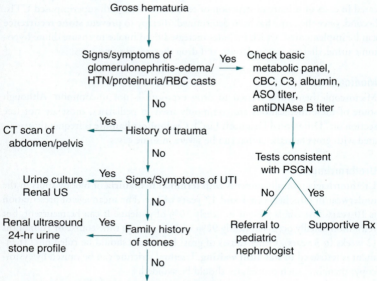

FIGURE 39-1   Evaluation of the pediatric patient with gross hematuria. *ASO,* antistreptolysin O titer; *C3,* third component of complement; *CBC,* complete blood count; *CT,* computed tomography; *Hb,* hemoglobin; *HTN,* hypertension; *PSGN,* poststreptococcal glomerulonephritis; *RBC,* red blood cells; *Rx,* prescription; *US,* ultrasound; *UTI,* urinary tract infection.

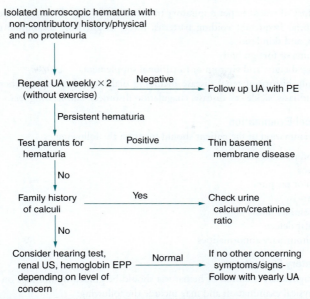

FIGURE 39-2   Evaluation of the pediatric patient with isolated microscopic hematuria.
UA, urinalysis; *US,* ultrasound.

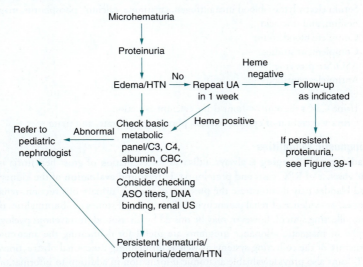

FIGURE 39-3   Evaluation of the pediatric patient with microscopic hematuria and other findings. *ASO,* antistreptolysin O titer; *C3,* third component of complement; *C4,* fourth component of complement; *CBC,* complete blood count; *HTN,* hypertension; *UA,* urinalysis; *US,* ultrasound.

- History of recent upper respiratory tract infections, sore throat, or impetigo
- Dysuria, frequency, voiding patterns, fever, weight loss, abdominal or flank pain, and skin lesions
- Trauma or foreign body
- Drug, dietary, and vitamin or nutritional supplements
- Family history of renal disease including dialysis and transplant, hematuria, urolithiasis, sickle cell disease, coagulation disorders, and hearing loss

Physical Examination

The examination of the patient should focus on the following:

- Blood pressure
- Edema
- Rash or purpura
- Arthritis
- Abdominal mass
- Ocular defects
- Genitourinary abnormalities

Laboratory Evaluation

The diagnostic evaluation of hematuria should be guided by findings on history and physical examination and may include the following:

- Fresh urinalysis with microscopic examination of sediment for RBCs, crystals, and casts
- Serum electrolytes—blood urea nitrogen, creatinine, calcium, phosphorus, magnesium, and uric acid
- Complete blood count
- Complement studies
- ASO/Streptozyme
- Antinuclear antibody
- Urine culture
- Urine Ca:Cr ratio or 24-hour urine calcium excretion
- Urinary excretion of cystine, oxalate, phosphorus, citrate, and urate

Diagnostic Modalities

Radiographic imaging is always indicated for evaluation of gross hematuria in the absence of RBC casts and proteinuria. **Ultrasound evaluation** of the kidneys and bladder may demonstrate the presence of tumors, urinary obstruction, renal stones, or evidence of renal parenchymal disease. Small stones or abnormalities of the collecting system, however, may be missed by ultrasound. Intravenous pyelography or magnetic resonance urograms are useful for delineating the anatomic structure of the collecting systems as well as for defining functional obstructions. CT scans also provide valuable anatomic information in addition to information about the presence of stones, tumors, or obstructions. Additional studies such as nuclear scans, cystoscopy, angiography, or renal biopsy should be considered in consultation with a subspecialist.

TREATMENT OF HEMATURIA

The treatment of hematuria is driven by the underlying pathophysiology and is in large part **conservative**. Hematuria with concurrent proteinuria, hypertension, renal failure, trauma, or severe hemorrhage may indicate the need for more **aggressive investigation and therapy**.

Suggested Readings

Diven SC, Travis LB. A practical primary care approach to hematuria in children. *Pediatr Nephrol.* 2000;14:65–72.

Feld LG, Meyers KE, Kaplan BS, et al. Limited evaluation of microscopic hematuria in pediatrics. *Pediatrics.* 1998;102(4):E42.

Feld LG, Waz WR, Perez LM, et al. Hematuria: an integrated medical and surgical approach. *Pediatr Clin North Am.* 1997;44(5):1191–1210.

Lieu TA, Grasmeder HM III, Kaplan BS. An approach to the evaluation and treatment of microscopic hematuria. *Pediatr Clin North Am.* 1991;38(3):579–592.

Mahan JD, Turman MA, Menster MI. Evaluation of hematuria, proteinuria, and hypertension in adolescents. *Pediatr Clin North Am.* 1997;44(6):1573–1589.

Meyers KEC. Evaluation of hematuria in children. *Urol Clin North Am.* 2004;31(3):559–573.

Roy S III. Hematuria. *Pediatr Ann.* 1996;25(5):284–287.

Hemolysis

INTRODUCTION

Hemolysis is **increased red blood cell (RBC) destruction with compensatory increased RBC production**. The patient with hemolysis usually presents with symptoms of **anemia and hyperbilirubinemia**. However, chronic hemolysis may be an incidental finding when a complete blood count (CBC) is obtained for other reasons.

The causes of hemolysis can be classified as intrinsic or extrinsic. **Intrinsic causes** are abnormalities that occur within the RBC (i.e., changes that involve the RBC membrane, enzymes, or hemoglobin). **Extrinsic causes** involve damage to normal RBCs by any external process. A second classification system categorizes the causes of hemolysis according to whether **RBC destruction occurs intravascularly or extravascularly** (Table 40-1). A third classification is according to whether the cause of hemolysis is inherited or acquired.

 DIFFERENTIAL DIAGNOSIS LIST

RBC Membrane Abnormalities
- Hereditary spherocytosis (HS)
- Hereditary elliptocytosis (HE)
- Hereditary pyropoikilocytosis
- Infantile pyknocytosis
- Paroxysmal nocturnal hemoglobinuria

Enzyme Defects
- Embden–Meyerhof pathway defects—pyruvate kinase deficiency
- Nucleotide metabolism defects—pyrimidine-5-nucleotidase deficiency
- Hexose monophosphate shunt defects—glucose-6-phosphate dehydrogenase (G6PD) deficiency

Hemoglobin Disorders
- Hemoglobinopathies— hemoglobin S, C, D, E
- Thalassemia syndromes— α-thalassemia, β-thalassemia
- Unstable hemoglobin syndromes— congenital Heinz-body hemolytic anemia, hemoglobin M disease

Alloimmune Causes
- Hemolytic disease of the newborn
- Hemolytic transfusion reaction

Autoimmune Causes
- **Warm-Reactive Antibodies**
  - Idiopathic
  - Neoplastic Causes
    - Immunodeficiency

TABLE 40-1	Intravascular and Extravascular Causes of Hemolysis

Intravascular Hemolysis
Disseminated intravascular coagulation (DIC)
Hemolytic uremic syndrome
Burns
Acute hemolytic transfusion reactions
Organ graft rejection
Prosthetic heart valves
Hemangiomata
March hemoglobinuria
Drugs
Venoms
Infections
Acute G6PD deficiency
Paroxysmal nocturnal hemoglobinuria

Extravascular Hemolysis
Alloimmune hemolysis
Autoimmune hemolysis
Red blood cell (RBC) membrane abnormalities
RBC enzyme abnormalities
Hemoglobinopathies
Thalassemia syndromes

G6PD, glucose phosphate dehydrogenase.

- Infectious Causes
  - Viruses (e.g., cytomegalovirus, hepatitis, influenza, coxsackievirus, HIV)
  - Bacteria (e.g., *Streptococcus, Escherichia coli, Salmonella typhi*)
  - Postimmunization (e.g., diphtheria-tetanus-pertussis, polio, typhoid)
- Toxic Causes
  - Antibiotics—penicillin, cephalothin, tetracycline, rifampin, and sulfonamides
  - Phenacetin
  - 5-Aminosalicylic acid
  - Quinine and quinidine
  - Insulin
  - Lead
  - Chlorpromazine
- Collagen Vascular Disease
  - Systemic lupus erythematosus
- Scleroderma
- Juvenile rheumatoid arthritis
- Polyarteritis nodosa
- Dermatomyositis
- **Cold-Reactive Antibodies**
  - Infectious Causes
    - Mycoplasma
    - Epstein–Barr virus (EBV)
    - HIV
  - Neoplastic Causes
    - Lymphoproliferative disease

Nonimmune Causes
- Microangiopathic Hemolytic Anemia
- Hypersplenism
- Toxic Causes
  - Drugs (e.g., vitamin K, phenacetin, sulfones, benzenes, phenylhydralazine)

- Lead
- Venoms
- Infectious Causes
  - Viruses (EBV, hepatitis)

- Bacteria (*Clostridium perfringens, E. coli, Streptococcus*)
- Parasites (malaria, histoplasmosis)

DIFFERENTIAL DIAGNOSIS DISCUSSION
Hereditary Spherocytosis
Etiology
Hereditary spherocytosis (HS), the most common **inherited RBC membrane defect,** is most often seen in patients of **northern European descent**. Genetic mutations in genes encoding RBC skeletal proteins lead to skeletal protein anomalies, membrane instability, and subsequent **hemolytic anemia** in affected individuals. Although HS is inherited in an autosomal dominant fashion, 10% to 25% of all cases are sporadic.

Clinical Features
The clinical severity depends on the severity of the hemolysis, which can be **mild to severe,** and on the degree of compensation by the patient. The classic clinical presentation of hemolytic anemia is **jaundice, pallor, and splenomegaly**. Patients may have hypersplenism, gallstones, worsening red cell destruction (hyperhemolysis) with infections, and transient red cell aplasia primarily caused by human parvovirus B19. Half of the patients have a history of **neonatal hyperbilirubinemia**.

Evaluation
The **peripheral blood smear** shows an **increased** number of **spherocytes** (i.e., small, round, dark-staining RBCs that lack central pallor). The mean corpuscular hemoglobin concentration is frequently elevated. Reticulocytosis is present. The **osmotic fragility test** demonstrates decreased resistance to osmotic lysis as compared with normal RBCs. The direct antibody test (DAT), often used to detect autoimmune hemolytic anemia (AIHA), is negative.

Treatment
Treatment of HS is **supportive**. Although transfusion of RBCs may be necessary for acute exacerbation of anemia, only a small number of patients depend on **RBC transfusions**. **Splenectomy** is used to decrease the extravascular red cell destruction and should be considered in children with poor growth or increased RBC transfusion requirements.

Hereditary Elliptocytosis
Etiology
Hereditary elliptocytosis (HE), more common in people of African or Mediterranean descent, is caused by genetic mutations that lead to red cell cytoskeleton instability. Similar to HS, HE is **inherited** in an autosomal dominant pattern, but sporadic mutations are not as common.

Clinical Features

Most children with HE are **asymptomatic,** but they may present for evaluation with a transient aplastic episode or a hyperhemolytic episode.

Evaluation

The **peripheral blood smear** reveals >15% elliptocytes (i.e., elongated, cigar-shaped, or oval RBCs). The peripheral blood smear in normal patients may contain up to 15% elliptocytes.

The differential diagnosis of HE includes **iron-deficiency anemia**.

Treatment

Splenectomy is curative but is not indicated unless anemia is profound.

G6PD Deficiency

Etiology

G6PD deficiency, **inherited** in an X-linked pattern, is the most common enzyme deficiency of the hexose monophosphate shunt. Affected patients are either heterozygous males or homozygous females. There is an increased incidence of G6PD deficiency in people of **African and Mediterranean descent**. Affected children may have **drug-induced hemolysis or a chronic hemolytic process**.

Medications and substances that can induce hemolysis in G6PD-deficient patients include acetanilid, doxorubicin, methylene blue, naphthalene, nitrofurantoin, primaquine, pamaquine, and sulfa drugs.

Clinical Features

Presentation depends on the type of G6PD deficiency variant inherited.

- **Patients with the African variant** of G6PD deficiency rarely present for evaluation with neonatal jaundice or chronic hemolytic anemia. They are usually identified when they present for evaluation following drug (or other substance) exposure. Drug-induced hemolysis can be severe, involving the sudden onset of pallor, malaise, scleral icterus, dark urine, and abdominal or back pain.
- **Patients with the Mediterranean variant** of G6PD deficiency usually have a more severe form of G6PD deficiency and may present for evaluation with signs and symptoms of neonatal hyperbilirubinemia, chronic hemolytic anemia, or drug-induced hemolysis.

Evaluation

If G6PD deficiency is suspected, a **blood sample** should be sent for analysis of G6PD enzyme activity. **"Bite" or "blister" cells** (RBCs with small outpouchings or blisters on the outer rim) may be identified on the **peripheral blood smear. Genetic testing is also available and included in the newborn screen in some states.**

Treatment

Drug-induced intravascular hemolysis is **self-limited and reversible** when the offending drug is discontinued. Children with **chronic hemolysis** may require **RBC transfusions** for exacerbations of anemia characterized by cardiovascular compromise.

Sickle Cell Disease

Etiology

Hemoglobin S (Hb S) is the predominant hemoglobin in the group of **genetic disorders** that encompass sickle cell disease (SCD). Hb S is an abnormal hemoglobin caused by a single nucleotide base substitution: Valine replaces glutamic acid in the sixth position of the β globin chain, resulting in structural changes in the RBC membrane. SCD variants include SCD-SS, SCD-SC, SCD-S β-thalassemia, and others. SCD is inherited in a recessive fashion with homozygous and compound heterozygous forms.

Clinical Features

Patients with SCD disorders have **hemolytic anemia and vaso-occlusive complications** and are at an **increased risk of infection**. People with **sickle cell trait** are generally **asymptomatic** but may have occasional hematuria, rarely splenic infarction, and possibly pregnancy-related complications. Currently, most patients are identified through **newborn screening** for hemoglobinopathies. Others, not identified through newborn screening, present with signs and symptoms of SCD complications:

- **Infection.** Children with SCD, especially those <3 years of age, are at an increased risk for the development of bacterial infections as a result of splenic hypofunction and other immunologic abnormalities. *Streptococcus pneumoniae* is the most commonly implicated microorganism; however, meningococcal organisms, *Haemophilus influenzae, E. coli, Salmonella* species, and *Staphylococcus aureus* are common pathogens in patients with SCD as well. Pneumococcal sepsis can be rapidly fatal in these patients, despite the use of penicillin prophylaxis and immunization with polyvalent pneumococcal vaccines.

- **Osteomyelitis.** Patients with SCD are at an increased risk of osteomyelitis; therefore, any child with SCD, bone pain, and fever, or soft tissue swelling should be evaluated for the presence of osteomyelitis. The most common organisms causing osteomyelitis in this patient population are *Salmonella* and *S. aureus*. It is difficult to discriminate between osteomyelitis and a vaso-occlusive episode in the child with SCD. Evaluation should include radiographic studies and orthopedic evaluation.

- **Stroke.** Children with SCD, particularly types SS and S β-thalassemia, may develop hemorrhagic or infarctive strokes. The clinical presentation includes seizures, hemiplegia, difficulty in speaking, or a change in mental status; however, subtle intermittent neurologic symptoms or severe headaches may indicate neurologic complications as well. Transcranial Doppler (TCD) ultrasonography screening identifies young children and adolescents who are at an increased risk of infarctive stroke.

- **Acute chest syndrome (ACS),** classically defined as a new infiltrate on chest radiograph, is one of the leading causes of morbidity and mortality in patients with SCD. The cause of ACS may be multifactorial in an individual patient and includes infection, pulmonary vascular damage, infarction, and cytokine release.

> **HINT:** Any patient who has experienced an episode of ACS is at an increased risk of recurrence. This risk may be decreased with hydroxyurea (HU) therapy or chronic transfusion therapy.

- **Painful episodes,** the most common complications of SCD, are unpredictable and often progressive. The exact pathophysiology is unknown but may be related to occlusion and damage of the microvasculature, leading to organ ischemia and infarction.
- **Splenic sequestration** is one of the leading causes of death in children with SCD. These children develop hypovolemic shock as a result of the loss of large volumes of blood into the spleen. Although the spleen in children with SCD-SS has usually autoinfarcted by the time the patient reaches 8 years of age, children with SCD-SC and SCD-S β-thalassemia can present with splenic sequestration at any age. Acute splenic sequestration episodes are characterized by splenic enlargement with evidence of hemoglobin levels below baseline and increased reticulocyte counts. Mild-to-moderate thrombocytopenia may also occur. Any child who has had one episode of splenic sequestration is at an increased risk of another.
- **Priapism** is a prolonged, painful penile erection and can occur in boys and men with SCD at any age. Priapism may be sustained over a long period of time or may be "stuttering" in nature (i.e., characterized by recurrent episodes within short periods of time).
- **Transient aplastic episode** (see also Chapter 57, "Pallor [Paleness]"). Any patient with chronic hemolytic anemia can experience aplastic episode (i.e., a transient arrest in erythropoiesis characterized by the sudden onset of pallor, frequently following a viral illness). Human parvovirus B19 infection is the most common cause. The anemia is often severe and reticulocyte counts are usually <2%.

Evaluation

Important historic information to be obtained from patients with SCD includes the following:

- Specific disease phenotype or genotype
- Baseline hemoglobin and reticulocyte counts
- Past disease complications
- Dates of last transfusion, transfusion-related complications, and red cell antigen genotype/phenotype

Appropriate laboratory tests in a child suspected of having SCD include a hemoglobin electrophoresis, CBC, and reticulocyte count.

Treatment

- **Suspected infection.** Any child with SCD and fever should be considered bacteremic or septic until proven otherwise. Blood cultures should be obtained promptly and parenteral antibiotics strongly considered, particularly in children with severe disease phenotypes (SS, S β-thalassemia).

- **Stroke.** Children at high risk of stroke based on abnormal TCD results should receive regular red cell transfusions to maintain a HbS% <30 because this significantly lowers initial stroke rates. Exchange transfusions are recommended for patients with acute strokes to decrease further cerebral damage. In children who have had a stroke, chronic transfusion therapy is strongly recommended to decrease the high risk of recurrent stroke.

- **ACS.** Because the underlying cause is often unclear, supportive care should include antibiotics, analgesics, aggressive pulmonary toilet, and supplemental oxygen as needed. Although transfusion therapy is beneficial, the clinical indications are not standardized. However, any child experiencing hypoxia or significant difficulty in breathing should receive an RBC transfusion, either simple or exchange. HU, an antimetabolite medication, has decreased ACS episodes and painful episodes in patients with SCD-SS and SCD-S β-thalassemia.

- **Painful episode.** Care is directed at pain control and close monitoring of patients for other disease complications and side effects of medications. Musculoskeletal pain can be managed acutely with analgesics and nonpharmacologic therapies (e.g., heat and relaxation). Dehydration should be avoided; ACS may be prevented by ambulation and frequent incentive spirometer use. HU should be used to decrease recurrent painful episodes.

- **Splenic sequestration.** If transfusions are necessary, it is important acutely to transfuse small aliquots of RBCs because the spleen releases the patient's RBCs as the sequestration episode resolves. Long-term management of these children is controversial; however, splenectomy should be considered for children who have experienced a life-threatening episode or repeated episodes requiring multiple transfusions.

- **Priapism.** If untreated, it may result in impotency. Initial management includes the use of intravenous hydration and analgesia. A urologist should be consulted, particularly if urinary retention develops or if detumescence does not occur promptly despite medical management.

- **Transient aplastic episode.** Because most children have human parvovirus infections, hospitalized patients should be admitted to single rooms with contact isolation and respiratory isolation. No pregnant caretakers should be permitted in the room. Children with congestive heart failure require RBC transfusion.

Hemoglobin C
Etiology
Hemoglobin C (Hb C) disease, an inherited hemoglobinopathy, results from a substitution of lysine for glutamic acid in the sixth position of the β-polypeptide chain. Variants of Hb C with α- and β-thalassemia exist as well.

Clinical Features and Evaluation
Patients with homozygous disease usually have mild chronic hemolytic anemia with splenomegaly, and the peripheral blood smear shows a marked number of target cells. Patients with Hb C trait are asymptomatic.

Hemoglobin E
Etiology
Hemoglobin E (Hb E) is a common hemoglobin variant, particularly in the **Asian population**. Variants of Hb E with α- and β-thalassemia exist as well.

Clinical Features and Evaluation
Patients with homozygous Hb E have mild hemolytic anemia with a mean corpuscular volume (MCV) that is usually <70 fL and target cells on the peripheral blood smear. Patients with Hb E trait are asymptomatic.

Thalassemia
Etiology
The thalassemia syndromes represent a group of **inherited disorders** caused by **decreased or absent** synthesis of the α or β **human globin chains**. The thalassemia syndromes occur more frequently in **Mediterranean, Asian, and African populations**. Because of unbalanced globin chain synthesis, unstable hemoglobin complexes are produced. Precipitation of the unpaired globin chains and subsequent RBC membrane damage cause **premature RBC lysis,** which leads to **hemolytic anemia** and a compensatory **increase in RBC production** in affected individuals.

Clinical Features of α-Thalassemia
There are four clinical classifications of the α-thalassemias:

- **One α gene mutation.** These patients, the silent carriers of α-thalassemia, have no clinical symptoms, a normal hemoglobin level, and a normal MCV.
- **Two α gene mutations.** Patients with α-thalassemia trait, caused by two α gene mutations, have mild microcytic hypochromic anemia. Because the degree of microcytosis is out of proportion to the degree of anemia, the likelihood of iron-deficiency anemia as a possible diagnosis is diminished.
- **Three α gene mutations.** Hemoglobin H (Hb H) disease, caused by three α gene mutations, is characterized by moderate-to-severe microcytic hypochromic anemia. The excess β chains form tetramers, a fast-migrating hemoglobin (seen on hemoglobin electrophoresis) referred to as "Hb H." Hemoglobin Bart's or γ globin chain tetramers can also be present in neonates with Hb H disease or α-thalassemia trait. In Hb H disease, anemia may be severe, with hemoglobin values ranging from 3 to 4 g/dL. Hemolytic episodes may be exacerbated by fever or infection.
- **Four α gene mutations.** Hydrops fetalis is caused by mutations of all four α genes. These infants fail to produce α globin in utero. They are severely anemic, develop congestive heart failure, and are usually stillborn unless treatment is initiated in utero.

Clinical Features of β-Thalassemia
The β-thalassemia syndromes are categorized according to three levels of clinical severity:

- **Thalassemia minor** (β-thalassemia trait). Patients are asymptomatic and have mild hypochromic anemia.

- **Thalassemia intermedia.** Patients have mild-to-moderate hypochromic anemia and are not transfusion dependent.
- **Thalassemia major (Cooley anemia).** Patients have severe hypochromic microcytic anemia (characterized by hemoglobin levels of 3 to 4 g/dL) and are transfusion dependent. Anemia develops frequently within the first 2 years of life, and patients may present for evaluation with pallor, lethargy, and hepatosplenomegaly. Bony expansion, a sign of heightened intramedullary hematopoiesis, may be found on physical examination.

Evaluation

Patients with **thalassemia major** may be diagnosed by **newborn screening for hemoglobinopathies**. **The presence of hemoglobin A may be low to absent.** For all patients suspected to have thalassemia, a **CBC** should be obtained from the patient and both parents. If **microcytic anemia** is present in either parent or both parents, then **hemoglobin electrophoresis studies** should be obtained.

α- and β-**Thalassemia trait** must be **distinguished from iron-deficiency anemia** because all patients with these disorders may have an MCV <75 fL. In patients with β-thalassemia trait, the MCV would be disproportionately low for the mild degree of anemia seen if the anemia were caused by iron deficiency, and the RBC mass would be increased.

- The RBC distribution width (RDW) index is increased in iron deficiency but normal in thalassemia trait.
- Hemoglobin electrophoresis shows an increased amount of Hb A2, Hb F, or both in patients with β-thalassemia trait but not in those with α-thalassemia trait or iron deficiency.

Iron-deficiency anemia and β-thalassemia trait can coexist and make diagnosis difficult. After treatment for iron deficiency, if the MCV remains low, then diagnostic studies for thalassemia traits should be pursued.

Treatment

Transfusion therapy in thalassemia major is directed at treating the anemia as well as suppressing endogenous RBC production. **Splenectomy** may be indicated in patients with an increasing need for RBC transfusions, in patients with significant growth retardation, or in patients in whom hypersplenism is associated with a worsening of the anemia.

Hemolytic Disease of the Newborn (Isoimmune Hemolytic Anemia)
Etiology

Hemolytic disease of the newborn results from **maternal sensitization to fetal RBC antigens** which differ from that of the mother.

- **In Rh hemolytic disease,** the Rh(D)-negative mother (previously exposed to the D antigen through pregnancy or transfusion) may produce anti-D. During each subsequent pregnancy, transplacental passage of maternal antibody may cause fetal hemolysis.

- **No previous exposure is necessary for ABO hemolytic disease** because anti-A and anti-B are naturally occurring isohemagglutinins. ABO incompatibility is the most common cause of hemolytic disease of the newborn, but Rh incompatibility is associated with the most severe hemolysis in the fetus or the newborn.
- **Hemolytic disease of the newborn can also develop when the mother lacks one of the so-called minor blood group antigens** (C, E, Kell, Duffy, or Kidd) that the fetus has inherited from the father.

Clinical Features

Newborns with hemolytic disease present for evaluation with **varying degrees of illness,** depending on the degree of anemia. Clinical manifestations result from the rate of RBC destruction and the degree of compensation. Newborns have **jaundice and anemia,** usually within the first 24 hours of life. Anemia may cause **congestive heart failure,** and, if the anemia is severe in utero, **hydrops fetalis** may develop. Neonates with hydrops fetalis usually die shortly after birth. **Hyperbilirubinemia** can also be severe and can lead to **kernicterus.**

Delayed anemia can occur in neonates who have been recognized as having isoimmune hemolytic anemia during the first few days of life or in those with mild hemolysis that was undetected initially. Hemoglobin levels may fall to 4 to 6 g/dL within the first 4 to 6 weeks of life.

Evaluation

If the patient's mother is Rh negative and the father Rh positive, then the infant is at risk for the development of hemolysis. The **Rh-negative mother** should be **screened routinely for the presence of anti-D** during gestation and should receive **RhoGAM** (anti-D immune globulin) in the last trimester of pregnancy, prophylactically at termination of pregnancy, or postpartum.

Antibody bound to the surface of the neonate's RBCs can often be demonstrated using a **DAT,** although a negative DAT does not rule out isoimmune hemolytic disease. The **maternal serum should be tested** for the presence of a specific antibody that may cause the hemolysis.

Treatment

Treatment is directed at reducing severe unconjugated hyperbilirubinemia and correcting severe anemia. **Exchange transfusion** should be considered if the hemoglobin level is <12 g/dL and falling within the first 24 hours of life or if the serum bilirubin level is >20 mg/dL within the first 24 hours of life. **Phototherapy** and **hydration** for hyperbilirubinemia may be the only treatments necessary.

Details regarding the management of women at risk of carrying a fetus with Rh disease can be found in standard obstetrics textbooks. Routine immunization of mothers at risk has succeeded in decreasing the incidence of Rh hemolytic disease of the newborn in the United States.

HINT: If the neonate has type O blood or is Rh negative, he is not at risk for development of major blood group incompatibility. However, he may still be at risk for development of minor blood group incompatibility.

Acute and Delayed Hemolytic Transfusion Reactions
Etiology
Acute hemolytic transfusion reactions result when a **recipient with preformed antibodies receives an ABO-incompatible RBC transfusion**. These **life-threatening reactions** are usually caused by the **misidentification** of the donor or recipient of the blood for transfusion and, thus, are avoidable. Delayed hemolytic transfusion reactions (DHTRs) occur 7 to 14 days following a RBC transfusion. These reactions are caused by the presence of preformed antibodies to **minor blood group antigens** in previously transfused patients.

Clinical Features
Patients with acute hemolytic transfusion reactions develop **fever, chills, and tachycardia** commensurate with the volume of blood that has been transfused. Increased scleral icterus, dark urine, and back pain are frequent clinical features at the time of DHTR diagnosis.

Evaluation
The **urine dipstick test** results may be positive for the **presence of heme** with an **absence of RBCs**. Laboratory findings include a **positive DAT** in both kinds of hemolytic transfusion reactions. **Disseminated intravascular coagulation (DIC) and renal failure** may develop.

Treatment
The first intervention when an acute hemolytic transfusion reaction is suspected is to **stop the blood transfusion**. Treatment should include **aggressive intravenous hydration** and the use of **diuretics** to prevent fluid overload. **Alkalinization** may be considered to prevent renal failure. Intravenous gamma globulin and steroids are used to decrease the hemolysis associated with DHTRs. Cautious re-exposure to red cell units is advised. Repeat transfusion should be considered only in patients with cardiovascular compromise.

Autoimmune Hemolytic Anemia
Etiology
Autoimmune hemolytic anemia (AIHA), which may be **idiopathic or second-ary,** can cause **acute, life-threatening anemia** in the pediatric population. The idiopathic diagnosis is more common in the pediatric population since specific causes are difficult to identify. Secondary AIHA may be caused by warm-reactive or cold-reactive antibodies and may result from infection, malignancy, collagen vascular diseases, drugs, or toxins.

Clinical Features
Children with AIHA may have a **sudden onset of pallor, fever, scleral icterus, and dark urine**. However, a more insidious onset of AIHA may be seen, particularly in

children >10 years. **Splenomegaly** is usually present on physical examination. The course of the disease varies from a limited single short episode to a more prolonged illness, with relapses associated with infections.

Evaluation

Laboratory findings include normochromic, normocytic anemia with spherocytes seen on peripheral blood smear, as well as reticulocytosis. Hyperbilirubinemia is present. The DAT is usually positive; however, a negative DAT does not eliminate the possibility of AIHA. Childhood AIHA is usually mediated by IgG. The presence of hemolysis with IgM may be associated with *Mycoplasma* or EBV infection.

Treatment

Treatment is directed at **cardiovascular support and decreasing the amount of RBC destruction**. **Prednisone** (2 mg/kg/day) is given orally if the child is stable, or the equivalent dose in a parenteral form can be given. **Urine output should be maintained** to avoid renal failure.

RBC transfusions should be avoided unless hypoxia or cardiovascular compromise is present because severe hemolytic transfusion reactions can occur. **If RBC transfusion is necessary,** the "least incompatible" donor unit of blood should be used. The **first 15 mL of blood should be administered under very close observation**. The urine should be checked for the presence of hemoglobin, and the plasma layer of a spun hematocrit should be checked for a pink tinge consistent with hemolysis.

Microangiopathic Hemolytic Anemia

Etiology

Microangiopathic hemolytic anemia is associated with a variety of conditions, including **DIC, prosthetic heart valves, cardiac disease** (e.g., coarctation of the aorta, severe valvular disease, endocarditis), **hemolytic uremic syndrome, thrombotic thrombocytopenic purpura, severe burns, march hemoglobinuria, renal transplant rejection, and hemangiomata**.

Clinical Features

The degree of anemia is **variable**. Thrombocytopenia may or may not be present, and **reticulocytosis** is usually present. DIC may occur.

Evaluation

The peripheral blood smear shows **prominent RBC fragments,** such as helmet cells and schistocytes.

Treatment

Treatment should be directed at the **underlying cause**.

EVALUATION OF HEMOLYSIS

History and Physical Examination

A well-focused history and physical examination can direct the physician in ordering appropriate tests and making a diagnosis (Table 40-2).

TABLE 40-2	Clinical Evaluation of Pediatric Patients with Suspected Hemolytic Anemia
Question	**If the Answer Is "Yes," Consider . . .**
History	
Is the patient a neonate?	Hemolytic disease of the newborn
Has the child had previous episodes of scleral icterus or dark urine, particularly with intercurrent illnesses?	Chronic (vs. an acute) hemolytic process
Is the patient currently taking medications or has he received medications recently?	G6PD deficiency or drug-induced hemolysis, depending on the type of medications and the ethnic background of the child
Are there mothball products in the household?	G6PD deficiency
Has the patient participated in very strenuous exercise recently, such as running a marathon?	March hemoglobinuria
Does the patient have cardiac disease or prosthetic heart valves?	Microangiopathic hemolytic anemia
Has the patient had a recent severe diarrheal illness or viral prodrome?	HUS and chronic hemolytic anemia
Is the patient an African-American?	G6PD deficiency, thalassemia, SCD
Is the patient of Mediterranean descent?	G6PD deficiency, thalassemia
Has the patient had a blood transfusion recently? Is the patient on a chronic transfusion protocol?	Acute or delayed hemolytic transfusion reaction, particularly if the patient is chronically transfused
Is there a family history of gallstones or splenectomy in early childhood? Is there a family history of anemia?	Chronic hemolytic anemia, inherited
Physical Examination	
Is there scleral icterus, jaundice, and splenomegaly?	Hemolytic anemia
Is there evidence of maxillary hyperplasia, towering forehead, or other evidence of bone marrow expansion?	Chronic hemolytic process

G6PD, glucose-6-phosphate dehydrogenase; *SCD,* sickle cell disease.

 HINT: Some patients with congenital hemolytic anemias present for evaluation during transient aplastic episodes without histories suggestive of chronic hemolysis.

Laboratory Studies

At minimum, the initial laboratory evaluation should include a CBC and reticulocyte count. Lactate dehydrogenase, aspartate aminotransferase, and indirect bilirubin levels are often high in hemolytic states with a low serum haptoglobin.

Review of the peripheral blood smear for spherocytes, schistocytes, and increased polychromasia is very important. A DAT can be revealing when RBC destruction is caused by antibody production against erythrocytes (e.g., in AIHA or hemolytic disease of the newborn).

 HINT: Three common conditions are frequently mistaken for hemolytic anemia: hemorrhage, recovering bone marrow (e.g., seen after chemotherapy or viral illness), and partially treated nutritional deficiencies. The reticulocyte count is often increased with evidence of anemia; however, this finding is not related to intrinsic or extrinsic causes of hemolysis.

APPROACH TO THE PATIENT (Figure 40-1)
Treatment of Hemolysis
Generally, treatment for hemolytic anemia is directed toward **managing cardiovascular compromise and treating the underlying cause** in patients with acquired disease.

Splenectomy
Splenectomy should be considered for children with **congenital hemolytic anemia** to reduce RBC transfusion requirements and to manage complications of hypersplenism (e.g., poor growth). All children who have had their spleens removed are at **greater risk for development of an infection,** particularly with *S. pneumoniae, H. influenzae, Neisseria meningitidis,* or *E. coli.* The risk of infection is greater after splenectomy in young children, particularly those aged 4 years, and in those who have underlying conditions associated with increased risk of infection. Immunizations against *H. influenzae, S. pneumoniae,* and *N. meningitidis* are recommended before splenectomy. Prophylactic use of oral penicillin is effective in reducing the incidence of bacterial sepsis.

Chronic Transfusion
Children with chronic hemolytic anemia, particularly children with β-thalassemia major or SCD with severe complications, often require **frequent transfusions** (i.e., every 3 to 6 weeks), either to maintain the hemoglobin level above a certain value or to keep the percentage of Hb S below a certain value. **Complications** of frequent blood transfusions include **iron overload, RBC alloimmunization, and viral infection**. Iron overload is treated with **chelation therapy,** usually with oral chelators such as deferasirox, parenteral chelators such as deferoxamine preparations, or **exchange transfusions** in appropriate patients with SCD.

Complications of Chronic Hemolytic Anemia
Generally, the complications of chronic hemolytic anemias are related to increased RBC destruction, increased RBC production, and anemia. These complications include **folic acid deficiency and gallstones** as a result of increased RBC turnover, **splenomegaly** as a result of increased RBC entrapment and extramedullary hematopoiesis, and **transient aplastic episode**.

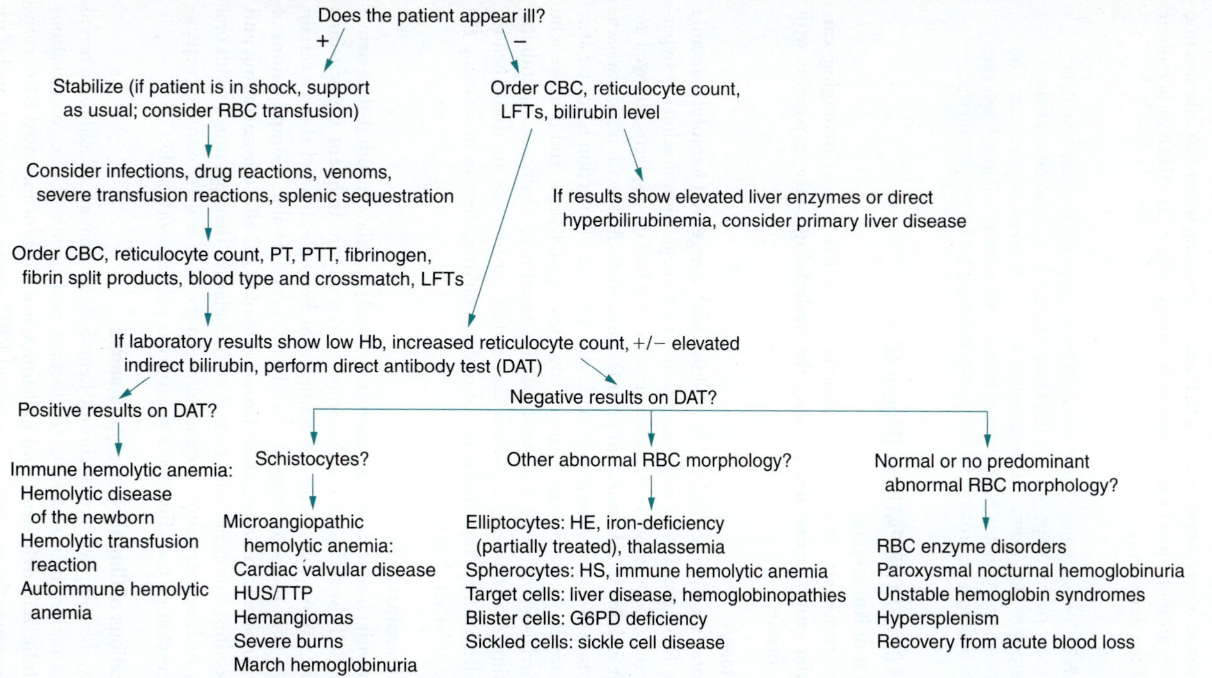

FIGURE 40-1 Evaluation of a pediatric patient with suspected hemolytic anemia. *CBC*, complete blood cell count; *G6PD*, glucose-6-phosphate dehydrogenase; *Hb*, hemoglobin; *HE*, hereditary elliptocytosis; *HS*, hereditary spherocytosis; *HUS*, hemolytic uremic syndrome; *LFTs*, liver function tests; *PT*, prothrombin time; *PTT*, partial thromboplastin time; *RBC*, red blood cell; *TTP*, thrombotic thrombocytopenic purpura.

Suggested Readings

Cohen AR. Pallor. In: Fleisher GR, Ludwig S, eds. *Textbook of Pediatric Emergency Medicine.* 3rd ed. Baltimore, MA: Williams & Wilkins; 1993:388–396.

Cunningham MJ. Update on thalassemia; clinical care and complications. *Pediar Clin North Am.* 2008;55(2):447–469.

Rees DC, Williams TN, Gladwin MT. Sickle-cell disease. *Lancet.* 2010;376(9757):2018–2031.

Hemoptysis

INTRODUCTION

Hemoptysis is the **expectoration or coughing up of blood from the respiratory tract**. Bleeding from the respiratory tract can range from blood-streaked sputum to coughing up of massive quantities of bright red blood. Although bleeding into the lungs and airways is uncommon in children, **massive hemoptysis** (loss of >8 mL blood/kg or 240 mL blood/24 hours) is a **life-threatening condition** requiring immediate evaluation and therapy. Hemoptysis may be the result of pulmonary hemorrhage and should be distinguished from hematemesis or bleeding from the nasopharynx. Pulmonary hemorrhage can be diffuse or focal; associated with underlying cardiopulmonary disorders including congenital heart disease or airway anomalies; related to underlying systemic conditions; infectious; or idiopathic. The most common cause of hemoptysis in children is infection or conditions complicated by infections (such as cystic fibrosis, lung abscess, tuberculosis and bronchiectasis). Inflammatory disorders which erode into the bronchial circulation or conditions that place the bronchial circulation under systemic vascular pressure are likely to cause severe hemoptysis.

 HINT: Patients with massive hemoptysis most likely have a single focus of bleeding.

 HINT: Wandering alveolar infiltrates found on chest radiograph in a child presenting with respiratory distress is highly suggestive of pulmonary hemorrhage (regardless of whether the patient presented with hemoptysis).

 DIFFERENTIAL DIAGNOSIS LIST

Diffuse
Isolated
- Lung immaturity
- Cow milk hyperreactivity (Heiner syndrome)
- Pulmonary capillary hemangiomatosis

- Idiopathic (pulmonary hemosiderosis)

Associated with Other Organ Dysfunction
- Nephritis (Goodpasture, nephritis with immune complexes, nephritis without immune complexes)

- Myocarditis
- Celiac disease
- Diabetes
- Collagen vascular disease
- Wegener granulomatosis
- Henoch–Schönlein purpura and other systemic vasculitis
- Lymphangioleiomyomatosis
- Tuberous sclerosis
- Systemic necrotizing vasculitis, hypersensitivity angiitis, mixed connective tissue disease, Behcet disease

Secondary

- Congestive heart failure
- Congenital heart disease (e.g., congenital pulmonary vein stenosis—pulmonary veno-occlusive disease)
- Tetralogy of Fallot with pulmonary atresia and multiple collaterals and pulmonary arterial stenosis
- Mitral stenosis with left atrial hypertension
- Clotting disorders
- Malignancy
- Immunosuppression (e.g., s/p bone marrow transplantation)
- Diffuse alveolar injury (penicillamine, propylthiouracil, cocaine, radiologic contrast agents, nitrofurantoin, cytotoxic agents, trimellitic anhydride, radiation, smoke inhalation, insecticide (paraquat) inhalation, acid aspiration, oxygen toxicity, sickle cell disease (acute chest syndrome))

Focal
Conducting Airways

- Bronchitis
- Bronchiectasis (e.g., cystic fibrosis)

- Airway anomalies (bronchogenic cysts, bronchial adenoma, unilateral pulmonary agenesis, bronchial artery aneurysm, Ehlers–Danlos syndrome)
- Vascular anomalies (hemangioma, angioma, arteriovenous malformation or fistula, hereditary hemorrhagic telangiectasia)
- Foreign body aspiration
- Tracheostomy complication
- Trauma (contusion, suctioning, intubation)

Parenchymal

- Trauma
- Pneumothorax
- Infection (**Bacterial:** *Pneumococcus, Staphylococcus, Meningococcus,* Group A *Streptococcus, Mycoplasma, Bordetella pertussis, Pseudomonas,* leptospirosis; **Viral:** influenza virus, varicella-zoster virus, hepatitis B virus, HIV; **Fungal:** *Aspergillus, Histoplasma, Coccidioides, Blastomyces;* **Parasitic:** visceral larva migrans, filariasis, toxoplasmosis, hydatidosis, **Arthropod Infestation:** hemorrhagic fevers)
- Infarction (pulmonary embolism)
- Cavitary lesions (e.g., tuberculosis, abscess, histoplasmosis)
- Neoplasms (**Benign:** hemangiomas, angiomas, pulmonary sequestration, inflammatory pseudotumor, enteric cysts; **Malignant:** bronchial adenoma, sarcoma, teratoma; **Metastatic:** sarcoma, Wilms tumor, osteogenic sarcoma)

Others

- Catamenial hemoptysis
- Factitious (Munchausen by proxy syndrome)

DIFFERENTIAL DIAGNOSIS DISCUSSION

> **HINT:** An inhaled foreign body must always be considered in any child with hemoptysis.

> **HINT:** Pneumonia, bronchitis, lung abscess, and laryngotracheitis can be associated with hemoptysis.

Cystic Fibrosis

Cystic fibrosis is the most common nontraumatic cause of pulmonary hemorrhage in the United States, which is typically due to endobronchial infection and inflammation and less commonly due to rupture of a bronchial artery that may be life threatening, and is discussed in Chapter 23, "Cough."

Bronchiectasis

Bronchiectasis is discussed in Chapter 23, "Cough."

Pulmonary Hemosiderosis

Etiology

Hemosiderosis may be primary or secondary.

- **Primary hemosiderosis.** Primary idiopathic hemosiderosis involves bleeding into the lungs, of unknown cause, and is a diagnosis of exclusion. The classification is as follows:
  - Isolated
  - With cardiac or pancreatic involvement
  - With glomerulonephritis (Goodpasture syndrome)
  - With sensitivity to cow's milk and milk-protein allergies (Heiner syndrome)
- **Secondary hemosiderosis** can result from cardiac disease, collagen vascular disease or systemic vasculitis, bleeding disorders, or granulomatosis.

Clinical Features

Patients may present not only with acute respiratory distress, recurrent episodes of cough, dyspnea, and wheezing, but also with chronic fatigue, pallor, and even failure to thrive. Recurrent pneumonia with associated microcytic anemia should also promote consideration.

Typically, the child appears ill (i.e., **lethargic, pale, tachypneic, tachycardic**) and is usually afebrile. The pallor results from **anemia,** which is caused by recurrent subclinical bleeding. **Sputum is frequently rust colored;** frank hemoptysis is less common as a presentation. **Infiltrates** on a chest radiograph may be **diffuse** and fluffy, and may be fleeting. **Increased work of breathing, decreased breath sounds, and crackles** may be noted on physical examination.

Evaluation

The diagnosis is confirmed by demonstrating **macrophages-containing hemosiderin**. A macrophage sample may be obtained via **gastric lavage** (performed three times in the morning before the patient has risen from the supine position) or more commonly via flexible fiber optic **bronchoscopy with bronchoalveolar lavage**.

 HINT: Primary idiopathic hemosiderosis is a diagnosis of exclusion and requires a comprehensive workup, including evaluation for immunologic, infectious, and cardiac causes. Milk-protein precipitin values should be obtained for any child with pulmonary hemorrhage of unknown cause.

Treatment

Blood transfusions may be required in the acute phase. Conventional therapy for idiopathic hemosiderosis includes prednisone (2 mg/kg per day for 4 to 6 weeks, tapered over 1 to 2 months in an attempt to wean the patient completely or to at least achieve an every-other-day regimen). **Azathioprine or cyclophosphamide** is used for patients who do not respond to steroid therapy or in place of steroids. Children who test **positive for milk precipitin values** should be placed on a **non-casein-based diet**. Although some children respond, many do not.

Goodpasture Syndrome

A pulmonary-renal immune complex disorder, Goodpasture syndrome is characterized by **deposits of anti-glomerular basement membrane (anti-GBM) antibodies in the kidneys and lungs**. Circulating anti-GBM antibodies are also found in the **serum**. The disorder is most common in **young white boys**. **Hemoptysis,** along with cough and dyspnea, is common and may occur prior to the development of renal disease. Isolated pulmonary disease often responds to corticosteroids, but renal involvement may also require plasmapheresis or dialysis.

Wegener Granulomatosis

Characterized by **vasculitis with granuloma formation,** Wegener granulomatosis involves both the **upper and lower respiratory tracts and the kidney**. The cause of this disease is unknown. Wegener granulomatosis is distinguished by necrotizing lesions of the upper and lower respiratory tract and necrotizing glomerulonephritis. The **sinuses, nasal septum, and nasopharynx** are usually involved. The disorder may present with nasal and sinus congestion, arthritis or arthralgia, and skin lesions in addition to cough and hemoptysis. **Massive hemoptysis** may be the presenting symptom and is secondary to **necrotizing pneumonitis** in the lower respiratory tract. **Acute glomerulonephritis and renal failure** usually precede the pulmonary manifestations, and radiographic abnormalities may be noted prior to the development of respiratory symptoms. Treatment involves prolonged high-dose corticosteroids and cyclophosphamide, and relapses may be seen.

EVALUATION OF HEMOPTYSIS
Patient History

A careful history of the patient is important to rule out an exogenous agent or an underlying cardiopulmonary disorder. A description of the **color of the blood,** the **duration of the bleeding,** and the **amount of blood** is helpful in defining the severity of the condition and making a specific diagnosis. Prior history of pulmonary symptoms or illnesses, as well as general symptoms of fatigue or malaise, pallor, exercise intolerance, or poor growth, should be reviewed. Recent history of cough, fever, chills, and exposures should also be elicited.

 HINT: It is important to distinguish hemoptysis (coughing of blood) from hematemesis (vomiting of blood). In hematemesis, the blood is often brown and has a low pH as a result of contact with gastric acid. Care must also be taken to differentiate hemoptysis from epistaxis, oral or nasopharyngeal bleeding, and bleeding caused by tonsillitis, sinusitis, gingivitis, or nasal trauma. In addition to a detailed nasopharyngeal examination, examination of the fingernails may illicit dried blood.

 HINT: The main features of alveolar hemorrhage, apart from hemoptysis, are shortness of breath, anemia, hypoxemia, and diffuse pulmonary densities on a chest radiograph.

 HINT: Primary tuberculosis commonly presents with hemoptysis.

Physical Examination

The physician should first ensure that the patient's **vital signs and hemodynamic status** are stable prior to any further evaluation. The upper and lower respiratory system should be completely examined, and one may note crackles or wheezing on auscultation. A cardiac examination may reveal a murmur or signs of heart failure. Hepatomegaly and/or splenomegaly may be noted on abdominal examination. Features of **systemic illnesses** (e.g., connective tissue disorders, vasculitides) should be sought, with attention to examinations of the skin and extremities (for digital clubbing). Specific findings that may be suggestive of the cause include the following:

- **Putrid sputum** suggests the presence of a lung abscess or bronchiectasis.
- **Acute pleuritic chest pain** raises the possibility of pulmonary embolism or another pleura-based lesion (e.g., abscess, fungal cavity, vasculitis).
- **Localized wheezing** occurs with an intramural lesion (e.g., foreign body, tumor).
- **Pleural rub** suggests the presence of pleural disease.
- **Clubbing and chronic hypoxemia** suggest the presence of a chronic pulmonary or cardiac disorder (e.g., cystic fibrosis, bronchiectasis, cyanotic congenital heart disease).
- **Pallor** may not be noticeable in severe anemia.

Laboratory Studies

A **complete blood count with differential and reticulocyte count, coagulation studies, and sputum culture** with **Gram stain** should be obtained in all patients with significant hemoptysis (more than a few teaspoons). Blood typing and cross-matching should be done if significant blood loss is considered. Stools should be guaiac or hemoccult tested. Other laboratory studies are ordered according to clinical suspicion for a particular condition. These studies may include the following:

- Urinalysis, urine microscopy, and serum blood urea nitrogen and creatinine levels (pulmonary-renal disorder)
- Erythrocyte sedimentation rate, complement, antinuclear antibodies, and rheumatoid factor (vasculitis and connective tissue disorders)
- Reticulocyte count (hemosiderosis, recurrent bleeding)
- Immunoglobulin E (IgE) level and eosinophil count (Heiner syndrome, autoimmune disorders)
- Serum anti-GBM antibody level (Goodpasture syndrome)
- Serum c-anti-neutrophil cytoplasmic antibody and perinuclear anti-neutrophil cytoplasmic autoantibody (Wegener granulomatosis)
- Bacterial, viral, fungal, and parasitic cultures (infection identification)
- Purified protein derivative analysis (tuberculosis)
- Chloride sweat test (cystic fibrosis)
- Endomysial IgA (celiac disease)
- ppd (tuberculosis)

Other Diagnostic Modalities

- **Chest radiograph.** A chest radiograph should be obtained for all patients with significant hemoptysis or clinical distress. The acute radiographic changes are usually diffuse and bilateral, often sparing the apices and costophrenic angles. Chronically, more nodular or reticulonodular densities may be seen. Unilateral hyperlucency may indicate a radiolucent foreign body; in that case, a lateral decubitus film should be evaluated for paradoxical asymmetry. As infiltrates may be wandering, a repeat chest radiograph in 24 to 48 hours may be useful.
- **High-resolution computed tomography (HRCT) of the chest with contrast or CT angiogram (CTA)** is more sensitive and specific than a chest radiograph for demonstrating the alveolar pattern in an intrapulmonary bleed. HRTC is also helpful in diagnosing sequestration and locating anomalous vessels. Pulmonary fibrosis may be seen in chronic or recurrent disease. CTA may not be sensitive enough to elucidate small vessel or alveolar bleeding.
- **Magnetic resonance imaging and magnetic resonance angiography** are valuable for detecting neoplasia **and anomalous vasculature**.
- **Pulmonary function testing** may reveal both obstructive (early) and restrictive (later) lung disease.
- **Radionuclide scanning** with technetium-99m-labeled sulfur colloid can detect perfusion defects caused by emboli and may be helpful in detecting a localized bleeding site.
- **Laryngoscopy** or **bronchoscopy** (or both) can differentiate upper from lower respiratory tract bleeding and focal from diffuse bleeding. These modalities can also localize the bleeding to a particular bronchopulmonary segment. A rigid

bronchoscope should be used for patients with severe bleeding because it enables the physician to ventilate the patient (if necessary), to control the airway, and to provide definitive treatment in some cases. A flexible bronchoscope is better suited for diagnostic purposes, bronchoalveolar lavage, and obtaining samples for culture.

- **Bronchoalveolar lavage** can be used for definitive cultures, and staining for hemosiderin-laden macrophages.
- **Lung biopsy** may be indicated if the workup is negative (consistent with idiopathic or primary pulmonary hemosiderosis) and suspicion of an underlying condition still exists.
- **Echocardiography** may allow exclusion of an underlying cardiac disorder.
- **Cardiac catheterization and angiography** can help delineate the bronchial and pulmonary vasculature, localize an isolated bleeding vessel, define the underlying cause (dilated tortuous bronchial vessels, increased number of vessels, bronchopulmonary anastomosis), and evaluate hemodynamics (in congenital heart disease and suspected pulmonary hypertension). Angiography can include treatment (coiling of collateral vessels) and guide surgical resection in large-vessel diffuse disease.

TREATMENT OF HEMOPTYSIS

In most cases, hemoptysis is self-limited and not life threatening. Definitive treatment, after stabilization, is directed at causative agents and underlying disorders if found.

Stabilization

An **aggressive approach** in an **intensive care setting** is indicated when a massive hemorrhage occurs. An airway must be **established immediately**. (Aspiration of blood and asphyxia are more likely to kill the patient than is exsanguination.) **Supplemental oxygen** should be used for hypoxemia or profound acidosis. One should be prepared to use **intubation and mechanical ventilation** for both airway maintenance and management of hypoxemia and respiratory failure. **Positive pressure ventilation with elevated positive end-expiratory pressure may be indicated to tamponade bleeding. Hypovolemia** requires **fluid resuscitation, blood transfusion, or both. Acidosis** requires the administration of **fluids** (e.g., 0.9% normal saline, lactated Ringer's solution) and blood.

Infants with intrapulmonary bleeding almost always have concomitant left-sided heart failure with pulmonary edema and may require positive-pressure ventilation with positive end-expiratory pressure, vasopressor administration (e.g., dopamine, dobutamine, epinephrine), and fluid restriction (except for blood transfusion, when necessary).

Termination of Bleeding

The effectiveness of conservative therapy is well established and is the mainstay except for in cases of massive hemoptysis. Methods of terminating bleeding include the following:

- **Bronchoscopic lavage** of a segment of the lung with iced saline can be successful in some cases, but is rarely used.
- **Endobronchial tamponade.** A balloon-tipped catheter is placed in the affected bronchus, inflated, and left in place for 24 hours.
- **Selective embolization** of the bronchial or pulmonary vessels with catheter-introduced coils is an effective way of stopping persistent or recurrent bleeding.
- **Electrocoagulation** is found to be useful by some authors.
- **Selective intubation** of a main bronchus with a cuffed tube may be useful in unilateral bleeding.
- **Surgical resection** of the focus of bleeding may provide definitive treatment in isolated bleeding segments or vascular anomalies.
- **Endobronchial thrombin and intravenous vasopressin** are the newer therapies.

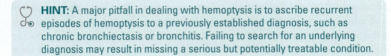

HINT: A major pitfall in dealing with hemoptysis is to ascribe recurrent episodes of hemoptysis to a previously established diagnosis, such as chronic bronchiectasis or bronchitis. Failing to search for an underlying diagnosis may result in missing a serious but potentially treatable condition.

Suggested Readings

Barben JU, Ditchfield M, Carlin JB, et al. Major haemoptysis in children with cystic fibrosis: a 20-year retrospective study. *J Cyst Fibros.* 2003;2(3):105–111.

Batra PS, Holinger LD. Etiology and management of pediatric hemoptysis. *Arch Otolaryngol Head Neck Surg.* 2001;127(4):377–382.

Boat TF. Pulmonary hemorrhage and hemoptysis. In: Chernick V, Boat TF, Wilmott RW, et al., eds. *Kendig's Disorders of the Respiratory Tract in Children.* 7th ed. Philadelphia, PA: WB Saunders; 2006:676–685.

Godfrey S. Pulmonary hemorrhage/hemoptysis in children. *Pediatr Pulmonol.* 2004;37(6):476–484.

Sidman JD, Wheeler WB, Cabalka AK, et al. Management of acute pulmonary hemorrhage in children. *Laryngoscope.* 2001;111(1):33–35.

Susarla SC, Fan LL. Diffuse alveolar hemorrhage syndromes in children. *Curr Opin Pediatr.* 2007;19:313–320.

Hepatomegaly

INTRODUCTION

Hepatomegaly is an important physical examination finding, which may reflect intrinsic liver disease or a wide array of systemic diseases. Determination of liver size may be achieved with a combination of techniques, including palpation, percussion, and auscultation. Among these, palpation is the most common approach. It is accomplished by applying gentle manual pressure to the right lower abdominal wall and advancing superiorly until the inferior border of the liver is appreciated with the fingertips. Extension of the liver below the xiphoid process and/or below the right costal margin in the midclavicular line by more than 3 cm in neonates or more than 2 cm in older children may suggest hepatomegaly. However, several pitfalls in this technique must be considered. Increased lung expansion, accumulation of air or liquid in the pleural or subdiaphragmatic space, and a narrow chest cavity (e.g., scoliosis or pectus excavatum) may all result in inferior displacement of the liver without actual hepatic enlargement. Presence of the Riedel lobe, a normal anatomic variant in which the right lobe of the liver extends far below the right costal margin, may also confound the examination. Thus, **determination of the liver span is recommended**. The span is measured by ascertaining the upper border via chest wall percussion and the lower border via one or more of the three aforementioned techniques. Auscultation is performed by placing the stethoscope below the xiphoid and "scratching" superiorly from the right lower quadrant until the lower edge of the liver causes a change in the transmitted sound. In neonates, the normal liver span is 4.5 to 5 cm. By 12 years of age, it measures 7 to 8 cm in boys and 6 to 7 cm in girls.

The differential diagnosis for pediatric hepatomegaly is expansive and is best organized by considering six broad mechanisms of liver enlargement (all beginning with the letter "I" for ease of recall): **I**nfection, **I**nflammation (noninfectious), **I**nappropriate accumulation of fat, **I**nfiltration, **I**mpaired outflow of blood or bile, and **I**nborn errors of metabolism resulting in abnormal cellular storage:

 DIFFERENTIAL DIAGNOSIS LIST

Infection (Infectious Hepatitis)
- **Viral Infections**
  - Hepatitis A to E

- Epstein–Barr virus (EBV) (infectious mononucleosis)
- Cytomegalovirus (CMV)

- Herpesvirus
- Varicella
- Enterovirus
- Adenovirus
- Rubella
- HIV
- **Bacterial Infections (± sepsis or abscess)**
  - *Bartonella henselae* ("cat-scratch" disease)
  - *Salmonella typhi*
  - *Streptococcus*
  - *Staphylococcus*
  - Tularemia
  - Brucellosis
  - *Listeria monocytogenes*
  - Actinomycosis
  - Ehrlichiosis
  - Tuberculosis
- **Spirochete Infections**
  - *Treponema pallidum* (syphilis)
  - *Borrelia burgdorferi* (Lyme disease)
  - Leptospirosis
- **Rickettsial Infections**
  - *Rickettsia rickettsii* (Rocky Mountain spotted fever)
  - *Coxiella burnetii* (Q fever)
- **Fungal Infections**
  - Aspergillus
  - Histoplasmosis
  - Coccidioidomycosis
  - Candidiasis
- **Parasite/Amoeba Infections**
  - *Entamoeba histolytica*
  - Toxocariasis
  - Schistosomiasis
  - Clonorchis sinensis
  - Leishmaniasis
  - *Plasmodium falciparum* (Malaria)

Inflammation (Noninfectious Hepatitis)

- Autoimmune hepatitis (AIH)
- Primary sclerosing cholangitis
- Juvenile idiopathic arthritis (JIA)

- Systemic lupus erythematosus
- Radiation
- Giant cell hepatitis (neonatal)
- Toxins
  - Organic (e.g., Amanita phalloides mushroom)
- Drugs (e.g., acetaminophen overdose)
- Alcohol

Inappropriate Accumulation of Fat

- Obesity (nonalcoholic fatty liver disease (NAFLD) or nonalcoholic steatohepatitis (NASH))
- Diabetes mellitus
- Ethanol (chronic use)
- Drugs (e.g., corticosteroids, valproic acid)
- Parenteral nutrition (PN)
- Protein malnutrition (kwashiorkor)
- Celiac disease
- Reye syndrome

Infiltration (Tumors and Other Cellular Infiltrates)

- **Tumors**
  - Hepatoblastoma
  - Hepatocellular carcinoma
  - Hemangioma
  - Hemangioendothelioma
  - Metastasis (e.g., neuroblastoma)
- **Cellular Infiltrates**
  - Extramedullary hematopoiesis (e.g., in sickle-cell disease)
  - Leukemia
  - Lymphoma
  - Langerhans cell histiocytosis (LCH)
  - Hemophagocytic lymphohistiocytosis (HLH)
  - Malignant histiocytosis

Impaired Outflow of Blood

- Veno-occlusive disease (VOD)
- Budd–Chiari syndrome
- Congenital hepatic vein web/stenosis

- Congestive heart failure
- Constrictive pericarditis
- Bile (extrahepatic cholestasis)
  - Biliary atresia
  - Choledochal cyst
  - Choledocholithiasis
  - Biliary ascariasis
- Bile (intrahepatic cholestasis)
  - PFIC
  - Alagille syndrome
  - Nonsyndromic bile duct paucity
  - Cystic fibrosis

Inborn Errors of Metabolism of Lipids and Sphingolipids
- Niemann–Pick disease
- Gaucher disease
- Wolman disease
- Cholesteryl ester storage disease

- Mucolipidoses
- Fatty acid oxidation disorders
- Proteins
  - Tyrosinemia
  - α-1 Antitrypsin deficiency
- Carbohydrates
  - Mucopolysaccharidoses (e.g., Hunter, Hurler)
  - GM1 Gangliosidosis
  - Glycogen storage disease
  - Hereditary fructose intolerance
  - Galactosemia
  - Peroxisomes (e.g., Zellweger syndrome)
- Metals
  - Iron (primary and secondary hemochromatosis)
  - Copper (Wilson disease)

DIFFERENTIAL DIAGNOSIS DISCUSSION
Viral Infection
It is not uncommon for children with viral syndromes to have modest hepatomegaly with mild elevations in transaminase levels. **In most cases, the course is benign, and only observation for resolution of the infection is required.** Certain hepatotropic viruses (listed above) may cause a more significant acute hepatitis, associated with tender hepatomegaly, jaundice, and marked elevations in liver transaminases. In rare cases, these findings may herald the onset of fulminant liver failure, and close observation with monitoring of liver synthetic parameters, including prothrombin time/international normalized ratio (PT/INR), albumin, and glucose levels, is warranted. Viral hepatitis is discussed in further detail in Chapter 45, "Jaundice."

Infectious Mononucleosis
Infectious mononucleosis is discussed in Chapter 50, "Lymphadenopathy."

CMV Infection
CMV Infection is discussed in Chapter 73, "Splenomegaly."

HIV Infection
HIV-related cholangiopathy, typically associated with CMV, *Microsporidia or Cryptosporidia* superinfection, is the most common hepatic manifestation of advanced HIV infection. Patients may present with **abdominal pain, diarrhea, icterus or jaundice, and hepatomegaly**. Widespread implementation of HAART therapy has reduced the incidence of this complication. The course of **chronic**

HBV and HCV infection may be more severe in the setting of HIV coinfection. HIV infection is discussed in further detail in Chapter 70, "Sexually Transmitted Diseases."

Liver Abscess
Etiology
In the United States and other developed countries, pediatric liver abscess is a rare phenomenon, primarily caused by bacteria. *Staphylococcus,* **anaerobes, and gram-negative rods are the predominant culprits**. Parasitic agents, including *Entamoeba histolytica and Echinococcus granulosa,* predominate in underdeveloped nations, where liver abscess is more common. Risk factors for liver abscess in the pediatric population include:

- Immunodeficiency (e.g., chronic granulomatous disease, history of bone marrow transplant)
- Congenital biliary obstruction (e.g., biliary atresia, choledochal cyst)
- Inadvertent portal vein cannulation with umbilical vein catheterization of the neonate
- Liver transplantation
- Inflammatory bowel disease

Clinical Features
Patients may present with fever, pain/tenderness in right upper quadrant, anorexia, nausea, vomiting, and, occasionally, jaundice. Signs can be subtle, particularly in the immunocompromised patient, and a **high index of suspicion may be required**.

Evaluation
The white blood cell count, alanine aminotransferase (ALT), aspartate aminotransferase (AST), and alkaline phosphatase levels are usually increased. Blood cultures identify a bacterial organism in 50% of cases. Amebic infection can be diagnosed with indirect hemagglutination (90% sensitivity) or IgG enzyme immunoassay (99% sensitive). Ultrasound, computed tomography (CT), and magnetic resonance imaging (MRI) are useful imaging modalities.

Treatment
Initial therapy involves empiric broad-spectrum intravenous antibiotic therapy. A typical regimen includes triple therapy with ampicillin, a β-lactamase inhibitor, and metronidazole. CT- or ultrasound-guided percutaneous aspiration with or without drain placement is generally advocated for abscesses ≥5 cm in diameter. Open surgical drainage is indicated in cases of spontaneous abscess rupture or failed percutaneous drainage.

Autoimmune Hepatitis
Etiology
Autoimmune hepatitis is a progressive inflammatory disease that is likely caused by dysregulated immune reactions to host liver antigens. Genetic and environmental factors have been implicated.

Clinical Features

Autoimmune hepatitis is **more prevalent in female patients**. A personal history or family history of other autoimmune disease may be elicited. The clinical **presentation may mimic acute viral hepatitis**. A subset of these patients will develop progression to acute liver failure within weeks of initial manifestations. The **presentation may also be more insidious**. In these cases, vague constitutional symptoms, such as fatigue, anorexia, and headache, predominate with or without relapsing icterus/jaundice. Approximately **10% of patients remain asymptomatic until signs of portal hypertension evolve**. Given the highly varied presentation, AIH should be considered in the differential diagnosis of both acute and chronic hepatitis, as well as more advanced cirrhosis.

Evaluation

Physical examination may reveal signs of acute hepatitis, including fever, icterus/jaundice, and tender hepatomegaly, or stigmata of chronic liver disease, including splenomegaly, ascites, dilated abdominal wall veins, spider nevi, and palmar erythema. In addition to transaminase elevation with or without conjugated hyperbilirubinemia, laboratory studies often reveal an elevated globulin fraction (i.e., total protein to albumin ratio). Levels of autoantibodies, including antinuclear, antismooth muscle, and anti-liver–kidney-microsomal antibodies, may be elevated. Liver biopsy is necessary to establish the diagnosis, and classically reveals interface hepatitis with plasma cell involvement. The PT/INR and albumin level should be evaluated in all patients to ensure preservation of liver synthetic function.

Treatment

Patients often respond to **treatment with corticosteroids** (e.g., prednisone), but symptoms may recur when steroids are withdrawn. Chronic immunosuppression with **azathioprine** is often helpful in maintaining remission. **Liver transplantation** may be necessary if liver failure and/or complications of portal hypertension evolve.

Toxin/Drug Hepatotoxicity

Drugs that can cause hepatitis and cholestasis through direct hepatotoxicity or inappropriate fat accumulation are summarized in Chapter 45, "Jaundice."

Primary Nonalcoholic Fatty Liver Disease
Etiology

The term NAFLD encompasses a broad spectrum of disease involving inappropriate accumulation of fat in the liver (steatosis), ranging from uncomplicated steatosis to steatosis with inflammation (steatohepatitis) with or without fibrosis and/or cirrhosis. **Primary NAFLD is associated with obesity and/or insulin resistance,** which may be seen in diabetes mellitus or "prediabetic" states.

Clinical Features

Primary NAFLD is rare before the age of 8 years. Children are typically asymptomatic, though some may complain of abdominal pain. Physical examination often reveals **obesity** (BMI ≥95th percentile in 90% of patients). **Tender or nontender hepatomegaly and acanthosis nigricans,** a sign of insulin resistance, may be present.

Diagnosis

Liver enzymes may be normal or elevated. Conjugated bilirubin levels are typically within normal range. Associated, albeit nondiagnostic, laboratory findings include elevated fasting glucose, insulin, and triglyceride levels. The **most common imaging technique used to identify steatosis is ultrasound**. **Liver biopsy is often performed to exclude steatohepatitis** and other causes of abnormal fat accumulation in the liver.

Treatment

Dietary and other lifestyle changes aimed at reducing obesity are the mainstay of treatment. No medical therapies have proven efficacy in treating pediatric NAFLD.

Parenteral Nutrition-Associated Liver Disease (PNALD)
Etiology

Chronic PN may be complicated by **cholestatic liver disease,** which commonly affects neonates and infants, **or steatosis/steatohepatitis,** which commonly affects older children. Both conditions can result in hepatomegaly. The **etiology of PNALD is poorly understood**. Nutritional components of the intravenous solution, including protein hydrolysate (vs. amino acid) solutions and soybean-derived lipid emulsions may contribute to the pathogenesis. Concomitant infections may compound PNALD.

Clinical Features

Patients often develop **hepatomegaly with or without icterus and jaundice within 2 to 3 weeks of total PN initiation**. Over time, signs of portal hypertension (e.g., splenomegaly, ascites, bleeding varices) and liver failure may develop.

Evaluation

Liver transaminase levels, conjugated bilirubin levels, and nutritional parameters should be followed closely. **Alternative treatable causes of liver disease** (e.g., biliary atresia in cholestatic infants <2 months) **should be excluded**. Liver synthetic function should be monitored closely with PT/INR and albumin determinations.

Treatment

Transition to enteral feeding is the most effective treatment and may reverse PNALD if implemented early. If enteral feeding is not possible, **cyclical rather than continuous administration of PN** may be helpful. Early/aggressive treatment of intestinal bacterial overgrowth and sepsis episodes is critical. Certain children with advanced PNALD and short-bowel syndrome limiting enteral nutrition may be candidates for **combined liver-small bowel transplantation,** which can be curative.

Protein–Calorie Malnutrition
Etiology

Starvation states are commonly associated with marked hepatomegaly, caused by mobilization of free fatty acids from adipose tissue and deposition in the liver.

Kwashiorkor, which is characterized by severe protein deficiency, is the most prevalent form of malnutrition in the world. In developed countries, kwashiorkor can be associated with extreme dietary regimens, such as excessive rice milk administration in the setting of milk protein allergy.

Clinical Features
In addition to hepatomegaly, children with kwashiorkor have a severely **wasted appearance, apathy, dermatitis, and edema**. Susceptibility to infection is increased. Severely ill patients may develop stupor and coma.

Evaluation
Laboratory testing abnormalities include **anemia, hypoglycemia, hypoalbuminemia, and hypoproteinemia**. **Vitamin and mineral deficiencies** are universal. Urinalysis (UA) reveals **ketonuria**. Bone age, measured by radiographic evaluation of the left hand and wrist, shows a delay in **skeletal maturation** with respect to chronologic age.

Treatment
Enteral "refeeding" with careful monitoring of laboratory nutritional indices and electrolytes is usually curative.

Celiac Disease
Patients with celiac disease may present with **elevated liver transaminase levels with or without hepatomegaly**. Liver disease is **typically asymptomatic**. Celiac disease is discussed further in Chapter 10, "Abdominal Pain, Chronic."

Reye Syndrome
Etiology
Reye syndrome is a rare, reversible, noninflammatory **encephalopathy associated with fatty degeneration of the liver**. This syndrome is caused by mitochondrial dysfunction, which occurs in the setting of salicylate treatment of influenza or other viral illness.

Clinical Features
Patients develop the **abrupt onset of vomiting following a prodrome of viral symptoms**. Hepatomegaly is common at presentation. Neurologic changes rapidly develop. The ensuing progressive encephalopathy is characterized by initial irritability and combativeness, followed by confusion, delirium, and eventually coma.

Evaluation
Laboratory studies reveal elevations in liver transaminases and ammonia. The **bilirubin level is typically normal**. The PT is typically elevated and serum glucose levels are depressed.

Treatment
Care is supportive. While the liver often recovers, cerebral edema can be lethal. Fluid restriction, hyperventilation, and mannitol are the mainstays of treatment.

Histiocytic Disorders

Etiology

Reactive disorders associated with proliferation and infiltration of mononuclear phagocytic cells are classified into three groups:

- Langerhans cell histiocytosis (LCH)
- Hemophagocytic lymphohistiocytosis (HLH)
- Malignant histiocytic disorders

Both LCH and HLH are **linked to an overstimulated, albeit ineffective, immune response to a viral or other infection**. LCH is characterized by tissue infiltration with cells similar to the Langerhans cells of the skin, which causes organ damage through the production of cytokines and prostaglandins. HLH is a macrophage-related disorder characterized by proliferation of erythrophagocytic histiocytes in the liver, bone marrow, spleen, lymph nodes, skin, or central nervous system (CNS). HLH has been reported in association with various viral, bacterial, fungal, and parasitic infections, as well as collagen vascular disorders and malignancies. Several familial forms of HLH can cause relapsing disease of variable severity.

Clinical Features

Patients with LCH may present with isolated bony lesions or with multisystem involvement of the skin, teeth, liver, bone marrow, lungs, liver, spleen, gastrointestinal tract, or CNS. Complications include pulmonary and hepatic fibrosis, liver and bone marrow failure, and neurologic abnormalities. Patients with HLH commonly present with fever, jaundice, fatigue, and hepatosplenomegaly. Complications include overwhelming infection, bleeding, and progressive CNS disease.

Evaluation

Complete blood count, coagulation studies, liver transaminases, and a chest radiograph are all important initial studies. A **skeletal survey is used in LCH** to search for bony lesions. **HLH is usually associated with cytopenias** (at least two of three cell lines), **hypertriglyceridemia, hypofibrinogenemia, hyperferritinemia (>500 μg/dL), and hepatitis. Bone marrow evaluation** is typically confirmatory, though identification of hemophagocytic infiltration in lymph node, or ascites fluid, may also be diagnostic.

Treatment

Underlying infection should be aggressively treated with broad-spectrum antibiotics and/or antifungals. **Chemotherapy, radiotherapy, immunotherapy** (etoposides, corticosteroids, cyclosporine, and intravenous immune globulin), and **bone marrow transplantation** have been used in histiocytic disorders with variable success.

Veno-Occlusive Disease

Etiology

Veno-occlusive disease is characterized by **progressive injury to the endothelial cells** lining the terminal hepatic venules, which culminates in hepatocyte necrosis, sinusoidal congestion, and ultimate obliteration of the central hepatic venules.

The process typically occurs in **patients undergoing bone marrow transplantation** (allogeneic > autologous) and is likely related to pre-transplantation conditioning with total body irradiation and chemotherapy.

Clinical Features

The onset of VOD is marked by **gradual weight gain and jaundice** in the 2 weeks following transplantation. Approximately 7 to 10 days later, patients develop **abdominal pain, hepatomegaly, and encephalopathy**. **Ascites** is common.

Evaluation

Laboratory studies reveal elevations in liver transaminase levels, conjugated bilirubin, and ammonia levels. **Doppler ultrasound** of the liver confirms the diagnosis.

Treatment

Treatment of VOD is supportive and primarily involves **sodium restriction, diuretic therapy, and paracentesis,** with the goal of minimizing extravascular fluid while maintaining robust intravascular volume to support liver and kidney perfusion. Experience with **defibrotide** has been promising.

Biliary Atresia

Biliary atresia is discussed in Chapter 46, "Jaundice, Newborn."

Tyrosinemia

Etiology

Tyrosinemia is an **autosomal recessive disorder caused by mutations in the** fumarylacetoacetate hydrolase **(FAH) gene,** which encodes FAH in the tyrosine degradation pathway. The **liver, kidney, and CNS** are primarily affected. Tyrosinemia is more common in patients of French–Canadian (Quebec) and Scandinavian descent.

Clinical Features

Irritability, vomiting, and failure to thrive typically develop in the first year of life. **Jaundice, hepatomegaly, and signs of liver failure,** including coagulopathy and hypoglycemia, are common. Additional signs include **rickets and developmental delay**. Patients with untreated tyrosinemia are at high risk of developing hepatocellular carcinoma.

Evaluation

Laboratory tests may show anemia, hyperbilirubinemia, elevated transaminase levels, and **severe coagulopathy,** which is out of proportion to the elevation in liver enzymes. Signs of **renal Fanconi syndrome,** including hypouricemia, hypophosphatemia, and aminoaciduria, may also be present. The **α-fetoprotein level is often markedly elevated**. Elevations in **urine and plasma succinylacetone are pathognomonic** for tyrosinemia and confirm the diagnosis.

Treatment

Treatment includes **dietary management** and therapy with **NTBC,** a novel compound that blocks the tyrosine metabolism pathway above FAH and thereby prevents the accumulation of toxic metabolites. **Liver transplantation** may be curative in advanced cases.

α-1 Antitrypsin Deficiency

α-1 Antitrypsin deficiency is discussed in Chapter 45, "Jaundice."

Galactosemia

Etiology

Classic galactosemia is **caused by galactose-1-phosphate uridyltransferase deficiency,** which leads to an **inability to metabolize galactose-1-phosphate** and the accumulation of this substance in the liver, kidney, and brain.

Clinical Features

Infants typically develop **irritability, lethargy, vomiting, and hypoglycemia** after introduction of breast milk or lactose-containing formulas. Liver manifestations generally evolve within the ensuing week and include **hepatomegaly** with **marked jaundice**, which may be **exacerbated by brisk hemolysis**. Undiagnosed patients ultimately develop failure to thrive, developmental delay, and **mental retardation**. **Cataracts** are common and may even be present at birth.

Evaluation

Timely diagnosis is critical to prevent permanent brain damage. UA reveals the presence of **reducing sugars,** and the diagnosis is confirmed with the measurement of galactose-1-phosphate uridyltransferase activity.

Treatment

Treatment involves dietary exclusion of galactose.

Wilson Disease (Hepatolenticular Degeneration)

Etiology

Wilson disease is an **autosomal recessive disease of copper metabolism** caused by a mutation in the ATP7B gene. This gene encodes a protein in the hepatocyte that (1) shuttles copper to the Golgi apparatus and (2) transports copper into the bile canaliculus. The defect **in ATP7B decreases copper excretion from the liver,** resulting in a vicious cycle of **hepatocyte death and copper release**. Over time, the **released copper accumulates in other organs** (e.g., the kidney and the brain) and may cause irreversible damage.

Clinical Features

Symptoms typically evolve during **late childhood or early adolescence**. Hepatic involvement predominates and is characterized by **wide spectrum of liver disease,** including asymptomatic transaminase elevation and/or hepatomegaly, cholestasis, cirrhosis, and fulminant liver failure. In those patients with a fulminant presentation, copper-induced **oxidative stress may induce a Coombs negative hemolytic anemia,** associated with an unconjugated hyperbilirubinemia, a reduced alkaline phosphatase level, and an elevated AST/ALT ratio. **Psychiatric and neurologic involvement is often subtle or absent** in children. A careful history may reveal mood swings and deterioration in school performance and/or handwriting.

Evaluation

Initial evaluation should include measurement of the serum ceruloplasmin level and 24-hour urine copper level. **Ceruloplasmin levels <20 mg/dL and 24-hour urine copper levels >100 µg/24 hours are suggestive, but not diagnostic, of Wilson disease.** If either test is abnormal, a **liver biopsy** should be performed. Classic histopathologic features of Wilson disease include steatosis, mitochondrial changes, and a quantitative hepatic copper level >250 µg/g. A **slit lamp examination** of the eyes can also confirm the diagnosis if copper granule deposits are identified in the ocular limbus. However, absence of this finding, known as the **Kayser–Fleischer ring,** cannot reliably exclude the diagnosis. Genetic testing for mutations in ATP7B is also available.

Treatment

Dietary copper should be limited, and copper chelation therapy with D-**penicillamine or trientine** is initiated. Patients with advanced chronic liver disease or fulminant presentation may require liver transplantation.

EVALUATION OF HEPATOMEGALY
Patient History

The following questions may help narrow the differential diagnosis:

- **Is there a history of preceding viral illness?** Mild hepatomegaly may be apparent with even benign viral illness.
- **Did a prodromal illness lead to jaundice?** Infectious etiologies (e.g., hepatitis A) and AIH should be considered.
- **Is there a history of poor feeding with respiratory distress?** Hepatomegaly in the setting of poor feeding and respiratory distress is a classic clinical triad for congestive heart failure in infants. Pneumonia should also be considered in the differential diagnosis.
- **Is there a history of trauma?** Abdominal trauma may result in liver laceration or hematoma, leading to *apparent hepatomegaly.*
- **Is the patient lethargic or irritable?** Sepsis and metabolic disorders may present with a history of lethargy or irritability.
- **Is there a history of vomiting with developmental delay or behavioral abnormalities?** Many of the inborn errors of metabolism may present with vomiting and nonspecific neurodevelopmental abnormalities.
- **Is there a family history of early death or neurologic disease?** Metabolic disorders, as well as the familial form of HLH, should be considered.
- **What is the patient's medication history?** Many drugs can cause liver abnormalities with hepatomegaly. Aspirin use is associated with Reye syndrome.
- **Is there a maternal history of perinatal illness or poor prenatal care?** Infectious etiologies, such as HIV, hepatitis, CMV, and syphilis should be considered.
- **Is there a history of umbilical vein catheterization?** Hepatic abscess is a known complication of umbilical vein catheterization.
- **Is there a history of foreign travel?** Malaria, as well as other infectious etiologies, should be considered if the patient has recently traveled abroad.

- **Is there a history of tick bite?** Rocky Mountain spotted fever, ehrlichiosis, and babesiosis are all concerns after tick bites.
- **Is there a history of animal contact?** Cats or kittens are the main culprits in *Bartonella henselae* infection ("cat scratch disease") and toxoplasmosis. Contact with cat or dog feces is also a risk factor for toxocariasis. Dogs are occasional carriers of *Echinococcus,* as are coyotes, wolves, and other canine species. Leptospirosis is usually transmitted by direct contact with water that has been contaminated with rat, dog, or cattle urine. Brucellosis should be considered if there has been contact with cattle or unpasteurized milk, goat, sheep, or swine. Exposure to infected dogs may also lead to brucellosis. Inhalation of spores containing the fecal droppings of birds or bats is associated with histoplasmosis.

Physical Examination

- **Jaundice** is often the presenting sign in patients with viral hepatitis, hemolytic anemia, anatomic pathologies, and drug hepatotoxicity.
- **Fever** supports an infectious or noninfectious inflammatory diagnosis (e.g., AIH), but may also be present in oncologic presentations.
- **Exudative pharyngitis** often accompanies EBV or CMV infection.
- **Adenopathy** raises suspicion for an infectious or oncologic process.
- An **abdominal mass** raises concern for neuroblastoma or other neoplastic processes.
- **Splenomegaly** occurs with metabolic, infectious, oncologic, and anatomic disorders, as well as with any process that causes hepatic fibrosis and portal hypertension.
- **Eye findings** may be seen in metabolic disorders (e.g., KF rings in Wilson disease, cataracts in galactosemia) or infectious disorders (e.g., CMV).
- **Facial dysmorphism** suggests a metabolic or genetic disorder, such as Alagille syndrome.

Laboratory Studies

Appropriate laboratory studies may include the following:

- **Liver transaminases.** Hepatocellular injury is marked initially by elevations in liver transaminases, including ALT and AST. The ALT level is more specific for liver disease because the AST level also rises with hemolysis and muscle disorders. Alkaline phosphatase (which is also nonspecific) and gamma glutamyltransferase levels are often elevated in cholestatic disorders. Lactate dehydrogenase is another nonspecific marker of liver injury.
- **Bilirubin.** Elevations in conjugated bilirubin are found in cholestatic disorders; elevations in unconjugated bilirubin are seen in hemolytic processes and congenital disorders of bilirubin metabolism.
- **PT, albumin, and glucose.** These studies reflect the synthetic function of the liver.
- **Complete blood count.** The white blood cell and platelet counts are useful when certain infections or infiltrative processes are suspected. The hemoglobin should be carefully monitored in hemolytic and traumatic processes.
- **Routine blood smear.** Evidence of hemolysis and certain infiltrative processes (e.g., leukemia) can be appreciated on the blood smear. Parasitic disease such as malaria can often be identified on the blood smear.

- **Ammonia level.** The ammonia level may be elevated in advanced liver failure, in Reye syndrome, and in certain metabolic disorders.
- **Viral serologies.** Serologic studies are confirmatory in cases of many viral infections (e.g., hepatitis A to E, EBV, CMV).
- **Blood cultures.** Blood cultures should be obtained in cases of suspected sepsis or liver abscess.
- **UA.** Hemoglobinuria is a common finding in hemolytic anemias. Metabolic disorders are sometimes associated with abnormalities in the UA (e.g., the presence of urinary-reducing sugars in galactosemia).
- **Plasma amino acids and urine organic acids.** Metabolic studies of the plasma and urine are warranted when metabolic disorders are suspected.

  Appropriate ancillary studies may include the following:

- **Ultrasound.** Ultrasound is useful to visualize the anatomy of the liver and surrounding structures noninvasively. Intrahepatic and extrahepatic masses are readily identified, and the anatomy of the biliary tree can be evaluated. Doppler studies add important information about the hepatic blood flow.
- **CT and MRI scans.** CT and MRI are useful to detect smaller masses and may better distinguish among tumors, cysts, and abscesses. CT is the most useful study when trauma is suspected.
- **Radionuclide scan.** Nuclear scintigraphy can help distinguish hepatitis from biliary atresia. Tracer uptake into the liver is impaired in the former entity, whereas excretion into the bowel is impaired in the latter entity.
- **Cholangiography.** Direct visualization of the intrahepatic and extrahepatic biliary tree is possible through cholangiography. This test is particularly useful in the diagnosis of biliary atresia.
- **Liver biopsy.** Biopsy of the liver is indicated in cases of suspected autoimmune or oncologic processes, metabolic disorders, and anatomic pathologies (e.g., biliary atresia, Alagille syndrome).
- **Bone marrow biopsy.** Bone marrow biopsy is confirmatory in many oncologic and metabolic (e.g., storage) disorders.

TREATMENT OF HEPATOMEGALY

Treatment of hepatomegaly first necessitates identification of the underlying cause. Suspected **treatable conditions should be aggressively pursued at the initial presentation,** particularly when acute liver failure is evident. Timely initiation of antibiotics to treat infection/abscess, corticosteroids to treat AIH, and D-penicillamine to treat Wilson disease can limit morbidity and obviate the need for liver transplantation in certain patients. In neonates, early identification of correctable causes of extrahepatic biliary obstruction, such as biliary atresia, can translate into improved long-term outcomes and survival. Likewise, a high index of suspicion for certain inborn errors of metabolism, such as galactosemia, hereditary fructose intolerance, and tyrosinemia, can prompt dietary restrictions that may preserve neurodevelopmental integrity and save lives.

In the patients with evidence of liver failure, careful fluid management is critical to limiting extravascular fluid accumulation, while maintaining intravascular volume to preserve renal and hepatic blood flow. A combination of sodium restriction, gentle diuresis, and paracentesis can often achieve this balance. **Blood glucose monitoring,** with supplementation as needed, can prevent the neurologic complications of hypoglycemia. Similarly, the PT/INR should be followed closely. **Vitamin K supplementation** is often necessary to restore normal coagulation in the setting of marked cholestasis, which may interfere with absorption of vitamin K and other fat-soluble vitamins. In advanced liver failure, inadequate hepatic production of clotting factors may necessitate the need for fresh frozen plasma and/or other supportive blood products. Finally, administration of lactulose and/or neomycin can help to expedite elimination of ammonia and limit encephalopathy.

Suggested Readings

De Kerguenec C, Hillaire S, Molinie V, et al. Hepatic manifestations of hemophagocytic syndrome. *Am J Gastroenterol.* 2001;96:852–857.

Elisofon SA, Jonas MM. Hepatitis B and C in children: current treatment and future strategies. *Clin Liver Dis.* 2006;10(1):133–148.

Emerick KM, Whitington PF. Neonatal liver disease. *Pediatr Ann.* 2006;35(4):280–286.

Lee CK, Jonas MM. Pediatric hepatobiliary disease. *Curr Opin Gastroenterol.* 2007;23(3):306–309.

Lipton JM, Westra S, Haverty CE, et al. Case records of the Massachusetts General Hospital. Weekly clinicopathological exercises. Case 28–2004. Newborn twins with thrombocytopenia, coagulation defects, and hepatosplenomegaly. *N Engl J Med.* 2004;351(11):1120–1130.

Misra S, Ament ME, Vargas JH, et al. Chronic liver disease in children on long-term parenteral nutrition. *J Gastroenterol Hepatol.* 1996;11:S4–S6.

Smith K. Hepatomegaly. *Clin Pediatr.* 2005;44(9):813–814.

Troy SB, Rickman LS, Davis CE. Brucellosis in San Diego: epidemiology and species-related differences in acute clinical presentations. *Medicine.* 2005;84(3):174–187.

Walker WA, Mathis RK. Hepatomegaly: an approach to differential diagnosis. *Pediatr Clin N Am.* 1975;22(4):929–942.

Wolf AD, Lavine JE. Hepatomegaly in neonates and children. *Pediatr Rev.* 2000;21:303–310.

Hypertension

INTRODUCTION

Normotension is defined as blood pressure (BP) (systolic, diastolic, or both) that is <90th percentile for the patient's age, height percentile, and sex. **Prehypertension** is defined as BP levels ≥90th percentile but <95th percentile. **Hypertension** is defined as average systolic and/or diastolic BP ≥95th percentile for gender, age, and height on three or more separate occasions (readings).

- **Stage 1 hypertension** is the designation for BP levels that range from ≥95th percentile to 5 mm Hg ≥99th percentile.
- **Stage 2 hypertension** is the designation for BP levels >5 mm Hg above the 99th percentile.
- **Hypertensive urgency** is severely elevated BP with no evidence for secondary end-organ damage.
- **Hypertensive emergency** is severely elevated BP with clinical evidence for end-organ damage (retinopathy, papilledema, encephalopathy, seizures, gastrointestinal bleed, cardiac failure, or renal insufficiency).

Labile blood pressure refers to BP (systolic, diastolic, or both) that is sometimes above and sometimes below the 95th percentile and does not result in hypertensive damage to organs. Labile BP is frequently found in teenagers. **White coat hypertension** is present when elevated BP readings are found in a medical setting with normal BPs measured elsewhere. **Masked hypertension** is present when the BP is normal or prehypertensive in the office but elevated when measured elsewhere (often confirmed by 24-hour ambulatory BP monitoring).

The prevalence of hypertension in the pediatric population is estimated to be between 1% and 5%. Younger children are more likely to have an underlying cause for hypertension than adolescents and adults. However, primary (essential) hypertension is now seen in children and adolescents and is associated with obesity, metabolic syndrome, and a family history of hypertension.

> **HINT:** The younger the patient and the higher the BP, the more likely a secondary cause for hypertension will be found.

DIFFERENTIAL DIAGNOSIS LIST

Primary Hypertension (Essential Hypertension)
Monogenetic Causes
- Gordon syndrome
- Liddle syndrome
- Syndrome of apparent mineralocorticoid excess
- Glucocorticoid remediable aldosteronism

Renoparenchymal Causes
- Glomerulonephritis—acute and chronic
- Hemolytic uremic syndrome
- Focal segmental glomerulosclerosis
- Lupus nephritis
- Pyelonephritis (acute or chronic) or reflux nephropathy
- Polycystic kidney disease—autosomal recessive, autosomal dominant
- Wilms tumor
- Obstructive uropathy
- Trauma

Vascular Causes
- Coarctation of the aorta
- Large arteriovenous fistula
- Mid-aortic syndrome (idiopathic, Williams syndrome, NF-1, tuberous sclerosis, Takayasu arteritis)
- Renal artery stenosis (fibromuscular dysplasia)
- Renal artery thrombosis
- Renal venous thrombosis

Endocrine Causes
- Cushing syndrome
- Hyperthyroidism or hypothyroidism
- Hyperparathyroidism
- Pheochromocytoma
- Neuroblastoma
- Congenital adrenal hyperplasia
- Conn syndrome (hyperaldosteronism)

Neurologic Causes
- Traumatic brain injury
- Intracranial hemorrhage (epidural, subdural, subarachnoid)
- Increased intracranial pressure
- Familial dysautonomia
- Guillain–Barré syndrome
- Pain

Drug-Related Causes
- Corticosteroids
- Calcineurin inhibitors
- Epinephrine
- Cocaine
- Amphetamines
- Sympathomimetics
- Oral contraceptives
- Caffeine
- Calcineurin inhibitors (Cyclosporin A, Tacrolimus)

Miscellaneous Causes
- Stress
- Orthopedic traction
- Burns
- "White coat" hypertension
- Masked hypertension
- Malignant hyperthermia
- Acute intermittent porphyria

APPROACH TO THE PATIENT
Patient History
- **Hypertension is often asymptomatic.** Are there symptoms of hypertension present (e.g., headache, blurry vision, epistaxis, chest pain, flushing, fatigue, and difficulty sleeping)?

- Was there a neonatal history of umbilical artery catheter placement, neonatal asphyxia, and/or bronchopulmonary dysplasia?
- Is there a history of renoparenchymal disease or symptoms of gross hematuria or edema?
- Is there a history of urinary tract infections with reflux nephropathy and/or renal scar formation?
- Is there a family history of hypertension, obesity, familial endocrinopathies, and/or renal disease?
- Is there a history of obesity or metabolic syndrome?
- Is the patient taking or has the patient taken any medications that may result in or contribute to hypertension?
- Does that patient have sweating, flushing, palpitations, and abdominal pain, which may be consistent with pheochromocytoma or neuroblastoma?

Physical Examination

Systolic, diastolic, and mean BP should be obtained in the upper extremity at the level of the heart while calm. BP should be checked in all four extremities and femoral pulses should be palpated to rule out coarctation of the aorta. Assess for retinal changes seen on funduscopic examination and cardiovascular changes (e.g., abdominal bruit, heart murmur, S3, or S4 gallop). Bell's palsy in children may indicate severe undiagnosed hypertension.

Stigmata for syndromes—café au lait, neurofibromas, malar rash, acanthosis, moon facies, short stature, obesity, virilization, ambiguous genitalia, proptosis, thyromegaly.

 HINT: Falsely high readings stem from using a cuff that is too small. The cuff should cover two-thirds of the upper arm from the tip of the acromion to the elbow, and the bladder width should cover 80% to 100% of the circumference of the arm.

Evaluation

A **24-hour ambulatory BP** monitoring may be helpful in diagnosing white coat hypertension, masked hypertension, or labile hypertension. Laboratory studies should include complete blood count, urinalysis, urine culture, serum electrolytes, blood urea nitrogen, serum creatinine, and fasting lipid profile. Ultrasound studies that may be performed to assist with diagnosis include renal ultrasound and echocardiogram. Further evaluation is based on history and physical examination, and/or to assess secondary causes: voiding cystourethrogram, nuclear renal scan, 3D *computed tomography angiography or magnetic resonance angiography,* serum metanephrines, plasma rennin activity, and aldosterone level. More extensive studies include renal angiogram, metaiodobenzylguanidine scan, renal biopsy, and genetic studies for monogenetic causes of hypertension.

Treatment

Hypertensive emergencies should be treated with intravenous BP medications, aiming to decrease the BP by 25% over the first 8 hours and gradually normalizing BP over 24 to 48 hours. **Hypertensive urgencies** can be treated by either

TABLE 43-1	Commonly Used Antihypertensive Agents in Children	
Category	**Agent**	**Common Side Effects**
Diuretics	Chlorothiazides	Hypokalemia, hypochloremic alkalosis, volume depletion, hyperuricemia, hyperlipidemia, hyperglycemia
	Metolazone	Hypokalemia, hyponatremia, hypochloremic alkalosis
	Furosemide	Volume depletion, hypokalemia, alkalosis, nephrocalcinosis
	Spironolactone	Hyperkalemia, mild acidosis, gynecomastia
	Eplerenone	Hyperkalemia, mild acidosis
Vasodilators	Hydralazine	Flushing, tachycardia, headaches
	Minoxidil	Hypotension, hirsutism
β-blockers	Atenolol	Bronchospasm, hypoglycemia
	Labetalol	Bronchospasm, hypotension, tingling in skin or scalp, headache
Calcium channel blockers	Nifedipine	Hypotension, peripheral edema, elevated liver enzymes
	Amlodipine	Peripheral edema, flushing, palpitations
	Diltiazem	Flushing
ACE inhibitors	Captopril, Enalapril, Lisinopril, Benazepril	Hyperkalemia, dry cough, increase in serum creatinine, angioedema
ATIIR blockers	Losartan, Valsartan, Candesartan, Irbesartan	Hyperkalemia, increase in serum creatinine
Renin inhibitors	Aliskiren	Hyperkalemia

ACE, angiotensin-converting enzyme; *ATIIR,* angiotensin II receptor.

intravenous or oral antihypertensives depending on symptomatology. **Mild primary hypertension** may be managed with nonpharmacologic treatment: weight reduction, exercise, and sodium restriction. **Pharmacologic therapy** should be directed to the cause of secondary hypertension when this is known or for severe, sustained primary or secondary hypertension. Chronic oral antihypertensive pharmacologic therapy is generally required for sustained primary or secondary hypertension. Medications may be needed in children with mild-to-moderate hypertension if nonpharmacologic therapy has failed or if end-organ changes are present. The physician should be familiar with potential medication interactions and side effects (Table 43-1). Drug doses should be maximized prior to adding a second agent.

Suggested Readings

Brady TM, Feld LG. Pediatric approach to hypertension. *Semin Nephrol.* 2009;29(4):379–388.

Flynn JT. Pediatric hypertension update. *Curr Opin Nephrol Hypertens.* 2010;19(3):292–297.

Meyers KEC, Falkner B. Hypertension in children and adolescents: an approach to management of complex hypertension in pediatric patients. *Curr Hypertens Rep.* 2009;11(5):315–322.

National Heart, Lung, and Blood Institute. The fourth report on the diagnosis, evaluation and treatment of high blood pressure in children and adolescents. *Pediatrics.* 2004;114(2):S555–S576.

Portman R, McNiece K, Swinford R, et al. Pediatric hypertension: diagnosis, evaluation, management, and treatment for the primary care physician. *Curr Probl Pediatr Adolesc Health Care.* 2005;35(7):262–294.

Hypotonia

INTRODUCTION

Hypotonia is defined as abnormally low resting muscle tone. It primarily manifests as decreased resistance to passive movement and abnormalities in resting posture. Hypotonia most commonly presents in infancy (often called "floppy babies"), although low tone may present acutely with a variety of illnesses at any age.

The first task when confronted with a patient with possible hypotonia is to **differentiate decreased tone from weakness or lethargy,** although some infants present with both problems simultaneously. Likewise, hyporeflexia is a separate finding with a distinct differential diagnosis.

It is critically important to localize the process within the nervous system— central hypotonia refers to suprasegmental disorders affecting brain, brainstem, and cervical spinal junction; lower motor neuron diseases affect anterior horn cell, peripheral nerve, neuromuscular junction, and muscle. A careful history and physical examination, including a thorough neurological examination, frequently narrows the differential diagnosis enough to necessitate only confirmatory diagnostic tests, sparing the patient a shotgun approach including unnecessary and often painful, costly, or invasive procedures.

DIFFERENTIAL DIAGNOSIS LIST

In Infants
Central Hypotonia

Infection (e.g., sepsis, meningitis, encephalitis)

Genetic abnormalities (e.g., Down syndrome, Prader–Willi syndrome, fragile X)

Metabolic disease (e.g., leukodystrophy, glycogen storage disease)

Trauma (e.g., birth trauma, nonaccidental trauma)

Hypoxic ischemic encephalopathy (e.g., decreased perinatal perfusion)

Vascular (e.g., stroke, intracranial hemorrhage)

Anatomic (e.g., congenital brain malformations)

Drug/toxin (e.g., narcotics)

Other causes (e.g., benign congenital hypotonia, hypothyroidism)

Peripheral Hypotonia

Spinal muscular atrophy (SMA)

Nerve injury (e.g., brachial plexus injury)

Myasthenia gravis

Medications/toxins (e.g., botulinum toxin, hypermagnesemia)
Congenital myopathies
Congenital myotonic dystrophy

In Children
Central Hypotonia

Infection (e.g., sepsis, encephalitis)
Metabolic disease (e.g., adrenoleukodystrophy, glycogen storage disease)
Neoplasm (e.g., brain tumor, infiltrative neoplasm)

Vascular (e.g., stroke)
Toxins/electrolyte abnormalities (e.g., ingestion)

Peripheral Hypotonia

Spinal muscular atrophy
Infection (e.g., myositis)
Trauma (e.g., nerve injury)
Neuropathy (e.g., Charcot–Marie–Tooth disease)
Guillain–Barré syndrome
Myasthenia gravis
Muscular dystrophy
Dermatomyositis
Tick paralysis

DIFFERENTIAL DIAGNOSIS DISCUSSION

Most "floppy babies" in the newborn period do not have hypotonia of a neurological etiology but are weak and/or lethargic from other causes, such as infection or dehydration. Likewise, older children with focal "decreased tone" can actually be manifesting orthopedic problems or joint laxity. The first step in considering the differential diagnosis of hypotonia for any patient, therefore, is to consider the possibility of nonneurological illness.

> **HINT:** The two most common pitfalls in diagnosing hypotonia are confusing weakness or lethargy for hypotonia and assuming a neurological etiology, without consideration for nonneurological causes.

Once careful history and physical examination confirm that the problem is truly hypotonia, the next step is to determine localization in the neuraxis (see later). Central hypotonia is caused by problems in the central nervous system; peripheral hypotonia is related to disturbance somewhere at the level of the spinal cord, nerve, neuromuscular junction, or muscle. There are myriad causes of hypotonia, and a full differential is often beyond the scope of the general pediatrician. Distinguishing central from peripheral hypotonia, however, is usually easily accomplished during the initial evaluation and can help guide appropriate evaluation and referral (see Table 44-1).

The differential diagnosis differs extensively between infants and children >1 year of age; therefore, they are divided accordingly here. Selected diagnoses are described here, but the full differential is extensive and beyond the scope of this book.

TABLE 44-1	**Features of Central Versus Peripheral Hypotonia**	
	Central Hypotonia	**Peripheral Hypotonia**
History	Encephalopathy Hypoxic ischemic injury Seizures	Joint contractures Normal mental status No seizures
Examination	No weakness Dysmorphic features Normal or brisk reflexes	Muscle weakness Sensory deficits Diminished or absent reflexes

INFANTS
Central Hypotonia
Etiology and Clinical Features
Central hypotonia is caused by problems in the **central nervous system** (i.e., the brain or upper motor neurons in spinal cord). Tone abnormalities are **global,** involving the whole body, and often accompanied by **encephalopathy,** or altered mental status. Seizures and sleep/wake cycle disturbances also may suggest a central problem. Babies with central hypotonia have low resting tone but usually have **preserved strength** when they do make effort with their limbs. The numerous causes of central hypotonia may be grouped into larger categories.

- **Infection.** Consider sepsis, meningitis, encephalitis, and toxoplasmosis, other, rubella, cytomegalovirus, herpes simplex (TORCH) infections.
- **Genetic abnormalities.** A number of genetic syndromes include hypotonia as a presenting feature in the neonatal period, even before dysmorphic features or other affected organs might be apparent. There are dozens of definable syndromes, and more are being identified with the availability of genome-wide microarrays that can show novel or familial disease-causing copy number variants.

   Important and common syndromes include:

- **Trisomy 21** (Down syndrome) is the most commonly observed chromosomal abnormality, occurring in approximately 1 in 1,000 births. Children with Down syndrome have characteristic facial features, dermatoglyphic and hand abnormalities, and are at higher risk for cardiac and gastrointestinal (GI) defects.
- **Prader–Willi syndrome** is usually the result of a paternally inherited deletion in chromosome 15, although other inheritance patterns can also lead to the same outcome. Affected neonates have severe hypotonia, feeding difficulties, and failure to thrive. Mental retardation, hypogonadism, and hyperphagia with obesity become prominent features later in childhood.
- **Turner syndrome** is caused by the 45 X0 genotype, occurring in 1 in 5,000 infants. It only occurs in females, who also may have short stature, broad chest, webbed neck, hearing loss, and coarctation of the aorta.
- **Fragile X syndrome** is caused by increased triplet nucleotide repeat in the region of the *FMR1* gene. Although girls may present with a milder phenotype,

the profound symptoms seen in infancy are usually only seen in boys. Mental retardation and autism are prominent features.

- **Metabolic disease.** A host of inborn errors of metabolism can cause hypotonia. This category should be suspected particularly in patients who are initially asymptomatic but fall ill after initiation of feeding or during intercurrent illness. Developmental regression raises special concern for metabolic disease. If metabolic disorders are suspected, a neurologist or geneticist with expertise in metabolic disorders should be consulted because effective dietary or gene replacement therapy is available for some conditions.

- **Trauma.** Birth trauma, either involving the brain or cervical spine, and the possibility of subsequent nonaccidental trauma must always be considered and evaluated by appropriate imaging. Spinal cord trauma, as in complicated delivery, may cause spinal shock, signaled by autonomic changes and acute deficits in bladder and bowel function; immediate neurological consultation is indicated.

- **Hypoxic ischemic encephalopathy** can result from any impairment in oxygenation and blood flow to the brain. This may include difficult delivery or be secondary to other disease, such as respiratory or cardiac failure.

- **Vascular insults.** Neonatal stroke may include arterial ischemic stroke, venous sinus thrombosis, and intracranial hemorrhage. Each of these may include focal symptoms that are mild and much less obvious than global hypotonia.

- **Anatomic abnormalities.** Neuroimaging may reveal congenital anomalies in brain and/or cord development causing hypotonia. Some of these abnormalities are quite dramatic such as schizencephaly, lissencephaly, or holoprosencephaly, but many others are less specific with submicroscopic migrational anomalies that may not be capable of demonstration until maturation and myelinization. Even then, one might only see a blurring of gray–white matter junction or unusual gyral pattern.

- **Drugs/toxins.** Medications given to the mother prior to delivery, particularly **narcotics, sedatives, and magnesium (to prevent preterm labor),** may lead to congenital hypotonia.

- **Other causes.** Benign congenital hypotonia is a diagnosis of exclusion. These children initially present with hypotonia in the newborn period or first months of life. Because motor milestones are so important in infancy, they may present with developmental delay but catch up by early childhood. Hypotonia usually resolves in the first years of life but can persist into adulthood. **Hypothyroidism** is treatable if identified early, so must always enter the differential.

Peripheral Hypotonia
Etiology and Clinical Features
Peripheral hypotonia is caused by problems at the level of the lower motor neuron, nerve, muscle, or neuromuscular junction. The characteristic findings are preserved mental status, accompanying weakness, and decreased or absent deep tendon reflexes.

- **SMA** is the result of a mutation in the *SMN1* gene on chromosome 5p. Affected patients have progressive degeneration of anterior horn cells. SMA type I

(Werdnig–Hoffmann disease) may present as early as the newborn period with hypotonia and weakness, and it progresses in the first year of life to include weakness of facial muscles. Tongue fasciculation may be present. The disease is universally fatal; although treatment trials show promise, supportive care is the current standard.

- **Nerve injuries** can lead to focal hypotonia and weakness. The most common type in neonates is brachial plexus injury (**Erb palsy**). It is caused by stretching of the nerves of the brachial plexus. This may occur with difficult deliveries of macrosomic neonates, especially if traction on the head or arm is required. The affected arm is adducted and internally rotated, with the forearm extended and the wrist flexed. The diagnosis is made clinically and may be confirmed with nerve conduction studies (NCS) and electromyography (EMG).

- **Myasthenia gravis** occurs when **antibodies against the acetylcholine** receptor cause blockade of signal transmission at the **neuromuscular junction**. Antibodies are transferred from the affected mother in 10% of neonates born to mothers with myasthenia gravis. Other forms of **congenital myasthenia** also result from impaired neuromuscular junction signaling and can be caused by a genetic defect in receptor, synaptic vesicle, or enzyme production. The diagnosis may be made via Tensilon test, NCS with EMG, and serum testing for specific antibodies.

- **Medications/toxins** may act on the nerves, muscles, or neuromuscular junction to cause hypotonia. A well-known example is **botulinum toxin**. In infants, disease is produced by an enteric-toxin mechanism (as opposed to ingestion of preformed toxin in tainted food seen in older children and adults). Spores of *Clostridium botulinum* may be ingested in contaminated honey, but they are also often ingested during contact with contaminated soil, as in homes near construction, or when parents have been involved in labor in contaminated soil. Germination leads to toxin production in the immature GI tract, which produces constipation. Absorption of toxin leads to disease, often beginning with diplopia and followed by progressive bulbar and extremity weakness. Pupils do not constrict in response to light, a characteristic finding that helps distinguish botulism from other causes of hypotonia. Diagnosis is made with NCS/EMG and detection of organism or toxin in stool sample. Treatment includes aggressive supportive care in the intensive care unit, avoidance of aminoglycoside antibiotics, and use of botulinum antitoxin.

- **Congenital myopathies** include central core and nemaline rod myopathy. Decreased muscle bulk and abnormal creatine kinase are suggestive of these diseases.

- **Congenital myotonic dystrophy.** Myotonic dystrophy is an inherited condition demonstrating anticipation (earlier age of onset or increased severity of symptoms in offspring of affected individuals). Affected mothers may only demonstrate weak handshake, mild facial diplegia, or prolonged labor, but their children may be much more severely affected, with arthrogryposis and profound weakness, including the need for mechanical ventilation.

IN CHILDREN

Although some of the disease categories in children are similar to infants, important differences are highlighted here.

Central Hypotonia

- **Infection.** Encephalitis should be considered if encephalopathy is a feature.
- **Metabolic disease.** Although many metabolic diseases present in infancy, several storage diseases do not become apparent until later in life. History of developmental regression, or repeated encephalopathy or profound weakness in times of illness, suggest this category.
- **Neoplasm.** In addition to brain tumor, infiltrative neoplasms of the spinal cord may cause hypotonia.
- **Vascular insults.** These include spinal cord infarction.
- **Toxin/electrolyte abnormalities.** Ingestions of medications, recreational drugs, and toxins can cause subacute onset of hypotonia. Inhalants should also be considered if encephalopathy occurs. Lead poisoning, although decreased in recent decades, remains of concern.

Peripheral Hypotonia

- **SMA,** types II and III, present later in life than Werdnig–Hoffmann disease (type I). Type II presents in toddlers; type III has a mean onset of 9 years of age. Each may present with weakness, most notably in the proximal muscles, as well as difficulty with motor skills. NCS and EMG or genetic testing can make the diagnosis.
- **Infection.** Although rare in infants, myositis in children can cause myalgias, weakness, and hypotonia.
- **Trauma.** A careful history can reveal recent trauma causing focal nerve injury in the area affected by hypotonia.
- **Neuropathy.** Hereditary neuropathy, such as Charcot–Marie–Tooth disease, can cause mild, diffuse hypotonia. Acquired neuropathy caused by toxins or infection (such as HIV) is also considered when sensory or motor deficits are present.
- **Guillain–Barré syndrome** is a postinfectious, autoimmune disease that causes demyelination of the peripheral nerves. Ascending, progressive weakness typically develops approximately 2 weeks following mild flulike or GI illness. Paresthesias are also common. Cerebrospinal fluid abnormalities with elevated protein and no leukocytosis may aid the diagnosis, but findings may not be seen until the second week of symptoms or later. NCS/EMG testing can also be helpful. Supportive treatment is essential, and the disease course may be modified with intravenous immunoglobulin.
- **Myasthenia gravis** is caused by **acetylcholine receptor antibodies** as described earlier. In children, myasthenia gravis is an acquired illness caused by the production of **autoantibodies**. Children have both hypotonia and fluctuating weakness, usually **worsened by activity** or at the end of the day.
- **Muscular dystrophy** is of many types and can present in childhood. Progressive weakness and decreased muscle bulk are clues toward this diagnosis.

- **Dermatomyositis** is an autoimmune illness with characteristic rash, myalgias, and weakness. The weakness comes in flares; diagnosis is aided by skin findings, elevation of creatine kinase, and abnormal erythrocyte sedimentation rate.
- **Tick paralysis** occurs when the patient has a tick attached to the affected limb. Careful inspection of skin reveals the causative insect, and removal results in quick recovery.

APPROACH TO THE PATIENT

Conditions that are amenable to rapid treatment (e.g., electrolyte imbalance, infection) must be excluded and treated first. Correction removes complicating factors from further evaluation and may even relieve symptoms alone.

Stabilization of the patient is the highest priority. A number of central and peripheral causes of hypotonia have the potential for rapid progression and life-threatening consequences. Constant attention must be paid to airway stabilization and respiratory function because these are commonly impaired in diseases causing hypotonia.

After the patient is stable, the evaluation may proceed as described next. Because the differential diagnosis of hypotonia is broad, care should be taken to ascertain all of the historical facts and to perform a complete examination. A neurology consult is generally necessary to help narrow the differential diagnosis after the preliminary categorization is performed.

EVALUATION OF HYPOTONIA
Patient History

- When did the symptoms first appear?
- Are the symptoms worsening or staying the same?
- Was the onset acute or gradual? Paroxysmal onset suggests an acute event, such as stroke or trauma. Ingestion or infection is more likely to be subacute; metabolic and degenerative diseases have more chronic progressions.
- Where are the symptoms? Clarify if the problem is global or affects only one limb.
- Are there any associated symptoms? Multisystem disease should raise the suspicion for a genetic syndrome. Encephalopathy points toward central hypotonia. Sensory deficits suggest nerve disease.
- What is the birth history? Decreased fetal movements prior to birth suggest problems existing before delivery. Prematurity should adjust the examiner's expectations for normal tone and strength. Traumatic delivery can point toward brachial plexus injury. Acidotic cord blood gas, neonatal seizures, and other evidence of birth depression may support hypoxic-ischemic encephalopathy.
- Is there a family history of hypotonia, nerve, or muscle problems? Affected parents may have a milder phenotype, so hereditary neuropathies or muscle disease may have never been diagnosed.

Physical Examination

In addition to a general physical examination, special care should be taken with the following points:

- **Mental status**—altered mental status strongly supports a central cause of hypotonia.
- **Posture** of trunk and extremities—the most accurate examination is performed with the child awake, relaxed, and (in infants) the head at midline. In older children, low truncal tone may manifest as slumped posture or poor head control.
- **A "frog-leg" position** (i.e., hips abducted, flexed, and externally rotated) is seen in hypotonic infants.
- **Head lag** when the infant is pulled from a supine to sitting position supports the diagnosis of hypotonia.
- **Vertical suspension** should be performed in all infants; in the hypotonic infant, there is a tendency to slip through the examiner's hands when held under the axillae.
- **Horizontal suspension** results in a hypotonic infant draping over the examiner's hands, rather than holding the head and extremities up in the air ("inverted comma sign").
- **Muscle bulk,** when decreased, is concerning for primary muscle disease.
- **Fasciculations** are concerning for SMA.
- **Deep tendon reflexes** are more likely to be normal or brisk in central hypotonia, diminished or absent in peripheral hypotonia.

Laboratory Studies

Care should be taken to gather as much information as possible with the history and physical examination before proceeding with laboratory assessment. **Complete blood count and urinalysis** can be helpful in evaluating infection. **Metabolic panel, bilirubin level** (in infants), and **thyroid function** testing can be helpful screening tests. If metabolic disease is suspected, **serum amino acids, urine organic acids, and ammonia** levels can be helpful screens. **Newborn screen** results should be obtained. **Creatine phosphokinase** can indicate muscle disease. Cerebrospinal fluid analysis can indicate infection or an autoimmune disease, such as Guillain–Barré syndrome. **Chromosome analysis** is helpful if genetic disease is suspected.

Diagnostic Modalities

- **NCS and EMG** are helpful in peripheral hypotonia and may even be diagnostic.
- **Magnetic resonance imaging** of the brain can identify structural abnormalities, vascular lesions, and evidence of genetic or metabolic disease in central hypotonia.
- **Muscle ultrasound** can help identify myopathic changes and identify those patients who might benefit from **muscle biopsy**.

Suggested Readings

Bodensteiner JB. The evaluation of the hypotonic infant. *Semin Pediatr Neurol.* 2008;15:10–20.
Chen C, Visootsak J, Dills S, et al. Prader-Willi syndrome: an update and review for the primary pediatrician. *Clin Pediatr.* 2007;46:580–591.

Chiang LM, Darras BT, Kang PB. Juvenile myasthenia gravis. *Muscle Nerve.* 2009;39:423–431.

Domingo RM, Haller JS, Gruenthal M. Infant botulism: two recent cases and literature review. *J Child Neurol.* 2008;23(11):1336–1346.

Dubowitz V. Evaluation and differential diagnosis of the hypotonic infant. *Pediatr Rev.* 1985;6:237–243.

Engel AG, Sine SM. Current understanding of congenital myasthenic syndromes. *Curr Opin Pharmacol.* 2005;3:308–321.

McNeely PD, Drake JM. A systematic review of brachial plexus surgery for birth-related injury. *Pediatr Neurosurg.* 2003;38:57–62.

Paro-Panjan D, Neubauer D. Congenital hypotonia: is there an algorithm? *J Child Neurol.* 2004;19:439–442.

Petersen MC, Palmer FB. Advances in prevention and treatment of cerebral palsy. *Ment Retard Dev Disabil Res Rev.* 2001;7:30–37.

Thompson CE. Benign congenital hypotonia is not a diagnosis. *Dev Med Child Neurol.* 2002;44:283–284.

Thompson JA, Filloux FM, Van Orman CB, et al. Infant botulism in the age of botulism immune globulin. *Neurology.* 2005;64:2029–2032.

Verma S, Anziska Y, Cracco J. Review of Duchenne muscular dystrophy (DMD) for the pediatricians in the community. *Clin Pediatr.* 2010;49(11):1011–1017.

Jaundice

INTRODUCTION

Jaundice is defined as a **yellow discoloration** of the skin, mucous membranes, and sclerae caused by **increased levels of circulating bilirubin**. The term "jaundice" is derived from the French word *jaune,* which means *yellow.* Typically, the concentration of bilirubin in the plasma must exceed 1.5 mg/dL to be easily visible. The first step in the evaluation of jaundice is laboratory determination of fractionated bilirubin, as the diagnostic approach differs significantly for unconjugated and conjugated hyperbilirubinemia. In unconjugated hyperbilirubinemia, elevations are due to one of the following:

- Increased production of bilirubin from the breakdown of heme proteins (largely hemoglobin)
- Decreased conjugation or excretion of bilirubin
- Increased enterohepatic circulation of bilirubin (which is less of an issue in an older child)

Conjugated hyperbilirubinemia is largely due to either hepatic dysfunction or obstruction of the biliary system.

Consideration of jaundice in the older child requires a different approach than that of a jaundiced neonate (described in Chapter 46, "Jaundice, Newborn").

 DIFFERENTIAL DIAGNOSIS LIST

Unconjugated Hyperbilirubinemia
Increased Production of Bilirubin
 (Hemolysis)
 Red blood cell (RBC) defects
 Hemoglobinopathies
 Autoimmune hemolytic
  anemia
 Hemolytic uremic syndrome
Decreased Bilirubin Conjugation
 or Excretion
 Gilbert syndrome (GS) and
  Crigler–Najjar syndrome
  (CN)

Mixed Unconjugated/Conjugated Hyperbilirubinemia
Rotor syndrome (RS) and Dubin–
 Johnson syndrome (DJS)
Hormonal deficiency (hypothyroid-
 ism, hypopituitarism)

Conjugated Hyperbilirubinemia
Infectious Causes
 Viral hepatitis: A, B, C, D, and
  E, cytomegalovirus (CMV),
  Epstein–Barr virus (EBV),
  enterovirus, and echovirus

Bacterial infection: Sepsis and liver abscess

Parasitic infections: Ascariasis

Infection of the biliary tree (cholangitis)

Toxic Causes

Drug-induced liver injury (DILI)

Acetaminophen overdose (and others, including numerous antibiotics and anticonvulsants)

Amanita mushroom ingestion

Disorders of Copper and Iron Storage

Wilson disease

Juvenile hemochromatosis (JHC)

Secondary iron overload (transfusion-related)

Genetic Causes

Alpha-1 antitrypsin deficiency

Cystic fibrosis

Autoimmune Causes

Autoimmune hepatitis (AIH)

Autoimmune sclerosing cholangitis overlap syndrome

Sclerosing cholangitis (primary or secondary)

Obstructive Causes

Cholecystitis

Choledocholithiasis

Tumor (hepatic, biliary, pancreatic, peritoneal, duodenal)

Choledochal cyst

Pancreatic disease

Vascular Causes

Budd–Chiari syndrome

Veno-occlusive disease (VOD) (hepatic sinusoidal obstruction syndrome)

SELECTED DIFFERENTIAL DIAGNOSIS DISCUSSION
Unconjugated Hyperbilirubinemia

Hemolysis can result from **hemoglobinopathies, RBC defects, and autoimmune processes**. Increased destruction of RBCs releases a heme moiety that is broken down to biliverdin by the heme oxygenase complex, and from biliverdin to unconjugated bilirubin through the activity of biliverdin reductase. Laboratory investigation will often show an **increased reticulocyte count, decreased haptoglobin, and increased lactate dehydrogenase levels**. In autoimmune processes, patients may be **Coombs positive**. There is often a positive family history of hemoglobinopathy. Hereditary spherocytosis is the most common congenital RBC membrane disorder, with a frequency of 1 in 5,000 and is inherited in an autosomal dominant fashion. A further discussion of hemoglobinopathies, RBC defects, and autoimmune hemolytic anemia can be found in Chapter 40, "Hemolysis."

GS is a heterogeneous group of at least four different disorders that all share at least a 50% decrease in hepatic *bilirubin UDP-glucuronosyltransferase* (BUGT). BUGT acts to conjugate bilirubin, which is then excreted into the enterohepatic circulation. The genetic isoform responsible for bilirubin conjugation is **UGT1A1**. GS is characterized by **recurrent, mild unconjugated hyperbilirubinemia in the presence of otherwise normal liver function tests**. Elevation is variable and ranges from 1 to 4 mg/dL. Unless it is coinherited with hemoglobinopathies or RBC defects, it is rarely clinically apparent until after puberty. Large-scale studies have suggested an incidence rate between 3% and 10%, with a strong male predominance. **GS is not associated with any negative implications for health or**

longevity. There have been reports of associated fatigue or abdominal pain, but studies of larger populations have suggested no significant difference from control populations.

CN Types I and II are caused by a profound decrease in BUGT levels. In CN I, **unconjugated serum bilirubin levels range from 25 to 35 mg/dL,** and affected patients can develop kernicterus even into adulthood, which can be prevented only with lifelong phototherapy, and in some cases, liver transplantation. **CN II is more frequent and less severe than CN I, with serum bilirubin levels ranging from 8 to 25 mg/dL.** CN I and CN II can be differentiated through phenobarbital treatment; in CN II, treatment leads to a significant decrease in serum bilirubin and increased biliary bilirubin conjugates, there is no change in bilirubin levels pre- and post-phenobarbital treatment.

RS and DJS are two similar but distinct disorders of hyperbilirubinemia. They are rare and inherited in an **autosomal recessive** fashion. In both syndromes, there is an elevation of both conjugated and unconjugated bilirubin in the presence of other liver function tests that are normal. Both conditions are asymptomatic, unassociated with morbidity or mortality, and require no therapy. DJS is more common than RS, and presents from birth to 40 years of age rather than in early childhood with RS. Liver examination in RS is completely normal, but in DJS, liver pathology shows distinctive brown-black pigmentation with storage located in the lysosomes microscopically.

Thyroid disorders affect bile flow and composition. Hypothyroidism has been shown in animal studies to be associated with decreased bile flow due to a decrease in bile salt-independent flow.

Conjugated Hyperbilirubinemia
Infectious Causes
The **most likely cause of acute onset of conjugated hyperbilirubinemia in older infants and children is an acute viral infection**. Hepatitis A, B, C, D, and E viruses, in addition to CMV and EBV are the most common causes of jaundice and hepatitis. Other hepatotropic viruses include adenovirus, arbovirus, coxsackievirus, yellow fever, herpes simplex virus, human immunodeficiency virus, paramyxovirus, rubella, and varicella.

Hepatitis A virus is contracted primarily through the fecal-oral route, and is widespread with ~25,000 cases yearly in the United States. The average incubation period is 28 days; however, **fecal shedding can occur for 3 weeks before and for 1 week after the onset of jaundice**. Clinically, examination can be significant for **jaundice, dehydration, and a mildly enlarged liver**. Serum aminotransferase values are usually **20 to 100 times the upper limit of normal,** and usually decrease within the first 2 to 3 weeks, remaining abnormal for up to 3 months. Hyperbilirubinemia occurs in 1 of 12 children and often resolves within 4 weeks. Adults are more likely to develop fulminant hepatitis, with a fatality rate of 1% versus 0.1% in children. Active prophylaxis is available in the form of hepatitis A vaccine, a formalin-inactivated virus that induces a protective immune response in 99% of children.

Hepatitis E virus is also spread by the fecal-oral route, and causes high mortality in pregnant women. It is mainly an issue in adults, but isolated childhood infections have been reported.

Hepatitis B virus (HBV) is a major worldwide cause of mortality. It can be transmitted **(1) parenterally through contaminated transfused blood products or intravenous drug use, (2) percutaneously or transmucosally from exposure to blood or other contaminated blood fluids, and (3) vertically during childbirth**. As many as 350 million individuals are chronically infected, and annually, 250,000 deaths are attributed to chronic hepatitis B and its complications. The presentation of acute HBV infection is dependent upon the age of acquisition. The route of transmission in the pediatric population can be divided into three groups: perinatal, infancy/childhood, and adolescent/young adult. In the adolescent/young adult population, the incubation period ranges from 28 to 180 days, with a prodrome of **fever, anorexia, fatigue, malaise, and nausea**. Extrahepatic manifestations including migratory arthritis, angioedema, Gianotti–Crosti syndrome (or popular acrodermatitis of childhood) are evident during the prodrome period. Typically, the prodromal symptoms last 1 to 2 weeks, begin to subside, and are followed by symptoms of jaundice, hepatosplenomegaly, and pruritus. Symptoms can persist for 1 to 2 months. In general, 90% will resolve symptoms and 10% will go on to chronic infection. **In perinatal, vertically acquired infections, the child is often asymptomatic, with 85% to 90% going on to develop chronic HBV infection.** Infants and children who do not become infected perinatally from their mothers still remain at high risk of infection during the first 5 years of life.

Treatment of acute hepatitis B is supportive, with the majority of affected individuals recovering without treatment. **Chronic infection is defined by detectable serum HBsAg for at least 6 months and evidence of active viral replication.** The goals of treatment of chronic HBV include cessation or decrease in viral replication, normalizing liver pathology and aminotransferases, and none of the currently available medications in the United States achieve these goals for all children. Chronically infected patients should be managed under the care of a pediatric hepatologist. Passive prophylaxis with hepatitis B immune globulin is indicated for single instances of exposure, such as perinatal exposure, needlestick accidents, and sexual contact. Active prophylaxis has been available since 1982. Mass hepatitis B vaccination programs in places such as Taiwan have led to a decreased mortality from fulminant hepatitis in infants and decreased incidence of childhood hepatoma.

Hepatitis D virus (HDV) causes disease only as a coinfection in patients with acute or chronic HBV infection. Mortality rate in coinfected HDV patients ranges from 2% to 20% as opposed to 1% in acute HBV alone. HDV is acquired parenterally.

Hepatitis C virus (HCV) is transmitted parenterally, with the large portion of cases transmitted percutaneously through blood transfusions and intravenous drug abuse, and the remainder transmitted sexually or perinatally. Skin tattooing and accidental needlestick injury have been associated with HCV transmission. The majority of initial HCV infections in children are asymptomatic, particularly in those children who contracted the disease in the perinatal period. The incubation period after transmission is 1 to 5 months, with slow, insidious onset and a mild clinical illness, causing jaundice in only 25% of patients. **In the pediatric population, where HCV is contracted perinatally, it is often asymptomatic with a >90% chance of developing chronicity and an increased risk of hepatocellular carcinoma and cirrhosis.**

Treatment of acute HCV with interferon-α-2β in adults prevents chronicity in nearly all cases when therapy is initiated within the first 3 months of exposure. Chronic HCV is treated with combination therapy with pegylated interferon-α and ribavirin, a nucleoside analogue. Patients should be considered for treatment if they are at least 3 years of age with evidence of chronic infection, and no contraindications to therapy, which include renal failure, severe heart disease, anemia (ribavirin), depression, and thyroid disease (interferon).

EBV is the principal cause of infectious mononucleosis, which is generally a mild disease in healthy children. Eighty percent of children will have elevated serum aminotransferase levels, in addition to the symptoms of fever, fatigue, and pharyngitis; 10% to 15% will have hepatomegaly. Treatment is supportive, with steroids administered in the presence of tonsilloadenoidal hypertrophy that threatens airway patency.

In immunocompetent individuals, **CMV** can cause an infectious mononucleosis-like picture with mild hepatic involvement. CMV can cause severe disease in immunocompromised children as well as in congenital infections.

When viral hepatitis is suspected, testing should be done for IgM antibody to hepatitis A, hepatitis B surface antigen, hepatitis C polymerase chain reaction (PCR), as well as EBV PCR, CMV PCR, and serologies. Additional viral panels should also be evaluated. See Table 45-1 for a summary of interpretation of antibody tests.

Drug-Induced Liver Injury

One of the most important functions of the liver is drug metabolism, which can be broadly described by two phases: activation (Phase I) and detoxification (Phase II). Hepatotoxicity is affected by the balance between the two phases. The spectrum of presentation of DILI is broad, with **hepatitis, cholestatic, or hepatitic-cholestatic** presentations. **Acetaminophen** toxicity, the most common cause of DILI, has a distinct clinical presentation—after an immediate symptomatic interval of nausea and vomiting, there is an asymptomatic period of 2 to 4 days, followed by clinically apparent liver injury: **jaundice, elevated liver function tests, coagulopathy, and, eventually, liver failure and progressive encephalopathic coma**. There are numerous other medications that have been associated with DILI, including various antibiotic and antifungal therapies, anticonvulsants, and hormonal therapies.

Diagnosis requires a high index of suspicion, screening carefully for potential exposure to environmental or industrial toxins. Treatment for DILI is stopping the responsible drug—most diseases will resolve spontaneously, but can persist up to 4 to 6 months. It is important to screen for other causes of childhood liver disease.

TABLE 45-1	Serologic Markers of Hepatitis Infection			
Virus	**Marker**	**Definition**	**Method**	**Significance**
Hepatitis A virus (HAV)	Anti-HAV Anti-HAV-IgM	Total antibodies to HAV IgM antibody to HAV	RIA/EIA RIA/EIA	Current or past infection Current or recent infection
Hepatitis B virus (HBV)	HBsAg Anti-HBS HBeAg Anti-HBe HBV DNA HBcAg Anti-HBc	Hepatitis B surface antigen Antibody to HBsAg Nucleocapsid-derived Ag Antibody to HBeAg HBV viral DNA Core Ag of HBV Antibody to HBcAg	RIA/EIA RIA/EIA RIA/EIA RIA/EIA PCR RIA/EIA	Ongoing HBV infection or carrier status Resolving or past infection Protective immunity Immunity from vaccination Active infection High infectivity Resolving or past infection Active infection Correlates with disease activity Loss indicates resolution Can be detected only in the liver Sensitive indication of replication Ongoing or past infection
Hepatitis C virus (HCV)	Anti-HCV HCV RNA	Antibody to multiple HCV antigens HCV viral RNA	ELISA RIBA PCR	Current or past HCV infection Active infection
Hepatitis D virus (HDV)	Anti-HDV Anti-HDV IgM	IgG/IgM to HDV antigen IgM to HDV antigen	RIA/EIA RIA/EIA	Acute or chronic infection Acute infection
Hepatitis E virus (HEV)	Anti-HEV IgM Anti-HEV IgG	IgM to HEV protein IgG to HEV protein	EIA	Early HEV infection Late HEV infection

EIA, electroimmunoassay; *ELISA,* enzyme-linked immunosorbent assay; *PCR,* polymerase chain reaction; *RIA,* radio-immunoassay; *RIBA,* radio-immunobinding assay.
Modified from Pall H, Jonas M. Acute and chronic hepatitis. In: Wyllie R, Hyams JS, Kay M, eds. *Pediatric Gastrointestinal and Liver Disease.* 3rd ed. Philadelphia, PA: Elsevier; 2006.

For acetaminophen, a specific antidote is available in the form of *n*-acetylcysteine, which, if used early, can prevent hepatic failure and death. Liver transplantation may be necessary in the presence of fulminant hepatic failure.

Wilson Disease
Wilson disease is the most common metabolic cause of fulminant liver failure in children >3 years of age. Diagnosis is suggested by **characteristic low alkaline phosphatase level, low ceruloplasmin, increased urine copper concentration, evidence of hemolysis, renal disease, and the presence of Kayser–Fleischer**

rings on ophthalmologic examination. Other hepatic presentations include asymptomatic elevations in liver enzymes, chronic hepatitis, hepatomegaly, or cirrhosis with portal hypertension. Patients with Wilson disease can present with neurologic involvement prior to the development of frank liver failure. Liver transplantation is indicated for advanced liver failure.

Iron Overload

There are several causes of liver damage associated with iron overload in the pediatric population. In the neonate, as the name suggests, **neonatal hemochromatosis** presents as frank liver failure. In the older child, liver damage from iron is more likely to be caused by **JHC and secondary iron overload. Hereditary hemochromatosis (HHC)** is one of the most common genetic diseases in the Caucasian population, particularly in those of Northern European descent. Typically, HHC does not cause liver disease prior to the age of 20 years. JHC is a rare iron-loading disorder that leads to severe iron load and organ failure prior to the age of 30 years. Treatment is similar to that of HHC with **periodic phlebotomy** to maintain normal iron balance. Secondary iron overload, also known as hemosiderosis, is a common issue for children who have transfusion-dependent diseases (thalassemia, sickle cell, and aplastic anemia). Clinical symptoms do not present until the second decade of life. Treatment centers upon **chelation therapy,** usually with **deferoxamine or deferasirox**.

Genetic Causes

α_1-**Antitrypsin deficiency is a relatively common genetic disorder,** with an incidence of 1 in 1,600 to 1 in 2,000 live births. Children with α_1-antitrypsin deficiency may develop **chronic liver disease** and premature pulmonary emphysema in adulthood secondary to decreased serum concentrations of α_1-antitrypsin, a protease inhibitor. **In 10% to 20% of patients, progressive liver disease leading to cirrhosis and hepatic failure develops by late childhood.** Diagnosis is made by determining the α_1-antitrypsin phenotype by isoelectric focusing (Pi typing). Individuals with homozygous **Pi-ZZ phenotype** are at risk for developing hepatic dysfunction. There is no specific treatment in the setting of progressive liver disease, and liver transplantation is indicated for liver failure.

Cystic fibrosis-associated liver disease has a broad range of presentation, can manifest as neonatal cholestasis, hepatomegaly, hepatitis, hepatic steatosis, and can progress to multilobular cirrhosis with portal hypertension and end-stage liver disease. Liver transplantation has achieved relatively good results in the presence of nutritionally replete patients without severe pulmonary compromise.

Autoimmune Causes

Autoimmune liver disease in the older child is most commonly caused by AIH, but also can present as an entity known as autoimmune sclerosing cholangitis overlap syndrome. AIH is **a chronic necroinflammatory hepatitis of unknown cause that can lead to fibrosis and cirrhosis**. It affects both children and adults, with peaks of incidence at 10 to 20 and 45 to 70 years of age. AIH is classified based on the presence of autoantibodies, with **AIH-I, or classic AIH, represented by positive antinuclear, antismooth muscle, and anti-F-actin antibodies. AIH-II**

represents about 20% of all cases, is associated with anti-LKM (liver-kidney-microsomal) and anti-liver cytosol-1 antibodies. AIH-II presents at an earlier age with more severe initial presentation and poor response to immunosuppressive therapy. Diagnosis is made by clinical features, histologic findings, and the presence of characteristic autoantibodies. **Hyperproteinemia and hyperglobulinemia have been described in association with AIH.** There are no current guidelines for the management of immunosuppressive treatment of AIH. Pediatric regimens can consist of a combination of corticosteroids and immunosuppressive agents such as mercaptopurine or azathioprine. A number of children will progress to cirrhosis and end-stage liver disease, and in these patients, liver transplantation has been successful, although AIH can occur following transplantation despite aggressive immunosuppression.

Obstructive Causes

Hepatobiliary tract diseases such as **choledocholithiasis** (common bile duct gallstones) and cholecystitis can rarely cause jaundice in the older child. In younger children, gallstones are often secondary to a predisposing disease, such as hemolytic disease or total parenteral nutrition. In adolescents, obesity and the use of oral contraceptives increase susceptibility to gallstone disease. Typically, right upper quadrant pain associated with jaundice in the presence of predisposing factors suggests choledocholithiasis. **Choledochal cysts are congenital dilations of the biliary systems that can cause intermittent biliary obstruction.** These cysts can present at any age. Diagnosis is through magnetic resonance cholangiopancreatography, but can require additional imaging with endoscopic retrograde cholangiopancreatography or percutaneous transhepatic cholangiography to fully define the lesion. Definitive treatment is surgical hepaticojejunostomy with removal of the biliary drainage system and formation of a Roux-en-Y loop. **Uncorrected cysts** will ultimately lead to **impaired bile outflow, chronic hepatic injury, biliary cirrhosis and liver failure**. There is a **high risk** of developing **malignancy (cholangiocarcinoma) in any residual tissue,** making **complete excision** of the cyst and any bile duct mucosa essential.

In addition, any anatomic abnormality or mass causing external compression can obstruct the biliary drainage and present with jaundice and pruritus. **Abdominal ultrasonography** is a noninvasive, sensitive and specific way to examine the pancreas and the biliary tree, and is the diagnostic procedure of choice.

Vascular Causes

Budd–Chiari syndrome (noncardiogenic hepatic venous outflow obstruction) presents with abdominal pain, abdominal distention from ascites, jaundice, and hepatosplenomegaly. It results from obstruction of the hepatic veins or inferior vena cava, and has been associated with hypercoagulable states, myeloproliferative states, tumors, and the use of contraceptives. Another form of hepatic venous outflow obstruction is VOD (also known as hepatic sinusoidal obstructive syndrome) where concentric narrowing of the terminal hepatic venules occurs. VOD is most commonly associated with bone marrow transplantation, but can also occur as a result of chronic ingestion of foods or teas containing pyrrolizidine alkaloids.

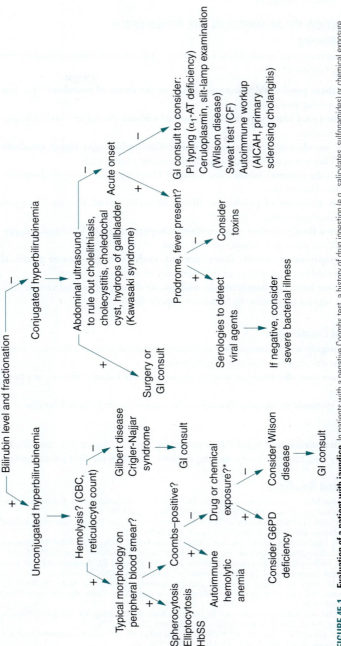

FIGURE 45-1 Evaluation of a patient with jaundice. In patients with a negative Coombs test, a history of drug ingestion (e.g., salicylates, sulfonamides) or chemical exposure (e.g., naphthalene moth balls, fava beans) should be sought because glucose-6-phosphate dehydrogenase (G6PD) deficiency can lead to hemolysis on exposure to these agents. G6PD deficiency is especially common in African-American boys. *AICAH,* autoimmune-type chronic active hepatitis; α_1-*AT,* α_1-antitrypsin; *CBC,* complete blood cell count; *CF,* cystic fibrosis; *GI,* gastrointestinal; *HbSS,* hemoglobin SS; *RUQ,* right upper quadrant.

EVALUATION OF JAUNDICE IN THE OLDER CHILD
Patient History

Important questions to ask when evaluating a patient with jaundice include the following (Figure 45-1):

- **Were there prodromal symptoms prior to the onset of jaundice?** This suggests an infectious cause.
- **Is there a past history or family history of a blood disorder?** This could suggest hemolysis.
- **Is the jaundice acute in onset and associated with right upper quadrant pain?** This is suggestive of choledocholithiasis or cholecystitis.
- **What is the patient's medication history?** There is a wide variety of drugs that can cause liver injury.
- **Is there a history of psychiatric illness or social stress?** This could suggest intentional ingestion.
- **Is there a family history of unexplained hepatic disease?** This could suggestive Wilson disease or another genetic cause.
- **Are symptoms of chronic illness present, such as weight loss or pruritus?** This would be suggestive of an inflammatory or metabolic process.
- **Has there been any hematemesis, melena, or change in mental status?** This would suggest progressive or fulminant hepatic failure.

Physical Examination

Hepatomegaly and splenomegaly are common and can suggest either viral hepatitis or the presence of portal hypertension.

Tenderness over the liver can suggest cholangitis, choledocholithiasis, or cholecystitis.

Signs of systemic or chronic disease can be present in progressive liver disease.

Imaging

Abdominal ultrasound is helpful in evaluating jaundice, because it can evaluate the biliary tree, the vessels surrounding the liver, as well as the liver parenchyma.

Suggested Readings

Fawaz R, Jonas MM. Acute and chronic hepatitis. In: Wyllie R, Hyams J, Kay M, eds. *Pediatric Gastrointestinal and Liver Disease.* 4th ed. Philadelphia, PA: Elsevier; 2011:811–828.

Gilger MA. Diseases of the gallbladder. In: Wyllie R, Hyams J, Kay M, eds. *Pediatric Gastrointestinal and Liver Disease.* 3rd ed. Philadelphia, PA: Elsevier; 2007:989–1002.

Gourley GR. Neonatal jaundice and disorders of bilirubin metabolism. In: Suchy FJ, Sokol RJ, Balistereri WF, eds. *Liver Disease in Children.* 3rd ed. New York: Cambridge University Press; 2007:270–310.

Knisely AS, Narkewicz MR. Iron storage disorders. In: Suchy FJ, Sokol RJ, Balistereri WF, eds. *Liver Disease in Children.* 3rd ed. New York: Cambridge University Press; 2007:661–666.

O'Connor JA, Sokol RJ. Copper metabolism and copper storage disorders. In: Suchy FJ, Sokol RJ, Balistereri WF, eds. *Liver Disease in Children.* 3rd ed. New York: Cambridge University Press; 2007:626–661.

Perlmutter DH. α-1 Antitrypsin deficiency. In: Suchy FJ, Sokol RJ, Balistereri WF, eds. *Liver Disease in Children.* 3rd ed. New York: Cambridge University Press; 2007:545–571.

Sullivan KM, Gourley GR. Jaundice. In: Wyllie R, Hyams J, Kay M, eds. *Pediatric Gastrointestinal and Liver Disease.* 4th ed. Philadelphia, PA: Elsevier; 2011:176–186.

Jaundice, Newborn

INTRODUCTION

Jaundice is a term used to describe the visible manifestation of elevated serum concentrations of bilirubin. The breakdown products of heme proteins, the most abundant of which is hemoglobin, are the major source of bilirubin. The heme moiety is broken down to biliverdin by heme oxygenase and reduced to unconjugated bilirubin via the action of biliverdin reductase. Unconjugated bilirubin travels to the liver through the bloodstream, mostly bound to albumin, where it is transformed into the conjugated form. Conjugated bilirubin enters the small intestine and is excreted in the stool. Enzymes in the small intestine convert a portion of this conjugated bilirubin back into unconjugated bilirubin, which can return to the bloodstream. Here, it can reenter the hepatic circulation and add to the bilirubin load. This process is called the **enterohepatic circulation of bilirubin**. Note that elevations of either conjugated or unconjugated bilirubin can cause jaundice, and each etiology has a distinct laboratory evaluation and treatment. For unconjugated hyperbilirubinemia, elevations may be caused by increased production, decreased conjugation or excretion, or increased enterohepatic circulation of bilirubin. Alterations in conjugated bilirubin are primarily caused by bile duct/excretion abnormalities or hepatic dysfunction. Figure 46-1 represents a basic schematic for the consideration of the broad differential diagnosis of hyperbilirubinemia.

DIFFERENTIAL DIAGNOSIS LIST

Unconjugated Hyperbilirubinemia: Physiologic

- **Increased Bilirubin Production**
  - Blood group incompatibility—Rh, ABO, and minor blood group
  - Red blood cell (RBC) enzyme abnormalities—glucose-6-phosphate dehydrogenase (G6PD), pyruvate kinase, and hexokinase deficiency
  - RBC membrane defects—hereditary spherocytosis, elliptocytosis, and pyknocytosis
  - Hemoglobinopathies—α-thalassemia, and sickle cell disease
  - Increased RBC load—cephalohematoma, polycythemia, and ecchymosis
  - Infants of diabetic mothers

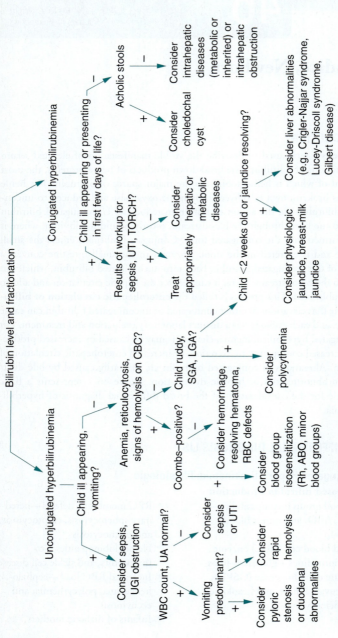

FIGURE 46-1 Evaluation of a newborn with jaundice. *CBC,* complete blood count; *LGA,* large for gestational age; *SGA,* small for gestational age; *TORCH,* toxoplasmosis, other infections, rubella, cytomegalovirus, herpes simplex; *UA,* urinalysis; *UTI,* urinary tract infection; *WBC,* white blood cell.

- **Decreased Bilirubin Conjugation or Excretion**
  - Hormonal deficiency—hypothyroidism and panhypopituitarism
  - Bilirubin metabolism disorders—Gilbert syndrome, Crigler–Najjar (types 1 and 2), and Lucey-Driscoll syndrome
  - Sepsis—bacterial, viral, and fungal
- **Increased Enterohepatic Circulation**
  - Breast-feeding failure jaundice
  - Breast-milk jaundice
  - Bowel obstruction or ileus
  - Pyloric stenosis

Conjugated Hyperbilirubinemia

The differential diagnosis of conjugated hyperbilirubinemia is an extensive list, encompassing more than a hundred distinct disease entities. The majority of the disorders causing conjugated hyperbilirubinemia in the neonates can be organized into obstructive, infectious, metabolic, and miscellaneous categories. Some of the most important etiologies are listed here.

- **Bile Duct Abnormalities**
  - Biliary atresia
  - Choledochal cyst
- **Infection**
  - Hepatic—toxoplasmosis, rubella, cytomegalovirus, herpes simplex (TORCH) infections, and enterovirus
  - Systemic—bacterial sepsis and urinary tract infection
- **Metabolic/Genetic Disorders**
  - Galactosemia
  - Tyrosinemia
  - α_1-Antitrypsin deficiency
  - Alagille syndrome
- **Miscellaneous**
  - Total parenteral nutrition (TPN)-related cholestasis
  - Neonatal hemochromatosis
  - Idiopathic neonatal hepatitis

SELECTED DIFFERENTIAL DIAGNOSIS DISCUSSION
Unconjugated Hyperbilirubinemia
Physiologic Jaundice

> **HINT:** Over 50% of infants have clinical jaundice in the first few days of life, but visible jaundice in the first 24 hours of life is pathologic until proven otherwise.

In utero, fetal unconjugated bilirubin easily crosses the placenta and is conjugated and excreted by the mother. Following birth, the neonate is solely responsible and somewhat ill-prepared for bilirubin metabolism. Because of this, jaundice develops in >50% of infants in the first few days of life. Physiologic jaundice never appears in the first 24 hours, and peaks at 4 days in term infants. Many physiologic factors contribute to this "physiologic hyperbilirubinemia," including a larger RBC mass, decreased RBC life span (70 to 90 days in neonates vs. 120 days in adults), reduced bilirubin uridine diphosphate-glucuronosyltransferase (UDPGT) activity (<1% that of adults in the first 10 days of life), and delayed meconium passage leading to increased enterohepatic circulation.

It is important to note that breast-fed infants have higher bilirubin levels, and with more neonates breast-feeding, clinicians have to reassess what "normal" levels of total serum bilirubin (TSB) are in these otherwise healthy neonates. Historically, 95% of term infants had bilirubin levels that did not exceed 12.9 mg/dL. However, recent studies have shown that in breast-fed infants, the normal mean peak TSB level is 8 to 9 mg/dL, with an upper limit of 17 to 18 mg/dL.

Increased Bilirubin Production
Blood Group Incompatibility
If a blood group incompatibility exists between the fetus and the mother, maternal IgG against fetal red cells can cross the placenta, resulting in hemolysis and increased bilirubin production in the fetus and newborn. An incompatibility can exist in the Rh, ABO, or minor blood group antigens.

 HINT: Rh incompatibility requires prior sensitization and therefore does not happen in a first pregnancy, whereas ABO incompatibility can occur in a first-born infant.

Rh Incompatibility
Rh incompatibility occurs when an Rh-negative mother carries an Rh-positive fetus. The mother must have had previous sensitization to the Rh antigen, usually via a prior pregnancy, which results in the production of antibodies directed against the Rh antigen. Rh-positive infants born to Rh-negative mothers display a wide spectrum of disease, ranging from unaffected (15% to 20%) to severe disease, including erythroblastosis fetalis, and fetal death (25%). The administration of blocking antibodies (RhoGAM) to pregnant Rh-negative mothers prevents Rh sensitization and has reduced the incidence of erythroblastosis fetalis caused by Rh sensitization to 1 per 1,000 live births in the United States.

ABO Incompatibility
ABO incompatibility occurs when a mother with type O blood carries a fetus with type A or B blood. This condition is confined to mothers with type O blood because these women carry anti-A and anti-B IgG antibodies that cross the placenta. Mothers with type A or type B blood produce mostly IgM antibodies against their respective antigens, and these IgM antibodies fail to cross the placenta. Because A and B antigens are common in nature, group O mothers are previously sensitized to these antigens and hemolysis may occur in the first pregnancy. Although ABO incompatibility occurs in 15% of all pregnancies, ABO hemolytic disease occurs in less than 5% of ABO-incompatible mother–infant pairs. Hemolysis tends to be less severe than with Rh incompatibility. The classic presentation is anemia, reticulocytosis, and hyperbilirubinemia occurring in the first 24 to 72 hours of life.

RBC Enzyme Abnormalities
Glucose is the primary metabolic substrate for the red cell, and because the mature red cell lacks organelles including mitochondria, glucose can only be metabolized

via anaerobic pathways. Defects in glucose metabolism or pathways that protect against red cell oxidation can result in hemolysis and hyperbilirubinemia.

Glucose-6-Phosphate Dehydrogenase Deficiency

HINT: Consider the diagnosis of G6PD in infants from the appropriate ethnic backgrounds who have severe hyperbilirubinemia or who are poor responders to phototherapy.

G6PD is the most common red cell enzyme deficiency, occurring most commonly in infants of Mediterranean, Middle Eastern, African, and Southeast Asian descent. This disorder occurs in up to 15% of African American newborns. The mode of inheritance is X-linked recessive. Presence of this deficiency confers resistance against *Plasmodium falciparum,* the infectious agent causing malaria. G6PD generates substrates that protect the red cell against oxidative stress. Erythrocytes lacking these substrates undergo hemolysis with oxidative stress. Important triggers in the neonate include sepsis or exposure to other stressors (naphthalene, sulfa drugs, acetaminophen, breast milk of a mother who has eaten fava beans, etc.). However, the pathogenesis of hyperbilirubinemia appears to be more complicated than simple hemolysis. Often, the offending agent is not identified, and infants with significant hyperbilirubinemia have no evidence of hemolysis, leading some authorities to postulate a concurrent impairment in bilirubin conjugation or clearance. Classically, hyperbilirubinemia appears between 24 and 96 hours postpartum, and it can be severe, even in the absence of significant anemia. Up to 50% of patients also have Gilbert syndrome (see later), and this combination increases the risk of hyperbilirubinemia and kernicterus. Many states include G6PD in the routine newborn screen. In the 2004 American Academy of Pediatrics (AAP) guidelines for hyperbilirubinemia, the committee emphasized the possibility for the underdiagnosis of G6PD deficiency in the newborn period, and encouraged practitioners to consider this diagnosis in infants with the appropriate ethnic backgrounds who are poor responders to phototherapy.

Pyruvate Kinase Deficiency

Deficiency in pyruvate kinase causes ineffective adenosine triphosphate generation from glucose, resulting in shortened red cell survival. This disorder is inherited in an autosomal recessive pattern and is most common in whites of northern European descent. Clinical expression ranges from severe neonatal jaundice to compensated hemolytic anemia.

RBC Membrane Defects

Defects that affect the red cell membrane and cytoskeletal structure alter the shape and deformability of the cell and result in hemolysis and hyperbilirubinemia. Conditions include hereditary spherocytosis, elliptocytosis, and pyknocytosis.

Hereditary Spherocytosis

With an incidence of 1 in 5,000, hereditary spherocytosis is the most common congenital RBC membrane disorder. This disease is inherited in an autosomal dominant manner, with 25% of cases arising from new mutations. Family history can be significant for splenectomy, gallstones, and anemia.

Increased RBC Load

Any condition that results in increased RBC load can result in hyperbilirubinemia secondary to breakdown of extravascular or sequestered erythrocytes. Common conditions include cephalohematoma, extensive bruising after traumatic delivery, and polycythemia.

Infants of Diabetic Mothers

Macrosomic infants of insulin-dependent diabetic mothers represent a unique group of patients at risk for hyperbilirubinemia. These infants have high levels of erythropoietin and increased erythropoiesis; thus ineffective red cell production and polycythemia are probably responsible for the resulting hyperbilirubinemia.

Decreased Bilirubin Conjugation or Excretion

Hormone Deficiency

The pathogenesis of hyperbilirubinemia in infants with hypothyroidism and hypopituitarism is poorly understood. Hypothyroidism results in unconjugated hyperbilirubinemia, whereas hypopituitarism can result in either unconjugated or conjugated hyperbilirubinemia.

Bilirubin Metabolism Disorder

Bilirubin uridine diphosphate-glucuronosyltransferase (UDPGT) is responsible for converting unconjugated bilirubin into the conjugated form. Defects in this enzyme can result in unconjugated hyperbilirubinemia.

Crigler–Najjar Syndromes, Types I and II

 HINT: Crigler–Najjar syndrome type II is less severe than type I and is uniquely responsive to phenobarbital, which induces enzymatic activity.

Type I is a rare disease that results from an autosomal recessive inheritance of a deficiency in UDPGT activity. These patients develop severe hyperbilirubinemia in the first 2 to 3 days of life and often require exchange transfusion. Patients with type II disease (also known as Arias syndrome) retain some UDPGT activity, and infants typically have less severe hyperbilirubinemia. Furthermore, infants with type II disease are also partially responsive to phenobarbital, which induces enzyme activity.

Gilbert Syndrome

Gilbert syndrome affects 5% to 10% of the general population, and both autosomal dominant and recessive patterns of inheritance are described. Infants may have mildly elevated levels of unconjugated bilirubin when compared to controls because of decreased UGT1 activity. Presentation with pathologic hyperbilirubinemia in the newborn period is rare, unless a concurrent condition such as G6PD deficiency or hereditary spherocytosis exists.

Lucey–Driscoll Syndrome

Lucey–Driscoll syndrome can be associated with significant hyperbilirubinemia and is thought to be related to a hormone or antibody from the maternal serum that inhibits the action of UDPGT. This is a self-limited process and should be considered in unexplained familial severe hyperbilirubinemia.

Sepsis

Sepsis results in hyperbilirubinemia secondary to hemolysis and impaired conjugation. Patients with sepsis may have both elevated unconjugated and conjugated bilirubin levels. The presence of a urinary tract infection has been specifically associated with jaundice presenting after 8 days of age or an elevated conjugated fraction of bilirubin.

Increased Enterohepatic Circulation of Bilirubin
Breast-Feeding Failure Jaundice and Breast-Milk Jaundice

 HINT: Breast-feeding failure jaundice is early onset of jaundice, occurring in the first 2 to 4 days of life, whereas breast-milk jaundice is responsible for later-onset or persistence of jaundice from the end of the first week through the first few weeks of life.

Multiple studies have indicated a link between breast-feeding and an increased incidence and severity of neonatal hyperbilirubinemia. Breast-fed infants are three times more likely to develop bilirubin levels of >12 mg/dL within the first week of life, and levels commonly peak at 10 to 30 mg/dL. Additionally, up to 10% to 30% of breast-fed infants continue to have elevated serum bilirubin levels into the second to sixth weeks of life. Jaundice that occurs in the first 2 to 4 days is called "breast-feeding failure jaundice" and that occurring later, from 4 to 7 days and continuing to cause prolonged jaundice, is termed "breast-milk jaundice." There is considerable overlap with these two conditions. Both maternal and newborn factors that lead to inefficient nutritional intake by the infant are thought to contribute to the etiology of breast-feeding failure jaundice. These include lack of proper technique, engorgement, cracked nipples, and ineffective suck or latch. Delayed meconium passage and increased enterohepatic circulation are thought to cause the indirect hyperbilirubinemia that appears under these conditions. Multiple factors found in breast milk are implicated in causing the prolonged unconjugated hyperbilirubinemia known as breast milk jaundice, including the presence of a glucuronidase enzyme that deconjugates bilirubin in the intestinal lumen allowing for increased enterohepatic circulation. However, the absolute etiology remains unclear.

Conjugated Hyperbilirubinemia
Conjugated hyperbilirubinemia is defined as a level ≥1 mg/dL if the total bilirubin is <5 mg/dL, or a conjugated fraction that accounts for >20% of the total bilirubin if the total bilirubin is >5 mg/dL. The differential diagnosis of conjugated hyperbilirubinemia, or cholestasis, is long, with both hepatocellular and ductal

disturbances of bilirubin excretion playing a role. However, after a full diagnostic workup is performed, between 70% and 80% of cases can be attributed to either biliary atresia or idiopathic neonatal hepatitis in term infants. In preterm infants, the most likely cause is TPN-related cholestasis.

Bile Duct Abnormalities
Biliary Atresia

 HINT: For biliary atresia, the Kasai portoenterostomy procedure is more successful if performed in the first 8 weeks of life. For this reason, infants with persistent jaundice into the second or third week of life require a fractionated bilirubin to ensure the conjugated fraction is not elevated.

Biliary atresia is one of the most common diagnoses responsible for cholestasis, occurring in 1 per 10,000 births and accounting for one-third of all cases of conjugated hyperbilirubinemia. A progressive, inflammatory sclerotic process results in extrahepatic obstruction of the bile ducts and ongoing inflammation of the intrahepatic bile ducts that can lead to biliary cirrhosis. Although multiple etiologies are proposed, the causative agent remains obscure. Infants often appear well at birth, but persistent jaundice develops in the first few weeks of life. Early diagnosis is critical because the definitive treatment to reestablish bile flow, the Kasai portoenterostomy, is most successful when done at <8 weeks of age. Despite treatment, most patients eventually require liver transplantation.

Infection
Several congenital infections can manifest as conjugated hyperbilirubinemia. These include the TORCH infections. Viral infections of the neonate, including hepatitis A and B, and enterovirus can cause liver failure and hyperbilirubinemia. Additionally, bacterial sepsis and urinary tract infections can cause conjugated hyperbilirubinemia.

Metabolic/Genetic Disorders
Multiple metabolic disorders, including tyrosinemia and galactosemia, may have conjugated hyperbilirubinemia and fulminant liver disease as part of their clinical presentation. α_1-Antitrypsin deficiency, inherited in an autosomal recessive fashion, affects 1 in 2,000 live births. Only 5% of these patients develop rapidly progressive liver disease requiring transplant within the first 4 years of life, with the remaining 95% manifesting variable symptoms extending into adult life. Alagille syndrome (arteriohepatic dysplasia) consists of dysmorphic facies and cholestasis associated with paucity of intrahepatic bile ducts. This disorder occurs in 1 in 70,000 live births.

Miscellaneous
Cholestasis Related to Total Parenteral Nutrition
TPN is essential in many conditions that require withholding enteral feeding from neonates. Prolonged administration of TPN results in liver injury, resulting in elevated transaminases, elevated gamma-glutamyltransferase, and jaundice. The

longer the duration of TPN administration, the higher the risk of cholestasis tends to be. The onset of cholestasis usually occurs following 2 weeks of TPN administration. In most patients, cholestasis slowly resolves with the initiation of enteral feeding and discontinuation of parenteral nutrition. This condition most commonly affects preterm infants because of their greater exposure to TPN.

Neonatal Hemochromatosis (NH)

Neonatal hemochromatosis is a condition of hepatic failure, including conjugated hyperbilirubinemia, in the newborn period and is associated with iron deposition in multiple organs, including the liver. Other affected organs can be the pancreas and the heart, for example. Experts postulate that this condition may be related to an alloimmune phenomenon with maternal antibodies directed at a substrate on the fetal liver. Affected infants can be treated successfully with double volume exchange transfusion and intravenous immunoglobulin (IVIG) infusion. Mothers with affected infants have been treated in subsequent pregnancies with IVIG resulting in near elimination of this disease in those offspring.

Idiopathic Neonatal Hepatitis

Idiopathic neonatal hepatitis is defined as conjugated hyperbilirubinemia without general viral illness or an etiology specific to a metabolic abnormality. Liver biopsy shows transformation of hepatocytes into multinucleated giant cells. Distinguishing this from biliary atresia, though difficult, is essential for proper clinical management. Jaundice frequently occurs in the first week of life, but can manifest as late as 4 months. Familial cases have poor prognosis, with <30% recovery. Sporadic cases resolve in 60% to 80% of patients.

CLINICAL FINDINGS
History
Family History

- Family history of hematological disorders, splenectomy, gallstones, and previously affected children: inherited causes of hyperbilirubinemia

Pregnancy, Labor, and Delivery

- Maternal blood type and Rh status: Rh and ABO incompatibility
- TORCH titers
- Maternal diabetes
- Maternal medications: sulfonamides, nitrofurantoins, antimalarials, and oxytocin
- Abnormal fetal anatomy ultrasound: gastrointestinal (GI) obstruction and choledochal cyst
- Traumatic delivery: hemorrhage and hematoma

Infant History

- Gestational age, postnatal age, and ethnicity of the infant
- Intrauterine growth restriction/small for gestational age—may be associated with inherited, metabolic, or infectious causes, as well as polycythemia

- Newborn screen results, if available
- Infant blood type and direct Coombs test results, often sent on cord specimen
- Nutrition—breast-feeding versus formula feeding; TPN exposure
- Voiding and stooling pattern

Physical Examination
Level of Jaundice

> **HINT:** Jaundice becomes clinically apparent at levels >5 mg/dL and progresses cephalocaudally. Studies show, however, that prediction of bilirubin levels by evaluating the progression of jaundice from head to toe is unreliable.

It has long been noticed that jaundice progresses in a cephalocaudal manner. Clinical jaundice appears at TSB >5 mg/dL and can be elicited by blanching the skin with slight pressure and evaluating the color of the underlying skin and subcutaneous tissue. It is best to evaluate for the presence of jaundice in natural light. The clinical use of cephalocaudal progression of jaundice to gauge TSB levels appears less reliable in darkly pigmented neonates and when TSB levels exceed 12 mg/dL.

General Physical Examination
- **Signs of extravascular blood**—cephalohematoma and ecchymosis
- **Plethoric infant**—polycythemia
- **Ascites, pleural effusion, and hepatomegaly**—Rh isoimmunization and α-thalassemia
- **Pallor and hepatosplenomegaly**—hemolysis
- **Fever, temperature instability, lethargy, respiratory distress, vomiting, and seizures**—sepsis or acute bilirubin encephalopathy
- **Microcephaly, petechiae, hepatosplenomegaly, and chorioretinitis**—TORCH infections
- **Abdominal mass**—choledochal cyst and intestinal obstruction
- **Dark urine and acholic stool**—cholestasis

Acute Bilirubin Encephalopathy and Kernicterus

> **HINT:** "Acute bilirubin encephalopathy" is the preferred term for the initial symptoms of neurological dysfunction associated with elevated levels of bilirubin. Kernicterus is reserved for the chronic manifestations.

The prevention of acute bilirubin encephalopathy that may progress to kernicterus is the main reason for timely diagnosis and appropriate treatment of hyperbilirubinemia in the newborn period. Unconjugated bilirubin, in the free or unbound form, that crosses the blood–brain barrier is toxic to neurons of the basal ganglia and various brainstem nuclei. Clinical manifestations of acute bilirubin encephalopathy are often mistaken for sepsis, asphyxia, or hypoglycemia.

In term babies, several phases of acute bilirubin encephalopathy are described. The early phase consists of lethargy, poor feeding, and hypotonia. The intermediate phase follows with stupor, irritability, and hypertonia and occasionally fever and high-pitched cry. The hypertonia may consist of backward arching of the neck (retrocollis) and trunk (opisthotonos). The advanced phase consists of opisthotonos, shrill cry, no feeding, apnea, coma, and occasionally seizures and death. "Kernicterus" is the term reserved for describing the chronic form of bilirubin encephalopathy. With survival, the infant may develop choreoathetosis, sensorineural deafness, dental enamel dysplasia, and paralysis of upward gaze.

The level of hyperbilirubinemia at which kernicterus occurs is unclear. In patients with Rh hemolytic disease, treatment of levels >20 mg/dL prevents long-term sequelae. Recent studies suggest that with hemolysis, both the level and duration of hyperbilirubinemia contribute to the development of kernicterus. It has been shown that otherwise healthy infants without hemolysis may develop marked hyperbilirubinemia (20 to 25 mg/dL), and this does not appear to lead to adverse neurologic outcomes; however, contradictory reports exist. Conditions that increase bilirubin deposition in the brain include low albumin, acidosis, hypercarbia, hypoxemia-ischemia, and systemic illness (shock, sepsis, respiratory distress syndrome). Relatively little is known about bilirubin levels and kernicterus in the preterm infant, although most experts recommend treatment at lower levels than those recommended for term infants. Only careful attention by the clinician to individual risk factors can ensure that neonates with hyperbilirubinemia are treated appropriately.

Data from the Kernicterus Registry suggest an increasing incidence of kernicterus, with 1 case per 624,000 live births in the United States. Some have postulated that early discharge with delayed follow-up, failure to check bilirubin levels in newborns with jaundice that presents in the first 24 hours of life, and an insufficient response to jaundice by clinicians may play a role in this phenomenon.

LABORATORY EVALUATION
Unconjugated Versus Conjugated Versus Indirect Versus Direct Hyperbilirubinemia

When ordering bilirubin levels, clinicians often have to choose between unconjugated, conjugated, indirect, and direct levels. These levels are determined via different laboratory methods and deserve mention here. Traditional methods of bilirubin measurement took advantage of the reaction between bilirubin and a diazo reagent. Direct bilirubin reflects the conjugated component that reacts directly with the diazo reagent. This includes delta bilirubin, which is the fraction of conjugated bilirubin covalently bound to albumin that appears after prolonged hyperbilirubinemia. Total bilirubin levels can be determined by adding an accelerant to the reaction, and the indirect component is calculated by taking the difference between total and direct bilirubin. Various nontraditional methods have been developed to assess conjugated and unconjugated bilirubin directly. Conjugated levels do not include delta bilirubin. Thus, direct bilirubin and conjugated bilirubin are slightly different, as are indirect and unconjugated levels. Often, conjugated and unconjugated levels are more quickly obtained and the tests of choice for evaluating newborn hyperbilirubinemia.

Transcutaneous Bilirubin Measurement

Transcutaneous bilirubinometry (TcB) is a noninvasive method of measuring total bilirubin levels. Some concerns have been raised regarding the accuracy of these readings at levels >15 mg/dL and in African American and Hispanic populations. However, this technique has gained widespread use as a screening tool to help detect early hyperbilirubinemia in the newborn nursery. The AAP has recently advocated the use of TcB to assist screening for hyperbilirubinemia in healthy newborn infants ≥35 weeks' gestation prior to discharge from the newborn nursery. However, elevated levels must be confirmed with serum measurements if the TcB value is at 70% of the TSB level recommended for the use of phototherapy or in the high-intermediate zone on the Bhutani risk nomogram (see Figure 46-2).

Unconjugated Hyperbilirubinemia

Any infant with clinically visible jaundice should have a TSB with unconjugated and conjugated levels determined. Serial TSB levels are helpful because special attention should be paid to the neonate whose bilirubin rises to ≥0.5 mg/dL/hr over 4 to 8 hours or is >5 mg/dL per day. Levels increasing this quickly may indicate active hemolysis. Further laboratory studies include checking a blood type and direct Coombs test (can be done on cord blood) in neonates born to mothers with type O blood. Of these patients, one-third have a positive Coombs test, and of those, only 15% have bilirubin ≥12.8 mg/dL. The result of this test alone should not be used to rule in or rule out ABO incompatibility as a cause of hyperbilirubinemia. A complete blood count, peripheral smear, and reticulocyte count can lead to the diagnosis of anemia secondary to hemolysis. If sepsis is suspected, blood culture, urine culture, and cerebrospinal fluid analysis may also be indicated. Measurement of serum albumin can assist the clinician in determining which infants may benefit from exchange transfusion. An albumin <3.0 g/dL is considered a risk factor for developing acute bilirubin encephalopathy, and an elevated bilirubin-to-albumin ratio may be considered when making treatment decisions regarding exchange transfusion. Newborn screen results should be checked (hypothyroidism), and G6PD enzyme activity should be determined in the correct clinical scenario. G6PD levels in the setting of hemolysis may be normal in a G6PD-deficient infant. If clinical suspicion remains, a repeat level should be drawn when the hemolysis has resolved.

The frequency of laboratory evaluation is based on the severity of hyperbilirubinemia and the pathologic process involved. TSB levels should be checked every 2 to 3 hours when levels are >25 mg/dL, every 3 to 4 hours when TSB is 20 to 25 mg/dL, every 4 to 6 hours when TSB is <20 mg/dl, and every 8 to 12 hours when TSB is decreasing on phototherapy.

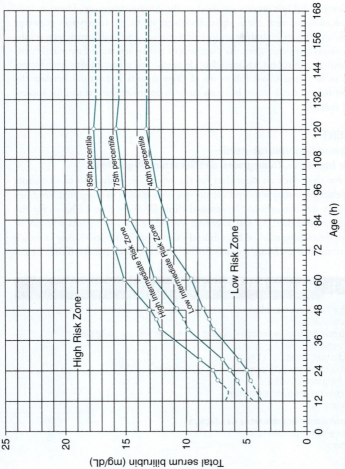

FIGURE 46-2 **Bhutani risk nomogram.** (Reprinted with permission from Bhutani VK, Johnson L, Sivieri EM. Predictive ability of a predischarge hour-specific serum bilirubin for subsequent significant hyperbilirubinemia in healthy term and near-term neonates. *Pediatrics.* 1999;103:6–14.)

Conjugated Hyperbilirubinemia

The North American Society for Pediatric Gastroenterology, Hepatology and Nutrition (see web address in Suggested Readings section) has developed clinical practice guidelines. Conjugated hyperbilirubinemia is never physiologic and requires immediate evaluation. Any infant with clinical jaundice at 2 weeks of age should be evaluated for cholestasis by checking TSB and conjugated or direct bilirubin levels. Multiple studies can lead to the correct diagnosis. These include blood/urine cultures, viral titers, ophthalmologic exam, α_1-antitrypsin genotyping, liver function tests including coagulation studies, and newborn screen results (galactosemia, tyrosinemia). For the diagnosis of biliary atresia and neonatal hepatitis, abdominal ultrasound, radionucleotide scans, and percutaneous liver biopsy may need to be done. Close follow-up of these infants is essential because the diagnosis of biliary atresia must be made early to optimize the chances for success of surgical therapy.

TREATMENT

Unconjugated Hyperbilirubinemia

Preventive Measures, Nomograms, and Screening Algorithms

The AAP has developed an algorithm for the systematic evaluation of all infants for the development of hyperbilirubinemia (see web address in Suggested Readings section). Every newborn should be assessed clinically every 8 to 12 hours for the development of jaundice. Special attention should be paid to infants who are at high risk for developing marked hyperbilirubinemia (see Table 46-1). Any jaundice occurring in the first 24 hours requires further workup. Additionally, if the clinical

TABLE 46-1   Important Risk Factors for Severe Hyperbilirubinemia
Predischarge TSB or TcB measurement in the high-risk or high-intermediate-risk zone
Lower gestational age
Exclusive breast-feeding, particularly if nursing is not going well and weight loss is excessive (>8%–10%)
Jaundice observed in the first 24 hr
Isoimmune or other hemolytic disease (e.g., G6PD deficiency)
Previous sibling with jaundice
Cephalohematoma or significant bruising
East Asian race[a]
Hyperbilirubinemia neurotoxicity risk factors
Isoimmune hemolytic disease
G6PD deficiency
Asphyxia
Sepsis
Acidosis
Albumin <3.0 mg/dl

G6PD, glucose-6-phosphate dehydrogenase; *TcB,* transcutaneous bilirubin; *TSB,* total serum bilirubin.
[a]Race as defined by mother's description.
Adapted with permission from Maisels MJ, Bhutani VK, Bogen D, et al. Hyperbilirubinemia in the newborn infant ≥35 weeks' gestation: an update with clarifications. *Pediatrics.* 2009;124(4):1193–1198.

assessment suggests significant jaundice, TSB should be checked. Once a TSB is obtained, multiple nomograms exist to assist the clinician with management. The hour-specific bilirubin nomogram developed by Bhutani (see Figure 46-2) is helpful in determining a neonate's risk of developing hyperbilirubinemia with the next measurement, and it is used mostly as a tool for determining the appropriate time for follow-up. The AAP has developed treatment nomograms for neonates born at ≥35 weeks of gestation that are stratified by gestational age and the presence or absence of risk factors associated with the development of acute bilirubin encephalopathy. These nomograms help the clinician decide whether a neonate should receive phototherapy (see Figure 46-3) or exchange transfusion (see Figure 46-4).

The AAP has recently updated their recommendations for screening healthy newborn infants ≥35 weeks' gestation prior to discharge from the newborn nursery. In addition to universally screening infants, using either TcB or TSB, for hyperbilirubinemia prior to discharge from the newborn nursery, specific algorithms for recommended follow-up have been developed. These algorithms take into consideration gestational age, with or without hyperbilirubinemia risk factors, and the risk zone of the predischarge bilirubin according to the Bhutani nomogram (see Figure 46-2) and provide suggested timing of follow-up and/or repeat bilirubin assessment. While this strategy will potentially increase the cost of newborn care, the goal of preventing kernicterus and long-term sequelae remain paramount.

Phototherapy

> **HINT:** Phototherapy is the mainstay of therapy for hyperbilirubinemia and works by converting unconjugated bilirubin, in a nonenzymatic fashion, into a polar, water-soluble, and, therefore, more-readily excretable form.

Phototherapy should be instituted as dictated by the AAP guidelines, which contain specific postnatal age and gestational age nomograms guiding therapy (see Figure 46-3). Unconjugated bilirubin absorbs light maximally in the blue portion of the visible spectrum (450 nm). The use of phototherapy results in the photoisomerization of bilirubin into a polar, water-soluble, and more readily excretable form. Both configurational and structural isomers are formed as a result, and the most common structural isomer is lumirubin. Multiple factors affect the efficacy of phototherapy, including spectrum of light, irradiance (dosage of light) of the phototherapy unit, exposed surface area of the infant, and the distance of the infant from the light source. Fiberoptic pads placed under the infant increase surface area exposure. The current AAP guidelines call for the use of intensive phototherapy, with an irradiance of at least 30 mW/cm^2 per nanometer for all infants with gestational age ≥35 weeks requiring phototherapy. Phototherapy should be discontinued when TSB reaches <13 to 14 mg/dL or when values reach <40th percentile on the Bhutani nomogram (see Figure 46-2). The utility of checking "rebound bilirubin" levels remains unclear but can be helpful when phototherapy was stopped before the peak bilirubin was suspected to occur (i.e., 4 days of life) or in the setting of possible ongoing hemolysis.

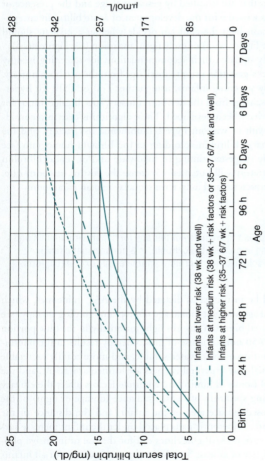

FIGURE 46-3 **Guidelines for phototherapy.** (Reprinted with permission from American Academy of Pediatrics. Management of hyperbilirubinemia in the newborn infant 35 or more weeks of gestation. *Pediatrics.* 2004;114(1):297–316.)

- Use total bilirubin. Do not subtract direct reacting or conjugated bilirubin.
- Risk factors = isoimmune hemolytic disease, G6PD deficiency, asphyxia, significant lethargy, temperature instability, sepsis, acidosis, or albumin < 3.0 g/dL (if measured)
- For well infants 35–37 6/7 wk can adjust TSB levels for intervention around the medium risk line. It is an option to intervene at lower TSB levels for infants closer to 35 wks and at higher TSB levels for those closer to 37 6/7 wk.
- It is an option to provide conventional phototherapy in hospital or at home at TSB levels 2–3 mg/dL (35–50 mmol/L) below those shown but home phototherapy should not be used in any infant with risk factors.

Within the figure:

Infants at lower risk (38 wk and well)

Infants at medium risk (38 wk + risk factors or 35–37 6/7 wk and well)

Infants at higher risk (35–37 6/7 wk + risk factors)

Y-axis left: Total serum bilirubin (mg/dL) — 0, 5, 10, 15, 20, 25

Y-axis right: μmol/L — 0, 85, 171, 257, 342, 428

X-axis: Age — Birth, 24 h, 48 h, 72 h, 96 h, 5 Days, 6 Days, 7 Days

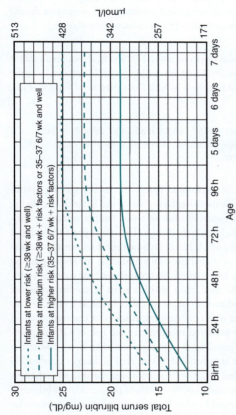

FIGURE 46-4 **Guidelines for exchange transfusion.** (Reprinted with permission from American Academy of Pediatrics. Management of hyperbilirubinemia in the newborn infant 35 or more weeks of gestation. *Pediatrics.* 2004;114(1):297–316.)

- The dashed lines for the first 24 hours indicate uncertainty due to a wide range of clinical circumstances and a range of responses to phototherapy.
- Immediate exchange transfusion is recommended if infant shows signs of acute bilirubin encephalopathy (hypertonia, arching, retrocollis, opisthotonos, fever, high pitched cry) or if TSB is 5 mg/dL (85 μmol/L) above these lines.
- Risk factors–isoimmune hemolytic disease. G6PD deficiency, asphyxia, significant lethargy, temperature instability, sepsis, acidosis.
- Measure serum albumin and calculate B/A ratio (See legend).
- Use total bilirubin. Do not subtract direct reacting or conjugated bilirubin.
- If infant is well and 35–37 6/7 wk (median risk) can individualize TSB levels for exchange based on actual gestational age.

Chart legend:
- Infants at lower risk (≥38 wk and well)
- Infants at medium risk (≥38 wk + risk factors or 35–37 6/7 wk and well)
- Infants at higher risk (35–37 6/7 wk + risk factors)

Side effects of phototherapy include disruption of the mother–baby unit, increased insensible water loss, retinal injury from ultraviolet light, and, in the setting of an elevated conjugated fraction, a brown discoloration of the skin called "bronze-baby syndrome." The presence of an elevated conjugated fraction or bronzing of the skin is not a contraindication to the use of phototherapy. The conjugated fraction should not be subtracted from the TSB in determining when to use phototherapy or perform exchange transfusion. However, if an infant's bilirubin increases during phototherapy and is associated with purpura or bullous eruptions on the skin, the diagnosis of congenital erythropoietic porphyria should be entertained (resulting from photosensitivity and induced hemolysis).

Intravenous Fluids

Administration of intravenous fluids does not lower TSB levels, although an infant receiving phototherapy may have increased insensible water losses that may be compounded by poor feeding and thus may benefit from parenteral fluid therapy.

Exchange Transfusion

 HINT: The bilirubin-to-albumin ratio can be used as an adjunct in determining the need for exchange transfusion because it emphasizes the risk factor of a low serum albumin.

Exchange transfusion should be performed based on the age-specific nomograms published in the AAP guidelines. Replacing twice the infant's circulating blood volume can rapidly correct hyperbilirubinemia and remove offending antibodies in the setting of isoimmune hemolytic disease. Typically, type O blood and AB+ plasma are used to reconstitute whole blood because time does not allow crossmatching infant blood. Presence of skilled personnel and close monitoring of the patient in an intensive care setting are required. Secure intravascular access is essential, and if umbilical lines are to be used, their position must be confirmed before starting the procedure. Slow withdrawal from umbilical catheters at a rate of ~1 to 2 mL/kg/minute is recommended with concomitant infusion of the reconstituted whole blood. Peripheral lines are preferred to minimize the risk of GI complications, but their use may be complicated by the limitations of their small caliber. An effective double-volume exchange transfusion (160 mL/kg) exchanges nearly 85% of the patient's blood volume while a single-volume exchange transfusion exchanges nearly 63%. A posttransfusion rebound to 60% to 80% of pre-transfusion bilirubin level is common, representing reequilibration between vascular and extravascular compartments. Complications include transfusion reaction, infection, ischemic bowel/necrotizing, enterocolitis, hypocalcemia (especially with packed RBC stored in sodium citrate), thrombocytopenia, and hemodynamic instability. Risk of death is 1% in healthy infants and may be as high as 12% in sick neonates.

Intravenous Immune Globulin for Isoimmune Hemolytic Hyperbilirubinemia

In the setting of an isoimmune hemolytic disease causing hyperbilirubinemia (Rh, ABO, or minor blood group antigens), IVIG attenuates hemolysis and, therefore, hyperbilirubinemia. Use of IVIG for this condition is recommended by the

AAP for hyperbilirubinemia unresponsive to phototherapy or levels approaching exchange transfusion criteria, based on studies demonstrating reduced need for exchange transfusion with fewer side effects. The current recommendation is for the administration of IVIG (0.5 to 1 g/kg over 2 hours) if the TSB is rising despite intensive phototherapy or is within 2 to 3 mg/dL of the exchange level. This dose can be repeated in 12 hours, if necessary.

Phenobarbital

Phenobarbital is used in certain populations to increase the conjugation and excretion of bilirubin by inducing the expression of the glucuronyl transferase enzyme. It has been studied for the treatment of both conjugated and unconjugated hyperbilirubinemia. Currently, phenobarbital is not a mainstay of therapy.

Synthetic Metalloporphyrins (Tin-Mesoporphyrin)

These compounds limit the production of bilirubin because they act as a competitive inhibitor of the heme oxygenase enzyme responsible for the first step in bilirubin production. Tin-mesoporphyrin is the best studied of these compounds and has been used with some success to avoid the need for exchange transfusion in certain populations (e.g., Jehovah's Witnesses), whose beliefs do not allow exposure to blood products. Currently, these products are not approved by the Food and Drug Administration.

Conjugated Hyperbilirubinemia

Treatment of conjugated hyperbilirubinemia depends on the ultimate diagnosis and should be coordinated with a pediatric gastroenterologist. Care should be made to optimize nutrition, with attention paid to fat-soluble vitamins (A, D, E, and K). Medical management is limited and believed to be purely supportive. Phenobarbital increases conjugation and excretion of bilirubin, but it is not routinely recommended because of sedative effects. Ursodeoxycholic acid may increase bile flow, but efficacy is not confirmed. For patients with biliary atresia, outcomes after Kasai portoenterostomy are improved if the surgery is performed in the first 8 weeks of life.

Suggested Readings

American Academy of Pediatrics. Management of hyperbilirubinemia in the newborn infant 35 or more weeks of gestation. *Pediatrics.* 2004;114(1):297–316. Available at: http://aapolicy.aapublications.org/cgi/content/abstract/pediatrics;114/1/297.

Bhutani VK, Johnson L, Sivieri EM. Predictive ability of a predischarge hour-specific serum bilirubin for subsequent significant hyperbilirubinemia in healthy term and near-term neonates. *Pediatrics.* 1999;103:6–14.

Dennery PA, Seidman DS, Stevenson DK. Neonatal hyperbilirubinemia. *N Engl J Med.* 2001;344(8):581–590.

Hartley JL, Davenport M, Kelly DA. Biliary atresia. *Lancet.* 2009;374(9702):1704–1713.

Mack CL. The pathogenesis of biliary atresia: evidence for a virus-induced autoimmune disease. *Semin Liver Dis.* 2007;27(3):233–242.

Maisels MJ, Bhutani VK, Bogen D, et al. Hyperbilirubinemia in the newborn infant ≥35 weeks' gestation: an update with clarifications. *Pediatrics.* 2009;124(4):1193—1198. Available at: http://pediatrics.aappublications.org/content/124/4/1193.short.

Moyer V, Freese DK, Whittington PF, et al. Guideline for the evaluation of cholestatic jaundice in infants: recommendations of the North American Society for Pediatric Gastroenterology, Hepatology, and Nutrition. *J Pediatr Gastroenterol Nutr.* 2004;39(2):115–128. Available at: http://www.naspghan.org.

Wong RJ, Stevenson DK, Ahlfors CE, et al. Neonatal jaundice: bilirubin physiology and clinical chemistry. *NeoReviews.* 2007;8(2):e58–e67.

Joint Pain

INTRODUCTION

Arthritis is defined as the limitation of motion of a joint with associated **swelling, pain with motion, tenderness, or warmth**. **Arthralgia** is joint pain in which there is **no limitation of range of motion** and in which **none of the other associated findings** are present. Arthritis or arthralgia may present as **polyarticular** (multiple joint), **pauciarticular** (few joints), or **monoarticular** (one joint).

DIFFERENTIAL DIAGNOSIS LIST

Traumatic/Structural Causes
- Recent trauma—fracture and sprain
- Foreign body synovitis
- Overuse syndromes—stress fracture, apophysitis (tendonitis), and Osgood–Schlatter disease
- Degenerative—Legg–Calvé–Perthes disease, slipped capital femoral epiphysis (SCFE), patellofemoral pain syndrome, osteochondritis dissecans, and chondromalacia patella

Infectious Causes
- Septic arthritis
- Osteomyelitis
- Viral arthritis
- Postinfectious arthritis—acute rheumatic fever (ARF), poststreptococcal arthritis, Lyme disease, and postdysenteric arthritis (Reiter syndrome)

Inflammatory Causes
- Transient (toxic) synovitis
- Reactive arthritis

- Kawasaki disease
- Systemic lupus erythematosus
- Dermatomyositis
- Polyarteritis nodosa
- Henoch–Schönlein purpura
- Behçet syndrome
- Psoriatic arthropathy

Immunologic Causes
- Serum sickness
- Erythema multiforme
- Inflammatory bowel disease
- Juvenile idiopathic arthritis (JIA)

Congenital Causes
- Hemophilia
- Sickle cell disease (SCD)
- Hypermobility syndromes
- Multiple epiphyseal dysplasias

Neoplastic Causes
- Bone tumors
- Leukemia and lymphoma
- Neuroblastoma

Miscellaneous Causes
- Functional (growing pains)

DIFFERENTIAL DIAGNOSIS DISCUSSION
Traumatic/Structural Causes of Joint Pain
Recent Trauma: Fractures and Sprains
Etiology

Fractures located **near the growth plate** are a common cause of posttraumatic joint pain.

Clinical Features and Evaluation

The growth plate is often the **weakest portion of the joint** in children. For this reason, in patients whose growth plates have not yet fused, it is difficult to diagnose anything other than the most minor joint injuries as "sprains." Fractures near the growth plate can be classified by their radiographic appearance and severity.

Treatment

Injuries that reveal **localized or "point" tenderness** at a child's joint require **immobilization and orthopedic follow-up, even if radiographs fail to reveal an obvious fracture site** (Salter I fracture classification).

 HINT: Salter I growth plate fractures may not present with abnormal radiographs. Thus, immobilization and orthopedic follow-up is warranted for all except the most minor traumatic joint injuries.

Foreign Body Synovitis
Etiology

Splinters, glass, or other **foreign material located near a joint space** can induce an **inflammatory response,** causing **synovitis or tendonitis.** This process can occur over a period of months, or it can develop earlier if complicated by infection.

Clinical Features and Evaluation

Diagnosis is based on a **high index of suspicion** and a **review of the history.** **Plain radiographs** are helpful **only with radiopaque foreign materials,** such as glass.

Treatment

Treatment consists of **surgical exploration and removal** of the foreign material.

Overuse Injury

Overuse injuries occur when a **small amount of stress** is placed on the joint **for a long period.** Although these injuries are **most common in the knee joint,** overuse injuries of other joints can occur secondary to exercise of inappropriate rate, intensity, or both (e.g., "Little Leaguer's elbow").

Stress Fractures

Stress fractures occur most commonly in the **lower extremity** and may be difficult to diagnose without a **bone scan.**

Apophysitis

Apophysitis is **inflammation of a tendon or ligament at its insertion site near the joint.** It occurs more commonly than pure tendonitis in children. In apophysitis, the tenderness is usually **localized to the area just above or below the joint,** and radiographs are generally normal.

Osgood–Schlatter Disease

Osgood–Schlatter disease is thought to be either an **apophysitis or an avulsion of the tibial tubercle secondary to recurrent traction of the patellar tendon**. The patient, usually an **active preadolescent or adolescent,** complains of **tenderness below the patella** and has **pain on extension of the knee against force. Radiographs** may be normal but can reveal **irregularity** and, possibly, **fragmentation** of the tibial tubercle. Treatment consists of **limiting activity until the natural fusion of the tubercle** occurs during midadolescence.

Degenerative Disease

Legg–Calvé–Perthes Disease

Legg–Calvé–Perthes disease is an avascular necrosis of the femoral head that can produce **hip or thigh pain**. The diagnosis should be considered in **5- to 10-year-old boys** with an **indolent presentation of limp** and with **painful abduction and internal rotation of the affected hip**. Plain **radiographs** might reveal changes in the femoral head on the affected side; a **bone scan** allows earlier detection of the disease. Other causes of avascular necrosis include SCD and **chronic steroid use**.

Slipped Capital Femoral Epiphysis

Slipped capital femoral epiphysis, **displacement of the femoral head from the femoral neck,** is most typically seen in **obese adolescents**. These children complain of **hip or thigh pain** and walk with the **affected leg externally rotated**. **Hip radiographs (both anteroposterior and frog-leg projections)** are diagnostic. **Orthopedic referral is mandatory**.

Patellofemoral Pain Syndrome

Patellofemoral pain syndrome results from **recurrent transmission of force onto a malaligned patella**. The common scenario is an adolescent girl who complains of pain on flexion of a previously rested knee joint, pain when traveling down an incline, or **weakness,** causing the **knee to** "**give out** from under her." **Damage to the articular cartilage** (i.e., idiopathic adolescent anterior knee pain syndrome) can occur. Radiographs are frequently normal. **Exercise that strengthens the medial quadriceps muscles** may help realign the patella. **Surgical realignment** may be necessary.

Osteochondritis Dissecans

Osteochondritis dissecans is a **degenerative** process in which **cartilage replaces bone at an articular surface,** usually the **lateral epicondyle of the distal femur, the radial capitellum, or the talus**. It can develop because of either **acute trauma or repeated application of smaller forces,** which cause a **small subchondral fracture**. Osteochondritis dissecans is most common in children undergoing a **growth spurt**. Radiographs may be normal early in the course of the disease. **Immobilization in a non-weight-bearing cast** frequently alleviates the problem. However, **surgical removal of the avulsed fragment** occasionally is necessary.

Infectious Causes of Joint Pain
Septic Arthritis
Etiology

The cause is predominantly **bacterial,** occurring by **hematogenous delivery, by direct extension from osteomyelitis, or from a penetrating injury** to the joint. *Staphylococcus aureus and Streptococcus pyogenes* are the most commonly involved organisms, though *Kingella kingae* has also been implicated in a significant portion of cases. Other bacterial causes to consider include group B streptococcus and Gram-negative organisms in neonates, *Neisseria gonorrhoeae* in adolescents, *Salmonella* in patients with SCD, and *Haemophilus influenzae* in unimmunized children. **Pyogenic infection** in the joint space causes increased pressure within the joint capsule, resulting in **derangements of the vascular and lymphatic supply**. **Bacterial and leukocyte proliferation** may also occur, causing the release of proteolytic enzymes. These changes can rapidly **damage cartilage and bone tissue**.

Clinical Features

Most patients with septic arthritis develop **fever** within the first few days of infection. If the **hip or shoulder joints** are involved, the patient holds the extremity **slightly flexed, abducted, and externally rotated** to relieve the pressure within the joint. The **knee and elbow,** if affected, are **slightly flexed,** and the **ankle** is **plantar flexed**. The **application of pressure** to the joint **or movement of the joint** through almost **any range of motion produces pain**. This finding contrasts with that found in purely traumatic injuries, which may be asymptomatic through a limited range of motion. **Erythema, heat, and swelling** may be present but are difficult to detect in the hip and shoulder joints as these joints are relatively deep beneath the skin surface.

Neisseria infections can produce either **monoarticular or polyarticular** disease. Gonococcal arthritis may begin as polyarthralgia, with a progression to monoarticular arthritis within a few days. These **symptoms** begin within 2 to 4 weeks of the initial urethritis and commonly **increase in severity 1 week following the menstrual period** in girls. Acute cases may be associated with **fever, malaise, or dermatitis**. **Tenosynovitis** (painful tendon sheaths) may also be present.

Evaluation

Plain radiographs may not be helpful early in the course of illness, but they may reveal distortion of the normal fat pads and evidence of a joint effusion. **Ultrasound** can be useful to identify the presence of a joint effusion.

Although the peripheral leukocyte count alone is not often helpful, laboratory data including an elevated C-reactive protein (CRP) and erythrocyte sedimentation rate (ESR) can be helpful in diagnosing septic arthritis. The joint fluid may appear turbid and reveals a large number of leukocytes and a low fluid-to-serum glucose ratio, as described in Table 47-1.

Joint fluid cultures identify the causative organism in about 60% of patients. In contrast, blood culture results are positive in only 30% of all patients. Joint fluid culture results are more likely to reveal the organism **within the first week**

TABLE 47-1	Characteristics of Synovial Fluid			
	Appearance	**WBC/mm³**	**% Neutrophils**	**Glucose Synovial Fluid to Blood**
Normal	Clear	<2,000	<40	>0.5
Infectious	Turbid	>75,000	>75	<0.5
Inflammatory (JIA, SLE)	Clear or turbid	5,000–75,000	50	>0.5
Traumatic	Bloody or clear	<5,000	<50	>0.5

JIA, juvenile idiopathic arthritis; *SLE,* systemic lupus erythematosus; *WBC,* white blood cell.

of infection. Chronic meningococcemia presents a **similar clinical picture** to gonococcal joint disease; however, **joint fluid cultures** are usually **sterile.**

Treatment

Septic arthritis is a **medical and surgical emergency**. Management of septic arthritis involves **evacuation of the purulent material** from the joint space **as soon as possible. Open surgical drainage** is preferred for the hip joint and remains an option for other joints that contain thick purulent material as well. **Parenteral antibiotic therapy** directed at the presumed causative organisms should be initiated immediately after the diagnosis is made. A combination of **intravenous therapy and oral therapy** is given for **2 to 4 weeks** after diagnosis.

Osteomyelitis

Etiology

Osteomyelitis in children can present with symptoms **similar** to those of **septic arthritis: fever, limp, refusal to use an extremity in younger children, or discrete localized pain in older children**. Although the pathophysiology of osteomyelitis differs from that of septic arthritis, the **predominant causative bacteria** are the same. Occasionally, **viral, fungal, and mycobacterial causes** are reported.

Clinical Features

Since osteomyelitis tends to affect the metaphyseal portion of the bone, symptoms can often be confused with joint pain. However, in contrast to septic arthritis, **isolated movement of the affected joint** in an older child with osteomyelitis **does not cause as much pain as does palpation of the affected portion of the bone**. The **CRP and the ESR are usually increased** and are helpful in monitoring the response to therapy.

Evaluation

The triple-phase bone scan is a sensitive and specific test of osteomyelitis, except in neonates.

Plain radiographs may reveal periosteal elevation or bone destruction 10 to 21 days after the onset of illness.

Magnetic resonance imaging can be used to detail the extent and degree of bone and soft tissue injury and to define the presence of a bone abscess ("Brodie abscess"). It is the study of choice for suspected pelvic or vertebral body osteomyelitis and provides better spatial resolution, which is helpful in cases where a surgical procedure is warranted (e.g., abscess drainage). However, it is more expensive than bone scan, and for younger children, sedation is often necessary to complete the study. Bone scan is the study of choice in suspected cases of multifocal infection.

Blood culture results identify the causative organism in ~50% of patients with osteomyelitis.

Needle aspiration of metaphyseal bone, in combination with a blood culture, can increase the yield of a microbiologic diagnosis to 80%.

 HINT: CRP >2 mg/dL and ESR >20 mm/hour have each been shown to be up to 95% sensitive in detecting acute osteoarticular infections.

Treatment
High-dose antibiotic therapy is required to ensure adequate penetration of the bone and complete eradication of the bacterial nidus. A **combination of intravenous and oral antibiotics** may be required for a longer total course than in patients with septic arthritis. However, recent evidence suggests that **shorter courses of intravenous antibiotics, followed by oral antibiotics** can be administered successfully to treat osteomyelitis caused by *S. aureus.* The decision to switch from parenteral to oral antibiotic therapy is based on the absence of signs and symptoms of inflammation, improvement in serum inflammatory markers, and the child's ability to comply with, and appropriately absorb, the oral regimen. The total duration of therapy should be no less than 3 weeks as the rates of chronic infection are highest in those receiving shorter courses of antibiotic therapy.

Viral Arthritis
Young children **<5 years** can often present with pain caused by **infection of the joint by viruses**. **Parvovirus and adenovirus** are two of the more common culprits, and the **fever, rash, and polyarthritis** are frequently **preceded by an upper respiratory infection**.

Postinfectious Arthritis
Acute Rheumatic Fever
The **arthritis** of ARF is **migratory** and involves **several large joints in quick succession**. Commonly, each joint is **affected for <1 week,** and the entire polyarthritis rarely lasts >1 month. The **arthralgia** is also **migratory,** but is differentiated from the arthritis by the **absence of swelling, redness, and decreased range of motion** in an otherwise **painful joint**. One **cannot use both the arthritis and the arthralgia as criteria** for diagnosis.

Since the joint manifestations of ARF occur **within 5 weeks** of the initial streptococcal infection, **antistreptococcal antibody levels** are almost always **increased** during this period. Children with **poststreptococcal reactive arthritis do not**

TABLE 47-2	Revised Jones Criteria (1992) for Diagnosis of Acute Rheumatic Fever	
Major Criteria	**Minor Criteria**	
Carditis	Fever	
Polyarthritis	Arthralgia	
Erythema marginatum	Elevated ESR, CRP	
Sydenham chorea	Prolonged PR interval on ECG	
Subcutaneous nodules		

CRP, C-reactive protein; *ECG,* electrocardiogram; *ESR,* erythrocyte sedimentation rate.
Diagnosis of ARF requires both of the following:
1. Evidence of a preceding group A streptococcal infection, defined as an elevated or a rising antistreptolysin O (ASO) titer, a positive throat culture, or a positive rapid antigen test.
2. Either **two major** or **one major and two minor** criteria listed above.
Adapted from Dajani AS, Ayoub E, Bierman FZ, et al. Guidelines for the diagnosis of rheumatic fever: Jones criteria, updated 1992. *Circulation.* 1993;87:302–307.

fulfill the Jones criteria for ARF (Table 47-2) but may still complain of **prolonged polyarthritis** after group A hemolytic streptococcal infection. These children may still develop **recurrent arthritis** and may carry a **greater risk** of development of a subsequent **"second attack" of rheumatic fever**. Some physicians, therefore, treat these patients similarly to those with ARF. Treatment consists of **antistreptococcal and anti-inflammatory medications**. The arthritis associated with ARF responds dramatically to treatment with **aspirin**.

Lyme Disease

Approximately 60% of patients with documented Lyme disease complain of **painful joints** at some point during their illness. The knee is the most frequently affected joint. Initially, many patients suffer from **polyarthralgias** within the first few weeks of illness. **Frank arthritis** of one or more large joints can occur **2 weeks to 2 years after the onset** of disease, and episodes of **arthritis and arthralgia** can recur over **subsequent years in untreated patients**. Each episode usually lasts a few weeks, but it can also last as long as 1 year.

 HINT: Monoarticular arthritis of the knee is a common presentation of Lyme disease in endemic areas.

Many patients **do not report a history of deer tick bite and do not exhibit the pathognomonic rash** of erythema migrans. The diagnosis, albeit difficult to confirm, is supported by the finding of **concurrent clinical manifestations and serologic evidence** of recent infection. Examination of **synovial fluid** for polymerase chain reaction to the *Borrelia* antigens can be diagnostic but is less sensitive than the blood test for Lyme exposure.

Intravenous therapy is warranted only for cases of arthritis that do not respond to treatment with **amoxicillin (or doxycycline in children >8 years)** for 1 month.

Postdysenteric Arthritis

Occasionally, patients who have recently suffered **acute gastroenteritis** experience **subsequent aseptic arthritis** affecting the large joints. This may occur days to weeks after the infection. It is most common after Yersinia, Campylobacter, and Shigella infections. In some patients, the **arthritis lasts for years** and may produce **destructive changes** in the joint. **Reiter syndrome,** the symptoms of which are **arthritis, urethritis, and uveitis,** may present similarly after gastrointestinal or chlamydial infections in HLA-B27–positive patients.

Inflammatory Causes of Joint Pain

Transient (Toxic) Synovitis

Etiology

The cause of transient synovitis is **unknown,** but it is associated with **upper respiratory infections**.

Clinical Features

The child with transient synovitis is most commonly a boy of **3 to 9 years** who has a **preceding or concurrent upper respiratory infection**. The **hip** is the most commonly affected joint, causing a **limp** as well as **hip, thigh, or knee pain**.

Evaluation

Differentiation from septic arthritis and osteomyelitis is based on the child's **nontoxic appearance, ability to move the hip through some range of motion without pain,** and, if obtained, **normal serum inflammatory markers**.

Treatment

Treatment of transient synovitis includes **rest** of the affected extremity, **administration of oral analgesic medications, and follow-up** to assure resolution within 1 week.

Reactive Arthritis

Reactive arthritis is a sterile inflammatory condition that occurs in response to an infection at a distant site in the body. This is often very difficult to distinguish from infectious causes of arthritis. Nonsteroidal anti-inflammatory medications may be beneficial in treating reactive arthritis.

Other Inflammatory Causes

Joint pain can be a minor manifestation of other known conditions, such as Kawasaki disease, systemic lupus erythematosus, dermatomyositis, polyarteritis nodosa, Henoch–Schönlein purpura, Behçet syndrome, and psoriatic arthropathy. The nonmusculoskeletal symptoms and signs of these conditions often overshadow the joint or bone involvement, and the musculoskeletal findings rarely contribute in a unique manner to the diagnosis.

Immunologic Causes

Serum Sickness

Serum sickness is an antigen–antibody mediated disease of **immune complex deposition**. It commonly occurs 1 to 2 weeks after **exposure to viral antigens** or to certain medications, such as cephalosporin or sulfa drugs. However, many other infectious or medicinal agents have been implicated. Symptoms consist of an urticarial rash, arthralgias in the large joints, and constitutional symptoms, such as fever. The rash may turn purple within a few days. Steroid treatment is reserved for the most severe cases.

Erythema Multiforme (see Chapter 64, "Rashes")
Erythema multiforme is an illness with causes similar to those of serum sickness, in which erythematous target lesions found over the entire body are accompanied by pauciarticular arthritis.

Inflammatory Bowel Disease (see Chapter 34, "Gastrointestinal Bleeding, Lower")
Inflammatory bowel disease can present initially as a form of arthritis. There are multiple forms of arthritic manifestations of inflammatory bowel disease. The most common is the pauciarticular enteropathic arthritis of large joints associated with erythema nodosum. The attacks can last up to 6 weeks and coincide with the acute exacerbations of inflammatory bowel disease.

Ankylosing Spondylitis
Ankylosing spondylitis is a less common form of arthritis associated with inflammatory bowel disease in HLA-B27-positive children.

Juvenile Idiopathic Arthritis
Juvenile idiopathic arthritis is a systemic illness with arthritis as one of its manifestations. It carries an incidence of ~3 in 100,000 children, with a female predominance of 2:1.

The clinical presentation of JIA may be divided into three types: pauciarticular, polyarticular, and systemic. Within these types, the age of onset and the presentation of illness may vary, as delineated in Table 47-3.

The key to the diagnosis of JIA is the presence of symptoms for at least 6 weeks, with a fluctuating clinical course. The diagnosis is made primarily from historical and physical examination findings. Laboratory analysis should be guided toward the evaluation of other illnesses that may be causing the joint pain, but antinuclear antibody testing can be included. Rheumatoid factor testing is usually not helpful, and it is positive only in older girls with polyarticular manifestations. The ESR is often normal in all patients except those with systemic JIA. A thorough search for other illnesses with similar manifestations should ensue before diagnosing this condition. Anti-inflammatory drugs are the mainstay of treatment for the arthritis of JIA. Intra-articular corticosteroid injections, low-dose methotrexate, and biologic agents that act as tumor necrosis factor blockers are successful in alleviating symptoms in children with JIA.

Neoplastic
Primary Bone Tumors
Etiology
Primary bone tumors are uncommon in children; however, they can cause joint pain if they are localized to the proximal or distal portions of the bone.

TABLE 47-3 Subgroups of Juvenile Idiopathic Arthritis

Subgroup	% of JIA at Onset	Gender Ratio	Age at Onset	Joints Affected	Serologic and Genetic Test	Extra-articular Manifestations	Prognosis
Rheumatoid-positive polyarticular	15	90% Female	Late childhood	Any joints, especially hands and wrists	ANA 75% RF 100%	Low-grade fever, anemia, malaise, and rheumatoid nodules	>50% Severe arthritis
Rheumatoid-negative polyarticular	20	70% Female	Younger onset	Any joints	ANA 50%	Low-grade fever, mild anemia, malaise, growth retardation	20%–40% Severe arthritis
Type 1 pauciarticular	45	80% Female	Early childhood	Few large joints (hips and sacroiliac joints spared)	ANA 50%	Few constitutional complaints, chronic iridocyclitis in 50%	Severe arthritis uncommon; 10%–20% ocular damage from iridocyclitis, if untreated
Type 2 pauciarticular	5	90% Male	Late childhood	Few large joints (hip and sacroiliac involvement common)	ANA negative, HLA-B27 75%	Few constitutional complaints, acute iridocyclitis in 5%—10% during childhood	Clinically similar to spondyloarthritis
Systemic onset	15	50% Female	Any age	Any joints	ANA negative, RF negative	High fever, rash, organomegaly, polyserositis, leukocytosis, growth retardation	30% Severe arthritis

ANA, antinuclear antibody; RF, rheumatoid factor; HLA-B27, histocompatability antigen-B27.
Adapted with permission from Fleisher GR, Ludwig S, eds. Textbook of Pediatric Emergency Medicine. 6th ed. Philadelphia, PA: Lippincott Williams & Wilkins; 2010:1128.

Osteogenic sarcoma (osteosarcoma) is the most common primary bone tumor in children and can spread to the joint space by direct extension or as a "skip" lesion.

Ewing sarcoma, another malignant bone tumor in children, involves the joint space less often than does osteogenic sarcoma.

Eosinophilic granuloma, a benign bone lesion that can cause joint pain, often mimics the more malignant tumors.

Osteoid osteoma, another benign bone lesion that can cause joint pain, has a predilection for the femur or tibia and may present as nighttime bone pain that awakens the child from sleep and responds dramatically to anti-inflammatory drugs.

Clinical Features

Frequently, the symptoms are **subtle,** with **progressive development of bone or joint pain,** a **soft tissue mass,** and possibly **recurrent fevers**. The patient or his parents may relate the symptoms to a **single episode of trauma, and pathologic fractures** may occur when minor trauma causes a break in a bone that is weakened by the presence of tumor.

Evaluation

The diagnosis is usually made after review of the **plain radiographs,** which reveal the tumor and corresponding bony changes.

Leukemia and Lymphoma

Leukemia and lymphoma can cause either **bone or joint pain** in children. Most often, the patient presents with **arthralgias** in conjunction with **other systemic problems**. The concomitant findings include **hepatomegaly or splenomegaly, petechiae, lymphadenopathy, anemia, and fever**. The joint pain is usually **chronic and remitting. Peripheral blood smear and bone marrow aspiration or lymph node biopsy** are diagnostic.

Miscellaneous

Limb Pain of Childhood

"Growing pains" should only be considered a diagnosis of exclusion. They are thought to result from **muscle overuse**. The pain lasts **less than a few hours,** frequently **awakens the child at night,** and usually **localizes to the muscles of bilateral lower extremities**. The pain is **rarely (if ever) localized to the joint**.

EVALUATION OF JOINT PAIN

Patient History

The medical history should include questions regarding the presence of **rash, fever, or recent illness**. In addition, the **time course** of the joint pain should be elicited. A **history of trauma** can account for any acute event or be the disclosing event in a more chronic problem, such as SCFE, chondromalacia patella, stress fractures, bone tumors, and hemophilia.

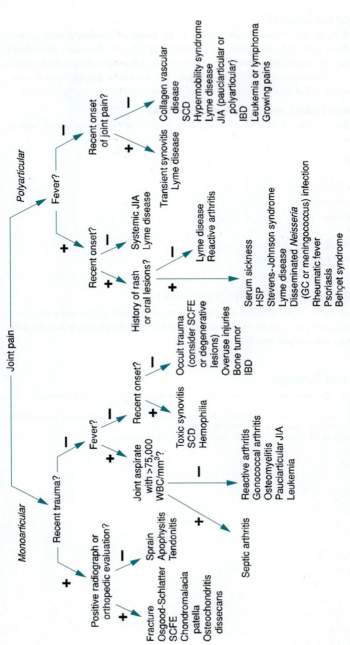

FIGURE 47-1   Approach to the child with joint pain. *GC*, gonococcus; *HSP*, Henoch–Schönlein purpura; *IBD*, inflammatory bowel disease; *JIA*, juvenile idiopathic arthritis; *SCD*, sickle cell disease; *SCFE*, slipped capital femoral epiphysis; *WBC*, white blood cell.

Physical Examination

Physical examination should concentrate on the **range of motion** of each joint in comparison with the corresponding contralateral joint. A thorough **neurologic examination** should be performed with attention to **muscle strength and tone** as well as careful observation of the **child's gait**. The remainder of the physical examination may reveal specific rashes, mucosal lesions, lymphadenopathy, or fever.

Laboratory Studies and Radiographic Evaluation

The following tests should be considered, as needed, in the evaluation of patients with joint pain:

- ESR
- CRP
- Joint fluid analysis
- Plain radiographs
- Bone scan
- MRI
- White blood cell count
- Ultrasound

APPROACH TO THE PATIENT (Figure 47-1)

Although many of the illnesses that cause joint pain can be diagnosed and treated by a pediatrician or a family physician, **referral to an orthopedist, a rheumatologist, or an oncologist** may be necessary.

Suggested Readings

Adebajo AO. Rheumatic manifestations of infectious diseases in children. *Curr Opin Rheumatol.* 1997; 9:68–74.

Caird MS, Flynn JM, Leung YL, et al. Factors distinguishing septic arthritis from transient synovitis of the hip in children. *J Bone Joint Surg Am.* 2005;88(6):1251–1257.

Sorokin R, Ward SB. Joint pain. *Med Clin North Am.* 1995;79:247–260.

Leukocytosis

INTRODUCTION

Leukocytosis is defined as an increase in the total number of white blood cells (WBCs). The normal WBC count varies by age, with infants having the highest total leukocyte count. Leukocytosis may result from an increase in any of the types of WBCs found in the bone marrow. Neutrophilia is most common, but lymphocytosis, monocytosis, basophilia, eosinophilia, and atypical lymphocytosis can also occur. Lymphoblasts or myeloblasts can be seen in abundance in the peripheral blood in leukemia, causing leukocytosis. Leukemoid reactions, which consist of benign but excessive leukocytosis (WBC counts that can be over 50,000/mm³) associated with an increase in the number of immature myeloid cells (blasts, promyelocytes, myelocytes, and metamyelocytes) in the peripheral blood, can also occur.

 DIFFERENTIAL DIAGNOSIS LIST

Neutrophilia
- **Infectious Causes**
  - **Bacterial Infection**
    - *Staphylococcus*
    - *Streptococcus*
    - *Gonococcus*
    - *Meningococcus*
    - *Escherichia coli*
    - *Pseudomonas*
    - *Corynebacterium diphtheriae*
    - *Pasteurella*
  - **Viral Infection**
    - Herpes zoster
    - Varicella
    - Rabies
    - Poliomyelitis
    - Epstein–Barr virus (infectious mononucleosis)
  - **Fungal Infection**
    - *Actinomyces*
    - *Coccidioides*
  - **Mycobacterial Infection**
    - Tuberculosis
  - **Rickettsial Infection**
  - **Spirochetal Infection**
    - Leptospira
    - Lyme disease
    - Syphilis
  - **Other Infections**
    - Kawasaki disease
- **Toxic/Drug/Hormonal Causes**
  - Corticosteroids, adrenocorticotrophic hormone
  - Mercury, lead, kerosene, camphor
  - Epinephrine, norepinephrine, serotonin, histamine, acetylcholine
- **Neoplastic Causes**
  - Eclampsia
  - Uremia
  - Anorexia

- **Inflammatory Causes**
  - Collagen vascular diseases (e.g., rheumatoid arthritis)
  - Acute rheumatic fever
- **Hematologic Causes**
  - Hemolysis—associated with both acute hemolysis, as in autoimmune hemolytic anemia, and chronic hemolysis, as in sickle cell anemia
  - Acute blood loss
  - Myeloproliferative disorders
  - Surgical or functional asplenia
  - Leukemoid reaction
- **Miscellaneous Causes**
  - **Physical Stimuli**
    - Burns
    - Pain
    - Electric shock
    - Trauma/surgery
  - **Physiologic**
    - Pregnancy/labor
    - Ovulation/menstruation
    - Vigorous exercise
    - Emotional stress

Eosinophilia (>4% of Total WBC Count)

- **Infectious Causes (Especially Parasites)**
  - *Ascaris* infestation
  - Hookworm infestation
  - *Strongyloides* infestation
  - Trichinosis
  - Visceral larva migrans
  - Filariasis
  - Malaria
  - Toxoplasmosis
  - *Pneumocystis carinii*
  - Schistosomiasis
  - Scabies
  - Scarlet fever
  - Aspergillosis
  - Coccidioidomycosis

- **Toxic Causes**
  - Drug hypersensitivity reaction
  - Postirradiation
- **Neoplastic Causes**
  - Leukemia
  - Hodgkin and non-Hodgkin lymphoma
  - Brain tumors
  - Myeloproliferative disorders
- **Inflammatory/Allergic/Immune Conditions**
  - Polyarteritis nodosa
  - Sarcoidosis
  - Goodpasture syndrome
  - Milk precipitin disease
  - Enteritis/ulcerative colitis
  - Environmental allergies
  - Asthma
  - Hay fever
  - Urticaria
  - Lymphoproliferative disorders
- **Miscellaneous Causes**
  - Hereditary eosinophilia
  - Tropical eosinophilia (syndrome of pulmonary infiltrates, asthma-like symptoms, lymphadenopathy, and eosinophilia thought to be secondary to an unidentified filarial parasite)
  - Peritoneal dialysis
  - Chronic renal or liver disease
  - Immune deficiency syndromes

Monocytosis (>8% to 10% of Total WBC Count in Childhood; >2% of Total WBC Count in Newborn Period)

- **Infectious Causes**
  - Tuberculosis
  - Syphilis
  - Brucellosis
  - Malaria
  - Bacterial endocarditis

- Rocky Mountain spotted fever
- Typhoid fever
- **Neoplastic Causes**
  - Preleukemia
  - Acute myelogenous leukemia (AML)—myelomonocytic and monocytic forms
  - Juvenile myelomonocytic leukemia
  - Chronic myelogenous leukemia
  - Hodgkin and non-Hodgkin lymphoma
- **Inflammatory Causes**
  - Systemic lupus erythematosus
  - Rheumatoid arthritis
  - Ulcerative colitis/Crohn disease
  - Sarcoidosis
- **Miscellaneous Causes**
  - Chronic neutropenia syndromes (e.g., Kostmann syndrome)
  - Postsplenectomy

Basophilia (>1% of Total WBC Count)
- **Infectious Causes**
  - Varicella
  - Tuberculosis
  - Influenza
- **Neoplastic Causes**
  - Chronic myelogenous leukemia
  - Hodgkin disease
- **Inflammatory Causes**
  - Ulcerative colitis
  - Rheumatoid arthritis
- **Miscellaneous Causes**
  - Asthma
  - Drug hypersensitivity reaction
  - Chronic hemolytic anemia
  - Postsplenectomy or postradiation

Lymphocytosis
- **Infectious Causes (Associated with an Increased Number of Atypical Lymphocytes)**
  - Bacterial infection
  - Pertussis*
  - Tuberculosis
  - Brucellosis
  - Typhoid fever
  - Viral infection
  - Infectious mononucleosis (Epstein–Barr virus)†
  - Cytomegalovirus†
  - Acute viral lymphocytosis (with common viral infections)*
  - Infectious hepatitis (A, B, or C)†
  - Rubeola
  - Rubella
  - Mumps
  - Varicella
- **Other Infections**
  - Syphilis
  - Toxoplasmosis
- **Miscellaneous Causes**
  - Physiologic lymphocytosis (percentage of lymphocytes is greater than percentage of polymorphonuclear leukocytes from 2 to 5 years of age)
  - Relative lymphocytosis (secondary to neutropenia)
  - Endocrine—thyrotoxicosis, Addison disease
  - Drug hypersensitivity reaction
  - Crohn disease/ulcerative colitis
  - Leukemia

---

*Frequently associated with very *high* lymphocyte counts.
†Frequently associated with high *atypical* lymphocyte counts.

DIFFERENTIAL DIAGNOSIS DISCUSSION
Neutrophilia

 HINT: Healthy newborn infants normally experience a period of neutrophilia associated with a "left-shifted" differential (an increase in the
percentage of early myeloid forms in the peripheral blood). The peak
WBC count occurs during the first few days of life and decreases to adult
levels within the first few weeks.

Neutrophilia is the **most common type of leukocytosis**. The cause of neutrophilia is **most frequently an infection,** although drugs, inflammation, and other
conditions listed in the differential diagnosis can be responsible. Neutrophilia is a
result of one or more of the following mechanisms:

- Increased neutrophil production by the bone marrow
- Increased release of neutrophils from bone marrow storage
- A shift of neutrophils from the marginating to the circulating pool
  Prolonged neutrophil survival owing to decreased neutrophil entry into tissue or
  decreased removal by the spleen

Some forms of neutrophilia develop within minutes of exposure to the
stimulus. For example, the neutrophilia that follows exposure to epinephrine is a
result of neutrophils shifting from the marginating to the circulating pool. Other
forms of neutrophilia take longer to develop as they occur by a combination of
these mechanisms. The **duration of neutrophilia is usually days to weeks,**
although in some instances it may persist for months.

Eosinophilia

 HINT: Allergy is the most common cause of eosinophilia in children in
the United States. Outside of the United States, parasites are the most
common cause.

Normal eosinophil counts vary with age, reaching the adult value by 6 to 8 years
of age. **Boys have slightly higher counts than girls,** and most individuals experience a **diurnal variation** in eosinophil count, with the **peak at night.** Most
eosinophils reside in the tissues (especially in areas exposed to the external environment, such as the gastrointestinal and respiratory tracts) and their **release into the
bloodstream is the primary cause** of eosinophilia. Histamine release in allergic
conditions or chronic inflammation tends to make the walls of blood vessels per-
meable, resulting in a release of eosinophils into the peripheral blood. Although
allergy is the most common cause, skin diseases, parasitic infections, and conditions associated with chronic inflammation can also be the factors. **Hypereosinophilic syndrome** is a rare myeloproliferative disorder characterized by persistent
profound, chronic eosinophilia (greater than $1,500/mm^3$ for at least 6 months),

leading to end-organ infiltration and damage. Hypereosinophilic syndrome most commonly results from mutations in FIP1L1-PDGFRA.

Acute Lymphoblastic Leukemia

Incidence
Acute lymphoblastic leukemia (ALL) is the **most common malignancy** seen in the pediatric population. The peak age for the development of ALL is ~4 years, although individuals of all ages can be affected. Certain individuals, such as those with **Down syndrome,** are at an **increased risk** for the development of this disorder.

Etiology
The **cause is unknown,** although genetic, environmental, infectious, and immune-mediated factors are all implicated.

Clinical Features
Symptoms at presentation may include **pallor, fatigue, fever, bleeding, or bruising**. Bone pain is common, and young children may present for evaluation with a **limp or refusal to walk**. Physical findings include **bruises, petechiae, lymphadenopathy, and hepatosplenomegaly**.

Evaluation
Laboratory evaluation may reveal **leukocytosis, anemia, and thrombocytopenia**. In ~50% of patients, the WBC count is 10,000/mm^3 at the time of diagnosis, and in 20% of patients, it is 50,000/mm^3. **Neutropenia** (absolute neutrophil count of 500/mm^3) is also frequently seen. **Lymphoblasts** can be found **in the peripheral blood,** but the inexperienced observer may report them as atypical lymphocytes. Definitive diagnosis of leukemia is made by a **bone marrow aspiration** that demonstrates at least **25% lymphoblasts**. **Flow cytometric staining for surface antigens, as well as cytogenetic and molecular analysis**, should also be performed to differentiate between ALL subtypes as the prognosis and therapy vary widely between the subtypes. The **spinal fluid** and testes need to be examined because the central nervous system is a sanctuary site of extramedullary disease.

Treatment
Prognostic factors, including initial WBC count, patient age, immunophenotype (pre-B vs. pre-T), and genetic tests dictate the treatment indicated. High-risk patients require more intensive therapy. Most treatment plans last **2 to 3 years** and begin with a **remission induction phase intended to decrease the detectable leukemic burden to less than 5%**. The following phases of therapy aim to decrease and eventually eliminate all leukemic cells from the body:

- **Central nervous system preventive therapy** is incorporated into all protocols.
- **Multiagent chemotherapy** is the mainstay of treatment, although irradiation to the central nervous system is used for some high-risk patients.
- **Bone marrow transplantation** is another treatment approach used for the child who has experienced a relapse in the bone marrow or in certain patients with very high-risk features at diagnosis.

Other sites of relapse include the central nervous system and the testes. The prognosis for long-term disease-free survival with current therapy is ~75% for all risk groups.

 HINT: Tumor lysis syndrome (a metabolic triad of hyperuricemia, hyperkalemia, and hyperphosphatemia) is a complication of therapy that occurs when leukemic cells lyse in response to cytotoxic chemotherapy and release their intracellular contents into the bloodstream. This occurs commonly in cells with a high-growth fraction (T-cell leukemia/lymphoma and Burkitt lymphoma). Aggressive hydration, alkalinization, and allopurinol administration before initiating chemotherapy may alleviate serious renal dysfunction. The first two maneuvers promote uric acid and phosphate excretion, and allopurinol reduces uric acid formation. Potassium should not be added to hydration fluids. By monitoring the electrolyte concentrations and renal function closely, one can often avoid the development of renal failure.

Acute Myelogenous Leukemia

Incidence

Acute myelogenous leukemia represents ~15% to 20% of all cases of leukemia seen in the pediatric population. It is slightly more common in older children but affects individuals of all ages. It affects both sexes equally. The **incidence is increased in** individuals with **Down syndrome, Fanconi anemia, Diamond–Blackfan anemia, Bloom syndrome, Li–Fraumeni syndrome, and severe congenital neutropenia**. It is also a **common "secondary malignancy"** resulting from **prior exposure to chemotherapy** (especially regimens that included alkylating agents and/or epipodophyllotoxins).

Etiology

The **cause is unknown**. Predisposing factors include the earlier-mentioned syndromes, exposure to large doses of **ionizing radiation,** and exposure to certain **chemicals**.

Clinical Features

Symptoms at presentation are similar to those of ALL and include **pallor, fatigue, fever, infection, bruising, and bleeding**. The physical examination may reveal **hepatosplenomegaly, lymphadenopathy, bruises, or petechiae. Leukemic infiltration of the skin** (leukemia cutis) may occur; it appears as colorless or slightly purple lesions. **Localized tumors or chloromas** can also be seen.

Evaluation

Laboratory evaluation typically reveals **neutropenia, anemia, and thrombocytopenia**. The WBC count is variable, although ~25% of children have a WBC count of >100,000/mm³ at the time of diagnosis. Blasts may be seen in the peripheral blood. The definitive diagnosis is made by the examination of **bone marrow aspirate,** which demonstrates >**25% blasts**. As in ALL, the **spinal fluid** must also be examined for evidence of leukemia. Up to 15% of patients have evidence of blasts in the spinal fluid at the time of diagnosis.

Until recently, AML was characterized by morphology and histochemical staining, using the FAB (French–American–British) classification system. In 1999, the classification system was revised by the WHO, using genetic alterations found in the myeloblasts to differentiate types. Morphology and histochemical staining remain important; however, genetic alterations, including chromosomal translocations, gains, and losses, and genetic mutations have been shown to be more predictive of response to therapy and overall prognosis.

Poor prognostic variables include having a high WBC count at the time of diagnosis, translocations involving 11q23, and monosomy 7. **Good prognostic variables** include t(8;21), t(15;17), and inv (16).

Treatment

Standard treatment consists of **multiagent chemotherapy** that includes central nervous system preventive therapy. **Allogeneic hematopoietic stem cell transplant (bone marrow transplant; HSCT) from a matched sibling donor during first remission** is the **treatment of choice** for the majority of patients. Most patients without a matched sibling are treated with chemotherapy alone. Some lower risk subtypes are treated with chemotherapy alone even if a matched sibling donor is available. Relapsed AML and some higher risk subtypes at diagnosis require HSCT with best available donor even if there is no sibling match. The **prognosis remains poor** with long-term disease-free survival rates of ~50%. In addition, AML therapy is far more toxic than the ALL therapy. **Serious infection rates** are especially high during the therapy, and the **late effects of treatment** can be problematic.

Complications

The following three complications of AML deserve mention:

- Disseminated intravascular coagulation (DIC)
- Leukostasis
- Tumor lysis syndrome (mentioned previously)

> **HINT:** DIC can occur with any subtype of AML but is especially common in the t(15;17) subtype (acute promyelocyte leukemia). Aggressive treatment with platelet and fresh-frozen plasma transfusions is often indicated. The initiation of chemotherapy frequently causes the coagulopathy to worsen before it improves.

> **HINT:** Leukostasis (intravascular WBC clumping) rarely occurs unless the WBC count is >200,000/mm³. Since myeloblasts are larger and more **"sticky"** than lymphoblasts, leukostasis occurs more frequently in AML than in ALL. The most commonly involved organs are the brain and the lungs. Central nervous system hemorrhage or stroke can occur. The pulmonary involvement is manifested by tachypnea and development of a need for supplemental oxygen. Treatment consists of leukapheresis and prompt initiation of cytotoxic therapy. Red blood cell transfusion should be used with caution as it can increase whole blood viscosity.

HINT: Children with Down syndrome deserve special mention. Neonates with Down syndrome may develop a transient myeloproliferative
syndrome that mimics congenital leukemia in every way except that it
regresses spontaneously without therapy. For older children with Down
syndrome and AML, there is also a better prognosis than for the average
child with AML. The reasons are unclear.

Chronic Myeloid Leukemia

Incidence and Etiology

Chronic myeloid leukemia (CML) accounts for ~3% of all pediatric cases of leukemia. Individuals of any age can be affected, though most cases occur in late
childhood. The disease is relatively **indolent** as compared with the acute leukemias.

Clinical Features

The patient is often **asymptomatic** and presents with a **high WBC count or
splenomegaly** discovered at a routine well-child visit. However, symptoms such as
fever, night sweats, abdominal pain, or bone pain can occur. Physical examination reveals impressive splenomegaly. **Hepatomegaly** can also be present.

Evaluation

Laboratory evaluation typically reveals impressive **leukocytosis, thrombocytosis,
and mild anemia**. The bone marrow is hypercellular but with normal myeloid
maturation. The characteristic cytogenetic hallmark of CML is the **Philadelphia
chromosome**. This is associated with the classic t(9;22) with translocation of the
ABL segment from chromosome 9 to the major breakpoint cluster region (BCR)
of chromosome 22.

Treatment

There are **three phases** of chronic myelocytic leukemia: **chronic phase, accelerated phase, and blast crisis**. The **chronic phase** is the most common in children
and may last for years and represents **hyperproliferation of mature myeloid elements with less than 10% leukemic blasts**. Treatment during this phase has
changed dramatically over the past decade. In the past, patients were treated with
cytoreductive therapy followed by HSCT. Molecularly targeted therapies using
tyrosine kinase inhibitors (TKIs) that target the BCR–ABL fusion product are
now the treatment of choice. HSCT is reserved for rare patients who fail TKIs
or relapse. Without treatment, **patients enter the accelerated and blast phases,**
developing frank leukemia. Accelerated phase is a poorly defined intermediate
phase with increasing leukemic blasts (10% to 19%), cytopenias, clonal karyotype evolution, constitutional symptoms, and basophilia. Blast phase is the most
aggressive with patients developing >20% myeloblasts (resembling AML) or lymphoblasts (resembling ALL). **Once the blast phase has begun, the prognosis is
poor**. Patients with accelerated phase are also treated with TKIs; however, they
are less likely to respond and often require HSCT. Patients in blast phase require
TKIs, cytoreductive chemotherapy, and HSCT.

General Therapy Guidelines for Leukemia (ALL, AML, CML)

- **Prevent bleeding.** Aim to keep the platelet count above 20,000/mm^3 by means of platelet transfusions. Watch for signs of DIC.
- **Treat anemia.** Most oncologists aim to keep the hemoglobin level >8 g/dL (but as low as tolerable and not more than 10 g/dL if hyperleukocytosis is present). Some oncologists treat anemia only if the patient is symptomatic.
- **Identify and treat infection.** Since all neutropenic patients are at an increased risk for the development of an infection, fever should be treated aggressively. Blood should be drawn for culture, and use of broad-spectrum antibiotics (to cover both Gram-positive and Gram-negative organisms) should be instituted. Prolonged fever in the neutropenic host raises the question of the existence of fungal disease.
- **Watch for tumor lysis.** This was described in the discussion of ALL.
- **Watch for complications of hyperleukocytosis.** This was described in the discussion of AML.
- **Begin definitive chemotherapy promptly** once the diagnosis has been established.

Leukemoid Reactions

Etiology

Leukocytosis that develops in **response to an infection** or other stimuli can occasionally become **exaggerated,** often with WBC counts of greater than 50,000/mm^3. If the **white cells are not malignant blasts,** this syndrome is termed as leukemoid reaction (Table 48-1). Frequently, there is an associated **increase in the number of immature myeloid or lymphoid precursors** in the peripheral blood. Examination of the bone marrow typically reveals **myeloid hyperplasia** with normal maturation. Myeloid leukemoid reactions (comprising two-thirds of all cases) most often occur in association with **bacterial infection.** The etiologic agents

TABLE 48-1	Features of Leukemoid Reactions, ALL, and CML (Chronic Phase)		
Feature	**Leukemoid Reaction**	**ALL**	**CML**
Common physical examination findings	Evidence of infection	Hepatosplenomegaly or lymphadenopathy	Splenomegaly
Predominant WBC morphologic characteristics	Myelocytes or lymphocytes	Lymphoblasts	Myelocytes
WBC count	>50,000/mm^3	Wide range	>100,000/mm^3
Other cell lines	Normal hemoglobin and platelet counts	Anemia and thrombocytopenia	Mild anemia and thrombocytosis

ALL, acute lymphoblastic leukemia; *CML,* chronic myelocytic leukemia; *WBC,* white blood cell.

most frequently involved are *Staphylococcus, Haemophilus, Neisseria meningitidis, Meningococcus, and Salmonella.* Lymphoid leukemoid reactions (which comprise a third of all cases) occur most commonly in individuals infected with *Bordetella pertussis* or in common acute viral infections. **Other causes** of a leukemoid reaction include **granulomatous disease, severe hemolysis, vasculitis, drugs, and the presence of a tumor that metastasizes to the bone marrow**.

Evaluation
Distinguishing a leukamoid reaction from chronic myelogenous leukemia may be difficult and require molecular analysis. The acute leukemias may also exhibit excessive leukocytosis, usually composed of predominantly blast forms.

Suggested Readings
Kelly KM, Lange B. Oncologic emergencies. *Pediatr Clin North Am.* 1997;44:809–830.

Pieters R, Carroll WL. Biology and treatment of acute lymphoblastic leukemia. *Pediatr Clin North Am.* 2008;55:1–20.

Pui CH, Robison LL, Look AT. Acute lymphoblastic leukemia. *Lancet.* 2008;371:1030–1043.

Rubnitz JE, Gibson B, Smith FO. Acute myeloid leukemia. *Hematol Oncol Clin North Am.* 2010; 24:35–63.

Suttorp M, Millot F. Treatment of pediatric chronic myeloid leukemia in the year 2010: the use of tyrosine kinase inhibitors and stem cell transplantation. *Hematol Am Soc Hematol Educ Program 2010.* 2010;368–376.

Leukopenia

INTRODUCTION

Leukopenia is defined as a **decrease in the total white blood cell (WBC) count, usually to <4,000/mm³**. **Neutropenia** is defined as a **decrease in the number of circulating neutrophils** (both segmented and band forms). An absolute neutrophil count (ANC) of **1,500/mm³** or less is typically considered neutropenia. **Severe neutropenia refers to an ANC of <500/mm³.** The ANC is calculated by multiplying the total WBC count by the sum of the percentage of segmented neutrophils plus the percentage of band forms in the differential count. For example, if the WBC count is 4,000/mm³, with 12% segmented neutrophils/polymorphonuclear leukocytes, 10% bands, 60% lymphocytes, and 18% monocytes, the ANC will be 880 [4000 × (0.12 + 0.10)]. The differential diagnoses of isolated leukopenia and neutropenia are similar; the two conditions are, therefore, considered one entity for the purpose of this chapter.

> **HINT:** In 3% to 5% of African-American children, the total WBC count normally may be as low as 3,600/mm³, and the ANC may be as low as 1,000/mm³.

 DIFFERENTIAL DIAGNOSIS LIST

Infectious Causes
Bacterial Infection
- Sepsis syndrome, bacteremia (especially group B streptococcal disease in neonates)
- Tuberculosis
- Brucellosis
- Tularemia
- Typhoid
- Paratyphoid

Viral Infection
- Hepatitis A or B
- Parvovirus B19
- Respiratory syncytial virus
- Influenza A or B
- Rubeola
- Varicella
- Rubella
- Infectious mononucleosis (Epstein–Barr virus)
- HIV
- Cytomegalovirus

Protozoal Infection
- Malaria
- Kala-azar (visceral leishmaniasis)

Rickettsial Infection
- Scrub typhus
- Sandfly fever

Toxic Causes

- Ionizing radiation
- Heavy metals (gold, arsenic, mercury)

Medications

See Table 49-1

Congenital Causes

- Kostmann syndrome
- Cyclic neutropenia
- Shwachman–Diamond syndrome (neutropenia and exocrine pancreatic insufficiency)
- Reticular dysgenesis
- Barth syndrome (neutropenia, cardiomyopathy, myopathy)
- Neutropenia associated with X-linked agammaglobulinemia
- Neutropenia associated with dysgammaglobulinemia type I (neutropenia, absent immunoglobulin A [IgA] and IgG, and increase in IgM)
- Neutropenia associated with metabolic disease (hyperglycemia, isovaleric acidemia, propionic acidemia, methylmalonic acidemia)
- Neutropenia as part of bone marrow failure syndrome (Fanconi anemia, dyskeratosis congenital, Blackfan–Diamond syndrome)

Immune-Mediated Causes

- Autoimmune neutropenia (owing to IgG-mediated destruction of neutrophils)
- Felty syndrome (triad of neutropenia, splenomegaly, and rheumatoid arthritis)
- Secondary to collagen vascular disease—juvenile rheumatoid arthritis or systemic lupus erythematosus (SLE) (lymphopenic common in SLE)
- Neonatal alloimmune neutropenia (antibody derived from mother)

Miscellaneous Causes

- Aplastic anemia
- Splenic sequestration
- Nutritional deficiency (B_{12} or folate deficiency)
- Copper deficiency
- Familial benign neutropenia
- Leukemia
- Bone marrow infiltration (with tumor, osteopetrosis, Gaucher disease)
- Chronic idiopathic neutropenia

DIFFERENTIAL DIAGNOSIS DISCUSSION
Neutropenia Associated with Infection

Infection, usually viral, is the most common cause of neutropenia in childhood. Typically, neutropenia develops during the first few days of infection and persists for 3 to 8 days. **Neonates** are at especially **high risk** for developing neutropenia because they have only a small neutrophil reserve in their bone marrow, and they release neutrophils too quickly into the circulation when stressed. The mechanism by which an infection causes neutropenia is most often caused by direct marrow suppression or viral-induced immune neutropenia. Leukopenia is common in patients with HIV. Management of neutropenia in patients with infections consists of **treating the underlying infection**.

TABLE 49-1	Drugs That Can Induce Neutropenia or Leukopenia

Cytotoxic Chemotherapeutics

Alkylating agents (e.g., cyclophosphamide), antimetabolites (e.g., methotrexate), anthracyclines (e.g., doxorubicin)

Antimicrobials
Sulfonamides, penicillin, cephalosporins, macrolides, ciprofloxacin, acyclovir, isoniazid, imipenem

Analgesics
Aspirin, ibuprofen, indomethacin, acetaminophen

Anticonvulsants
Valproic acid, Dilantin, carbamazepine

Antithyroid Drugs
Thiouracil, thiocyanate

Antirheumatic Agents
Gold, penicillamine, phenylbutazone

Antihistamines
Cimetidine, ranitidine

Cardiovascular Drugs
Procainamide, captopril, nifedipine, hydralazine, propranolol

Antipsychotics, Antidepressants, and Neuropharmacologic Agents
Phenothiazines, risperidone, barbiturates, benzodiazepines

Miscellaneous
Allopurinol, retinoic acid, metoclopramide, spironolactone, intravenous immunoglobulin

Drug-Induced Neutropenia

Etiology

Drug-induced neutropenia may be caused by a cytotoxic effect, an immunologic effect, or may be an idiosyncratic reaction. Neutropenia can be a result of the following:

- **Increased sensitivity** of myeloid precursors to appropriate drug concentrations.
- **Altered drug metabolism** resulting in toxic levels of the drug in the bone marrow.
- An **immunologic response** that occurs after exposure to the drug, resulting in neutrophil destruction. In some cases, the drug serves as a hapten in promoting antibodies that can destroy neutrophils. In other cases, the drug causes the formation of circulating immune complexes that attach to the surface of the neutrophil and lead to its destruction.

Clinical Features

Fever, chills, and fatigue may occur in patients with **immune-mediated drug-induced neutropenia**. These symptoms typically develop **7 to 14 days after exposure** to the drug. The duration of the neutropenia is usually brief (1 to 2 weeks) after cessation of the drug.

Drug-induced neutropenia that is **not immune mediated is less predictable**. It may present several days to more than a month after exposure to the drug. The duration may be brief, or it may last months or years.

Table 49-1 shows a partial list of drugs that may cause neutropenia.

Treatment
Treatment consists of **prompt discontinuation** of the offending drug.

Kostmann Syndrome
Etiology
Kostmann syndrome, or **severe congenital neutropenia,** is a rare disorder that most commonly arises as a result of new autosomal dominant mutations in the gene *ELA2,* which encodes the neutrophil elastase. The gene responsible for many cases of autosomal recessive forms is HAX1.

Clinical Features
Children with this disorder frequently present for medical care in the **first few months of life. Fever, cellulitis, stomatitis, and perirectal abscesses** are the most common findings. These children are **at risk for** developing severe bacterial infections, which may be **life threatening**.

Evaluation
Laboratory test results reveal **profound neutropenia** (ANC of **<200/mm³**) with or without leukopenia. The differential count may reveal **monocytosis and eosinophilia**.

Bone marrow biopsy findings are variable. Usually, there is normal myeloid maturation up to the promyelocyte or myelocyte stage but **no evidence of mature neutrophils** (maturational arrest). Erythroid precursors and megakaryocytes are present in normal numbers, with a normal maturational sequence noted.

Treatment
The natural course of this disease is **death at an early age secondary to overwhelming infection**. Prophylactic antibiotics are not beneficial. Therapeutic use of the **cytokine granulocyte colony-stimulating factor (G-CSF)** has resulted in an improvement in the neutrophil count, decreased risk of development of serious infections, and improved survival in many patients with Kostmann syndrome. **Definitive treatment is hematopoietic stem cell transplant (HSCT; bone marrow transplant).** HSCT should strongly be considered for patients who are poor responders to G-CSF and/or have a history of severe and/or life-threatening infections. Patients who respond robustly to G-CSF can be closely monitored and may not need HSCT.

Autoimmune Neutropenia

 HINT: Autoimmune neutropenia is the most common cause of chronic neutropenia in children.

Etiology

Autoimmune neutropenia is a **benign and self-limited condition in the majority of patients**. Children with this disorder develop **antibodies against their own neutrophils, often after a recent viral infection**. This disorder affects individuals of all ages, but the highest incidence occurs in infants and young children.

Clinical Features

The majority of patients are asymptomatic. A small percentage of patients develop **skin infections, oral ulcerations, and pharyngitis**. Serious infections are uncommon. Some children have mild to moderate **splenomegaly** on physical examination.

Evaluation

Laboratory testing results reveal neutrophil counts that are often <250/mm³. Monocytosis is common. Bone marrow examination typically reveals normal cellularity with **myeloid hyperplasia** and a **paucity of mature neutrophils**. Diagnosis is made by demonstrating **antineutrophil antibodies** in the serum or on the surface of the neutrophil, although this is not necessary for the diagnosis in patients with the typical clinical features.

Treatment

In most children with this disorder, the neutrophil count usually increases in response to infection. Although the prognosis is good, **aggressive treatment of bacterial infections** is important. In many children, the WBC count completely normalizes within 1 to 3 years.

Cyclic Neutropenia

Etiology

Cyclic neutropenia, a **rare** diagnosis, is characterized by regular **oscillation in the number of circulating neutrophils** in the peripheral blood. The periodicity is usually every 21 days, with the period of neutropenia spanning 3 to 6 days. Cyclic neutropenia is the result of dominantly inherited mutations in the neutrophil elastase gene (ELA2).

Clinical Features

Symptoms usually appear before 10 years of age. Diagnosis is made from analysis of **serial complete blood counts (CBCs) and differential counts** (two to three times a week for 4 to 6 weeks). Clinical findings include **stomatitis, oral ulcers, pharyngitis with lymph node enlargement, and skin infection**. Laboratory test results reveal **severe neutropenia. Monocytosis and eosinophilia** occur in some patients. The **platelet and reticulocyte counts may also fluctuate,** although not consistently in the same direction. The **morphological characteristics of the bone marrow change** according to the time in the cycle, varying from normal to hypocellular, with maturational arrest of the myeloid line. The **ANC is low for 3 to 10 days and then begins to increase**.

Symptoms disappear as the ANC returns to normal. The **severity of infection varies** with each child and with the ANC. Some children do not have infections despite profound neutropenia, although there are reports of death in up to 10% of patients.

Treatment
Therapeutic use of G-CSF has been demonstrated to decrease the risk of infection.

Shwachman–Diamond Syndrome
Etiology
Shwachman–Diamond syndrome is a **rare congenital form of neutropenia** inherited as an autosomal recessive trait. The syndrome consists of neutropenia with **exocrine pancreatic insufficiency**. Some children also have metaphyseal **chondrodysplasia and dwarfism**. Greater than 90% of patients have mutations in the *SBDS* gene.

Clinical Features
The symptoms of **weight loss, diarrhea, steatorrhea, and failure to thrive** usually develop in infancy, resembling the **clinical presentation of cystic fibrosis**. Patients experience **recurrent infections;** the mortality rate from infection or bone marrow failure is 15% to 25%.

Evaluation
The sweat electrolyte values are normal in this syndrome. The neutrophil count is usually 200 to 400/mL. Genetic testing for SBCS mutations should be performed. Yearly bone marrow evaluations with cytogenetics are often recommended to assess bone marrow failure and malignant transformation.

Treatment
Treatment is aimed at: (1) correcting pancreatic insufficiency with pancreatic enzyme replacement, fat-soluble vitamins, and a low-fat diet; (2) fever management as described in treatment of leukopenia; (3) consideration of G-CSF for neutropenia; (4) orthopedic support to prevent and treat orthopedic deformities; and (4) transfusions of red cells and/or platelets if indicated for anemia and/or thrombocytopenia. Definitive treatment is HSCT; however, these patients do not tolerate conditioning chemotherapy and have a high rate of transplant-associated morbidity and mortality. Recent protocols using **reduced-intensity conditioning HSCT** approaches appear promising.

Chronic Idiopathic Neutropenia
Chronic idiopathic neutropenia of childhood is a **poorly understood** disorder. Symptoms of **skin infections** may appear in early childhood and vary with the degree of neutropenia. Laboratory test results reveal **neutropenia and associated monocytosis**. The diagnosis is essentially one of **exclusion** and should be considered in any child with **persistent chronic neutropenia, a benign clinical course, and no evidence of another neutropenic disorder**. The prognosis is good.

EVALUATION OF LEUKOPENIA
Patient History
- **Does the child have a fever?** This raises the question of infection, especially in a neutropenic patient. It may also give a clue to the cause because some infections can cause neutropenia.

- Does the child have any skin infections? Abscesses and cellulitis require prompt treatment in the setting of neutropenia.
- Has the child previously had a normal CBC? If so, this will exclude congenital causes of neutropenia, such as Kostmann syndrome.
- Has the child recently taken any medication (e.g., sulfonamides, penicillin, phenothiazines)?
- Does the child have any symptoms of a systemic infection, such as fever, rash, and upper respiratory symptoms? This could indicate infectious mononucleosis, rubeola, rubella, or varicella.
- Does the child have any symptoms of the following infections: tuberculosis, brucellosis, tularemia, or malaria?
- Is there a history of jaundice (seen in hepatitis A and B)?
- Is the child a sick neonate? This could indicate group B streptococcal infection or isoimmune neonatal neutropenia.
- Does the child have a history of recurrent skin infections or oral ulcerations? This suggests a more chronic, perhaps congenital neutropenia such as cyclic neutropenia or Kostmann syndrome.
- Does the child have an unusual diet or look malnourished? This could indicate malnutrition or an isolated B_{12}, folate, or copper deficiency.
- Is there a family history of neutropenia, recurrent infection, or death at an early age from infection? This would be seen in any of the congenital neutropenia syndromes—Kostmann syndrome, chronic benign neutropenia, or familial aplastic anemia.
- Is there any bruising or bleeding? Is the child pale or fatigued? If the answer is yes, this suggests that other cell lines are involved, such as in aplastic anemia, leukemia, or megaloblastic anemia.

Physical Examination
- **Is the child ill appearing?** Infection, either as the cause or as the result of neutropenia, is likely and should be treated promptly.
- **Is there evidence of cellulitis, perirectal abscesses, labial abscesses, or pharyngitis?** All are seen in neutropenic patients and require prompt treatment.
- **Are there oral ulcerations or swollen red gums** common in many neutropenic disorders?
- **Are there bruises, petechiae, or pallor** suggesting leukemia or aplastic anemia?
- **Is there splenomegaly** (found in hypersplenism, Felty syndrome, and leukemia?)
- **Is there hepatomegaly** (occurring in hepatitis, leukemia, and infectious mononucleosis)?
- **Are there phenotypic abnormalities,** such as thumb anomalies (Fanconi anemia), dwarfism (Shwachman–Diamond syndrome or cartilage-hair hypoplasia), or skin hyperpigmentation (Fanconi anemia, dyskeratosis congenita)?
- **Are there joint findings suggesting arthritis** (seen in juvenile rheumatoid arthritis, SLE, or Felty syndrome)?
- **Is there fever or rash?** See corresponding list in "Patient History."

Laboratory Studies

 HINT: In infants, the total WBC count is higher than in later childhood. Lymphocytes are the predominant WBC form in children 2 to 5 years of age. Neutrophils are the predominant WBC form in infants and in children over 5 years of age.

- CBC, differential count (sometimes serially)
- Bone marrow aspirate with or without biopsy
- Antineutrophil antibodies

Factitious Causes of Leukopenia (False-Positive Test Result)
- Delay in testing blood sample drawn from the patient
- Excessive leukocyte clumping (in the presence of cold agglutinins, increased immunoglobulin levels, or certain paraproteins)
- Leukocyte fragility (owing to certain drugs or leukemia)

Note: Results of a WBC count determined manually should identify the last two conditions.

TREATMENT OF LEUKOPENIA
Antibiotics
Prompt treatment of infection with antibiotics is indicated.

Cytokines
Cytokine Granulocyte Colony-Stimulating Factor
G-CSF is a **hematopoietic growth factor** produced by recombinant DNA technology that stimulates the growth of committed neutrophil progenitors. G-CSF is approved for use in treating the neutropenia that results from **cancer chemotherapy**.

Granulocyte Transfusions
Granulocyte concentrates are usually prepared by **leukapheresis of a single donor**. The indications for a granulocyte transfusion are few and include the following:

- Gram-negative sepsis not responding to antibiotics in a neutropenic host
- Life-threatening infections in a neutropenic patient who shows no sign of bone marrow recovery

Complications are many and include the **risks of infection, allergic or febrile transfusion reactions, and graft-versus-host disease**. A hematologist or blood bank physician should be involved in this decision.

 HINT: WBC concentrates should not be run through a leukoreduction filter.

APPROACH TO THE PATIENT

- If the child is ill appearing, the workup should be delayed while administration of appropriate antibiotics is started. If the cause of the fever is not evident, broad-spectrum antibiotics should be chosen.
- If a recent infection or drug exposure is noted in the history and the child is clinically well with isolated neutropenia, close follow-up with performance of several repeat CBCs and differentials may be all that is indicated.
- If the neutropenia is chronic or if there is a history of recurrent infection, a more extensive workup should be initiated that includes: (a) antineutrophil antibody testing; (b) serial CBCs and differential counts two to three times a week for 3 to 4 weeks; and (c) bone marrow aspirate and biopsy. More specific testing (i.e., gene mutation analyses for congenital syndromes) is dictated by the history and physical examination findings.

Suggested Readings

Bernini JC. Diagnosis and management of chronic neutropenia during childhood. *Pediatr Clin North Am.* 1996;43:773–792.

Calhoun DA, Christensen RD. Recent advances in the pathogenesis and treatment of nonimmune neutropenias in the neonate. *Curr Opin Hematol.* 1998;5:37–41.

Segel GB, Halterman S. Neutropenia in pediatric practice. *Pediatr Rev.* 2008;29:12–24.

Shastri KA, Logue GL. Autoimmune neutropenia. *Blood.* 1993;81:1984–1995.

Zeidler C, Boxer L, Dale DC. Management of Kostmann syndrome in the G-CSF era. *Br J Haematol.* 2000;109:490–495.

Lymphadenopathy

INTRODUCTION

Healthy children frequently have palpable lymph nodes, most commonly in the cervical, axillary, and inguinal areas. There is a broad differential diagnosis for lymphadenopathy in children. This enlargement can be suggestive of underlying disease, so it is important to have an organized and thoughtful approach to the evaluation of a child with lymphadenopathy. Lymph nodes can enlarge secondary to proliferation of normal lymphocytes (infection or lymphoproliferative process) or from migration and infiltration of nodal tissue by extrinsic inflammatory or metastatic malignant cells.

There are a number of factors to consider that will help narrow the differential diagnosis. These include:

- Patient age: Lymph nodes in the **cervical, axillary, and inguinal** region are frequently palpated in early childhood.
- Size: Anterior cervical and axillary nodes >1 cm or inguinal nodes >1.5 cm require further investigation. Enlarged **supraclavicular** nodes can reflect mediastinal or abdominal pathology and should always be considered pathologic.
- Location: Important to understand the patterns of drainage in order to carefully look for infection or inflammation. Examples include:
  - Anterior cervical nodes drain the mouth/pharynx: Upper respiratory infection
  - Occipital and posterior cervical nodes drain the scalp: Tinea capitis
  - Preauricular: Conjunctivitis, external ear infections
  - Axillary: Cat-scratch disease
  - Submental: dental infections, gingivostomatitis
- Quality (tender, warm, firm, erythematous): Requires further evaluation for infectious process.
- Area: localized versus generalized
- Length of time: Differential diagnosis varies for acute nodal enlargement (usually <3 to 4 weeks) versus chronic enlargement (>4 to 6 weeks).
- Presence of systemic symptoms: Weight loss, rash, fever, night sweats

> **HINT:** Supraclavicular nodes are normally not palpable and enlargement should be considered pathologic because of their association with mediastinal malignancy.

🔬 DIFFERENTIAL DIAGNOSIS LIST

Lymphadenopathy in Children
Infectious Causes
Bacterial Infection
Localized:
- *Staphylococcus aureus*
- Group A *Streptococcus* (pharyngitis)
- Anaerobes
- Tularemia
- Diphtheria
- Chancroid
- Atypical mycobacterium
- Cat-scratch disease (*Bartonella henselae*)

Generalized:
- Lymphogranuloma venereum
- Leptospirosis
- Bacteremia
- Scarlet fever
- Syphilis
- Tuberculosis (TB)
- Subacute bacterial endocarditis
- Brucellosis
- Leptospirosis
- Typhoid fever
- Plague
- Lyme disease
- Tularemia

Viral Infection
- Epstein–Barr virus (EBV)
- HIV
- Varicella
- Cytomegalovirus (CMV)
- Rubeola
- Rubella
- Infectious hepatitis
- Influenza
- Upper respiratory viral infection such as parainfluenza, rhinovirus, respiratory syncytial virus

Fungal Infection
- Histoplasmosis
- Coccidioidomycosis

Parasitic Infection
- Toxoplasmosis
- Malaria

Neoplastic
Primary Lymphoid Neoplasm
- Lymphoma
- Leukemia

Metastatic Neoplasm
- Neuroblastoma
- Rhabdomyosarcoma
- Thyroid carcinoma
- Nasopharyngeal carcinoma

Metabolic
- Gaucher disease
- Niemann–Pick disease

Immunologic
- Systemic lupus erythematosus
- Juvenile rheumatoid arthritis
- Vasculitis syndromes
- Serum sickness
- Autoimmune hemolytic anemia
- Chronic granulomatous disease
- Autoimmune lymphoproliferative syndrome

Medications
- Dilantin
- Isoniazid
- Immunizations

Endocrine
- Hyperthyroidism

Histiocytoses
- Langerhans cell histiocytosis
- Hemophagocytic syndromes
- Malignant histiocytosis

Sinus histiocytosis with massive lymphadenopathy (Rosai–Dorfman disease)

Miscellaneous
Kawasaki syndrome
Skin disorders

Atopic dermatitis
Sarcoidosis
Castleman disease (benign giant lymph node hyperplasia)
Kikuchi-Fujimoto disease

DIFFERENTIAL DIAGNOSIS DISCUSSION
Lymphadenitis
Etiology

Acute infective lymphadenitis is a problem frequently encountered in the pediatric population. It represents a primary infection of the lymph node. The causative organism frequently gains entry into the body through the pharynx, nares, dentition, or a break in the skin. The etiology is most often bacterial, with *S. aureus* being the most frequently isolated organism. Other pathogens that may be found include group A streptococci, *Mycobacterium tuberculosis,* atypical mycobacteria, gram-negative bacilli (such as *B. henselae*), *Haemophilus influenzae,* anaerobic bacteria, *Francisella tularensis, and Yersinia pestis.*

Clinical Features

Physical examination usually reveals a unilateral, tender, warm, often fluctuant lymph node with erythema of the overlying skin. Fever and elevated white blood cell count occur occasionally, most often in the younger child.

Evaluation and Treatment

Aspiration often reveals the cause and may provide symptomatic relief if the lymph node is large or in an awkward position. In uncomplicated cases, treatment with an oral antibiotic is frequently all that is needed. Recent increases in antibiotic resistance such as methicillin-resistant *S. aureus* may impact the choice of antibiotics. Infants, children who appear clinically ill or have an underlying immunodeficiency, those who do not improve or progress on oral antibiotics and those who develop associated cellulitis should be admitted to the hospital for intravenous antibiotics and further evaluation.

Reactive Lymphadenopathy
Etiology

Reactive hyperplasia of lymph nodes represents a response to antigenic stimuli (foreign material, cellular debris, or infectious organisms and their toxic products).

Clinical Features

The resulting lymphadenopathy can be acute or chronic. The cervical, axillary, and inguinal nodes are most commonly involved and can sometimes grow to be quite large. The nodes clinically enlarge secondary to infiltration with histiocytes or plasma cells. Acute cellular infiltration and edema causes distention of the capsule, producing tenderness when the lymph node is palpated.

Evaluation

- **In the acute setting:** Careful history and physical examination, with attention to symptoms of upper respiratory infections (influenza or adenovirus are commonly associated with cervical lymphadenopathy), symptoms of EBV or CMV, local infections of the ear, nose, teeth, or skin, or Kawasaki disease.

- **In chronic situations:** Chronic lymph node hyperplasia can pose a diagnostic dilemma (see section on "Evaluation of Lymphadenopathy"). Lymph node biopsy may be helpful and usually recommended when the lymph node has been enlarged for more than 4 to 6 weeks without a clear cause. In children who undergo lymph node biopsies, the majority (~75%) are reactive or benign. Lymph nodes infiltrated with malignancy are more likely to be supraclavicular in location, chronic (present for >4 weeks), >3 cm, and in patients with some abnormality on laboratory testing or imaging.

Treatment

Since reactive hyperplasia represents the body's normal response to stimuli, treatment is not indicated in most cases. The nodes usually regress with time.

Infectious Mononucleosis

Etiology

EBV, a member of the herpesvirus group, is the causative agent in infectious mononucleosis. The virus, transmitted by saliva, gains entry through the pharynx and spreads throughout the lymphatic system.

Clinical Features

The primary infection is frequently asymptomatic. Individuals who experience primary infection in adolescence or young adulthood are more likely to develop the clinical syndrome. After an incubation period of 4 to 8 weeks, the patient begins to experience fatigue, anorexia, headache, and malaise. Fever and sore throat usually develop within 1 week, bringing the patient to medical attention.

Physical findings at presentation include pharyngitis, lymphadenopathy, and hepatosplenomegaly. Not uncommonly, the patient is misdiagnosed with streptococcal pharyngitis and treated with amoxicillin. For reasons that are unclear, 80% to 100% of patients with EBV treated with amoxicillin or ampicillin develop a pruritic maculopapular rash, which can be helpful in making the diagnosis. Symptoms usually persist for several weeks, although fatigue and malaise may persist for months. Central nervous system complications include aseptic meningitis, encephalitis, Bell palsy, and Guillain–Barré syndrome. Other complications include splenic rupture, autoimmune hemolytic anemia, thrombocytopenia, neutropenia, myocarditis, interstitial pneumonitis, and airway obstruction.

Evaluation

Diagnosis is suggested by the clinical triad of **fever, lymphadenopathy, and pharyngitis** combined with the laboratory finding of atypical lymphocytosis. If the clinical presentation is unclear, serologic testing is available. Heterophile antibodies (e.g., **Monospot**) are usually positive in patients >4 years. EBV titers are a quantitative measure and more useful in younger children.

Treatment

Treatment is supportive because the disease is self-limiting. Patients should be advised to avoid contact sports for 6 to 8 weeks to decrease the risk of splenic rupture. The lymphadenopathy may persist for as long as 6 months after diagnosis.

Cat-Scratch Disease

Etiology

Cat-scratch disease is a benign self-limited regional adenitis that develops 1 to 2 weeks after a cat scratch or bite. Cervical, axillary, or epitrochlear nodes are most commonly involved. The etiologic agent is a gram-negative bacillus (*B. henselae*).

Clinical Features

The presenting symptom is usually a large swollen, erythematous, painful solitary lymph node. History and examination may reveal an erythematous papule that appeared ~2 weeks earlier in the area drained by the lymph node. Most patients recall a cat scratch or bite ~10 days before papule formation. Suppuration of the involved node occurs in 30% of cases. Atypical presentations of the disease include encephalitis, **Parinaud oculoglandular syndrome** (granulomatous conjunctivitis and unilateral preauricular node enlargement), erythema nodosum, osteolytic lesions, and thrombocytopenic and nonthrombocytopenic purpura.

Evaluation

Diagnosis is established by serologic detection of antibodies to *B. henselae*.

Treatment

In most instances, the nodes regress within 8 weeks without intervention. Occasionally, drainage is required. Antibiotic treatment may be considered for acutely ill patients who are immunocompromised.

Non-Hodgkin Lymphoma

Incidence

Non-Hodgkin lymphoma (NHL), the third most common pediatric cancer, is a heterogeneous group of lymphomas whose incidence increases with age. The incidence of NHL also varies with geographic area. Africa and the Middle East have the highest rates of NHL, with **Burkitt lymphoma** especially prevalent in Africa.

Etiology

In developing countries, EBV has been recovered from many of these tumors and researchers continue to investigate the role of EBV in tumor pathogenesis. Risk factors for development of NHL include inherited immunodeficiency syndromes (ataxia-telangiectasia, Wiskott–Aldrich syndrome, severe combined immunodeficiency disease, and X-linked lymphoproliferative disease) and acquired immunodeficiency syndromes (AIDS and posttransplant).

Clinical Features

The most common types of childhood NHL include three main histologic patterns: lymphoblastic (40%), Burkitt (40%), and large cell (20%). The clinical presentation can include constitutional symptoms (fever, weight loss) and any specific symptoms related to the enlarged lymph nodes, which include, but are not limited to, airway obstruction, mediastinal mass or visceral compression, obstruction, or perforation.

- **Lymphoblastic.** Most are of T-cell origin. Patients commonly present with cervical adenopathy and respiratory distress secondary to a mediastinal mass with or without pleural effusions. **Superior vena cava syndrome** is a life-threatening emergency that may arise in this setting. The mediastinal mass compresses the superior vena cava and/or trachea, impeding blood return and air flow. Symptoms include cough, dyspnea, and difficulty lying down secondary to respiratory distress. Physical findings include edema, plethora or cyanosis of the face, neck, and upper extremities, and wheeze or stridor. Immediate treatment with chemotherapy may obscure the diagnosis, but be lifesaving.
- **Burkitt.** Most patients in developed countries present with abdominal findings such as pain, swelling, intussusception, or obstruction. Abdominal pain and acute swelling are common complaints given the extremely rapid dividing time of this tumor. Because of the rapid tumor growth, patients are also at risk for tumor lysis syndrome and renal insufficiency if they have a high tumor burden at presentation.
- **Large cell lymphomas.** Large cell lymphomas have various clinical presentations that include constitutional symptoms such as fever, a mediastinal mass, inguinal adenopathy, bone, or skin involvement.

Evaluation

Workup should include a complete blood cell count (CBC) with differential, serum lactate dehydrogenase, uric acid, and chemistry panel to evaluate for metabolic abnormalities resulting from a rapidly dividing tumor. The diagnosis requires obtaining tissue from an enlarged lymph node, mass, or involved fluid (pleural, pericardial, ascites). Evaluation for extent of tumor spread includes computed tomography scan from neck through pelvis, PET scan, and examination of the bone marrow and spinal fluid.

Treatment

Since some of the NHL types can grow rapidly, prompt diagnosis is vital so that treatment can be initiated. Combination chemotherapy is the mainstay of treatment. These patients are at increased risk for **tumor lysis syndrome** (see discussion of leukemia in Chapter 48, "Leukocytosis"), as a result of the tumor's high growth rate and sensitivity to chemotherapy. In general, prognosis is good, even in patients with advanced disease (bone marrow or central nervous system involvement).

Hodgkin Lymphoma

Etiology

Hodgkin lymphoma is most frequently seen in adolescence. Although it can occur at other ages, it is especially rare in those <5 years. The etiology is unknown, but there are data to suggest EBV as a contributing factor to the pathogenesis in some cases.

Clinical Features

The patient usually presents with painless cervical or supraclavicular adenopathy, although other nodes may be involved. Systemic symptoms can include fever, weight loss, night sweats, anorexia, itching, and fatigue. Fever, night sweats, and weight loss are symptoms included in the staging system and are seen in about 20% of patients.

Evaluation

Physical examination most commonly reveals firm, rubbery nontender lymph nodes in the cervical or supraclavicular region. Most patients are well appearing.

If Hodgkin lymphoma is suspected, a chest radiograph should be obtained promptly because two-thirds of patients have some degree of mediastinal involvement and may be asymptomatic. The airway should be assessed for evidence of tracheal compression before any procedures are performed. Lymph node biopsy establishes the definitive diagnosis, revealing the characteristic **Reed–Sternberg cell** and one of the four histologic patterns (nodular sclerosing, lymphocyte predominant, lymphocyte depletion, and mixed cellularity). Further workup is necessary for staging purposes and to establish a baseline for following response to treatment. In addition to an excisional lymph node biopsy (if possible), additional studies should include a CBC, erythrocyte sedimentation rate, chemistry panel, computed tomography scans from neck through pelvis, PET scan, and bilateral bone marrow aspirate/biopsy.

Treatment

Treatment consists of combination chemotherapy and/or radiation therapy based on the patient's stage, risk group, and response to therapy. Long-term survival is excellent even for patients with advanced disease.

Tuberculosis

Incidence

The incidence of TB has risen in recent years. Early detection and prompt treatment are becoming increasingly important for preventing the spread of the disease. The highest rates of infection are currently seen in minority populations, urban settings, and crowded living conditions. Patients with HIV infection are especially likely to present with active disease. Transmission of the etiologic agent *M. tuberculosis* is by inhalation of infected droplets. The incubation period from the time of infection to the development of a positive skin test is 2 to 10 weeks. Clinical disease develops in a minority of infected patients. When disease does develop, it is usually within the first 2 years after infection.

Clinical Features

Patients most commonly present with either an asymptomatic infection or a pulmonary disease. Those with a positive skin test and no evidence of clinical disease should have a screening chest radiograph. Any patient with pneumonia, pleural effusion, or a cavitary lesion in the lung that does not improve with antibiotics should be evaluated for TB. Individuals with pulmonary disease may have symptoms that include fever, weight loss, failure to thrive, and cough. TB should be considered in any child with unexplained lymphadenopathy. Extrapulmonary disease (miliary, meningitis, lymph node involvement [i.e., Scrofula], bone/joint disease or rare sites such as middle ear, GI tract, skin, kidneys, and eye) can also occur in a minority of patients.

Evaluation

An infection is diagnosed by a positive skin test or by culture (which takes months to grow) from infected body fluids (sputum, gastric washings). The tuberculin preparation recommended for skin testing is the purified protein derivative (PPD). The standard dose is 5 tuberculin units in 0.1 mL of solution, which should be injected intradermally on the forearm. A positive reaction is defined as an induration >10 mm after 48 to 72 hours. Tine tests should not be used for definitive diagnosis and are of questionable value for screening.

Treatment

Treatment for children with TB infection consists of isoniazid and rifampin for 6 months. Most advocate for a third agent, pyrazinamide for the first 2 months of therapy.

EVALUATION OF LYMPHADENOPATHY

Patient History

> **HINT:** Since infections are the most common cause of acute and chronic lymphadenopathy, the history should focus on the presence of or exposure to infections.

- How long have the lymph nodes been enlarged?
- Are they getting larger? (in general, the larger the node, the more worrisome)
- Is the node red, tender, or painful? (lymphadenitis)
- Has there been fever, weight loss, or night sweats? (lymphoma, TB)
- Is there any bruising, bleeding, pallor, or fatigue? (leukemia)
- Is there fever, rash, or systemic symptoms? (scarlet fever, rubeola, rubella, EBV, Kawasaki disease)
- Are there joint complaints? (juvenile rheumatoid arthritis, systemic lupus erythematosus)
- Is there a history of a cat scratch (cat-scratch disease), tick bite (Lyme disease), or other animal exposure (tularemia)?
- Has there been exposure to an individual with TB?
- Is there a history of high-risk sexual behavior, substance abuse, or transfusion? Does a parent have any of these risk factors? (HIV)
- Is there a history of travel? (malaria)

Physical Examination

- Are the nodes generalized or regional? (see section on "Differential Diagnosis")

>  **HINT:** There are certain benign entities that may be confused with cervical adenopathy including:
>
> - Thyroglossal cyst
> - Brachial cleft cyst
> - Epidermal cyst
> - Cystic hygroma
> - Ectopic thyroid tissue
> - Neonatal torticollis

- What size are the nodes? (baseline measurement is important to ensure proper follow-up)
- Are the nodes erythematous, tender, warm, or fluctuant? (lymphadenitis)
- Are the nodes firm/hard and fixed in position? (malignancy)
- Is there fever or rash? (scarlet fever, rubeola, rubella, infectious mononucleosis, Kawasaki disease)
- Is there pharyngitis? (streptococcal disease, EBV)
- Is there hepatosplenomegaly? (EBV, CMV, leukemia, lymphoma)
- Are there bruises, petechiae, or pallor? (leukemia)
- Are there joint findings? (juvenile rheumatoid arthritis, systemic lupus erythematosus)
- Is there a palpable abdominal mass? (neuroblastoma)
- Is there any skin infection and/or inflammation? (tinea, atopic dermatitis)

Laboratory Studies

- CBC, differential count.
- Peripheral blood smear (atypical lymphocytes).
- Lactate dehydrogenase, uric acid (for suspected malignancy).
- Screening for specific infectious diseases. Examples include:
  - *B. henselae*
  - EBV
  - CMV
  - HIV
  - Toxoplasmosis
- PPD skin test.
- Chest radiograph.
- Ultrasound (distinguish suppurative from nonsuppurative lymphadenitis).
- Needle aspiration (may identify organism in suppurative lymphadenitis). Note: Should not perform if concern for malignancy or atypical mycobacterium.
- Open lymph node biopsy or excision is the preferred approach for patients with presumed malignancy or atypical mycobacterium.

APPROACH TO THE PATIENT

- Do you have a probable diagnosis (e.g., fever, sore throat, cervical lymphade-nopathy, exudative pharyngitis, likely streptococcal pharyngitis) after complet-ing the history and physical examination? If so, perform appropriate diagnostic tests (throat culture) and begin treatment with antibiotics if indicated.

- Are you unsure of the diagnosis in a patient who looks ill or is febrile without a clear cause? Consider admission to the hospital and a more extensive laboratory screen for infectious or malignant causes.

- Does the patient exhibit any worrisome symptoms or physical findings, such as the following?
  - Supraclavicular adenopathy
  - Hard, rubbery, or matted adenopathy
  - Fever, constitutional symptoms >1 week without infectious cause identified
  - Cervical nodes that continue to increase in size despite adequate antibiotic therapy
  - A node that continues to increase in size after 1 to 2 weeks
  - An enlarging node that does not regress in size after 4 weeks

- If the answer to one or more of these questions is yes, consider obtaining a CBC with differential, chemistry panel, uric acid, LDH, PPD skin test, and a chest radiograph. Open lymph node biopsy should be considered in the absence of a diagnosis for a patient with chronic lymphadenopathy. Fine needle aspiration is not recommended for pediatric patients with possible malignancy given the high false-negative rate, lack of preservation of nodal architecture, and pau-city of malignant cells, especially in patients with Hodgkin lymphoma. Chest radiography should be performed before the patient undergoes anesthesia for a lymph node biopsy. Assessing the possibility of a mediastinal mass in association with the lymphadenopathy is critical prior to anesthesia.

- In cases where the diagnosis is unclear in a patient who looks well and does not have any high-risk symptoms or physical findings, consider empiric antibiotics to cover common staphylococcal and streptococcal infections and close follow-up with serial examinations.

Suggested Readings

Friedmann AM: Evaluation and management of lymphadenopathy in children. *Pediatr Rev.* 2008;29: 53–60.

Nield LS, Kamat D. Lymphadenopathy in children: when and how to evaluate. *Clin Pediatr.* 2004;43: 25–33.

Twist CJ, Link MP. Assessment of lymphadenopathy in children. *Pediatr Clin N Am.* 2002;49:1009–1025.

Macrocephaly

INTRODUCTION

The skull provides a fixed space for the brain, blood vessels, and cerebrospinal fluid (CSF) in adults and older children, thus causing symptoms of increased intracranial pressure (ICP) in the case of a space-occupying lesion. However, in **infants** it has the capability of growth that can accommodate expansion of any intracranial compartment. Macrocephaly is defined by **head circumference greater than two standard deviations from the mean for gender** (i.e., 98th percentile). Large head size arises from the enlargement of any of the four major constituents of the head: **ventricles** (hydrocephalus), **brain parenchyma** (megalencephaly), **skull** (osteodysplasia), or **extracerebral fluid collections** (subdural, subgaleal, or subperiosteal).

Hydrocephalus is typically described as **communicating** (with free flow of CSF between the ventricles and the subarachnoid space) or **noncommunicating** (obstructive). Either type can be congenital or acquired. Communicating hydrocephalus is usually caused by **overproduction of CSF or blockage of CSF reabsorption** at the arachnoid villi. Common causes include intraventricular hemorrhage, infection, or inflammation (e.g., bacterial, tuberculous or cryptococcal meningitis, viral encephalitis), meningeal infiltration by tumor, and metabolic conditions (e.g., Hurler syndrome with associated mucopolysaccharidosis deposition at the leptomeninges).

Congenital hydrocephalus presents with enlarged head at birth, but it is increasingly being diagnosed *in utero* by routine ultrasonography (US). It usually presents during the newborn period or in early infancy with lethargy or irritability, vomiting, poor feeding, or poor weight gain. **Acquired hydrocephalus** shows a rapid rate of head growth crossing percentiles. Common findings include developmental delay, hypertonia, and hyperreflexia. Hydrocephalus of any etiology can show signs of increased ICP including apnea, bradycardia, a tense and bulging fontanelle, split sutures, the "setting sun sign" (i.e., downward deviation of the eyes showing sclera superiorly), vomiting, sixth nerve palsies, and increased blood pressure with bradycardia. Scalp veins may be prominent and tortuous.

- Diagnosis is made by serial head measurements (see Table 51-1) and neuroimaging.
- In patients with progressive hydrocephalus, treatment includes ventriculoperitoneal (VP) shunting.

TABLE 51-1	Expected Head Growth Velocity		
Full Term		**Preterm**	
Age	Rate of Growth	Age	Rate of Growth
0–3 mo	2 cm/mo	0–2 mo	1 cm/wk
3–6 mo	1 cm/mo	2–4 mo	0.5 cm/wk
7–12 mo	0.5 cm/mo	>4 mo	1 cm/mo

DIFFERENTIAL DIAGNOSIS LIST

Congenital
- Infectious—cytomegalovirus, toxoplasmosis, mumps, rubella
- Anatomic—Chiari malformation, hydranencephaly, aqueductal stenosis
- Neoplasm—medulloblastoma, choroid plexus papilloma, meningioma

Acquired
- Neoplasm—posterior fossa tumor: medulloblastoma, ependymoma, cerebellar astrocytoma

- Intraventricular tumor—ependymoma, choroid plexus papilloma, giant cell astrocytoma, meningioma
- Intraparenchymal mass—cyst, abscess, tumor
- Trauma—cephalohematoma, subdural or subgaleal fluid collections
- Vascular—aneurysm of the vein of Galen, intraparenchymal bleed, intraventricular hemorrhage

> **HINT:** Papilledema is uncommon in infancy because open fontanelles and unfused sutures allow skull expansion, thus relieving pressure.

DIFFERENTIAL DIAGNOSIS DISCUSSION
Congenital Infection
Congenital infections are discussed in detail in Chapter 56, "Neonatal Infections." Calcification seen on other neuroimaging techniques (especially CT) increases the suspicion for congenital infection.

Chiari Malformations
There are four types of Chiari malformations. The most common is **type II** (also called the "Arnold–Chiari malformation"), usually associated with **spina bifida**. In this variant, the cervical canals of both the brainstem and the cerebellum are displaced downward, the fourth ventricle is elongated, and hydrocephalus results from obstruction of the flow of CSF through the foramina of Magendie and Luschka. At birth, some patients already have advanced hydrocephalus; others show rapid head enlargement during the first weeks of life. Patients with Chiari malformations may exhibit signs and symptoms related to brainstem dysfunction (lower cranial nerve findings, breathing difficulty, apnea, poor feeding, swallowing

problems, poor gag, and tongue fasciculations) as well as symptoms of increased ICP.

- Serial head circumference measurements need to be performed.
- US, CT, or magnetic resonance imaging (MRI) of the head can confirm the diagnosis. MRI is recommended to optimally evaluate brain anatomy.
- Brainstem auditory evoked responses complement the MRI assessment.

> **HINT:** A child who presents with headache that worsens with cough or other Valsalva maneuvers should be evaluated for Chiari malformation.

Genetic Syndromes

Hydrocephalus is seen in many genetic disorders. Fifty percent of patients with trisomy 13 syndrome have meningomyelocele with hydrocephalus. **Warburg syndrome,** an autosomal recessive disorder, includes findings of hydrocephalus, retinal lesions, Dandy–Walker cyst, occipital encephalocele, agyria, and pachygyria. **Klippel–Feil syndrome,** with many modes of inheritance, causes malformation of the skull and cervical vertebrae that can be associated with Chiari malformation and hydrocephalus.

Hydranencephaly

Hydranencephaly is caused by the replacement of cortex by enlarged ventricles, presumably secondary to *ex vacuo* dilation following massive intrauterine infarctions. The infant may initially appear normal, with a normal head circumference and intact primitive reflexes, but developmental arrest and long tract signs make the absence of cortex evident as the child grows. Many patients die in early infancy, but prolonged survival is possible. Positive transillumination and percussion of the skull strongly support the diagnosis, which is made by prenatal ultrasound or neuroimaging after birth.

Congenital Aqueductal Stenosis

Cerebral aqueductal atresia or stenosis can occur following intrauterine hemorrhage, infection, brain tumor, venous malformation, or as an isolated developmental anomaly. Diagnosis is made by prenatal US or postnatal neuroimaging. Management includes placement of a VP shunt.

Acquired Hydrocephalus
Neoplasm

The most common tumors in children <2 years are choroid plexus papilloma, ependymoma, and medulloblastoma. Children with posterior fossa masses (e.g., medulloblastoma, ependymoma, cerebellar astrocytoma) present to medical care with signs of increased ICP, ataxia, papilledema, and meningismus. Persistent torticollis in a child should raise the suspicion of tumor. Intraventricular tumors (e.g., choroid plexus papilloma) can lead to hydrocephalus by increased CSF production or blockage of CSF pathways. Diagnosis is made by CT or MRI scans. Treatment of hydrocephalus is by surgical resection of the tumor with or without VP shunt.

Intraventricular Hemorrhage

Intraventricular hemorrhage is common in low-birth-weight infants because of immaturity of the germinal matrix vessels. Perinatal and neonatal stresses (e.g., sepsis, respiratory distress syndrome, hyperglycemia and hypoglycemia, hypoxemia, and shock) trigger hemorrhage. Low-grade intraventricular hemorrhage is usually asymptomatic. Grade III or IV hemorrhages (significant subependymal involvement, intraparenchymal extension) may result in obstructive hydrocephalus by compression of critical pathways or communicating hydrocephalus by blocking the CSF reabsorption in the arachnoid villi.

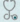 **HINT:** US is the preferred neuroimaging modality to screen for hydrocephalus in infants with open fontanels because it is easier and quicker to obtain than MRI and avoids exposure to radiation with CT.

Infection and Inflammation

Inflammation and meningeal seeding (from tumor cells) may result in communicating hydrocephalus. In addition, irritation or entrapment of the nerves throughout their course in the brain may cause patchy cranial nerve abnormalities. Massive subdural effusion or empyema complicating bacterial meningitis may contribute to head enlargement. Diagnosis is made by MRI with gadolinium enhancement.

Trauma

Cephalohematoma and subdural collections may result from traumatic delivery, either spontaneously or as a result of a forceps or vacuum delivery. Patients with a large subdural collection may experience rapid head enlargement associated with an acute **encephalopathy** characterized by lethargy, poor feeding, vomiting, and seizures.

- CT of the head should be performed immediately in all symptomatic infants with a history of traumatic birth injury because diagnostic delay can be fatal.
- Large symptomatic subdural collections may require neurosurgical intervention.

Megalencephaly or parenchymal enlargement is caused by anatomic or metabolic abnormalities including the following:

Benign familial macrocephaly, in which the head circumference grows rapidly from normal at birth to above the 98th percentile within the first year of life. Typically, there is a family history of large head with normal intelligence, and the infant has normal development and a normal neurologic examination. Although the head circumference is greater than two standard deviations above the mean, it remains parallel to the expected growth line over serial measurements. No workup is necessary, although if neuroimaging is performed, one finds top normal size of the ventricles and subarachnoid spaces.

 HINT: Even if head growth velocity is crossing percentiles, measuring the head circumference of the parents can be helpful in diagnosing benign familial macrocephaly and quickly reducing anxiety.

- **Sotos syndrome** (megalencephaly with gigantism) is characterized by cerebral gigantism with excessive somatic growth, advanced bone age, megalencephaly, and mild mental retardation.
- **Symptomatic megalencephaly** is a description for a group of diseases associated with megalencephaly, for example, degenerative diseases (e.g., Tay–Sachs disease, Canavan disease, Alexander disease) and neurocutaneous syndromes (e.g., neurofibromatosis, tuberous sclerosis).
- **Osteodysplasia** presents with increased skull thickness caused by anemia, osteochondrodysplasia, or rickets and can also lead to macrocephaly.
- **Autism** should be a consideration when macrocephaly is present. Enlarged head occurs in up to one-third of children with autistic spectrum disorders, and is usually most obvious between 1 and 3 years of age. One theory is that macrocephaly is caused by lack of normal pruning of ineffective synapses (apoptosis) in the autistic toddler. MRI rarely shows any migrational abnormality or other structural problem.
- **Idiopathic megalocephaly** is a diagnosis of exclusion when there are no identifiable causes, associated syndromes, or a family history of macrocephaly. MRI shows normal or mildly dilated ventricles.

Suggested Readings

Alper G, Ekinci G, Yilmaz Y, et al. Magnetic resonance imaging characteristics of benign macrocephaly in children. *J Child Neurol.* 1999;12(10):678–682.

Archibald SL, Fennema-Notestine C, Gamst A, et al. Brain dysmorphology in individuals with severe prenatal alcohol exposure. *Dev Med Child Neurol.* 2001;43(3):148–154.

Charney E. Management of Chiari II complications. *J Pediatr.* 1989;3(3):364–371.

Mercuri E, Ricci D, Cowan FM, et al. Head growth in infants with hypoxic-ischemic encephalopathy: correlation with neonatal magnetic resonance imaging. *Pediatrics.* 2000;105(2 Pt 1):235–243.

Sniderman A. Abnormal head growth. *Pediatr Rev.* 2010;31:382–384.

Vertinsky AT, Barnes PD. Macrocephaly, increased intracranial pressure and hydrocephalus in the infant and young child. *Top Magn Reson Imaging.* 2007;18(1):31–51.

Williams CA, Dagli A, Battaglia A. Genetic disorders associated with macrocephaly. *Am J Med Genet Part A.* 2008;146A:2023–2037.

Mediastinal Mass

INTRODUCTION

The mediastinum is a potential space within the thoracic cavity, between the two pleura. It is divided into anterior, middle, and posterior regions. The etiology of a mediastinal mass is often suggested by its regional location because it likely formed from the normal structures in that area.

- **Anterior Mediastinum**

  Anatomy: The anterior mediastinum is bounded by the first rib superiorly, the posterior surface of the sternum anteriorly, the anterior border of the upper dorsal vertebra posteriorly, and by an imaginary curved line that follows the cardiac border and extends backward until it reaches the border of the dorsal vertebra.

  Structures: This area contains structures anterior to the pericardium including the thymus, lymph nodes, and, rarely, extension of the thymus gland. The superior vena cava (SVC) is an easily compressible, thin-walled vessel with a low intraluminal pressure that is surrounded by the lymph nodes and thymus.

> **HINT:** SVC syndrome is generally associated with anterior mediastinal masses.

- **Posterior Mediastinum**

  Anatomy: The posterior mediastinum is bounded posteriorly by the anterior surface of the curve of the ribs, anteriorly by the posterior border of the pericardium, and inferiorly by the diaphragm.

  Structures: The primary structures in this area are the sympathetic ganglia, descending aorta, thoracic duct, and esophagus.

- **Middle Mediastinum**

  Anatomy: The middle mediastinum is the area between the anterior and the posterior regions with the diaphragm as its base.

  Structures: This region contains the trachea, bronchi, heart, great vessels, and the majority of the mediastinal lymph nodes.

DIFFERENTIAL DIAGNOSIS LIST

Anterior Mediastinum
- Germ cell tumor
- Hemangioma
- Histiocytosis
- Leukemia
- Lipoma
- Lymphangioma (cystic hygroma)
- Lymphoma—non-Hodgkin lymphoma (NHL), Hodgkin lymphoma (HL)
- Substernal thyroid
- Teratoma
- Thymic hyperplasia or cyst
- Thymoma

Middle Mediastinum
- Bronchogenic cyst
- Castleman disease
- Fibromatosis histoplasmosis
- Pericardial cyst
- Sarcoidosis
- Tuberculosis (TB)
- Vascular anomalies

Posterior Mediastinum
- Esophageal duplication cyst
- Thoracic meningocele
- Tumors of neurogenic origin—neuroblastoma, ganglioneuroblastoma, ganglioneuroma, neurofibroma, and schwannoma

Note: Ewing sarcoma and rhabdomyosarcoma can form masses in **any** of the mediastinal regions.

DIFFERENTIAL DIAGNOSIS DISCUSSION
Anterior Mediastinum

 HINT: Most (70%) anterior mediastinal masses in children are malignant.

Superior Vena Cava Syndrome/Superior Mediastinal Syndrome

SVC and superior mediastinal (SM) syndromes are **life-threatening complications of anterior mediastinal masses**. **SVC syndrome** implies **venous obstruction** from compression or thrombosis. When **coupled with tracheal compression,** the syndrome is called **SM syndrome**. Tracheal compression without signs of venous obstruction is more common and equally worrisome. The mediastinal mass compresses the SVC, the trachea, or both, impeding blood return and air flow and producing the signs and symptoms summarized in Table 52-1.

These are rare syndromes; only 10% to 15% of pediatric patients with malignant anterior mediastinal tumors have SVC syndrome or SM syndrome. However, it is **critical to recognize these patients** because their condition can **deteriorate dramatically** and quickly. **Immediate consultation with an oncologist** is always appropriate.

Leukemia

Patients with lymphoblastic leukemia (most often T-cell) can present with a mediastinal mass. This is the most likely diagnosis when there are concurrent abnormalities in the complete blood count (anemia, thrombocytopenia, neutropenia,

TABLE 52-1	Signs and Symptoms of Superior Vena Cava Syndrome or Superior Mediastinal Syndrome
History	**Physical Examination**
Cough, especially when supine	Retractions
Dyspnea or orthopnea	Wheezing or stridor
Headache	Papilledema
Dizziness or syncope, especially when symptoms are exacerbated with Valsalva maneuver	Prominence of neck or chest veins
Facial swelling	Suffusion or edema of face, neck and conjunctiva
Visual changes	Anxiety or confusion
Sense of fullness in ears	Quiet heart sounds, hypotension or pulsus paradoxus if cardiac tamponade
	Cyanosis or plethora

or leukocytosis) or circulating peripheral blasts. In these patients, the diagnosis is most easily made by bone marrow aspirate. In patients with hematologic malignancies, lumbar puncture may be combined with other diagnostic procedures in order to simultaneously assess malignant involvement of the spinal fluid.

Lymphoma

 HINT: Lymphoma is the most common cause of SVC and SM syndromes in children.

Non-Hodgkin Lymphoma
Mediastinal masses in patients with NHL are often caused by lymphoblastic lymphoma; however, it can also be secondary to diffuse large B-cell lymphoma (see Chapter 50, "Lymphadenopathy"). Approximately 60% of patients with lymphoblastic lymphoma present with a mediastinal mass, and they often have associated pleural or pericardial effusions.

Hodgkin Lymphoma
Although NHL has a slightly higher incidence than HL, the mediastinum is more often the primary site of involvement in HL. **Cervical adenopathy** is the most common clinical presentation, but approximately two-thirds of patients with HL also present with a mass consisting of **anterior mediastinal, paratracheal, and tracheobronchial lymph nodes**. **Tracheobronchial compression** has been observed on chest radiographs in 50% of children with newly diagnosed HL. Only 20% of patients with HL have systemic symptoms of including **fever, night sweats, and weight loss** of >10% in the previous 6 months. (HL is discussed in detail in Chapter 50, "Lymphadenopathy.") Patients can be asymptomatic with their mediastinal mass. In addition, they may not have systemic symptoms at the time of presentation. It is therefore critical to consider chest imaging in those

with suspicious lymphadenopathy in the cervical and supraclavicular areas even in asymptomatic patients.

Germ Cell Tumors

The **anterior mediastinum** is the second most common site of extragonadal germ cell tumors.

 HINT: Up to 20% of boys with mediastinal germ cell tumors have Klinefelter syndrome.

There are three types of extracranial germ cell tumors: mature teratomas, immature teratomas, and malignant germ cell tumors.

- **Mature teratoma.** The most common type of extracranial germ cell tumor. It is composed of well-differentiated tissues derived from the three germinal layers of the embryo (i.e., endoderm, mesoderm, and ectoderm). They are benign tumors and unlikely to develop into cancer.
- **Immature teratoma.** In addition to mature elements, the mass contains embryonic-appearing elements. In infants, immature teratomas are often noted secondary to their mass effect on normal structures, but in adolescents, they behave as highly malignant tumors.
- **Malignant germ cell tumors (yolk sac tumors, germinomas, and choriocarcinomas).** Extragonadal germ cell tumors form in areas other than the testicles and ovaries. They often develop along the midline of the body in areas such as the sacrum, coccyx, mediastinum, posterior abdomen, and neck. If a patient is suspected to have a mediastinal germ cell tumor, serum markers can be sent to evaluate for this and include α-fetoprotein or β-human chorionic gonadotropin.

Thymic Hyperplasia

An enlarged thymus is the most common cause of a widened anterior mediastinum in neonates. This is a **benign incidental finding** that does not cause symptoms unless the hyperplastic thymus is located in an abnormal position. Thymic enlargement is sometimes the result of a **thymic cyst,** which can be delineated by computed tomography (CT).

Lymphangioma (Cystic Hygroma)

Lymphangiomas are **rarely localized to the mediastinum** but can extend into the mediastinum from a neck lesion and cause symptoms. Lymphangiomas are almost always noted by the time the patient reaches 3 years of age. **If possible, surgical resection** is the treatment of choice.

Hemangioma

Like lymphangiomas, hemangiomas are reported in all portions of the mediastinum, but ~**75% of mediastinal hemangiomas occur in the anterior region**. Many are **asymptomatic,** but they may cause **airway compression** or, rarely, **bleeding into the pleural cavity**. Mediastinal hemangiomas are associated with hemangiomas at other sites in the body. Generally, hemangiomas **grow during the first and second year of life and then slowly regress**.

Histiocytosis

Histiocytosis is an increase in the number of mononuclear phagocytic cells (histiocytes). Rarely, patients with Langerhans cell histiocytosis (which is caused by immunologic stimulation of the normal antigen-processing Langerhans cell in an uncontrolled manner) present with a mediastinal mass.

Lipoma

Lipomas are benign tumors composed of aberrant fat cells. They grow very slowly and generally do not undergo malignant transformation.

Thymoma

A neoplasm of the thymus is not considered a thymoma unless it contains **neoplastic epithelial components**. Such tumors are rare in adults and even rarer in children. Thymomas are slow-growing tumors that extend locally and rarely metastasize. Rarely, **autoimmune disorders** (e.g., myasthenia gravis, systemic lupus erythematosus, rheumatoid arthritis, cytopenias, and thyroiditis) are reported in **association with thymomas**.

Middle Mediastinum
Histoplasmosis

This disease is caused by the fungus *Histoplasma capsulatum.* It is endemic in the Mississippi, Ohio, and Missouri River valleys where up to 80% of the population has a positive histoplasmin skin test by 20 years of age. The diagnosis is best made by either noting a fourfold increase in the complement fixation titer between acute and convalescent sera (using *Histoplasma* yeast and mycelial antigens) or by performing a tissue diagnosis.

Tuberculosis

TB, a mycobacterial disease, commonly affects **mediastinal lymph nodes** in children. Infection of nodes without significant pulmonary involvement is more common in primary pulmonary TB than in reactivation of the disease. Of note, as many as 20% of patients with culture-proven TB have negative Mantoux skin test reactions during the early phase of their illness (even when the skin testing is performed with 250 tuberculin units). A definitive diagnosis requires **histologic and bacteriologic confirmation**.

Sarcoidosis

This **chronic, multisystemic disease** of obscure origin is uncommon in patients <10 years of age and is more common in **African-American children**. The pathologic lesion is a noncaseating granuloma; the **lung** is the most frequently affected organ. **Hilar and paratracheal adenopathy** is often found in association with parenchymal infiltrates and may be far more dramatic than the parenchymal lesions. **Biopsy** of the affected tissue is the most valuable diagnostic tool.

Bronchogenic Cysts

These cysts, which are lined with ciliated epithelium, can be found in any portion of the mediastinum but most often are found **near the carina in the middle mediastinum**. Cysts can become **symptomatic** either **by becoming infected or**

by enlarging in size, thereby compromising the function of an adjacent airway. **Surgical excision is curative.**

Pericardial Cysts

Pericardial cysts are benign mediastinal lesions. They are usually unilocular cystic lesions with a thin connective tissue wall and clear fluid contents. Although they are considered developmental anomalies, they can be acquired. They are very rare in children.

Posterior Mediastinum

 HINT: Most posterior mediastinal masses in children are neurogenic in origin.

Tumors of Neurogenic Origin

Neuroblastoma, a malignant tumor, may arise **anywhere along the sympathetic nervous system chain.** Approximately 20% of neuroblastomas arise in the paraspinal ganglion of the thorax. **Thoracic neuroblastomas** are almost always attached to the **intervertebral foramina** and thus can cause **spinal cord compression.**

Differentiation of neuroblasts into benign ganglion cells occurs both **spontaneously and after therapy.** The term "ganglioneuroma" refers to such differentiated lesions. **Ganglioneuroblastoma** refers to **lesions containing malignant cells and benign ganglion cells.**

Thoracic Meningocele

Anterior spinal meningoceles are rare and associated with neurofibromatosis type 1 or Marfan syndrome.

Esophageal Duplication Cysts

Approximately 10% of alimentary tract duplications are esophageal, and two-thirds are **right sided.** The **duplication does not communicate with the esophagus** unless there is ulceration of the gastric mucosa within the cyst. Neurenteric cysts are esophageal duplication cysts that **contain glial elements;** vertebral anomalies usually accompany these cysts.

Ewing Sarcoma

This **small, round, blue-cell tumor** rarely occurs in children <5 years. Ewing sarcoma most frequently involves the **axial skeleton,** and some "mediastinal" masses actually originate from the chest wall (or a rib). True mediastinal involvement rarely occurs at diagnosis but is not infrequent in advanced cases.

Ewing sarcoma must be **differentiated from** other small, round, blue-cell tumors, including **neuroblastoma, lymphoma, and rhabdomyosarcoma.**

Rhabdomyosarcoma

This sarcoma, which arises from **primitive mesenchymal cells,** is the **most common soft tissue sarcoma in children.** However, in large series, only 1% of these tumors arise in the mediastinum, and these series do not stratify masses into the anterior, posterior, or middle mediastinum. Most patients with mediastinal rhabdo-myosarcomas are **boys (65%)** with a mean age of 10 years. Metastatic disease may be seen in the **lungs (including pleura), bone, and bone marrow** of these patients.

EVALUATION OF MEDIASTINAL MASS

 HINT: As many as a third of masses in the mediastinum are found incidentally when radiographs are performed to evaluate fever or other complaints.

History and Physical Examination

Table 52-1 lists the important features of the history and physical examination that should be specifically addressed to **rule out SVC or SM syndromes**. The **presence or absence of hepatosplenomegaly, adenopathy, systemic signs of a malignant tumor** (e.g., fever, weight loss, night sweats, fatigue), **or neurologic signs** (e.g., Horner syndrome, signs of cord compression) are equally important.

Laboratory Studies

Laboratory tests are tailored to the individual, but the following may be appropriate:

- **Complete blood count with differential.** The presence of lymphoblasts on smear, cytopenias from marrow infiltration or leukocytosis may allow the physician to consider diagnostic bone marrow aspirate without biopsying tissue from the mediastinal mass.
- **Chemistry panel, including uric acid.** A high uric acid level, lactate dehydrogenase level, or both are often seen in patients with high tumor burden and can be used as a screen for tumor lysis.
- α-**Fetoprotein** and β-human chorionic gonadotropin **levels** are helpful in suggesting the diagnosis of germ cell tumor, and useful in following the response to therapy.
- **Quantitative vanillylmandelic and homovanillic acid analysis.** Elevations of these substances in the urine are suggestive of neuroblastoma.
- Purified protein derivative skin test for TB.
- **Histoplasma complement fixation titers** should be obtained in endemic areas.

Other Diagnostic Modalities

- **CT and magnetic resonance imaging (MRI).** A CT scan can delineate the cystic nature of a lesion and reveals calcifications in 95% of patients with neuroblastoma and 35% of patients with germ cell tumors. Visualization of a tooth is pathognomonic of a teratoma. CT is more sensitive for bony erosion than MRI, but MRI is more helpful for detecting intraspinous extension and should be considered for patients with posterior mediastinal masses. Note: Only consider if the patient can tolerate recumbent positioning. If the patient has increased symptoms when lying flat, such as orthopnea, cough, chest pain, or anxiety, *do not perform* the scan.
- **Bone marrow aspirate.** Is indicated for patient with an abnormal CBC in whom the diagnosis of lymphoma or leukemia is suspected.

- **Pleurocentesis or pericardiocentesis.** It is usually possible to make a definitive diagnosis of some diseases (lymphoblastic lymphoma or leukemia) by assessing cells collected during these procedures.
- **Biopsy** may be necessary to make a definitive tissue diagnosis. Consultation with general anesthesia is critical. If it is not safe to perform diagnostic procedures with anesthesia, some patients may require biopsy, pleurocentesis, or bone marrow aspirate under local anesthesia.

> **HINT:** Before performing CT or MRI, a careful history should be taken for orthopnea because having a patient with SM syndrome lie supine can lead to decreased blood return to the heart or airway compromise.

> **HINT:** Before considering a biopsy to make a tissue diagnosis definitively, an echocardiogram (preferably upright and supine) should be obtained. If possible, the extent of tracheal compression by the tumor should be assessed as this is also correlated to risk while under anesthesia. Cardiopulmonary changes associated with general anesthesia can aggravate SVC syndrome and SM syndrome, leading to total airway obstruction, cardiac arrest, or both. These complications can develop in patients with mild or no preoperative symptoms.

TREATMENT OF MEDIASTINAL MASS

If a patient is critically ill and cannot tolerate a definitive diagnostic procedure, empiric chemotherapy, emergency radiation therapy (RT), or both are indicated. One must be aware, however, that **steroids or even low-dose radiotherapy** (200 cGy) **may render definitive diagnosis impossible**—even if a biopsy is done only 24 hours later. Biopsy of a node that is out of the field or intentionally shielded is, of course, still possible after the patient is stabilized.

Historically, RT was used as emergent therapy with or without concurrent systemic steroids given the tendency of some patients to transiently worsen afterward. This increase in symptoms was presumed to be secondary to edema from the RT. For a patient with suspected leukemia or lymphoma, it is now standard of care to use emergent steroid with or without additional chemotherapy. Examples include **cyclophosphamide in combination with vincristine or an anthracycline (depending upon the most likely diagnosis)**. This is a reasonable **alternative approach,** although this too may result in difficulty establishing the diagnosis. Even when the histologic diagnosis is lost, **continued treatment of the diagnosis that best fits the clinical picture** usually results in long-term disease-free survival.

Suggested Readings

Fisher MJ, Rheingold SR. Oncologic emergencies. In: Pizzo PA, Poplack DG, eds. *Principles and Practice of Pediatric Oncology.* 6th ed. Philadelphia, PA: Lippincott Williams & Wilkins; 2011:1124–1151.

Franco A, Mody NS, Meza MP. Imaging evaluation of pediatric mediastinal masses. *Radiol Clin North Am.* 2005;43:325–353.

Murmurs

INTRODUCTION

A murmur is an **auditory vibration produced by turbulent flow within the cardiac structures**. A murmur may be **physiologic** (i.e., a normal finding) or **pathologic**.

Heart Sounds

Variations in the normal heart sounds, as well as **adventitious** heart sounds, may be associated with murmurs and are essential clues to diagnostic interpretation of the murmur.

First Heart Sound (S_1)

The S_1 is produced by **closure of the mitral and tricuspid valves,** in that order. The mitral component and tricuspid component are **best heard at the apex and the lower sternal border region,** respectively.

- The intensity of the S_1 is accentuated in conditions characterized by increased cardiac output and a short PR interval because in these circumstances maximal excursion of the leaflets occurs during closure.
- Wide splitting of the S_1 with a delayed tricuspid component may be noted in patients with tricuspid stenosis, Ebstein anomaly, right bundle branch block, or when there is pacing of the left ventricle.

Second Heart Sound (S_2)

The S_2 is produced by **closure of the aortic valve (A_2) immediately followed by closure of the pulmonic valve (P_2)** and is best heard at the base of the heart. The P_2 is normally softer than the A_2 and is less widely transmitted. **Splitting of the S_2** is normally appreciated during quiet respiration. Inspiration results in two physiologic phenomena: an **increased capacitance of the lung vasculature,** with a greater period of systole for the right ventricle relative to the left ventricle, and **increased venous return to the right-sided structures**. Both of these phenomena result in **delayed closure of the pulmonic valve**.

- In mild forms of aortic or pulmonic stenosis, the A_2 or the P_2 may be soft.
- The S_2 is single and loud in the following circumstances: when there is fusion of the two components, such as in severe pulmonary hypertension; when there is only one semilunar valve, such as in atresia of either the aortic or the pulmonic

TABLE 53-1	Common Causes of Abnormally Wide Splitting of the Second Heart Sound (S_2)

Atrial septal defect
Mild pulmonic stenosis
Complete right bundle branch block
Left ventricular paced beats
Massive pulmonary embolus

valves or truncus arteriosus; and when the P_2 is inaudible because of an anteriorly positioned aorta, such as in tetralogy of Fallot or transposition of the great arteries.

- Abnormally wide splitting of the S_2 is noted in the conditions listed in Table 53-1.

Third Heart Sound (S_3) and Fourth Heart Sound (S_4)

Heart sounds are occasionally heard during ventricular diastole. **Early rapid filling of the ventricle,** which follows the opening of the atrioventricular valve, **may produce the third heart sound (S_3); ventricular filling related to the forceful expulsion of blood from the atrium into the ventricle** with atrial contraction **may produce the fourth heart sound (S_4). These sounds are best heard at the apex with the bell of the stethoscope. An audible S_3 may be normal in infants and young children,** whereas an **audible S_4 is distinctly abnormal**.

- Conditions that cause ventricular volume overload produce an abnormally prominent S_3 and are summarized in Table 53-2.
- Conditions that result in ventricular hypertrophy produce an S_4 and are summarized in Table 53-3.

Characteristics of a Murmur

- **Phase.** Murmurs are described as being **systolic** (occurring during systole following S_1, corresponding with ventricular contraction), **diastolic** (occurring during diastole following S_2, corresponding with ventricular relaxation), or **continuous** (occurring throughout the cardiac cycle).

TABLE 53-2	Conditions Causing a Prominent Third Heart Sound (S_3)

Physiologic (infants and children)
Congestive heart failure
Ventricular septal defect, with large pulmonary to systemic flow (Qp-to-Qs) ratio
Mitral insufficiency
Tricuspid insufficiency
Hyperdynamic ventricle with high output (e.g., anemia, thyrotoxicosis, arteriovenous fistula)

TABLE 53-3	Conditions Causing a Prominent Fourth Heart Sound (S₄)

Left ventricular outflow tract obstruction (e.g., aortic stenosis)
Right ventricular outflow tract obstruction (e.g., pulmonic stenosis)
Hypertrophic cardiomyopathy
Heart block (atrium contracting against a closed valve)

- **Length and timing.** Murmurs are described as having a short, medium, or long duration and occurring in the early, mid-, or late part of the cardiac cycle. The terms "holosystolic" and "pansystolic" refer to a murmur that begins with S_1 and ends with S_2.
- **Peak intensity (grade)** is summarized in Table 53-4.
- **Variation in intensity.** The term "crescendo" implies that the murmur starts low and builds to a peak; "decrescendo" implies that the murmur starts at its greatest intensity and subsequently diminishes. The term "crescendo–decrescendo" is used to describe a murmur that starts low, builds to a peak, and then diminishes over the course of the murmur (i.e., a "diamond-shaped" murmur).
- **Location and radiation.** The location of the murmur is described in relation to a chest wall landmark such as the sternum or intercostal spaces (e.g., the left upper sternal border of second intercostal space). The direction of projection (i.e., the radiation) is also noted (e.g., originating at the apex of the heart and radiating toward the left axilla).

Physical Maneuvers

The following maneuvers can alter the characteristics of a murmur:

- **Supine position.** Having the patient lie supine increases venous return to the heart and augments murmurs that are volume dependent (e.g., those associated with aortic stenosis or pulmonic stenosis; functional murmurs). Pericardial rubs are

TABLE 53-4	Grading of Murmurs

Grade	Description
I	Very soft, no thrill
II	Easily audible, of moderate intensity, no thrill
III	Prominent intensity but no thrill
IV	Loud murmur accompanied by a thrill
V	Very loud murmur accompanied by a thrill; heard with the stethoscope partially off the chest wall
VI	Very loud murmur accompanied by a thrill; heard with the stethoscope completely off the chest wall

diminished when the patient is supine because the visceral and parietal membranes move away from each other when the heart shifts posteriorly in the chest.

- **Valsalva maneuver.** Forced exhalation against a closed glottis or straining with the mouth and nose closed increases the intrathoracic pressure and reduces venous return to the heart. During the Valsalva maneuver, the two components of S_2 become single, and volume-dependent murmurs are attenuated.

 ## DIFFERENTIAL DIAGNOSIS LIST

Heart murmurs can be categorized into three groups: **functional or innocent** murmurs, which are **normal; physiologic** murmurs, which are caused by an **abnormality of flow not of primary cardiac origin; and pathologic** murmurs, which are caused by an **abnormality of primary cardiac origin**.

Functional or Innocent Murmurs
- Still murmur
- Cervical venous hum
- Peripheral pulmonic stenosis

Physiologic Murmurs
- High cardiac output states
- Arteriovenous fistula

Pathologic Murmurs
- Ventricular septal defect (VSD)—nonrestrictive and restrictive
- Atrial septal defect (ASD)
- Patent ductus arteriosus (PDA)
- Pulmonic stenosis
- Aortic stenosis
- Coarctation of the aorta

DIFFERENTIAL DIAGNOSIS DISCUSSION
Still Murmur (Innocent "Flow" Murmur)
Etiology
This sound, described in the early 20th century by Dr. George Frederick Still of Great Ormond Street Children's Hospital, London, is **one of the most common findings in the physical examination of a normal child**. It is heard in children **between 2 years of age and early adolescence** and may even persist into adulthood. Although its **cause is uncertain,** some evidence points to turbulent flow across the left ventricular outflow tract as the source.

Clinical Features and Evaluation
The Still murmur is a **systolic murmur, grade II to III** (never associated with a thrill), and **heard best at the left lower sternal border**. It is described as **vibratory, scratchy, or musical,** and it is **accentuated when the patient is supine** (i.e., with increased venous return to the heart). The **intensity and splitting of the S_2 are always normal**. Additional testing is usually not indicated if the murmur fits this description.

Cervical Venous Hum
Turbulent flow may occur **at the junction of the subclavian vein and head vessels as they join to form the superior vena cava,** resulting in a **continuous murmur**

called a venous hum. It is **low-pitched and heard best just beneath the right clavicle** while the child is **sitting up**. **Turning the patient's head to either the extreme right or the left,** placing the patient in **a supine position,** or **applying gentle pressure in the supraclavicular fossa** may dramatically **eliminate the murmur** and is **pathognomonic**. This murmur **may be confused with a PDA,** although the latter does not change with position and is best heard in the left clavicular region. Venous hums **usually disappear during adolescence** but may persist in thin adults.

Murmurs Associated with a High Cardiac Output State
Etiology
Murmurs secondary to a high cardiac output state (e.g., **fever, anemia, thyrotoxicosis**) are usually caused by a **relative stenosis of normal-size structures** in relation to increased blood flow.

Clinical Features
These murmurs are usually located at the **left mid- to upper sternal border,** are **grade II to III,** and of **medium pitch**. These are typically called ejection murmurs because the timing and intensity of the murmur follow the upstroke and downstroke of the systolic pressure curve. An S_3 **may be audible,** creating a gallop sound.

Evaluation
A **chest radiograph** may show **cardiac enlargement secondary to an increased end-diastolic volume,** but the electrocardiogram (ECG) **should be normal**. In patients with **chronic anemia** (e.g., those with sickle cell disease), high-output physiology may lead to **compensatory left ventricular hypertrophy,** which will be evident on ECG.

Treatment
Because the murmur is caused by an increased volume of flow, **treatment of the primary problem** (e.g., with **antipyretics or blood transfusion**) diminishes the intensity of the murmur.

Arteriovenous Fistula
Etiology
Congenital anomalous connections between arteries and veins may occur in the **lung, head, or liver**. Because of the constant pressure differential between the artery and vein, the **potential exists for a torrential amount of shunting** to occur, leading to **increased venous return to the right chambers** of the heart.

Clinical Features
A **continuous murmur** is heard over the site of the anomalous arteriovenous connection. In addition, increased flow across the pulmonic and aortic outflow tracts results in a **systolic murmur,** usually of **grade II to III,** along the **left mid- or upper sternal border**.

Evaluation
Auscultation over the liver and the head should be a routine part of the **evaluation of all newborn infants with a heart murmur**. **Chest radiographs** may reveal a **giant heart with increased pulmonary arterial markings**.

Peripheral Pulmonic Stenosis
Etiology
This murmur is **heard only in newborn infants,** primarily **premature** ones, and involves a **relative stenosis of the branch pulmonary arteries** in relation to the amount of pulmonary blood flowing across them.

Clinical Features
The murmur of peripheral pulmonic stenosis is a **low-pitched systolic** murmur with **occasional decrescendo run-off into diastole,** and it is heard **loudest in the back over both the right and the left lung** fields. At times, the murmur is heard **equally in both the right and the left axillae**. **No thrill** is present and the S_2 is normal.

Evaluation
Most infants **outgrow this murmur by 12 to 18 months of age,** but if it persists, an ECG may be indicated **to rule out a fixed anatomic stenosis of the branch pulmonary arteries**.

Nonrestrictive (Large) Ventricular Septal Defect
Etiology
In a **nonrestrictive VSD,** a **large communication between the lower pumping chambers** exists and allows blood to flow from the left to the right ventricle, resulting in **increased blood flow to the lungs and increased pulmonary venous return to the left atrium and the left ventricle**. Hence, in a large VSD, **the left ventricle pumps a significantly larger volume of blood than normal**.

> **HINT:** In a large nonrestrictive VSD, the right and left ventricular pressures are equal. As a result, a murmur related to a large VSD is not heard until there is a significant difference in the pulmonary and systemic vascular resistances. As pulmonary vascular resistance decreases, increasing amounts of blood shunts across the VSD from left to right. A murmur related to a large VSD may not become evident until pulmonary vascular resistance falls at 1 month of age.

Clinical Features
The murmur of a large VSD is **holosystolic,** reflecting the movement of blood between the right and left ventricles throughout systole. It is **heard best at the left lower sternal border,** frequently **radiating to the right lower sternal border**. A **thrill is not palpable** because the defect is large and nonrestrictive, producing little turbulence. **As the pulmonary vascular resistance continues to drop during the first 3 months of life, a greater amount of blood flow ("shunt") across the defect occurs,** so that **two to three times the amount of blood exiting the aorta** may end up **circulating through the lungs**.

A **low-pitched diastolic rumble murmur** may be **heard at the apex**. This rumble murmur is caused by a **relative mitral stenosis secondary to the increased blood volume returning to the left atrium** via the normal-size mitral valve.

Evaluation

In patients with a large VSD, the **ECG reveals left ventricular hypertrophy initially and biventricular hypertrophy over time**. A **chest radiograph** reveals a **large heart with increased pulmonary vascular markings**. If a large VSD is suspected, an **echocardiogram** to assess the location and anatomy of the defect is indicated. **Cardiac catheterization** may be necessary if complete anatomic detail is not satisfactorily delineated on the echocardiogram or if hemodynamic information is needed to aid in the decision making.

Treatment

A large VSD does not undergo spontaneous closure; therefore, **surgery is required**. A VSD with a **pulmonary to systemic flow (Qp-to-Qs) ratio 2:1** (as calculated by cardiac catheterization) is considered physiologically large and **requires closure**.

Restrictive (Small) Ventricular Septal Defect

By definition, small defects are **not hemodynamically significant** but **may produce a very prominent murmur**.

Clinical Features

Small defects in the muscular portion of the ventricular septum produce a **short, high-pitched, systolic** murmur **heard best along the left lower sternal border or apex** of the heart. The murmur may be **truncated**—not extending to the end of systole—and may even **abruptly stop at midsystole**. This occurs when the defect is closed off by its muscular borders at the peak of ventricular contraction. Because of the potential for tremendous turbulence across a restrictive narrow orifice in small muscular defects, a **thrill** may be appreciated, and the murmur **may be as loud as grade VI**. The natural tendency is for **muscular defects to become smaller with time,** and hence it is not uncommon for the **murmur to get louder with subsequent examinations**.

A small defect may also be noted in the **inlet portion of the ventricular septum adjacent to the septal leaflet of the tricuspid valve;** this is called a **perimembranous or conoventricular VSD**. A small conoventricular VSD produces a **high-pitched holosystolic** murmur, **heard best at the left lower sternal border and radiating to the right lower sternal border**. The septal leaflet of the tricuspid valve may fill in the defect, and **aneurysmal tissue may develop,** surrounding the VSD. This may produce an **early systolic click** that precedes the onset of the murmur. Additional **growth of aneurysmal tissue** adjacent to a perimembranous VSD **may result in its spontaneous closure**.

Evaluation

In a small VSD, the S_2 **is normal, as are the ECG and chest radiographs**. More than 50% of small VSDs undergo **spontaneous closure** by the time the patient reaches **2 years of age**.

Atrial Septal Defect

Etiology

ASD allows for **passive low-pressure flow of blood from the left atrium to the right atrium,** resulting in a volume load on the right ventricle and causing a **relative**

pulmonic stenosis (i.e., normal-size pulmonic structures but increased flow) and a **murmur similar to that heard in** patients with **pulmonic stenosis**. The murmur in an ASD is therefore not caused by flow at the defect site; rather, it is a **physiologic consequence of increased flow at the pulmonic valve level**.

Clinical Features

The murmur is **systolic, ejection type, usually grade II to III, and low to medium pitched**. It is **heard best at the left upper sternal border and second intercostal space,** with **occasional radiation to the lung fields in the back**.

A **widely split S₂ caused by the large right ventricular ejection volume is frequently found in patients with an ASD**. The S_2 **does not vary with respiration** because the usual effect of inspiration on right-sided volume is not as great in the presence of a large atrial communication.

In the presence of a **large shunt,** a **diastolic rumble murmur** may be heard at the **right lower sternal border** relating to **increased flow across the tricuspid valve** (normal flow returning via the superior and inferior vena cavae plus flow across the ASD).

Evaluation

Typically, the **ECG shows a mild right ventricular conduction delay** (i.e., a regular sinus rhythm prime [rSR'] pattern in the anterior precordial leads—V_{3R}, V_{4R}, and V_1). A **chest radiograph** reveals a **normal to slightly enlarged heart** with a **prominent pulmonary artery shadow along the left heart border. Pulmonary vascular markings are normal or slightly increased.** An **echocardiogram** is sufficient to confirm the diagnosis; cardiac catheterization is rarely indicated.

Patent Ductus Arteriosus
Etiology

Persistence in patency of the ductus arteriosus is a common cause of murmurs within the **first year of life**. In utero, the ductus arteriosus functions as the **conduit through which blood from the right ventricle is shunted away from the lungs to the descending aorta**. This structure is **highly sensitive to oxygen** and **usually undergoes spontaneous closure within 24 hours of birth**. In some infants, a stimulus (e.g., **prematurity, sepsis, volume overload**) may be identified as the **cause of the PDA**.

Clinical Features

Classically, the murmur heard in a PDA is a **continuous rumbling murmur,** at times even **harsh and machinelike**. It is **best heard in the left upper sternal border area and under the left clavicle**. The continuity of the murmur is caused by the **persistent pressure differential** that exists **between the aorta and pulmonary artery,** both in systole and in diastole, leading to **continuous left-to-right shunting** throughout the cardiac cycle. The **S₂ is normal** and may be **masked by the murmur**.

When **patients present** at the nadir of the pulmonary vascular resistance decrement (**at ~3 months,** earlier in premature infants), the **amount of shunting from** aorta to pulmonary artery may lead to **left ventricular volume overload and congestive heart failure**. In these patients, a **diastolic rumble** may be apparent at the **apex** as a result of increased flow across the mitral valve, and the **ECG** may show left **ventricular hypertrophy**. The diagnosis is confirmed on **echocardiogram**.

Treatment

Treatment consists of **close observation during the first 6 months** because **spontaneous closure** in this period is **still possible**. In patients who are <**6 months**, or in whom **congestive heart failure is present** and is **poorly controlled** with anticongestive medication (e.g., digoxin, diuretics), **surgical ligation** is recommended. In **premature infants, indomethacin treatment** is reported as extremely successful, although it is less effective after 2 weeks of age.

Pulmonic Stenosis

Etiology

Dysplasia of the pulmonary valve leaflets or a bicuspid pulmonary valve may cause pulmonic stenosis.

Clinical Features

When **stenosis is severe,** the infant may present with **cyanosis** from **impedance of flow** out of the right ventricle **and right-to-left shunting** at the level of the foramen ovale. **Emergent intervention** in this circumstance is necessary.

In patients with **mild to moderate** pulmonary stenosis, the typical presentation is a murmur noted on physical examination in a child without symptoms. The murmur is **systolic, low-pitched, crescendo–decrescendo and best heard at the second intercostal space at the left upper sternal border.** An **early, dull-sounding systolic ejection click** may be appreciated at the **left upper sternal border.** Frequently, the murmur **radiates along the course of the branch pulmonary arteries** and may be **heard over the lungs in the right and left back.** The S_2 **may split widely,** with normal respiratory variation, but the P_2 **component is soft.**

Evaluation

The **ECG and chest radiograph** may be **normal** in patients with **mild to moderate** pulmonic stenosis.

Treatment

In cases of **mild stenosis, treatment is not necessary;** however, in **moderate or severe stenosis, cardiac catheterization with balloon valvuloplasty** is required. Although pulmonic insufficiency is always created at the time of balloon valvuloplasty, the insufficiency is well tolerated as long as the tricuspid valve remains competent.

Aortic Stenosis

Etiology

Dysplasia, or more commonly, fusion, of the aortic leaflets may cause aortic stenosis. A **bicuspid aortic valve** is the **most common form of congenital heart "disease" in the older child** and adult and often results in **very mild or no obstruction**.

Clinical Features

> **HINT:** Severe aortic stenosis seen in infancy may not cause a murmur if obstruction to aortic outflow is of such a degree that a PDA is present to supply the systemic circulation.

In an **older child,** aortic stenosis **always produces a murmur**. The murmur is typically **systolic crescendo–decrescendo,** at times **harsh, and heard best at the right upper sternal border at the second intercostal space radiating along the course of the aortic arch up into the carotid vessels**.

A **thrill** may be palpable in the **suprasternal notch**. The **S$_2$ is softer than normal** and may be **single**. In patients with **mild to moderate cases** of aortic stenosis, a **high-pitched ejection click** may be heard in **early systole,** just preceding the onset of the murmur. Of note is that the click is best appreciated at the **apex of the heart,** not at the base, and its cause may relate more to inertial forces in the left ventricular outflow tract than to the opening of the aortic valve.

> **HINT:** Aortic stenosis may be a progressive disease. Increased harshness of the murmur as well as disappearance of the click may indicate an increased gradient across the aortic valve.

Evaluation

ECG findings of left ventricular hypertrophy and cardiac enlargement on the chest radiograph are present when the aortic stenosis is hemodynamically significant.

Coarctation of the Aorta

Etiology

Coarctation of the aorta is a **narrowing or shelf-like protuberance in the aortic arch distal to the left subclavian artery**. In **infancy,** coarctation is usually a **diffuse narrowing** of the area just **proximal to the insertion of the ductus arteriosus** (isthmus of the aortic arch). In **older children,** a **discrete shelf** is more commonly found and is thought to relate to remnants of ductal tissue within the aorta.

Clinical Features

A long systolic murmur **heard best along the left upper sternal border is most commonly noted in patients with coarctation of the aorta**. It is **loudest in the interscapular region in the back**. Bicuspid aortic valve is found in 80% of patients with coarctation of the aorta. As a result, an **early systolic ejection click may be heard at the base of the heart in patients with coarctation of the aorta** because of the presence of a bicuspid aortic valve.

In **older patients** with long-standing coarctation, **continuous murmurs** may be appreciated along the **lateral chest wall**. These are caused by intercostal collateral flow to the portion of the aorta distal to the narrowing.

Evaluation

On physical examination, a blood pressure gradient is noted between the right upper and lower extremities. Diminished femoral pulses may also be present. An **ECG** may show **left ventricular hypertrophy**. A **chest radiograph** is either **normal or reveals mild cardiomegaly**. Occasionally, **poststenotic dilation of the descending aorta distal to the coarctation** can be seen.

Suggested Readings

Allen HD, Phillips JR, Chan DP. History and physical examination. In: HD Allen, HP Gutgesell, EB Clark, et al., eds. *Moss and Adams' Heart Disease in Infants, Children, and Adolescents*. 6th ed. Philadelphia: Lippincott Williams & Wilkins; 2001:143–152.

Menashe V. Heart murmurs. *Pediatr Rev.* 2007;28(4):e19–e22.

Park MK. Routine cardiac evaluation in children. In: *The Pediatric Cardiology Handbook*. 3rd ed. Philadelphia, PA: Mosby; 2003:1–51.

Sivarajan VB, Vetter VL, Gleason MM. Pediatric evaluation of the cardiac patient. In: VL Vetter, ed. *Pediatric Cardiology: The Requisites in Pediatrics*. Philadelphia, PA: Mosby Elsevier; 2006:1–30.

Neck Mass

INTRODUCTION

Neck masses are a common clinical problem in children. Although the list of potential causes is extensive, most are due to **benign processes** that can be readily diagnosed after a complete history and physical examination. **Close follow-up** is important to ensure that less common causes in children such as malignancy are not overlooked.

 DIFFERENTIAL DIAGNOSIS LIST

Infectious Causes
Cervical Adenitis
- Bacterial infection—*Streptococcus pyogenes, Staphylococcus aureus,* Group B *Streptococcus,* oral anaerobes, and *Pasteurella multocida*
- Cat scratch disease (*Bartonella henselae*)
- Tularemia
- *Nocardia*
- *Mycobacterium tuberculosis*
- Atypical *mycobacterium*
Reactive Adenopathy
- Viral infection—upper respiratory viruses, mumps, measles, herpes virus, Epstein–Barr virus, cytomegalovirus, HIV
- Bacterial infection—syphilis, brucellosis
- Fungal infection—histoplasmosis, coccidioidomycosis
- Parasitic infection—toxoplasmosis, filariasis
- Other infections—head and neck infections (tonsillitis, otitis media, tinea capitis)
Lemierre's Syndrome

Congenital or Vascular Causes
- Thyroglossal duct cyst (TGDC)
- Branchial cleft cyst
- Cystic hygroma
- Laryngocele
- Dermoid
- Cervical thymic cyst
- Arteriovenous fistula

Neoplastic Causes
- Malignant neoplasms—leukemia, Hodgkin lymphoma, non-Hodgkin lymphoma, rhabdomyosarcoma, fibrosarcoma, thyroid/parathyroid carcinoma, neuroblastoma, metastatic deposits
- Benign neoplasms—lipoma, fibroma, neurofibroma, teratoma, osteochondroma, hemangioma

Metabolic or Genetic Causes
- Goiter
- Thyroid nodule

Traumatic Causes
- Hematoma
- Congenital muscular torticollis
- Subcutaneous emphysema
- Cervical spine fracture

Inflammatory Causes (Cervical Adenopathy)

- Kawasaki syndrome
- Systemic lupus erythematosus
- Sinus histiocytosis
- Sarcoidosis
- Periodic fever, aphthous stomatitis, pharyngitis, and adenitis (PFAPA) syndrome

Toxic Causes

- Drug-related adenopathy (e.g., phenytoin)

DIFFERENTIAL DIAGNOSIS DISCUSSION
Reactive Adenopathy

Familiarity with regional anatomy helps to narrow the differential diagnosis in a child who presents with a neck mass. Because **most neck masses in infants and children are enlarged lymph nodes,** it is important to be familiar with areas of lymphatic drainage. In addition, certain masses present in typical locations that help to identify the cause. The neck is divided into the anterior and posterior triangles, with the sternocleidomastoid muscle (SCM) forming the posterior border of the anterior triangle (Figure 54-1).

It is **important to distinguish adenopathy from adenitis. Adenopathy is defined by nodal enlargement. In adenitis, the swelling is usually accompanied by signs of inflammation** such as warmth, tenderness, and erythema. The vast **majority of children with adenopathy** have a **benign viral or easily treatable bacterial cause**. However, **follow-up is important** to assess resolution of symptoms and progressive reduction in size so as not to miss unusual infectious, inflammatory, or oncological processes. Moreover, any node >2 cm in diameter warrants further attention, as it falls outside the range of benign hyperplasia. A more detailed review of this topic is covered in Chapter 50, "Lymphadenopathy."

> **HINT:** Epitrochlear, popliteal, supraclavicular, or occipital nodes in children <2 years are rarely due to benign lymph node hyperplasia. These nodes, as well as any palpable nodes in the newborn infant, deserve further investigation.

Lemierre's Syndrome

Lemierre's syndrome (also known as necrobacillosis or postanginal sepsis) is a rare disease characterized by sepsis secondary to an anaerobic infection of the tonsillar or peritonsillar region and **superficial thrombophlebitis of the internal jugular vein**. It typically presents with prolonged pharyngitis or tonsillitis followed by lateral neck pain, swelling, and subsequent pulmonary symptoms. The most common bacteria isolated is *Fusobacterium necrophorum*. The key to diagnosis is having appropriate index of suspicion and confirmation by ultrasound, computed tomography (CT), or MRI demonstrating phlebitis of the internal jugular vein. Management consists of appropriate antibiotics and possible anticoagulation.

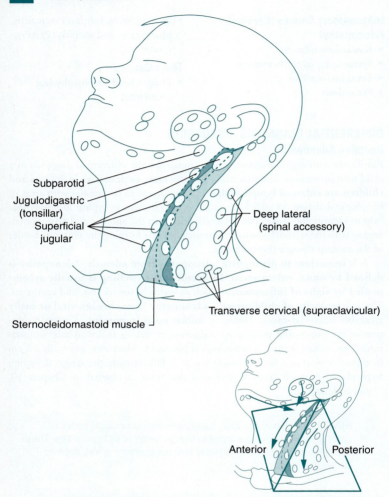

Subparotid

Jugulodigastric
(tonsillar)

Superficial
jugular

Deep lateral
(spinal accessory)

Transverse cervical (supraclavicular)

Sternocleidomastoid muscle

Anterior

Posterior

FIGURE 54-1 Division of the neck into anterior and posterior triangles.

Congenital Malformations
Thyroglossal Duct Cyst
Etiology

TGDC results from the cellular proliferation of **embryonic remnants of the thyroglossal duct**.

Clinical Features and Evaluation

TGDC is the **most common congenital neck mass** and usually presents in the **first decade of life**. TGDC may become apparent during an upper respiratory infection that causes cyst inflammation. Physical examination is best done with the **neck fully extended** and will reveal a **midline or paramedian swelling of the anterior neck**. The location can be anywhere along the embryonic pathway from the base of the tongue to the thyroid cartilage. The **mass is round and changes position when the child swallows or sticks out his tongue**. Children with TGDC should be **referred to an otorhinolaryngologist** for further evaluation. When suspected, it is important to differentiate TGDC from ectopic thyroid. The surgeon may consider further testing to confirm normal thyroid function and location.

Treatment
Almost all TGDC require **surgical excision** for definitive diagnosis and to prevent recurrent infections of the cyst.

Branchial Cleft Cyst/Fistula/Sinus
Etiology
The embryological branchial clefts give rise to the structures of the face and neck. Cysts result from the **proliferation of the remnants of these clefts, usually involving the second cleft**.

Clinical Evaluation
Branchial cleft remnants are the **second most common congenital neck mass**. A fistula or sinus will be obvious in the newborn; however, a cyst often does not become clinically apparent until early school age. Second branchial cleft cysts are found **anterior to the lower third of the SCM as a small, round, nontender, soft mass**. An upper respiratory infection or infection of the cyst itself may lead to an **inflammatory appearance**. Diagnosis should be suspected if a **mass lateral to the SCM persists or recurs despite antibiotic treatment** for an adenitis and can be further delineated by CT or MRI.

Treatment
If there is evidence of cyst infection, an **antibiotic** that covers skin flora should be initiated. Definitive treatment requires **surgical excision,** which can be done electively.

Cystic Hygroma
Etiology
Cystic hygromas arise from the **nonmalignant proliferation of lymphatic tissue that does not connect with normal lymphatic drainage**. These sacs become **filled with lymphatic fluid** secreted by the endothelial lining. They can compress or stretch surrounding tissues.

Clinical Evaluation
Cystic hygromas are the **third most common congenital neck mass**. The vast majority of hygromas are found in the **posterior cervical triangle** and most are diagnosed within the first year of life. The mass is **soft, easily compressible, and, if not secondarily infected, will transilluminate**. Upper respiratory infections or trauma may cause a rapid increase in size. **Encroachment on the airway may**

lead to respiratory symptoms such as stridor. Diagnosis is usually clinical, but **ultrasound or CT imaging** may be necessary to delineate the extent of the lesion.

Treatment

Spontaneous regression is rare. Currently, **staged surgical excision** is the mainstay of therapy. **Sclerosing agents** and other therapies may have an adjunctive role. Timing of surgery will depend on the location of the lesion, age of the child, and involvement of vital structures. **Tracheostomy and gastric tube feedings** are sometimes required.

Dermoid

Dermoids consist of ectoderm and mesoderm and are considered **true developmental neoplasms**. This rare midline mass is often **doughy, nontender, mobile,** and is found **above the level of the hyoid bone**. It may initially be confused with a TGDC; however, it **will not change position with tongue protrusion**. Signs of **inflammation** may occur with cyst infection. **Ultrasound and CT imaging** will help delineate the nature and extent of the lesion. **Surgical excision** is required.

Laryngocele

Laryngocele is an **extremely rare** congenital anomaly. It is an **air-filled mass that arises from the larynx**. External extension through the thyrohyoid membrane will result in a **compressible mass,** lateral to midline, which will **increase in size with a Valsalva maneuver**. Hoarseness, cough, dyspnea, or dysphagia may be suggestive of a laryngocele. Lateral radiographs may demonstrate the air-filled sac. **Surgical excision** is required.

Oncological Masses

See Chapter 50, "Lymphadenopathy," Chapter 52, "Mediastinal Mass," and Chapter 36, "Goiter" for more details on this topic.

 HINT: Fortunately, neck masses in children are rarely due to an oncological process. A mass that is rapidly growing, found in a neonate, adherent to underlying tissues, ulcerated, >3 cm in size, or located in the posterior triangle is more of a concern for malignancy.

Lymphoma

Hodgkin's lymphoma is the **most frequent malignant neck mass** in children. Hodgkin's lymphoma often presents with a **unilateral slowly enlarging mass of the neck,** whereas **non-Hodgkin's lymphoma is more often bilateral**. Systemic symptoms of **fatigue, fever, weight loss, night sweats ("B symptoms"), and respiratory distress** may be present. Findings related to **bone marrow dysfunction, mediastinal involvement, and spinal cord impingement** may also be found. **Node biopsy** is necessary for diagnosis. **Immediate referral to a pediatric oncologist** is indicated to plan the diagnostic and therapeutic evaluation.

Neuroblastoma

Neuroblastoma of the cervical region may present in a child **5 years old or younger with a neck mass and Horner syndrome** (miosis, ptosis, and anhidrosis). Neuroblastoma may also **metastasize** from other regions to the neck, but neurologic symptoms will be absent until the mass causes nerve compression.

Thyroid Masses

See Chapter 36, "Goiter."

Traumatic Causes

Congenital Muscular Torticollis (Fibromatosis of Infancy)

Etiology

Although the exact etiologic mechanism of this condition is unclear, **birth trauma causing injury and bleeding into the SCM** with subsequent fibrosis and contracture has been implicated. An **intrauterine position that obstructs SCM venous outflow** may also cause muscle injury and contracture.

Clinical Evaluation

Parents usually notice a neck mass or torticollis in the baby's **first month of life**. Physical examination reveals a **nontender, firm, mobile mass within the SCM**. The **head will be in lateral flexion** and the **chin will be pointed away from the mass**. Diagnosis can usually be made clinically. **Cervical spine radiographs** and **ultrasound** may assist in ruling out other less common causes.

Treatment

The vast majority of children improve with **passive stretching exercises. Delayed diagnosis and treatment may lead to irreversible asymmetric development of facial features**. If the torticollis persists past 6–12 months, a **surgical release of the muscle** may be necessary.

Inflammatory Causes

These disease processes may have **associated cervical adenopathy**. It is rare that cervical adenopathy is the first or only presenting finding.

Kawasaki Disease (Mucocutaneous Lymph Node Syndrome)

In Kawasaki disease, the lymph node must be 1.5 cm or larger. When present, it is usually found in the cervical chain. However, it is the least common finding of the five criteria. (discussed in more detail in Chapter 64, "Rashes".)

Sinus Histiocytosis (Rosai–Dorfman Syndrome)

This is an **extremely rare disorder** of unknown etiology. The typical patient is a young **African-American child** who presents with **prolonged fever** and **massive, nontender, bilateral cervical adenopathy**. Diagnosis depends on characteristic findings on **lymph node biopsy**. Treatment may include **chemotherapeutic agents,** and these patients should be **referred to an oncologist**.

APPROACH TO THE PATIENT

Most neck masses in children are benign. A thorough history and physical examination coupled with a follow-up visit will be sufficient to diagnose most masses. **Systemic symptoms, persistence or recurrence of a mass, or a history of exposure to an infectious agent** such as tuberculosis should prompt **further evaluation**. Further evaluation may include a **CBC, purified protein derivative tuberculin test, other pathogen-specific assays, or imaging with ultrasound or CT**. **Biopsy** should be considered in a patient whose mass has increased in size at 2 weeks, unchanged in size in 4–6 weeks, or not returned to normal at 8–12 weeks. **Inpatient evaluation and treatment** will often be necessary for neonates or for patients who are ill appearing, have signs of impending airway compromise, are immunocompromised, or have failed outpatient oral antibiotic treatment.

SUGGESTED READINGS

Do TT. Congenital muscular torticollis: current concepts and review of treatment. *Curr Opin Pediatr.* 2006;18(1):26–29.

Gosche JR, Vick L. Acute, subacute, and chronic cervical lymphadenitis in children. *Semin Pediatr Surg.* 2006;15(2):99–106.

Karkos PD, Asrani S, Karkos D, et al. Lemierre's syndrome: a systematic review. *Laryngoscope.* 2009; 119(8):1552–1559.

Niedzielska G, Kotowski M, Niedzielski A, et al. Cervical lymphadenopathy in children-incidence and diagnostic management. *Int J Pediatr Otorhinolaryngol.* 2007;71(1):51–56.

Rosa PA, Hirsch DL, Dierks EJ. Congenital neck masses. *Oral Maxillofac Surg Clin N Am.* 2008; 20(3):339–352.

Rozovsky K, Hiller N, Koplewitz BZ, et al. Does CT have an additional diagnostic value over ultrasound in the evaluation of acute inflammatory neck masses in children? *Eur Radiol.* 2010;20(2):484–490.

Tracy TF, Muratore CS. Management of common head and neck masses. *Semin Pediatr Surg.* 2007; 16(1):3–13.

Turkington JRA, Paterson A, Sweeney LE, et al. Neck masses in children. *Br J Radiol.* 2005;78(10):75–85.

Neck Pain/Stiffness

INTRODUCTION

In children, the chief complaint of neck pain often may represent neck stiffness or torticollis. **Torticollis** describes a **characteristic malpositioning of the head and chin** in which the head is tilted to one direction and the chin points oppositely. It is a sign of an underlying disease process and does not imply a specific diagnosis. The head and neck regions are highly complex anatomically, and many structures within these areas can give rise to symptoms. **Pain or stiffness can arise from structures within the neck** such as the cervical musculature, the vertebral bones, or lymph nodes. Alternatively, **pain from the scalp, ear, oropharynx, or mandible** can refer and be perceived in the neck region. **Pressure** originating from the head either external to the dura or from within the brain or spinal cord can cause neck pain or stiffness. Finally, processes involving the upper thorax can also cause pain that might radiate to the neck region.

DIFFERENTIAL DIAGNOSIS LIST

Trauma
- Fracture of cervical spine
- Subluxation of cervical spine
- Spinal cord injury without radiographic abnormality (SCIWORA) syndrome
- Atlantoaxial rotary subluxation
- Muscular contusions/spasm
- Subarachnoid hemorrhage
- Epidural hematoma of cervical spine
- Clavicular fracture

Infectious
- Meningitis
- Retropharyngeal abscess
- Peritonsillar abscess
- Epiglottitis
- Osteomyelitis
- Diskitis
- Epidural abscess
- Cervical adenitis
- Pharyngitis
- Upper respiratory tract infection
- Upper lobe pneumonia
- Viral myositis
- Otitis media/mastoiditis

Inflammatory
- Atlantoaxial rotary subluxation
- Grisel syndrome
- Collagen vascular diseases
- Juvenile intervertebral disk calcification (JIDC)

Congenital
- Congenital muscular torticollis (CMT)
- Skeletal malformations
- Klippel–Feil syndrome
- Atlantoaxial instability

Toxic Metabolic
- Dystonic reaction
- Tetanus

Neurologic
- Space-occupying lesions
- Brain tumor

- Spinal cord tumor
- Arnold–Chiari malformation
- Syringomyelia
- Arteriovenous malformation
- Strabismus
- Cranial nerve palsies
- Myasthenia gravis
- Migraine headaches

Miscellaneous
- Benign paroxysmal torticollis
- Gastroesophageal reflux (Sandifer syndrome)
- Psychogenic

DIFFERENTIAL DIAGNOSIS DISCUSSION
Major Trauma
Etiology
Cervical spine fracture, subluxation of the vertebral bodies, or **SCIWORA** syndrome may result from high-risk mechanisms of injury (e.g., motor vehicle collision, pedestrian struck by motor vehicle, falls from heights, or high-impact sports activities). The larger head size, weaker neck muscles, and increased ligamentous laxity render children more likely to sustain injury in the **upper cervical area** as compared with adults, who are more likely to sustain lower cervical injuries.

Clinical Features
Cervical spine injury should be **suspected in the patient with a high-risk mechanism of injury or suggestive signs or symptoms:** pain on neck palpation, neck muscle spasm, limited range of motion, torticollis, transient or persistent sensory changes, hyporeflexia, muscle weakness or flaccidity, priapism, bladder or bowel dysfunction, or hypotension with bradycardia (spinal shock). In addition, in the **nonverbal or uncooperative child** or the child who has an **altered mental status** or an **associated severe head injury,** the physical examination may be difficult or unreliable. In these children, the possibility of cervical spine injury should be considered at the outset of the evaluation and **spinal immobilization and precautions maintained until proved otherwise**.

Evaluation
Suspected cervical spine injury generally requires emergent evaluation. The child should be immobilized with a rigid cervical collar. The evaluation should begin by assessing the patient's respiratory and hemodynamic status. Then, a complete sensory and motor neurologic exam should be performed. In some alert, verbal, and cooperative children, an attempt to "clinically clear" the cervical spine may be made through a careful physical examination. **A careful examination of the cervical spine with the collar removed,** but with manual immobilization maintained, should yield no tenderness or deformity. At this point, the patient may be

allowed to attempt **active** (not passive) **neck flexion, extension, and lateral rotation**. Any limitation or complaint of pain with range of motion should prompt the immediate reinstitution of cervical spine immobilization followed by cervical radiography. The **radiographic evaluation** should include a minimum of three views: the lateral, anteroposterior, and open-mouth (odontoid) radiographs. Flexion and extension views are used to assess for ligamentous injury in a child with persistent neck pain after a normal three-view series. **Computed tomography (CT) scan** provides excellent bone detail, whereas magnetic resonance imaging (**MRI**) **scan** is used to evaluate the soft tissues and spinal cord.

Treatment
In addition to **supportive care,** a treatment adjunct for spinal cord injury with associated neurologic abnormality is the administration of **methylprednisolone,** 30 mg/kg over 15 minutes, followed by 5.4 mg/kg/hour for 23 hours. Based on studies in adults, this treatment is most effective if given within 8 hours of the injury.

Atlantoaxial Rotary Subluxation
Etiology
The odontoid process of the second cervical vertebrae is normally positioned squarely within the ring of C1, and the two vertebrae are secured by the transverse and alar ligaments. The increased laxity and longer lengths of the ligaments renders **children more susceptible** to traumatic cervical spine injury than their adult counterparts.

As the name implies, in patients with rotary subluxation, **C1 and C2** are **rotationally malpositioned**. This commonly results from a **minor traumatic mechanism,** as might occur during light wrestling or gymnastics. Some conditions such as **tonsillectomy** (Grisel syndrome), **upper respiratory infections, or juvenile rheumatoid arthritis** may cause inflammation and laxity of the transverse ligament, resulting in C1—C2 instability with rotary subluxation. In addition, certain conditions such as **Down syndrome or congenital odontoid dysplasias** may predispose to rotary subluxation.

Clinical Features
Patients commonly present with **neck pain or stiffness**. Physical examination reveals **torticollis, tender paracervical muscles, and decreased range of motion** of the neck. The torticollis results as the ipsilateral sternocleidomastoid muscle attempts to reestablish normal positioning. Rotary subluxation is a **stable cervical spine injury,** rarely causing spinal cord impingement, and neurologic signs are infrequently encountered.

The lateral radiograph may be normal or show distorted anatomy. Particular attention should be paid to check the **predental space** that may be widened. The diagnostic modality of choice, however, is the **static and dynamic neck CT scan**. A static CT scan usually shows the asymmetric location of the dens within the anterior arch of C1. In the dynamic CT, the rotation of C2 on C1 is fixed, persisting despite lateral rotation of the head to both directions.

Treatment

Most patients have resolution of symptoms with **supportive care with a soft collar** and the administration of nonsteroidal **anti-inflammatory drugs**. Orthopedic referral is suggested for the patients with persistent symptoms who may require reduction and stabilization with traction.

Meningitis

Meningitis is discussed in Chapter 21, "Coma."

Retropharyngeal Abscess, Peritonsillar Abscess, Epiglottitis, Cervical Adenitis, and Pharyngitis

Retropharyngeal abscess, peritonsillar abscess, epiglottitis, cervical adenitis, and pharyngitis are discussed in Chapter 72, "Sore Throat."

Diskitis
Etiology

Infectious diskitis is a **rare illness** with an unclear etiology. In ~50% of patients with diskitis, an aspirated culture of the affected area yields a bacterial pathogen (*Staphylococcus aureus* in most, also coagulase-negative *Staphylococcus, Kingella,* and *Salmonella*), which has led some to believe that the process is **infectious** in etiology. Yet the outcome in patients is the same with or without antimicrobial treatment. Others suggest a **traumatic or inflammatory** etiology, theorizing that a preceding traumatic event induces the release of tissue enzymes from the disk, resulting in inflammation. Diskitis more commonly affects the **lumbar area** but can occur in the cervical region.

Clinical Features

The clinical presentation is **gradual in onset** with few constitutional symptoms. The patient may present with mild irritability or more obvious pain. The physical examination is often near normal except that the child may refuse to move his neck.

The peripheral white blood count and differential are usually normal. Nonspecific indicators of inflammation (erythrocyte sedimentation rate [ESR], C-reactive protein) are almost always elevated. Blood cultures are rarely positive. Radiographs are usually normal early in the course of the illness but may demonstrate erosion of the adjacent vertebral plates by 4 to 8 weeks after the onset. Repair and residual sclerosis is the typical progression. Bone scan may detect disease earlier, showing increased uptake in the disk and vertebral bodies.

Treatment

The management of diskitis is **controversial**. Supportive treatment with immobilization and analgesia generally renders patients free of discomfort in about 48 hours. The role of parenteral antibiotics remains unclear.

Epidural Abscess

Epidural abscess is discussed in Chapter 58, "Paraplegia."

Congenital Muscular Torticollis

Etiology

CMT is a relatively common entity, occurring with a prevalence of 3 to 19 per 1,000 newborns. The **etiology is unknown,** although several theories exist. The **intrauterine theory** suggests that abnormal fetal positioning results in a shortened sternocleidomastoid muscle. Another theory contends that **birth trauma** during difficult deliveries leads to bleeding into the sternocleidomastoid muscle with subsequent compartment syndrome, fibrosis, and contracture. There is no genetic predisposition.

Clinical Features

CMT is **often undetected** in the **immediate newborn period**. The head tilt becomes more obvious, however, as the infant develops head control. The **head tilts** toward the shorted muscle and the chin points away. A **mass** can be palpated in the inferior portion of the sternocleidomastoid muscle in about a third of cases. Rarely, other musculoskeletal anomalies are associated, including hip dysplasia, metatarsus adductus, and talipes equinovarus.

Evaluation

A thorough **physical examination** to eliminate other causes of torticollis should be performed. **Radiographic evaluation** of the cervical spine can identify rare congenital vertebral anomalies such as Klippel–Feil syndrome (congenital fusion of any number of cervical vertebrae).

Treatment

Treatment is usually **nonsurgical** with **strengthening and stretching exercises**. Early **physical therapy** referral correlates with improved outcome. **Recurrence** of torticollis may occur in 11% of patients and can happen years later.

Paroxysmal Torticollis

Etiology

The etiology is unclear but felt to be either a **migraine** variant or related to **vestibular dysfunction**.

Clinical Features

The syndrome, generally presenting in the **first few months of life,** is characterized by **recurrent episodes of head tilt,** often alternating in sides. Torticollis is rarely the only finding. Other **associated symptoms** may include **vomiting, pallor, irritability, and ataxia**. Although frightening for the parents to witness, paroxysmal torticollis is a **benign, self-limited process**. The frequency of attacks progressively decreases and ultimately it resolves in 1 to 5 years.

Evaluation and Treatment

Evaluation of the initial episode consists of a careful history and physical examination to **rule out other causes of vomiting and ataxia** such as central nervous system (CNS) processes or intoxication. Subsequent attacks are managed by **supportive therapy** including intravenous fluid hydration if necessary. Pharmacologic treatment has not been well studied.

Dystonic Reactions

Etiology

Antiemetics, neuroleptics, and other medications with dopamine receptor antagonism can cause dystonia when taken either in overdose or in therapeutic doses.

Clinical Features

Patients with dystonic reactions experience a **severe, uncomfortable contraction of the sternocleidomastoid muscle**. Often the **facial muscles,** and sometimes the muscles of the **extremities and trunk,** are also involved.

Evaluation and Treatment

The administration of **diphenhydramine** (1.25 mg/kg) can be both diagnostic and therapeutic. The response is **rapid and dramatic**. The offending agent should be discontinued and diphenhydramine continued every 6 to 8 hours for several days to avoid recurrence.

Neurologic Causes

CNS processes can induce torticollis via a variety of mechanisms. **Space-occupying lesions** exerting pressure on the dura can cause irritation that can cause neck stiffness. Alternatively, **tonsillar herniation** may cause stretching or irritation of the accessory nerve, which then induces sternocleidomastoid spasm. In addition, a child with diplopia secondary to **cranial nerve dysfunction or strabismus** may attempt compensation through tilting his head to realign the visual axis. This head tilt may be perceived by the examiner as torticollis. The evaluation of the child with neck stiffness or torticollis must include a **careful neurologic examination** to assess for the presence of a neurologic cause.

Atlantoaxial Rotary Subluxation

Inflammatory conditions involving the transverse ligament of C1 and C2 can result in torticollis as described earlier.

Juvenile Rheumatoid Arthritis

The **cervical spine** is involved in 50% of patients with juvenile rheumatoid arthritis. It is rarely an early complication of the disease and is usually found in patients with >6 months of illness.

Juvenile Intervertebral Disk Calcification

Etiology

The uncommon disease entity of JIDC has an **unknown etiology** but has been postulated to arise from developmental changes in the water content, blood supply, and cellular matrix of the nucleus of the disk. There are several distinguishing features of JIDC, and therefore it is believed to be a **different** entity **than adult intervertebral disk calcification. The location of involvement in children is distinct from that in adults.** In JIDC, the cervical region is most commonly involved and the calcification occurs within the nucleus. In adults, the annulus of the disks in the thoracic or lumbar regions is affected. Childhood disease may be either asymptomatic or transiently symptomatic. Adults generally have asymptomatic, permanent calcification.

Clinical Features

Patients with JIDC may be divided into **symptomatic and asymptomatic** groups, depending on clinical features. It is unknown what triggers the development of symptoms. Many asymptomatic patients never develop symptoms, but resolution does not occur without a symptomatic period. In most symptomatic patients, symptoms develop over 24 to 48 hours and most commonly consist of **neck pain, torticollis, and fever**. Neurologic symptoms and signs are rare.

Evaluation and Treatment

In the symptomatic patient, **nonspecific laboratory evidence of inflammation** is apparent in one-third to one-half of patients (leukocytosis, elevated ESR). Blood cultures are negative. Radiographs of the spine demonstrate **intervertebral disk calcification** of the nucleus pulposus. During the acute episode, the involved **interspace may widen** and then normalize as the symptoms resolve. **Extruded calcified disk material** may be seen posteriorly within the spinal canal or within the prevertebral soft tissues. There is no destruction of the adjacent vertebral bodies and the retropharyngeal space is not enlarged. MRI can be used to evaluate for canal compromise that is secondary to disk herniation.

Given that the disease is usually benign and self-limited, treatment is generally **supportive** with bed rest, analgesics, heat, and muscle relaxants. Operative removal of the disk is usually not indicated. Symptoms resolve in 3 weeks (67%) to 6 months (95%). **Complete radiographic resolution** is the rule.

EVALUATION OF NECK PAIN

A child who presents with neck pain may have a **potentially life-threatening illness**. The immediate priority is to ensure the adequacy of the **airway, breathing, and circulation**. The possibility of **cervical spine injury** is **considered early,** and spinal immobilization and precautions are instituted if warranted. Most diagnoses are made based on the history and physical examination findings alone. Further evaluation with laboratory and radiographic tests are based on these findings.

History

In the history, it is important to characterize the nature of the chief complaint, **distinguishing neck pain from stiffness or torticollis**. Is the pain acute or chronic in nature? Is it constant or intermittent? Has there been any response to any home therapies? It is particularly important to elucidate any evidence of acute or chronic **CNS pathology** such as weakness, paresthesias, loss of bowel or bladder continence, or loss of developmental milestones. There should be a careful probing for any **symptoms of increased intracranial pressure** such as headaches, vomiting, or changes in school performance. Preceding **major trauma** is usually evident, but the possibility of **minor trauma** should be explored. Has the patient had fever, sore throat, cough, upper respiratory symptoms, or ear or mouth pain? Is the patient, or are any household contacts, taking any medications, either prescription or over the counter?

Physical Examination

A **general review of all systems** should occur. The diagnosis of meningitis usually can be excluded by physical examination. When in doubt, a **lumbar puncture** should be performed. The examination of the neck begins with **observation of positioning**. If **palpation** of the cervical spinous processes yields **localized tenderness or deformity,** a **cervical collar** should be placed and no further manipulation done until a **radiographic evaluation** shows the absence of fracture, subluxation, or ligamentous injury. Barring this, the rest of the neck should be carefully palpated for masses and muscle spasm. At this point, the child should be allowed to attempt **active (not passive) neck flexion, extension, and lateral rotation**.

Diagnostic Evaluation

The diagnostic evaluation is selective and based on history and physical examination clues to the diagnosis. **Laboratory studies** such as a complete blood count, ESR, C-reactive protein, and blood culture may provide nonspecific evidence for an infectious or inflammatory etiology. **Radiographic studies** such as plain films, CT, MRI, and nuclear medicine scans can be useful in selected circumstances.

TREATMENT OF NECK PAIN

Until the cause of the neck pain is established, treatment is **supportive** and may entail the following:

- Administration of analgesics, usually in the form of nonsteroidal anti-inflammatory drugs
- Application of warm compresses
- Administration of antipyretic agents

SUGGESTED READINGS

Ballock RT, Song KM. The prevalence of nonmuscular causes of torticollis in children. *J Pediatr Orthop.* 1996;16(4):500–504.

Bredenkamp JK, Maceri DR. Inflammatory torticollis in children. *Arch Otolaryngol Head Neck Surg.* 1990;116:310–313.

Dias MS, Pang D. Juvenile intervertebral disc calcification: recognition, management, and pathogenesis. *Neurosurgery.* 1991;28(1):130–135.

Do TT. Congenital muscular torticollis: current concepts and review of treatment. *Curr Opin Pediatr.* 2006;18(1):26–29.

Fernandez M, Carrol CL, Baker CJ. Discitis and vertebral osteomyelitis in children: an 18 year review. *Pediatrics.* 2000;105(6):1299–1304.

Galer C, Holbrook E, Treves T, et al. Grisel's syndrome: a case report and review of the literature. *Int J Pediatr Otorhinolaryngol.* 2005;69(12):1689–1692.

Gupta AK, Roy DR, Conlan ES, et al. Torticollis secondary to posterior fossa tumors. *J Pediatr Orthop.* 1996;16(4):505–507.

Hadjipavlou AG, Mader JT, Necessary JT, et al. Hematogenous pyogenic spinal infections and their surgical management. *Spine.* 2000;25(13):1668–1679.

Hall DE, Boydston W. Pediatric neck injuries. *Pediatr Rev.* 1999;20(1):13–19.

Khanna G, El-Khoury GY. Imaging of cervical spine injuries of childhood. *Skeletal Radiol.* 2007; 36(6):477–494.

Lewis D, Pearlman E. The migraine variants. *Pediatr Ann.* 2005;34(6):486–488, 490–492, 494–497.

Pang D. Spinal cord injury without radiographic abnormality in children, 2 decades later. *Neurosurgery.* 2004;55(6):1325–1342.

Parker C. Complicated migraine syndromes and migraine variants. *Pediatr Ann.* 1997;26:417–421.

Robin NH. In brief: congenital muscular torticollis. *Pediatr Rev.* 1996;17(10):374–375.

Singer JI. Evaluation of the patient with neck complaints following tonsillectomy or adenoidectomy. *Pediatr Emerg Care.* 1992;8(5):276–279.

Neonatal Infections

NEONATAL SEPSIS

Overview

The most common classification of neonatal sepsis is by age at onset.

- **Early-onset infection.** Clinical manifestations of early-onset infection occur **within the first 7 days of life** (95% present within the first 72 hours). Frequently, **maternal complications of labor or delivery** lead to these infections. Organisms from the maternal genital tract during the intrapartum period colonize the infant's skin and gastrointestinal and respiratory tracts. The reasons for progression from colonization to infection are not well understood. The most common organisms causing early-onset infection are group B streptococci (GBS), *Escherichia coli,* and, occasionally, *Listeria monocytogenes.*

- **Late-onset infection.** Clinical manifestations of late-onset infection occur **between 7 and 30 days of life**. Infection may be the result of **colonization during birth or during hospitalization** in the intensive care unit. Although most infants do not become ill as a result of this colonization, necessary invasive procedures put them at increased risk for infection. The most common organisms causing late-onset infection are coagulase-negative staphylococci, *Staphylococcus aureus, Enterococcus* spp., GBS, *E. coli, Klebsiella pneumoniae,* and *Candida* spp.

- **Late, late-onset infection.** The improved survival rate of **very-low-birth-weight infants** (<1,500 g) has prompted the addition of this third category: late, late-onset infection (generally between 31 and 90 days of life). Although these infants are no longer neonates, their "corrected" gestational age (usually 28 to 34 weeks) and continued need for hospitalization because of complications of prematurity accord them "newborn" status. A quarter of all very low birthweight infants who survive beyond 3 days of life have at least one episode of late-onset or late, late-onset sepsis. These infants usually have **central venous catheters or endotracheal tubes** in place. Infection in this group is **nosocomially acquired** and often caused by coagulase-negative staphylococci, *Pseudomonas aeruginosa, Enterobacter* spp., *Klebsiella* spp., *Serratia marcescens,* and *Candida* spp.

Common Pathogens

Group B *Streptococcus* Infection

The maternal colonization rate for GBS is 15% to 30%, and 50% of these women deliver infants who are **colonized at birth;** 1% of colonized infants develop invasive

TABLE 56-1	Select Risk Factors for Group B Streptococcal Infection
Maternal Risk Factors	
Prior infant with group B streptococcal sepsis	
Group B streptococcal bacteriuria	
Prolonged rupture of membranes (≥18 hr)	
Premature rupture of membranes (<37 wk of gestation)	
Preterm labor (<37 wk of gestation)	
Intrapartum fever >100.4°F (37.9°C)	

GBS infection. Women with prenatal colonization are 25 times more likely to deliver an infant with early-onset GBS disease. Table 56-1 shows other risk factors for infection. The most common clinical manifestations for **early-onset infection are sepsis, pneumonia, and, less often, meningitis** (5% to 10% of early-onset GBS cases). Early-onset GBS infection has a fulminant presentation; 50% of infected infants are symptomatic at birth. Initial manifestations include **respiratory distress, hypoxia, and shock**. The mortality rate of early-onset GBS infection is 5% to 10%. Late-onset infections typically occur within the first month of life, but a small subset of infants develops GBS infection 3 to 6 months after birth. **Late-onset infections** include **sepsis, meningitis** (30% to 40% of late-onset GBS cases), and, occasionally, **skin or soft tissue infections, osteomyelitis, or septic arthritis**. The mortality rate of late-onset GBS infection is 2% to 6%. **Permanent neurologic sequelae** occur in ~50% of patients with meningitis caused by GBS infection.

The use of **intrapartum antibiotics** to treat GBS colonized women has decreased the incidence of early-onset GBS infection in neonates by about 30%; the incidence of late-onset disease remains unchanged because intrapartum antibiotic administration does not effectively eradicate neonatal colonization. Currently, half of all cases of invasive GBS disease are late onset. American Academy of Pediatrics (AAP) and American College of Obstetrics and Gynecology recommendations include vaginal and rectal GBS screening of all pregnant women at 35 to 37 weeks of gestation. **Intrapartum penicillin is administered** in the following situations: previous infant with GBS; GBS bacteriuria; positive GBS screening culture; and unknown GBS status if there is preterm labor, membrane rupture >18 hours, or intrapartum temperature >100.4°F (38°C). Cefazolin, clindamycin, erythromycin, or vancomycin may be given to penicillin-allergic women based on results of GBS isolate susceptibility testing. Other **factors that increase the risk** of neonatal sepsis include a **multiple gestation pregnancy and maternal chorioamnionitis**.

E. coli Infection

E. coli, like GBS, is passed from **mother to infant,** and the ratio of infected to colonized babies is similar. **Early-onset and late-onset infections** occur. Organisms that have the K1 surface antigen are more apt to cause infection, especially meningitis.

Coagulase-Negative Staphylococcal Infection

Coagulase-negative staphylococci (primarily *S. epidermidis*) are most commonly associated with nosocomial infection. Risk factors include **prematurity** and the use of **indwelling catheters**. The organism produces a slime coating that allows it to adhere to the surfaces of synthetic polymers used to make central venous catheters and also enables it to evade the immune system. **Clinical manifestations** of staphylococcal sepsis are **often subtle,** and a **high index of suspicion** is needed to diagnose the infection early.

Fungal Infection

Candida albicans has been the most common cause of neonatal fungal infection; however, *C. parapsilosis* and other non-*albicans Candida* species (*C. tropicalis, C. glabrata*) are becoming more prevalent. Risk factors for fungal infection include gestational age <32 weeks, indwelling intravascular catheter, endotracheal intubation >7 days, receipt of intralipids or parenteral nutrition, and broad-spectrum antibiotic use, especially third-generation cephalosporins. Systemic infection occurs after hematogenous dissemination. Infants with persistently positive blood cultures for *Candida* spp. (>3 days) with a central venous catheter in place are three times more likely to have disseminated disease. The most commonly involved sites are the **heart** (15%), **retina** (6%), **kidneys** (5%), and **liver** (3%). *Malassezia furfur* **bloodstream infection** is associated with intralipid infusion.

DIFFERENTIAL DIAGNOSIS

Neonatal sepsis may present with a variety of clinical presentations. These same presentations can have a variety of other causes simulating or accompanying sepsis. Table 56-2 summarizes the differential diagnosis for sepsis.

Evaluation of Sepsis

All infants with suspected sepsis should receive antibiotics while awaiting blood culture results. The remainder of the evaluation, including lumbar puncture (LP), can be completed once the infant is stabilized.

Patient History

- Are there maternal factors that place the infant at risk for sepsis (see Table 56-1)?
- Is there a family history of infection or other diseases (e.g., galactosemia) in newborns?
- Does the infant have poor feeding, feeding intolerance (e.g., vomiting, abdominal distention), decreased activity, lethargy, or irritability?

Physical Examination

Signs of infection in the newborn infant are nonspecific and include the following disturbances:

- **Temperature**—fever (>100.2°F [37.9°C]) or hypothermia (<96.8°F [36.0°C])
- **Neurologic**—bulging fontanel, lethargy, irritability, weak suck or cry, hypotonia, hypertonia

TABLE 56-2 Differential Diagnosis of Sepsis

Category	Disorder	Associated Symptoms and Signs	Differentiating Features
Metabolic	Hypoglycemia	Respiratory distress, jitteriness, lethargy, seizures	Hypoglycemia can occur with sepsis; check blood glucose in sick infants; especially common in infants of diabetic mothers and small for gestational age infants.
	Hypocalcemia	Respiratory distress, jitteriness, seizures	Check calcium; especially common in infants of diabetic mothers and preterm infants.
	Inborn error of metabolism	Lethargy, vomiting, seizures, tachypnea	Urea cycle defects and organic acidemias often present after the first few feedings.
Pulmonary	Respiratory distress syndrome	Respiratory distress in preterm infant	CXR shows hazy, "ground-glass" appearance; often indistinguishable from bacterial pneumonia.
	Meconium aspiration	Respiratory distress in term infant	Classic CXR shows diffuse, patchy interstitial infiltrates with hyperinflation; may have severe cyanosis from pulmonary hypertension and right-to-left shunting.
	Transient tachypnea of the newborn	Tachypnea without significant respiratory distress	CXR clear or with fluid in fissures; usually minimal supplemental oxygen requirement; usually seen after cesarean section delivery.
Cardiac	Cyanotic congenital heart disease: tetralogy of Fallot, TGA, tricuspid atresia, truncus arteriosus, TAPVR	Tachypnea, cyanosis unresponsive to oxygen, cardiac murmur, extra heart sounds, or abnormal S_2	CXR without infiltrates but with abnormal pulmonary vasculature or cardiac silhouette; difference in pre- and postductal pulse oximetry; lack of response to hyperoxia test (Pa_{O_2}, 100 mm Hg breathing 100% O_2).
	Congestive heart failure (VSD, patent ductus arteriosus, myocarditis, AVM—especially hepatic or cerebral)	Poor feeding, tachypnea, poor perfusion, hepatomegaly, S_2	Congestive heart failure from a left-to-right shunt is unusual in the immediate newborn period when the pulmonary vascular resistance is high; onset is gradual.

	Ductal-dependent lesions (aortic coarctation, hypoplastic left heart, critical pulmonic stenosis)	Poor perfusion, tachypnea, metabolic acidosis, cyanosis	Often sudden in onset, from hours to weeks after birth; check arterial blood gas, four-extremity blood pressures, and pre- and postductal pulse oximetry.
Neurologic	Hemorrhage	Pallor, hypotonia, tachycardia, hypotension	Especially common in preterm infants and following traumatic vaginal delivery.
	Cerebral infarct	Seizures	May be associated with polycythemia or cocaine exposure; often idiopathic.
Gastrointestinal	Necrotizing enterocolitis	Feeding intolerance, abdominal distention, bloody stools	Usually associated with prematurity; abdominal radiograph may show pneumatosis, portal venous air, or free air; associated laboratory findings may include metabolic acidosis and thrombocytopenia.
	Malrotation, volvulus	Bilious emesis, abdominal distention, bloody stools, and shock	All newborns with bilious emesis should be evaluated for GI obstruction; **volvulus is a surgical emergency.**
Hematologic	Profound anemia	Pallor, tachycardia, jaundice (if caused by hemolysis)	Hemolysis, perinatal bleeding (vasa previa, placental abruption), or postnatal hemorrhage.

AVM, arteriovenous malformation; *CXR*, chest radiograph; *GI*, gastrointestinal; *PaO₂*, arterial oxygen tension; S_2, second heart sound; S_3, third heart sound; *TAPVR*, total anomalous pulmonary venous return; *TGA*, transposition of the great arteries; *VSD*, ventricular septal defect.

TABLE 56-3	Standard Sepsis Workup
Complete blood count with differential	
Blood culture	
Lumbar puncture (LP) and cerebrospinal fluid (CSF) analysis[a]	
Urinalysis and urine culture[b]	
Chest radiograph[c]	

[a]If the infant is clinically stable and has a platelet count >50,000/mm^3, an LP can be performed to obtain CSF for analysis of cell count, protein level, and glucose level, and for Gram stain and culture.
[b]If infant is >72 hr of life.
[c]If respiratory symptoms are present.

- **Respiratory**—tachypnea (respiratory rate >60/minute), grunting, nasal flaring, retractions, hypoxemia, apnea
- **Cardiovascular**—tachycardia, bradycardia, hypotension (systolic blood pressure <60 mm Hg in term infants), delayed capillary refill (<2 seconds)
- **Cutaneous**—jaundice, mottled skin, cyanosis, or petechiae
- **Skeletal**—focal bone tenderness

Laboratory Studies

Table 56-3 lists the studies included in a standard sepsis workup.

Complete blood count (CBC). The range of normal values for the white blood cell (WBC) count and differential changes with the gestational and chronological age of the baby. The normal WBC count is 10,000 to 30,000/mm^3 at birth and decreases to 5,000 to 15,000/mm^3 by the second week of life. Although elevated total WBC and absolute neutrophil counts (ANCs) are not helpful as single indicators of sepsis, neutropenia (ANC <1,500/mm^3) and an elevated immature-to-total WBC ratio >0.2 are more often associated with infection. Positive and negative predictive values in large enough studies have not been established to use these values for treatment decisions. The initial WBC count may be normal in an infected newborn, with abnormalities developing 24 to 48 hours later.

 HINT: Remember that several noninfectious conditions can cause neutropenia in newborns, including pregnancy-induced hypertension, asphyxia, intraventricular hemorrhage, hemolytic disease, and alloimmune neutropenia.

- **Cerebrospinal fluid (CSF) analysis.** The CSF sample should be evaluated for the cell count and differential and protein and glucose levels. Newborns have higher CSF cell counts and protein levels than older children and adults. The average CSF WBC count in an uninfected newborn is 6 WBCs/mm^3, and several studies have determined the normal range to be up to 20 WBCs/mm^3. The average value for protein in the CSF is 90 mg/dL in full-term infants and 120 mg/dL in preterm infants. Normal babies may have CSF protein of 150 mg/dL. Traumatic ("bloody") LPs can give results that are difficult to interpret. The correction factor applied to a traumatic LP is based on the WBC-to-RBC ratio in the CSF and in the peripheral blood. Unfortunately, it is often inaccurate in determining the true WBC and protein counts of the CSF.

- **Other studies.** Additional tests to consider include C-reactive protein, procalcitonin, d-dimers, hepatic function panel, serum electrolytes, glucose, CSF viral testing (e.g., enterovirus, parechovirus, herpes simplex virus [HSV]) by polymerase chain reaction (PCR), and viral cultures of nasopharyngeal secretions, rectal swabs, or CSF.
- **C-reactive protein and procalcitonin.** The level of C-reactive protein, an acute phase reactant, is often increased in response to infection. The negative predictive value of two C-reactive protein measurements <1 mg/dL measured 24 hours apart and within 48 hours of birth was >97% in one study. Serum procalcitonin measurements are also elevated in neonatal sepsis; values >40 ng/mL are reported in infected infants compared with values <5 ng/mL in uninfected infants. However, routine use of C-reactive protein and procalcitonin to guide initiation of antibiotic therapy in the asymptomatic newborn infant is not advocated because of insufficient data.

Treatment of Sepsis
Stabilization and Monitoring
One must always remember the ABCs: **airway, breathing, and circulation**. Close monitoring of the **respiratory status, perfusion, and urine output** is necessary in all newborns with sepsis.

Initial Empirical Antibiotic Therapy
Empirical antimicrobial therapy for suspected bacterial infections is guided by knowledge of pathogens suspected, associated focus of infection, and the antimicrobial susceptibility patterns in a particular intensive care unit. The standard therapy for suspected early-onset sepsis is **ampicillin** (which is effective against GBS, *L. monocytogenes,* most enterococci, and 50% of *E. coli* strains) plus **gentamicin** (provides good gram-negative coverage and is synergistic with ampicillin against many organisms). For hospital-acquired infections, **Vancomycin plus an aminoglycoside** (e.g., gentamicin, amikacin, tobramycin) is appropriate. **Imipenem** should be added for empiric treatment of gram-negative meningitis or when resistance to aminoglycosides is suspected. Obviously, the therapy should be altered appropriately when an organism is isolated and susceptibilities are available.

Specific Antibiotic Therapy
- **Group B *Streptococcus*.** Bacteremia or pneumonia can be treated with administration of ampicillin alone. If meningitis is present, aminoglycoside administration should be continued.
- **_L. monocytogenes._** Ampicillin plus an aminoglycoside is recommended.
- **_E. coli_ and _K. pneumoniae_.** Cefepime is preferred as empiric therapy. Alternate agents include imipenem. For susceptible organisms, cefazolin or cefotaxime are appropriate. Meningitis requires combination therapy with an aminoglycoside.

- **Other gram-negative organisms.** Therapy is more complicated because of development of strains resistant to gentamicin and cephalosporins. Administration of a carbapenem and amikacin (or tobramycin) should be considered. This decision should be made in conjunction with a specialist in pediatric infectious diseases. Cephalosporins should not be used as monotherapy to treat certain gram-negative rod bloodstream infections (e.g., *Serratia* spp., *P. aeruginosa, Citrobacter* spp., *Enterobacter* spp.) because of the risk of inducing resistant strains.
- **Coagulase-negative staphylococci.** Vancomycin is generally used; however, oxacillin can be used if sensitivity to this agent is demonstrated *in vitro.*
- **C. albicans.** Treat with amphotericin B. For meningitis, add oral flucytosine. For severe amphotericin B-associated toxicity (e.g., renal insufficiency), consider lipid amphotericin B, fluconazole, or caspofungin. Removal of the infected catheter is an important part of treatment of candidemia. Failure to remove the catheter as soon as candidemia is detected results in prolonged duration of candidemia and increased mortality rates.

Duration of Antibiotic Therapy

Expected duration of therapy depends on many variables, including **virulence of pathogen, rapidity of clinical response, removal of infected catheter, and adequacy of drainage of purulent foci,** if present. Table 56-4 presents the approximate duration of therapy for selected infections.

In cases of **bacterial meningitis,** a LP should be repeated several days into therapy to document sterilization of the CSF for gram-negative meningitis and meningitis caused by highly resistant bacteria. Therapy should continue **2 weeks**

TABLE 56-4	Approximate Duration of Therapy for Selected Infections in the Newborn Infant
Site of Infection	**Duration of Therapy (d)**
Skin/soft tissue	7–10
Bacteremia	10
Bacteremia with CVC	10–14[a]
Necrotizing enterocolitis	10–14
Pneumonia	10–14
Meningitis (gram-positive)	14
Meningitis (gram-negative)	21
Osteomyelitis/septic arthritis	28–42
Endocarditis	28–42
Fungemia (CVC removed)	14
Fungemia (disseminated)	>28

CVC, central venous catheter.
[a]Duration also depends on causative organism and whether or not the CVC was removed. In general, *Staphylococcus aureus* requires 14 d of therapy while other pathogens such as *Enterococcus* spp. may require shorter therapy.

after obtaining a negative culture result for gram-positive meningitis and 3 weeks after obtaining a negative culture result for gram-negative meningitis.

Other Treatment Modalities

- **Blood products.** Some centers treat coagulation disorders with administration of fresh-frozen plasma (15 mL/kg) to replenish clotting factors. Platelets should be given to maintain a count of >20,000/mm^3 (or >50,000/mm^3 if there is evidence of bleeding).

- **Alternative therapies.** Various strategies for prophylaxis or treatment of sepsis in the newborn have been studied, including exchange transfusion, neutrophil transfusion, administration of intravenous immuno-globulin, and cytokine therapy. Unfortunately, none has consistently proven effective for routine use. Hemopoietic colony-stimulating factors in recent trials increased ANC and decreased mortality rates in critically ill neutropenic neonates.

Approach to the Asymptomatic Patient with Risk Factors for Sepsis

The decision on whether to evaluate an asymptomatic newborn for infection should be based on **maternal and fetal risk factors,** such as those listed in Table 56-1. In asymptomatic infants with gestational age >35 weeks, the duration of intrapartum prophylaxis before delivery determines subsequent management. If **two or more doses of maternal prophylaxis** were given before delivery, **no laboratory evaluation or antimicrobial treatment** is required. These infants should be **observed in the hospital for at least 48 hours**. If **fewer than two doses** were given, the AAP and American College of Obstetrics and Gynecology recommend a **limited evaluation** (CBC with differential and blood culture) and **at least 48 hours of observation** before discharge from the hospital.

Premature neonates have at least a **10-fold higher risk for early-onset GBS sepsis** compared with term neonates. Furthermore, as the degree of prematurity increases, clinical evaluation for signs and symptoms of sepsis are less reliable. Therefore, asymptomatic infants <35 weeks of gestation should receive **limited evaluation** (CBC with differential and blood culture) and **at least 48 hours of observation** prior to hospital discharge. Empirical antibiotic therapy is not required. If, during the period of observation, the clinical course **suggests systemic infection, complete diagnostic evaluation and administration of empiric antibiotic therapy** are indicated. This degree of surveillance and treatment is justified by the high morbidity and mortality rates associated with neonatal infection.

CONGENITAL (TORCH) AND PERINATAL INFECTIONS
Overview

A congenital infection is acquired by the infant transplacentally during the first, second, or early third trimester. Table 56-5 lists the clinical features associated with these infections. The classic acronym for the agents that cause these congenital infections is TORCH. Infections that are acquired in the perinatal period are frequently included in this group:

TABLE 56-5	**Clinical Features Suggesting Infection with TORCH Agents**

Intrauterine growth retardation

Hydrops

Microcephaly, hydrocephalus, intracranial calcifications

Eye abnormalities (chorioretinitis, cataracts, glaucoma)

Cardiac malformations, myocarditis

Pneumonitis

Hepatosplenomegaly

Anemia, thrombocytopenia, petechiae

Jaundice (especially conjugated hyperbilirubinemia)

Bone abnormalities (osteochondritis, periostitis)

TORCH, toxoplasmosis, other (congenital syphilis and viruses), rubella, cytomegalovirus, and herpes simplex virus.

- **T**oxoplasmosis
- **O**ther (includes HIV, syphilis, enterovirus, parvovirus, hepatitis B virus, varicella-zoster virus)
- **R**ubella
- **C**ytomegalovirus (CMV)
- **H**erpes simplex virus

Common Infections
Cytomegalovirus Infection

CMV is the **most common viral cause** of congenital infection. Approximately 50% to 80% of women of childbearing age are seropositive for CMV, but the risk of reactivation during pregnancy causing fetal infection is small (<1%). Primary CMV infection occurs in 1% to 4% of pregnancies and the fetus is infected in 40% of these cases. Most affected infants are **asymptomatic at birth** and develop normally. Approximately **10% to 15% of infected infants have symptoms at birth,** and 90% of these infants develop sequelae (e.g., **mental retardation, hearing loss, seizures**).

Congenital CMV infection is diagnosed by **detection of the virus from the urine** (PCR rather than culture is used at some hospitals) within 2 weeks of birth; after this time, a detection of the virus could indicate intrapartum or postnatal infection, which is usually not clinically significant unless the baby is premature.

Treatment of congenital CMV infection usually involves **supportive care** and close follow-up. **Ganciclovir** treatment for 6 weeks reduces the progression of hearing loss in affected infants. Criteria for ganciclovir use include evidence of neurologic involvement such as intracranial calcifications, microcephaly, or CSF pleocytosis.

Syphilis

Congenital syphilis results from **transplacental passage** of the spirochete *Treponema pallidum;* rarely, infant contact with a maternal chancre results in perinatal transmission. Maternal syphilis in any stage can lead to fetal infection.

Fetal or perinatal death occurs in 40% of congenital syphilis infections. The **surviving infants** are **asymptomatic at birth** but, if not treated, **develop symptoms within the first few weeks of life**. The most common manifestations of early congenital syphilis are **hepatosplenomegaly, bone abnormalities, hemolytic anemia, and jaundice**. Less common findings include ocular involvement, bloody nasal discharge (snuffles), mucocutaneous rash, and pneumonia alba.

Maternal testing for syphilis involves **nontreponemal serology** using either the Venereal Disease Research Laboratory (VDRL) or the rapid plasma reagent (RPR) test. Treponemal test (i.e., the microhemagglutination-*T. pallidum* test or the fluorescent treponemal antibody absorbed test) are positive for life; therefore, they indicate disease history, not activity at the time of the blood study. In many cities, the health department keeps records of previous infection and treatments.

Indications for treatment of the infant vary; consult the latest AAP Committee on Infectious Disease report, the *Red Book,* for recommendations. Maternal history of treatment and response to treatment by a fourfold drop in titers are major factors to consider in management plans. Testing of the newborn infant includes the following:

- **Serum RPR.** Umbilical cord testing can show false-positive results.
- **LP.** Send CSF for VDRL; CSF analysis reveals pleocytosis and elevated protein.
- **Radiographs of the long bones.**

In the newborn period, the normally high CSF protein and infrequency of abnormal bone findings make the criteria just listed less absolute. Pregnancy can slightly elevate the RPR. Infants should be treated for congenital syphilis, if

- They were born to a mother with untreated syphilis.
- There is evidence of maternal relapse or reinfection.
- There is physical, radiologic, or laboratory evidence of syphilis.
- Their CSF VDRL is reactive.
- Their serum quantitative nontreponemal titer is at least fourfold greater than the mother's titer.

Treatment of early asymptomatic infection prevents long-term clinical sequelae. **Penicillin G** (50,000 U/kg given intravenously every 12 hours for 10 to 14 days) is the treatment of choice. **Infants born to mothers treated in the last month of pregnancy** should be evaluated; if the workup is normal, they may receive a single dose of **intramuscular benzathine penicillin G**. Detailed recommendations for the treatment of syphilis in pregnancy and infancy can be found in the *2006 Red Book: Report of the Committee on Infectious Diseases,* published by the AAP.

 HINT: False-positive VDRL tests occur in patients with lupus. Patients with Lyme disease have positive treponemal tests (microhemagglutination-*T. pallidum* or fluorescent treponemal antibody absorbed) and negative VDRL.

Hepatitis B

In utero infection with the hepatitis B virus rarely occurs; **perinatal transmission** is more common. Overall, there is a 60% to 70% chance of perinatal transmission if the mother has acute symptomatic infection. If the mother is seropositive for hepatitis B e antigen, the perinatal transmission rate is 90%, as opposed to only 10% if the mother is negative for hepatitis B e antigen.

Infected infants are asymptomatic at birth but may develop antigenemia and an increased level of transaminases by 2 to 6 months of age.

Hepatitis B can be **prevented by either active or passive immunization**. Current recommendations include treating all infants born to mothers who are hepatitis B surface antigen positive with hepatitis B immune globulin and hepatitis B vaccine.

 HINT: Mothers with hepatitis B may breast-feed their infants.

Herpes Simplex

Approximately 75% of neonatal HSV infections are caused by HSV type 2. Congenital infection with this organism is extremely rare; usually, the baby is infected via the maternal genital tract shortly **before or during delivery**. Primary maternal infection results in neonatal HSV infection in ~50% of cases, whereas recurrent infection poses a risk of ~5%. Transmission of HSV may be **prevented by cesarean delivery** when the mother has active genital lesions and the membranes have been ruptured for <4 hours.

Neonates with HSV infection manifest in three distinct clinical groups:

- Disease localized to the skin, eye, and/or mouth (SEM disease)
- Encephalitis with or without skin involvement (central nervous system [CNS] disease)
- Disseminated disease that involves multiple organ systems, including the CNS, lung, liver, adrenals, SEM

Disease onset occurs at <24 hours of life in 9%, at days 1 to 5 in 30%, and at >5 days in 60% of infants.

Skin lesions are seen in approximately two-thirds of infants **with CNS or disseminated disease. Seizures** occur in 50% with CNS disease and in 20% with disseminated disease. **Pneumonia** occurs in 35% to 40% of infants with disseminated disease. **Disseminated infection** appears **clinically similar to bacterial sepsis** (e.g., lethargy, poor feeding, temperature instability). As the disease progresses, **jaundice, disseminated intravascular coagulation, hepatosplenomegaly, and shock** develop. Common CSF findings include **pleocytosis** (with a lymphocyte predominance), an **increased RBC count,** and an **increased protein level**. A positive CSF HSV PCR test confirms the diagnosis of meningitis. The CSF HSV PCR test has a high sensitivity (>98%) and specificity. Skin or conjunctival cultures are positive in >90% of neonates with any type of HSV infection. HSV is difficult to isolate from CSF culture.

Neonatal HSV infection is treated with **high-dose acyclovir** (60 mg/kg/day, divided, every 8 hours). Duration of treatment is **14 days for SEM disease and at least 21 days for CNS or disseminated disease**.

HIV

The risk of transmission of HIV from a seropositive mother to her fetus is ~25%, although **treatment of the infected mother during pregnancy and delivery reduces the transmission** dramatically. The **risk increases** to ~50% **if the mother has AIDS or if she previously had a child who was infected**. It is not known whether cesarean section delivery reduces the probability of transmission. Because the virus can also be **transmitted through breast milk,** the current recommendation in the United States is to counsel HIV-positive mothers not to breast-feed.

For babies of mothers with **unknown HIV status,** the infants' HIV-exposure status should be determined by antibody testing; HIV antibody detection at this stage indicates HIV-exposure, but additional tests are needed to determine the presence or absence of neonatal HIV infection. Infants born to HIV-positive mothers (including infants with detectable antibody) require **HIV qualitative RNA PCR of the blood at birth, 2 weeks, 4 weeks, and 4 months** of age; 20% of infected infants have a positive test at birth and 95% of infants test positive by 2 weeks of age. **Infants with negative HIV DNA PCR** (at birth, 1 month, and 4 months of age) should undergo **HIV antibody testing at 12, 15, and 18 months** of age to confirm that maternal HIV antibody is no longer present. HIV-exposed infants should receive zidovudine (ZDV) for the first 6 weeks of life.

Opportunistic infections are reported in young infants; therefore, **trimethoprim-sulfamethoxazole prophylaxis** is usually **started at 6 weeks of age and discontinued at 4 months of age,** if testing reveals that the infant does not have HIV. Clinical trials have shown that **treatment of HIV-positive women** with **zidovudine** during the **second and third trimesters** of pregnancy and **intrapartum,** followed by **treatment of the newborn** for the first 6 weeks of life, **decreases the rate of transmission** of infection from mother to infant to ~8%.

Evaluation of Congenital Infection

Patient History

Confirm the results of maternal serologic screening for rubella, hepatitis B, syphilis, and HIV.

Physical Examination

Examine the baby for organ system involvement, including funduscopic examination. Table 56-6 lists the findings suggestive of particular infections.

Laboratory Studies

It is not necessary to perform a complete TORCH evaluation for every baby with suspected congenital infection. A **thorough history and physical examination** of the baby and **knowledge of maternal prenatal laboratory studies** (rubella, syphilis, hepatitis, and HIV serologies) can narrow the differential diagnosis. Table 56-7 lists the studies to consider in the evaluation of an infant with a suspected TORCH infection.

- **Serology.** Maternal IgG antibody crosses the placenta; therefore, the absence of rubella- or *Toxoplasma*-specific IgG in the infant excludes congenital

TABLE 56-6   Clinical Findings in Specific TORCH Infections

Toxoplasmosis
Hydrocephalus with generalized calcifications
Chorioretinitis, microphthalmia
Deafness

Rubella
Cataracts, glaucoma, pigmented retinopathy, microphthalmia
Deafness
Cardiac malformation (PDA, pulmonary artery stenosis)
"Blueberry muffin" appearance (extramedullary hematopoiesis)

CMV
Microcephaly with periventricular calcifications
Chorioretinitis
Inguinal hernias (boys)
Petechiae with thrombocytopenia

Herpes
Acute CNS findings
Keratoconjunctivitis
Skin, eye, mucous membrane vesicles

Syphilis
Interstitial keratitis, pigmentary retinopathy
Snuffles (persistent and often bloody nasal discharge)
Fissures (lips, nares) and mucous patches (mouth, genitalia)
Eczematoid skin rash
Osteochondritis and periostitis

CMV, cytomegalovirus; *CNS,* central nervous system; *PDA,* patent ductus arteriosus.
Modified with permission from Stagno S, Alford CA. Perinatal infections and maldevelopment. In: Bloom AD, James LS, eds. *The Fetus and the Newborn.* Volume 17, Series 1. New York: Wiley-Liss; 1981.

---

infection. However, positive IgG titers in the infant for rubella or *Toxoplasma* are not diagnostic of congenital infection. If the serology is positive, check specific IgM titers. In suspected congenital syphilis, serum RPR and CSF VDRL should be tested.

- **Viral culture.** All infants with suspected HSV should have surface viral cultures performed. Urine CMV PCR testing should be performed to assess for congenital CMV infection; shell-vial culture is occasionally used in lieu of PCR. Testing for CMV must be sent within 2 weeks of birth, otherwise postnatal acquisition cannot be excluded. Enteroviral culture of nasopharyngeal and rectal swabs and CSF may be indicated for a baby with myocarditis, hepatitis, or aseptic meningitis.

- **Other laboratory studies** include a CBC, bilirubin (conjugated and unconjugated), and transaminases. Darkfield examination of nasal discharge in patients with "snuffles" may reveal syphilis.

TABLE 56-7   **Evaluation of the Infant with a Suspected TORCH Infection**

Cerebrospinal Fluid
CSF cell count, protein, glucose (enterovirus, rubella, syphilis)
CSF PCR (enterovirus, HSV)
CSF VDRL (syphilis)

Blood
IgG (specify *Toxoplasma* or rubella—if positive, send IgM)
RPR (syphilis)
Hepatitis B surface antigen
PCR (enteroviruses, HIV)

Skin Lesions
Darkfield examination (syphilis)
Direct fluorescent antibody (HSV, varicella)[a]
PCR (HSV, varicella)
Tzanck smear (HSV)[a]
Culture (HSV)

Urine
PCR (CMV, enteroviruses)
Culture (CMV)

Mucosa
Conjunctiva culture (HSV)
Mouth or nasopharynx culture (HSV, enterovirus)[b]
Rectum culture (enterovirus, HSV)[b]

Other Studies
Audiologic evaluation (CMV, rubella, toxoplasmosis)
Head CT (CMV, toxoplasmosis)
Ophthalmologic examination (toxoplasmosis, rubella, CMV, HSV, varicella, syphilis)
Radiograph of long bones (rubella, syphilis)

CMV, cytomegalovirus; *CSF*, cerebrospinal fluid; *CT*, computed tomography; *HSV*, herpes simplex virus; *IgM*, immunoglobulin M; *PCR*, polymerase chain reaction; *RPR*, rapid plasma reagent; *VDRL*, Venereal Disease Research Laboratory.
See text for evaluation of an infant for HIV.
[a]Tzanck smear rarely used. PCR is preferred though direct fluorescent antibody testing is acceptable.
[b]Enteroviral cultures rarely performed given the high sensitivity of enteroviral PCR for detection of enterovirus in blood, urine, and stool specimens.

SUGGESTED READINGS

Bassler D, Stoll BJ, Schmidt B, et al. Using a count of neonatal morbidities to predict poor outcome in extremely low birth weight infants: added role of neonatal infection. *Pediatrics.* 2009;123:313–318.

Centers for Disease Control and Prevention. Trends in perinatal group B streptococcal disease, United States, 2000–2006. *MMWR. Morb Mortal Wkly Rep.* 2009;58(5):109–112.

Gozzo YF, Gallagher PG. Congenital TORCH infections. In: SS Shah, ed. *Pediatric Practice: Infectious Diseases.* New York: McGraw-Hill Professional; 2009:504–519.

Kimberlin DW, Lin CY, Jacobs RF, et al. Natural history of neonatal herpes simplex virus infections in the acyclovir era. *Pediatrics.* 2001;108:223–229.

Kimberlin DW, Lin CY, Sanchez PJ, et al. Effect of ganciclovir therapy on hearing in symptomatic congenital cytomegalovirus disease involving the central nervous system: a randomized, controlled trial. *J Pediatr.* 2003;143:16–25.

Phares CR, Lynfield R, Farley MM, et al. Epidemiology of invasive group B streptococcal disease in the United States. *JAMA.* 2008;299:2056–2065.

Read JS and The Committee on Pediatric AIDS. Diagnosis of HIV-1 infection in children younger than 18 months in the United States. *Pediatrics.* 2007;120:e1547–e1562.

Saiman L, Ludington E, Pfaller M, et al. Risk factors for candidemia in Neonatal Intensive Care Unit patients: The National Epidemiology of Mycosis Survey study group. *Pediatr Infect Dis J.* 2000;19:319–324.

Schrag SJ, Stoll BJ. Early-onset neonatal sepsis in the era of widespread intrapartum chemoprophylaxis. *Pediatr Infect Dis J.* 2006;25(10):939–940.

CHAPTER 57

Kim Smith-Whitley

Pallor (Paleness)

INTRODUCTION

Pallor (paleness) results from a **decreased amount of circulating hemoglobin or vasoconstriction of dermal blood vessels**. Causes can be classified as hematologic or nonhematologic.

DIFFERENTIAL DIAGNOSIS LIST

Hematologic Causes

Increased Red Blood Cell (RBC) Destruction—see Chapter 40, "Hemolysis"

- Isoimmune or alloimmune hemolytic anemia (hemolytic disease of the newborn)
- Autoimmune hemolytic anemia
- RBC membrane defects
- RBC enzyme defects
- Qualitative hemoglobin disorders
- Quantitative hemoglobin disorders
- Microangiopathic hemolytic anemia
- Drugs
- Toxins
- Infections

Bone Marrow Failure

- Transient erythroblastopenia of childhood
- Aplastic crisis with underlying congenital hemolytic anemia
- Diamond–Blackfan anemia
- Anemia associated with systemic illness
- Drug-related anemia
- Infection

- Aplastic anemia—idiopathic or secondary to drugs, chemicals, viruses, radiation, pregnancy
- Transient bone marrow suppression—caused by viral or bacterial infection, drugs, pregnancy, radiation
- Fanconi anemia
- Dyskeratosis congenita
- Pure red cell aplasia
- Congenital dyserythropoietic anemia
- Pregnancy

Bone Marrow Infiltration

- Leukemia or neoplasm metastatic to bone marrow
- Infection
- Osteopetrosis
- Histiocytosis
- Myelofibrosis
- Storage diseases

Nutritional Deficiencies

- Iron deficiency
- Folate deficiency
- Vitamin B_{12} deficiency

Blood Loss
- Hemorrhage
- Bleeding disorder

Nonhematologic Causes
Infectious Causes
- Bacterial process leading to shock, anemia, or both

Toxic Causes
- Lead poisoning

Neoplastic Causes
- Pheochromocytoma

Traumatic Causes
- Head trauma resulting in a closed head injury or cerebral hemorrhage

Congenital Causes
- Constitutional skin color

Metabolic or Genetic Causes
- Hypoglycemia

Inflammatory Causes
- Atopic dermatitis
- Other chronic systemic diseases

Miscellaneous Causes
- Shock
- Skin edema (myxedema, as in thyroid disease)
- Uremia
- Cystic fibrosis
- Seizures
- Syncope
- Lack of sun exposure

DIFFERENTIAL DIAGNOSIS DISCUSSION
Blood Loss
Etiology

Blood loss, acute and chronic, is one of the most common causes of anemia in the pediatric patient. Chronic blood loss may be caused by **gastrointestinal bleeding, excessive menstrual bleeding, or a bleeding disorder** characterized by frequent bleeding episodes.

Clinical Features

Patients with chronic blood loss may present with **pallor,** usually noted by an observer who has not seen the child recently. **Chronic blood loss** may be **difficult to recognize** because the hemoglobin level diminishes slowly.

Evaluation

Initial laboratory studies should include a **complete blood count (CBC), blood type and cross-match, prothrombin time, and partial thromboplastin time**. In a patient with anemia secondary to **chronic blood loss,** a peripheral smear shows **hypochromic, microcytic RBCs** from iron deficiency. In a patient with **acute blood loss,** it shows **normocytic, normochromic RBCs**.

Treatment

If bleeding is **massive or life threatening, intravenous access should be established, active bleeding controlled, and type O-negative, uncross-matched packed RBCs should be transfused**. Rarely, in the previously transfused, alloimmunized child, minor blood group antigen incompatibility results in **severe delayed hemolytic transfusion reactions** following the administration of O-negative uncross-matched packed cells.

Iron-Deficiency Anemia

 HINT: Nutritional deficiencies may be caused by decreased oral intake, increased requirements, decreased absorption, or ineffective transport or metabolism of the element. The specific deficiency should be determined as well as the underlying cause to provide optimal treatment.

Etiology
Iron deficiency, which is the most common cause of anemia in childhood, can occur at any age, although children between 6 and 36 months of age and girls between 11 and 17 years of age are at increased risk. Iron deficiency in childhood is caused by **rapid growth in the presence of inadequate dietary intake, chronic or massive blood loss, or poor gut absorption**. Infants with iron deficiency, usually have a history of **consuming large amounts of cow's milk** and other food substances low in iron.

 HINT: Iron deficiency is less common in breast-fed infants. Although the iron content of breast milk is lower than that of a formula based on cow's milk, iron absorption is improved.

 HINT: Pica may be a symptom of iron deficiency or a risk factor for iron deficiency. Children who eat dirt should be evaluated for lead poisoning.

Clinical Features
Children with severe iron deficiency are commonly **pale, irritable, and have little appetite**. In addition to signs of anemia, **spooning of the nails, angular stomatitis, and splenomegaly** may be present.

Laboratory Evaluation
The degree of iron deficiency can be estimated by the abnormalities found on laboratory studies. The following laboratory abnormalities occur progressively: **decreased serum ferritin, decreased serum iron, increased microcytosis, and decreased hemoglobin with a normal or decreased reticulocyte count**. The RBC distribution width (index) is increased. The **platelet count** may be markedly **increased**. The peripheral blood smear shows **hypochromic, microcytic RBCs with increased variation in RBC size** (anisocytosis) **and shape** (poikilocytosis). **Increased** numbers of **elliptocytes and ovalocytes** may be noted.

Treatment
Treatment of iron deficiency includes **iron supplementation,** as well as **treatment of the underlying cause** with **nutritional counseling** when appropriate. Oral iron replacement is achieved with **ferrous sulfate** (3 to 6 mg/kg/day of elemental iron in two or three divided doses). Although absorption is better on an empty stomach, gastric irritation is lessened if the iron is given **with meals**.

In patients with severe anemia, the hematologic response to ferrous sulfate administration can be documented by obtaining a **reticulocyte count within 7 to 10 days**. The reticulocyte count increases earlier than the hemoglobin level, which may not reach a normal level until 2 months after starting iron therapy, depending on the degree of anemia.

Many physicians believe that because iron deficiency is so common, the healthy child or adolescent with a **microcytic, hypochromic anemia** is appropriately managed using a **trial of iron supplementation without additional laboratory evaluation**. If a patient is managed this way, **close follow-up** should be provided. If the microcytic anemia persists, a comprehensive evaluation for other causes (e.g., thalassemia, anemia of chronic disease, chronic blood loss, sideroblastic anemia) should be performed.

Megaloblastic Anemias
Etiology
Megaloblastic anemias are often caused by **folate and vitamin B_{12} deficiencies,** which result in **abnormal DNA synthesis**. **Folate deficiency** in the United States is **primarily caused by malabsorption of folate, increased RBC turnover, and drugs**. **Vitamin B_{12} deficiency** may be **caused by malabsorption or pernicious anemia,** a rare disease caused by an inability to secrete the intrinsic factor required for normal vitamin B_{12} absorption.

Evaluation
Megaloblastic anemias are characterized by **macrocytic RBCs and a mean corpuscular volume (MCV) value >95 fL**. The **reticulocyte count is low,** and in advanced cases **pancytopenia** may exist. Analysis of a **bone marrow aspirate and biopsy** shows **dyssynchrony** between **nuclear and cytoplasmic maturation** with increased cellularity.

Serum folate may be decreased, but measurement of **RBC folate levels** provides a more accurate picture of chronic folate deficiency. In pernicious anemia, **serum vitamin B_{12} levels are reduced and intrinsic factor antibodies may be positive**.

Therapy
Therapy includes **supplemental folate or vitamin B_{12}** administration, as well as **treatment of the underlying cause** of the deficiency.

Transient Erythroblastopenia of Childhood
Clinical Features
Transient erythroblastopenia of childhood is characterized by the **acute onset of anemia** in a previously healthy child **between 6 months and 4 years of age**. There may be a history of a **viral prodrome**. The physical examination is normal except for signs of anemia.

Evaluation
The hemoglobin and reticulocyte values vary according to the stage of disease. **Early in the illness,** the **hemoglobin and reticulocyte count are low,** whereas **in the recovery stage** the hemoglobin may be low but the **reticulocyte count is increasing**. Therefore, **serial reticulocyte counts** should be used **in conjunction with serial hemoglobin values** to clarify the stage of disease.

Other laboratory findings include **neutropenia** (25% of patients) and a **normal platelet count**. The bone marrow aspirate shows a marked **decrease in erythroid precursors** early in the disease.

Treatment
Because of the potential severity of the anemia and the need for serial testing, these patients are initially managed more appropriately in a **hospital inpatient setting**. Transient erythroblastopenia of childhood usually **resolves in 1 to 2 months**. No medications accelerate bone marrow recovery. **RBC transfusion** is sometimes necessary.

Diamond–Blackfan Anemia (Congenital Hypoplastic Anemia)
Etiology
Diamond–Blackfan anemia is a **congenital disorder** characterized by **pure RBC aplasia**.

Clinical Features
Most patients become anemic within the first 6 months of life. **Congenital anomalies** occur in 25% of patients, including **radial anomalies** (triphalangeal thumbs); **short stature; and eye, palate, heart, and kidney anomalies**.

Evaluation
The disease is characterized by a **macrocytic anemia,** although a normocytic anemia with a decreased reticulocyte count is seen early in life. Bone marrow aspirate may show **normal cellularity** with isolated **decreased RBC precursors**. **Hemoglobin F is increased** in a heterogeneous fashion and erythrocyte adenosine deaminase levels are elevated. Some patients have RPS19 gene mutations.

Treatment
Approximately 60% to 70% of patients with Diamond–Blackfan anemia respond to corticosteroids and do not require chronic transfusions. Steroid-unresponsive patients receive **RBC transfusions** each month and have a poorer prognosis because of the long-term complications associated with chronic blood transfusion (e.g., iron overload). **Splenectomy** has also been attempted in steroid-unresponsive patients with mixed success. Some patients are cured by **bone marrow transplantation**.

Congenital Hemolytic Anemia with Aplastic Crisis
Etiology
Children with congenital hemolytic anemias can experience a **transient aplastic crisis as a result of human parvovirus B19 infection**.

Evaluation
Transient erythroblastopenia of childhood, Diamond–Blackfan anemia (congenital pure red cell aplasia), **and an aplastic episode** in the presence of a previously undiagnosed hemolytic anemia can be **difficult to distinguish** from one another. Children with congenital hemolytic anemia may have the following:

- A history of intermittent scleral icterus with intercurrent illnesses.
- **Family members with anemia** or those **who have required splenectomy or cholecystectomy** before adulthood. Children with transient erythroblastopenia

of childhood or Diamond–Blackfan anemia do not have this history as frequently.

- **Splenomegaly** on physical examination, which is absent in patients with transient erythroblastopenia of childhood but may be present in those with Diamond–Blackfan anemia.
- Peripheral RBC morphology that suggests the diagnosis of hereditary spherocytosis, hereditary elliptocytosis, or sickle cell disease (SCD).

If the RBC morphology is normal but the history is suspicious for a congenital hemolytic anemia, hemoglobin electrophoresis, measurement of RBC enzyme levels, and evaluation of membrane abnormalities should be performed (prior to transfusing the patient).

Children with congenital hemolytic anemia and aplastic crisis usually have a **febrile viral prodrome** and may have **profound anemia and reticulocytopenia**. Serum should be obtained for human parvovirus B19 titers (see Chapter 40, "Hemolysis").

Aplastic Anemia
Etiology
Aplastic anemia (i.e., bone marrow failure characterized by decreased bone marrow cellularity and pancytopenia) is **usually acquired**. However, congenital causes are not uncommon in children. Acquired aplastic anemia may be idiopathic or secondary to a number of processes (Table 57-1). Idiopathic aplastic anemia is more common because 30% to 50% of the patients have no antecedent cause. Most reported pediatric cases of aplastic anemia with definable causes result from **exposure to drugs, chemicals, or other toxic substances**. The criteria for severe aplastic anemia includes an absolute neutrophil count below 500/μL, a reticulocyte count <1%, a platelet count <20,000/μL, and decreased bone marrow cellularity.

Clinical Features
Patients with aplastic anemia usually present with signs of **thrombocytopenia** (e.g., petechiae, ecchymoses, abnormal bleeding); however, signs of **anemia** may be present as well. Hepatosplenomegaly and lymphadenopathy are usually absent on physical examination.

Evaluation
Laboratory findings demonstrate **moderate to severe anemia, thrombocytopenia, and neutropenia**. **Reticulocytopenia** occurs with corrected reticulocyte counts <2%.

Analysis of a bone marrow aspirate and biopsy sample is necessary to establish a diagnosis. Bone marrow aspirate shows a paucity of RBC, white blood cell (WBC), and platelet precursors, as well as an absence of bone marrow infiltration with malignant cells. Bone marrow biopsy shows a decrease in overall bone marrow cellularity and replacement with fatty tissue. A bone marrow biopsy that demonstrates normal cellularity does not eliminate the possibility of aplastic anemia because these patients may have patchy foci of normal bone marrow activity. In these patients, magnetic resonance imaging may be useful for demonstrating bone marrow replacement with fat, especially in the spine. Evaluation should include tests to determine congenital causes of bone marrow failure as well.

TABLE 57-1	Causes of Severe Aplastic Anemia

Drugs
Chloramphenicol
Sulfa drugs
Anticonvulsants
Cancer chemotherapeutic agents

Chemicals
Benzenes
Gold
Insecticides (DDT)
Lindane (active ingredient in shampoos used to treat pediculosis)

Pregnancy

Viral Infection
Hepatitis A, hepatitis B, hepatitis C
Epstein–Barr virus

Radiation

Paroxysmal Nocturnal Hemoglobinuria

Inherited Disorders
Fanconi anemia
Dyskeratosis congenital
Reticular dysgenesis
Shwachman–Diamond syndrome

Immunologic Disorders
Severe combined immunodeficiency disorder with graft-versus-host disease
Systemic lupus erythematosus
Eosinophilic fasciitis
Thymoma
Hypogammaglobulinemia

Treatment

Once the diagnosis of aplastic anemia is established and a full evaluation performed to identify possible causes, potential treatment options should be evaluated. Initial management of the pediatric patient with pancytopenia should be directed toward **treating life-threatening bleeding, infection, and anemia-related congestive heart failure**. Supportive measures include **irradiated RBC and platelet transfusions** (when necessary) and **antimicrobial administration** to treat or prevent severe infections.

The majority of cases of severe aplastic anemia can be **cured by bone marrow transplantation or pharmacologic regimens**. Any patient with severe aplastic anemia and an **HLA-identical sibling** should first be evaluated for bone marrow transplantation. If there is no HLA-identical sibling, pharmacological treatment includes the administration of immunosuppressive agents such as **antithymocyte globulin, cyclosporine, and corticosteroids**. Other options include **androgens and growth factors**. Despite therapeutic interventions, a small number of patients with aplastic anemia do not respond or they develop leukemia.

Bone Marrow Infiltration
Etiology
Malignant diseases that can infiltrate or replace bone marrow include **leukemia, rhabdomyosarcoma, neuroblastoma, retinoblastoma, Ewing sarcoma, lymphoma, and histiocytosis syndromes**. **Nonmalignant diseases** that infiltrate and replace bone marrow include **storage diseases, osteopetrosis, infections** such as tuberculosis, **and fibrous tissue replacement**.

Evaluation
Bone marrow infiltration with malignant or abnormal cells can cause **pancytopenia**. Peripheral blood smears may show predominant **teardrop-shaped RBCs and increased RBC and white blood cell precursors**.

Treatment
Treatment is directed toward **management of the causative disorder**. Supportive measures include **antibiotic therapy and RBC and platelet transfusions**.

EVALUATION OF PALLOR
A well focused history and physical examination can direct the provider in making a diagnosis (Table 57-2).

Patient History
The following information should be sought:

- Patient's age. The differential diagnosis is slightly different for neonates (Table 57-3)
- A complete prenatal history, birth history, and family history, including information regarding the need for transfusion, a childhood history of splenectomy or cholecystectomy, or abnormal bleeding (if excessive blood loss is the cause of anemia)
- Signs of anemia (e.g., pallor with or without scleral icterus)
- Symptoms of cardiovascular compromise (e.g., easy fatigability; shortness of breath, at rest or with exercise; orthopnea; headache; mental status changes)
- Presence of other systemic symptoms (e.g., fever)
- History of chronic disease
- History of seizures, syncope, or head trauma
- Dietary history

Physical Examination
In addition to a general physical examination, care should be taken to **examine the skin and mucosa**. In a dark-skinned child, pale conjunctivae, palmar creases, nail beds, and oral mucosa help confirm the presence of pallor (Table 57-2).

Cardiovascular findings often include tachycardia and a systolic ejection (flow) murmur. Signs of congestive heart failure caused by severe anemia include extreme tachycardia, a third heart sound (S_3) cardiac gallop, rales, hepatomegaly (possibly accompanied by splenomegaly), pedal edema (rare), and shock. Congenital anomalies suggest a congenital bone marrow failure syndrome.

Laboratory Studies
Appropriate laboratory studies (see Table 57-2) may include the following:

- CBC
- Reticulocyte count

TABLE 57-2	**Clinical Evaluation of Pediatric Patients with Pallor**
Question	**If the Answer Is "Yes," Consider ...**
History	
Has the child been lethargic with a sudden onset of pallor?	An acute process such as head trauma, bacterial infection, hypoglycemia, or an acute anemia
Has the child had a slow onset of pallor with other major systemic symptoms?	A chronic illness such as cystic fibrosis, nephrotic syndrome, malignancy
Does the child have a known chronic disease?	Anemia of chronic disease
Is the child an infant whose diet primarily consists of cow's milk?	Iron-deficiency anemia
Is the child African-American?	G6PD deficiency, SCD, thalassemia syndromes
Is the child of Mediterranean or Asian descent?	G6PD deficiency, thalassemia syndromes
Are the child's parents pale without a history of anemia?	Constitutional pallor
Is the child a neonate?	Acute or chronic blood loss, hemolytic disease of the newborn
Physical Examination	
Are there tongue abnormalities?	Nutritional deficiencies
Are there congenital anomalies?	Fanconi anemia, Diamond–Blackfan anemia, congenital infections
Is the child ill appearing with lymphadenopathy and hepatosplenomegaly?	Chronic systemic illness, congenital infection, malignancy
Does the child have jaundice and hepatosplenomegaly?	A hemolytic process
Does the child have petechiae, ecchymoses, or excessive bleeding?	A platelet or coagulation disorder
Does the child have hepatomegaly or a gallop on cardiovascular examination?	Congestive heart failure
Laboratory Studies	
Is the MCV low for age?	Iron-deficiency anemia, thalassemia, sideroblastic anemia, anemia of chronic disease
Is the MCHC low with microcytic, hypochromic RBC morphology?	Iron-deficiency anemia, thalassemia, sideroblastic anemia, anemia of chronic disease
Is the MCV elevated?	Megaloblastic anemia, reticulocytosis, hypothyroidism, trisomy 21, liver disease
Is there a normocytic, normochromic anemia?	Acute or chronic blood loss, hemoglobinopathies, early iron-deficiency anemia, infection, RBC membrane or enzyme abnormalities, hypersplenism
Is there an elevated RDW?	SCD, iron-deficiency anemia, megaloblastic anemias, thalassemia

(continued)

TABLE 57-2	Clinical Evaluation of Pediatric Patients with Pallor (*Cont.*)
Question	**If the Answer Is "Yes," Consider …**
Are the BUN and creatinine levels elevated?	Uremia, hemolytic uremic syndrome
Are there prominent target cells?	Liver disease, thalassemia, hemoglobinopathies
Are there prominent burr cells?	Liver disease, renal disease, dehydration, pyruvate kinase deficiency, artifact
Are there prominent schistocytes?	Severe hemolytic anemia, microangiopathic hemolytic process, Kasabach–Merritt syndrome, hemolytic uremic syndrome, thrombotic thrombocytopenic purpura
Are there prominent elliptocytes?	Hereditary elliptocytosis, iron-deficiency anemia, normal variant
Is there prominent basophilic stippling?	Consider iron-deficiency anemia, lead poisoning, thalassemias, unstable hemoglobins
Are there prominent blister cells?	G6PD deficiency
Are there prominent Howell–Jolly bodies?	Postsplenectomy patient, megaloblastic anemia

BUN, blood urea nitrogen; *G6PD,* glucose-6-phosphate-dehydrogenase; *MCHC,* mean corpuscular hemoglobin concentration; *MCV,* mean corpuscular volume; *RBC,* red blood cell; *RDW,* red (blood cell) distribution width (index); *SCD,* sickle cell disease.

- Peripheral blood smear
- Blood type and cross-match
- Bone aspirate and/or biopsy
- Serum electrolyte panel
- Blood urea nitrogen (BUN) and creatinine levels
- Glucose level
- Blood culture

 HINT: Pallor caused by anemia (i.e., a decrease in RBC mass) can only be confirmed by a CBC, which includes estimates of the RBC mass: the volume of packed RBCs, the hematocrit, and the hemoglobin level. Because expansion of the intravascular volume can decrease the hematocrit or hemoglobin levels, these values should be interpreted with the patient's intravascular volume status in mind.

APPROACH TO THE PATIENT

A child who presents with pallor and appears ill could have a **potentially life-threatening illness**. Most patients with **shock** are **pale, lethargic, and often have cool extremities**. After the patient is stabilized, **routine blood work** should be

TABLE 57-3	**Causes of Anemia in Neonates**

Blood Loss
Fetomaternal hemorrhage
Placental abnormalities
    Abruptio placentae
    Placenta previa
Twin-to-twin transfusion
Excessive blood loss caused by a coagulation disorder
Cord abnormalities
Hemorrhage
    Cephalohematomas
    Hepatic hematomas
    Intracerebral hemorrhage
    Delivery trauma involving the placenta, the umbilical cord, or both

Hemolytic Anemia
Blood group incompatibility
Red blood cell membrane or enzyme abnormalities
Hemoglobinopathies
Microangiopathic processes

Hypoplastic Anemia
Infections
    Cytomegalovirus infection
    Syphilis
    Toxoplasmosis
    Rubella
    Severe bacterial infections
Diamond–Blackfan anemia

obtained, including a CBC; serum electrolyte panel; serum BUN, creatinine, and glucose levels; blood culture; and blood type and cross-match. The brief history should **focus on head trauma** and the presence of **seizures, syncope, prior illness, or fever**. A more extensive history should be obtained after the child is stable.

A child who is pale and well appearing should also have a **CBC, reticulocyte count, and a serum chemistry panel, including bilirubin**. If the hemoglobin is low, the reticulocyte count is high, and the indirect bilirubin fraction is high, then a hemolytic anemia is very likely. A **Coombs or direct antibody test** should be obtained to determine whether the hemolysis is immune-mediated.

A **peripheral blood smear** should be examined in all children with anemia. Variations in the RBC shape (poikilocytosis) and size (anisocytosis) should be documented. Laboratory values such as the **MCV and mean corpuscular hemoglobin** should be included in the assessment. The **RBC distribution width** confirms the degree of anisocytosis and is increased in patients with iron-deficiency anemia, SCD, and megaloblastic anemias.

Once the differential diagnosis is narrowed (Figure 57-1), specific tests should be obtained as necessary. For example, iron studies should be obtained for a

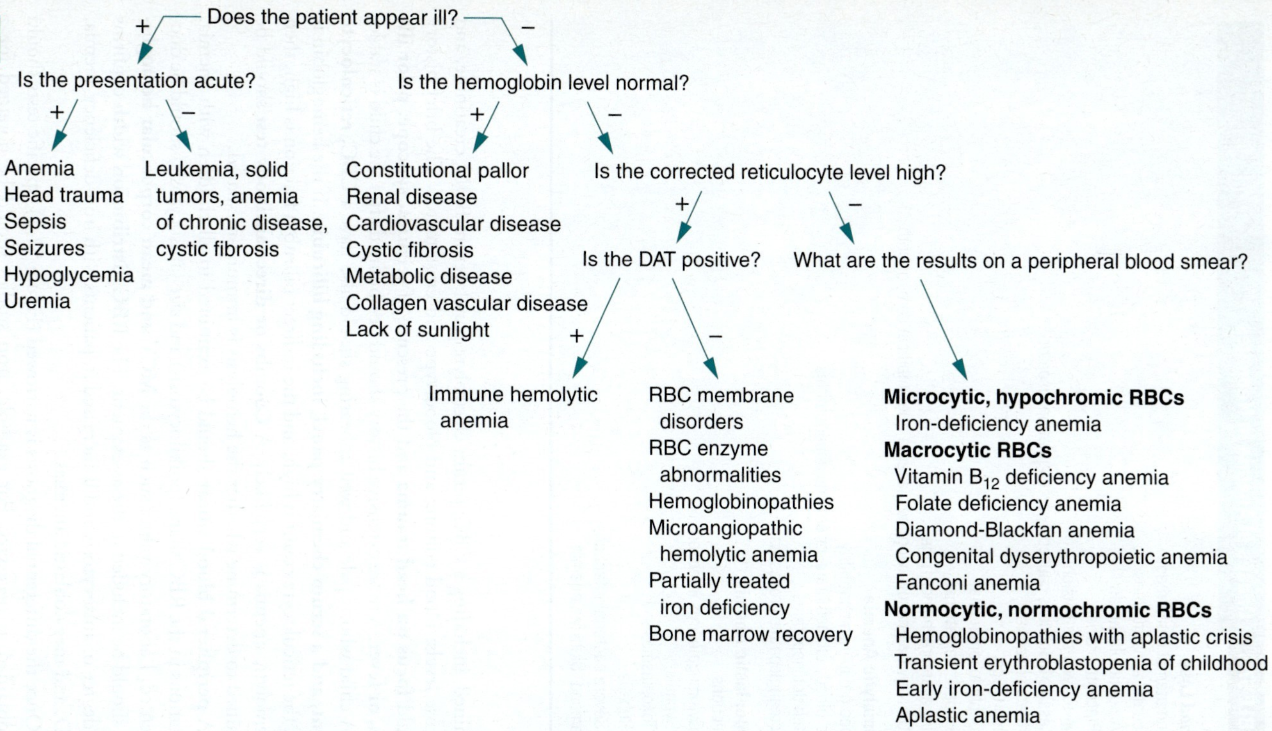

FIGURE 57-1 Evaluation of a patient with pallor. *DAT,* direct antibody test; *RBC,* red blood cell.

Is the presentation acute?

+

Anemia
Head trauma
Sepsis
Seizures
Hypoglycemia
Uremia

— Does the patient appear ill? —

+

Leukemia, solid
tumors, anemia
of chronic disease,
cystic fibrosis

—

Is the hemoglobin level normal?

+

Constitutional pallor
Renal disease
Cardiovascular disease
Cystic fibrosis
Metabolic disease
Collagen vascular disease
Lack of sunlight

—

Is the corrected reticulocyte level high?

+

Is the DAT positive?

+

Immune hemolytic
anemia

—

RBC membrane
disorders
RBC enzyme
abnormalities
Hemoglobinopathies
Microangiopathic
hemolytic anemia
Partially treated
iron deficiency
Bone marrow recovery

—

What are the results on a peripheral blood smear?

Microcytic, hypochromic RBCs
Iron-deficiency anemia
Macrocytic RBCs
Vitamin B_{12} deficiency anemia
Folate deficiency anemia
Diamond-Blackfan anemia
Congenital dyserythropoietic anemia
Fanconi anemia
Normocytic, normochromic RBCs
Hemoglobinopathies with aplastic crisis
Transient erythroblastopenia of childhood
Early iron-deficiency anemia
Aplastic anemia

well-appearing, milk-drinking toddler with a microcytic, hypochromic anemia. Children with a **chronic anemia,** a **severe anemia** with no cause, or an **anemia that is unresponsive** to definitive therapy should be referred to a **pediatric hematologist**.

Suggested Readings

Graham EA. The changing face of anemia in infancy. *Pediatr Rev.* 1994;15:175–183.
Molteni RA. Perinatal blood loss. *Pediatr Rev.* 1990;12:47–54.
Richardson M. Microcytic anemia. *Pediatr Rev.* 2007;28:5–14.
Segel GB, Hirsh MG, Feig SA. Managing anemia in pediatric office practice: part 1. *Pediatr Rev.* 2002;23:75–83.
Segel GB, Hirsh MG, Feig SA. Managing anemia in pediatric office practice: part 2. *Pediatr Rev.* 2002;23:111–121.
Shah S. Pallor. In: Fleisher GR, Ludwig S, eds. *Pediatric Emergency Medicine.* 6th ed. Baltimore: Lippincott, Williams & Wilkins; 2010:483–490.

CHAPTER 58

Lawrence W. Brown

Paraplegia

INTRODUCTION

Paraplegia is any **weakness of the lower extremities** caused by dysfunction of the nervous system at the level of the peripheral nerves, spinal cord, or brain. Some paraplegias have **congenital causes** (tethered cord, syringomyelia, familial spastic paraparesis, spastic diplegia). Those that are **acquired** are grouped by timing of onset:

- **Acute** (evolving over minutes to hours)—trauma, spinal cord infarction
- **Subacute** (evolving over hours to days)—transverse myelitis, viral myelitis, epidural abscess, Guillain–Barré syndrome
- **Chronic** (evolving over weeks to months)—tumors

 DIFFERENTIAL DIAGNOSIS LIST

Infectious Causes
- Epidural abscess
- Viral myelitis
- Diskitis
- Polyradiculoneuropathy
- Tubercular osteomyelitis

Neoplastic Causes
- Astrocytoma
- Ependymoma
- Neuroblastoma
- Other (e.g., glioma, ganglioglioma, meningioma, neurofibroma)

Traumatic Causes
- Contusion
- Transection
- Epidural hematoma

Congenital or Vascular Causes
- Spastic diplegia
- Cord infarction

- Arteriovenous malformation
- Congenital malformations— myelomeningocele, tethered cord, syringomyelia

Genetic/Metabolic Causes
- Familial spastic paraparesis
- Adrenal myeloneuropathy (rarely presents in childhood)

Inflammatory Causes
- Transverse myelitis
- Guillain–Barré syndrome (acute inflammatory demyelinating polyneuropathy)
- Chronic inflammatory demyelinating polyneuropathy

Psychosocial Causes
- Conversion disorder

DIFFERENTIAL DIAGNOSIS DISCUSSION
Trauma
Etiology
Spinal cord injury is usually associated with major force, such as occurs with **significant trauma**. The most common causes of traumatic paraplegia are **motor vehicle accidents and sports-related injuries,** although **gunshot injuries** are increasingly more common. Trauma can result in contusion, acute edema, compression secondary to epidural hematoma, or actual transection.

Clinical Features
Initial examination shows **weak, flaccid muscles, absent reflexes, and sensory loss** below the level of the lesion (spinal shock). **Bowel and bladder dysfunction** is typical. **Autonomic disturbance** (e.g., sweating, piloerection) is usually found below the level of the lesion. Over a period of weeks to months, **flaccidity evolves into spasticity, hyperreflexia, and extensor plantar responses**.

Evaluation
The **neck must be stabilized** in a cervical collar until the stability of the cervical spine is established. **Magnetic resonance imaging (MRI)** should be done to differentiate contusion or transection from epidural hematoma. Plain radiographs or **computed tomography (CT)** of the spine may also be helpful to evaluate for vertebral fractures and dislocations.

Treatment
- **Spinal-dose steroids** (i.e., intravenous methylprednisolone, 30 mg/kg over 1 hour) should be initiated immediately (within 8 hours of injury). The initial dose is followed with 5.4 mg/kg/hour for 24 hours (if treatment is initiated <3 hours after injury) or 48 hours (if treatment is initiated 3 to 8 hours after injury).
- **Neurosurgical intervention** may be required for decompression of epidural hematomas or reduction and stabilization of vertebral fracture.
- **Meticulous supportive care,** including good bowel and bladder management and deep venous thrombosis (DVT) prophylaxis with sequential compression stockings, is essential. Subcutaneous heparin, 5,000 U twice a day, or low-molecular-weight heparin may be added in patients at particularly high risk for DVT.

Spinal Cord Infarction
Etiology
Spinal cord infarction is usually the result of **occlusion** of the **anterior spinal artery,** which supplies blood to the ventral two-thirds of the cord. The most common causes in children are dissection secondary to **trauma, infection, emboli** in patients with cardiac disease, or **thrombosis** in patients with hypercoagulable states.

Clinical Features
Patients with spinal cord infarction present with **flaccid motor paralysis, areflexia, and dissociated sensory loss** (loss of pain and temperature sensation with sparing of vibration and position sense) below the level of arterial occlusion.

Bowel and bladder dysfunction are usual. **Back pain** is sometimes present. Over weeks to months, **flaccidity evolves** into **spasticity,** with hyperreflexia, clonus, and extensor plantar responses.

Evaluation

An **MRI** of the spine should be performed to look for evidence of cord infarction. A **spinal arteriogram** should also be considered. Evaluations for cardiac disease and hypercoagulable states should be performed if there is no obvious cause for the occlusion.

Treatment

Intravenous corticosteroids should be administered early to minimize cord edema, which may result in additional ischemia. **Anticoagulation** should be considered in **selected patients,** including those with hypercoagulable states, cardiogenic emboli, or vascular dissection.

Transverse Myelitis

Etiology

Transverse myelitis is an **acute inflammatory, demyelinating disorder** of the cord. It can occur as a complication of systemic **viral infections** (infectious mononucleosis [Epstein–Barr virus], varicella, mumps, rabies, rubella, rubeola, influenza, HIV) or **bacterial infections** (cat-scratch disease, *Mycoplasma pneumoniae*), **autoimmune disorders** (lupus), **immunizations** (rare), and **multiple sclerosis**.

Clinical Features

The mean age of onset is 9 years. The patient presents with **thoracic back pain, lower extremity numbness, leg weakness** (symmetric or asymmetric), and **progressive urinary retention or incontinence**. Initial findings include weak, flaccid muscles (symmetric or asymmetric); absent reflexes; and sensory loss below the level of the lesion. Optic disc swelling and decreased vision or vision loss are often present in patients with Devic disease (i.e., transverse myelitis accompanied by optic neuritis), although the ocular symptoms may occur after the onset of spinal symptoms. Spasticity, hyperreflexia, clonus, and extensor plantar responses are seen later in the course of the disease.

Evaluation

A **lumbar puncture (LP)** should be performed to check for cerebrospinal fluid (CSF) opening pressure (normal to slightly elevated), protein level (usually increased) and electrophoresis (looking for oligoclonal bands), and cell count (usually a mixed pleocytosis of <200 cells/mm^3). **Spinal MRI** often shows swelling and abnormal signal at the level of the lesion. **Head MRI** should also be performed to look for other areas of demyelination suggestive of MS. **Viral serologies** (including HIV) may be helpful in identifying a triggering viral infection. **Antinuclear antibody panel and complement levels** should be considered as a screen for an autoimmune disorder.

Treatment

Usual therapy is a 3- to 5-day course of **high-dose intravenous methylprednisolone** (15 mg/kg/day, maximum 1 g/day) followed by a **4-week prednisone**

taper. Use of intravenous immunoglobulin is also reported. **Supportive care** and intensive **physical therapy** are critical.

Viral Myelitis
Etiology
Viral myelitis is the **acute segmental infection of anterior horn cells**. Viruses most commonly responsible include poliovirus, group B coxsackievirus, and echoviruses.

Clinical Features
The patient usually has a history of **malaise, myalgias, low-grade fever,** and **upper respiratory tract symptoms progressing to severe headache and nuchal rigidity**. **Areflexia and flaccidity** and weakness of the muscles (usually asymmetric) are often heralded by pain in the spine and affected limbs. **Bulbar weakness** may also be present. There are usually no sensory symptoms.

Evaluation
The **most important diagnostic test is the LP,** which demonstrates pleocytosis (50 to 200 cells/mm^3). The predominance of polymorphonuclear cells is replaced by lymphocytes after the first week. CSF protein may be normal or slightly elevated, and CSF glucose is usually normal. **Viral isolation from CSF, stool, and nasopharyngeal swabs,** as well as **acute and convalescent viral titers,** can help confirm the diagnosis.

Treatment
Treatment of viral myelitis is **supportive**.

Epidural Abscess
Etiology
Epidural abscess is most commonly caused by the hematogenous spread of **bacteria,** usually *Staphylococcus aureus* in older children. The most common location is the **dorsal surface** of the **midthoracic** or **lower lumbar spine**.

Clinical Evaluation
Characteristically, the history includes **severe, localized back pain** (worse with cough or flexion) and **fever,** often associated with **headache, vomiting,** and a **stiff neck**. **Radiating pain** begins 3 to 6 days after the onset of back pain, followed by progressive **paraplegia and bladder dysfunction**. Examination shows localized spinal tenderness, lower extremity hyperreflexia, and spasticity (in patients with thoracic lesions) or hyporeflexia and decreased tone (in patients with lower lumbar lesions).

Evaluation
If epidural abscess is suspected, LP should not be performed because it can result in iatrogenic meningitis. **MRI,** however, is safe and demonstrates the lesion well.

Treatment
Initial treatment is with a **broad-spectrum intravenous antibiotic** with antistaphylococcal activity. Once a specific organism has been identified and sensitivities established, antibiotic therapy can be tailored to the patient. **Surgical drainage** may be required if there is evidence of cord compression.

Guillain–Barré Syndrome

Etiology

Guillain–Barré syndrome is an immune-mediated, acute, **inflammatory demyelinating polyneuropathy**. Approximately 50% of patients with Guillain–Barré syndrome have a history of antecedent viral infection.

Clinical Features

The syndrome can present at any age, but is **uncommon in children <3 years**. Often the first symptoms are **transient dysesthesias and muscle aches**. A typical feature is rapidly progressive, symmetric motor weakness beginning distally and ascending proximally. **Areflexia** is the rule and may precede significant weakness (e.g., biceps and triceps jerks may be lost while the arms are only minimally weak). **Facial weakness** and other cranial nerve involvement may be present in up to half of patients. Weakness can progress to include **respiratory muscles** with resultant hypoventilation. Although mild, symmetric, length-dependent sensory changes are common, extensive sensory loss or a sensory level should not be present. **Autonomic instability** (e.g., unstable blood pressure, cardiac arrhythmia) may occur.

Evaluation

On **LP**, patients with Guillain–Barré syndrome demonstrate **elevated CSF protein** with a paucity of cells (seen after the first week of illness). **Nerve conduction studies** show **reduced nerve conduction velocities and motor conduction block**. **Vital capacity and negative inspiratory potentials** should be monitored closely as indicators of impending respiratory failure.

Treatment

Meticulous **supportive care** (particularly of **respiratory function**) is critical. **Plasmapheresis or intravenous immune globulin** (2 g/kg divided over 2 to 5 days) is indicated if the patient loses the ability to ambulate independently.

 HINT: Initially, it can be very difficult to distinguish transverse myelitis, viral myelitis, epidural abscess, and Guillain–Barré syndrome from one another. It may not be possible to get a good sensory examination in an uncooperative child, and all four disorders can initially present with flaccid weakness and areflexia in the lower extremities. Furthermore, many of the diagnostic tests are not helpful until ~1 week into the course of the disease; for example, nerve conduction studies and CSF protein levels can both be normal for up to 1 week in Guillain–Barré syndrome. Although the following clues may help, ultimately the "tincture of time" and repeating studies after 1 week may be required to make a definitive diagnosis.

- **A high fever, severe back pain or tenderness,** and an **increased peripheral white blood cell count** are suggestive of epidural abscess.
- **Reflexes.** If the reflexes are down in the arms as well as the legs, think Guillain–Barré syndrome. Mild symmetric facial weakness (facial diplegia) and diminished gag reflex may also be present in Guillain–Barré syndrome but should not be seen in a spinal cord process.

- **Distribution of weakness.** The weakness in viral myelitis is often asymmetric, whereas Guillain–Barré syndrome and transverse myelitis usually cause symmetric weakness. In transverse myelitis, there is often a complete, uniform paralysis below the level of the lesion; in Guillain–Barré syndrome, the distal muscles tend to be weaker than the proximal muscles.
- **Bowel and bladder dysfunction** are suggestive of epidural abscess or transverse myelitis first, but remember that patients with Guillain–Barré syndrome occasionally also have bowel and bladder involvement.

Tumors
Etiology
Astrocytomas and ependymomas are the most common intrinsic spinal cord tumors, and **neuroblastoma** is the tumor that most commonly results in extrinsic cord compression (from extension of a paraspinal tumor through the neural foramen).

Clinical Features
Paraplegia caused by tumors presents with **slowly progressive leg weakness, gait difficulty, and sensory loss**. Often there is associated **back pain and bowel and bladder dysfunction**. Findings on physical examination depend on the location of the tumor: Thoracic lesions produce spastic paraplegia with hyperreflexia; tumors involving the conus medullaris and cauda equina produce weak, flaccid muscles with decreased or absent reflexes. **Sensory loss** is present below the level of the tumor. **Scoliosis** is frequently seen in association with intrinsic cord tumors.

Evaluation
Spinal MRI is the diagnostic test of choice for detection of tumors.

Treatment
Initial therapy consists of **dexamethasone** (0.25 mg/kg every 6 hours) to decrease surrounding edema. Definitive treatment depends on the type, extent, and location of the tumor but usually consists of some combination of **surgery, radiation,** and **chemotherapy**.

Tethered Cord
Etiology
In pediatric patients with tethered cord, the **conus medullaris** is **anchored** to the **base of the vertebral column** by a thickened filum terminale, lipoma, dermal sinus, or other site of traction. As the child grows, the spinal cord is stretched and lumbosacral segments become increasingly ischemic.

Clinical Features
Symptoms can occur at any time between infancy and young adulthood. Typical symptoms are **progressive clumsiness of gait, constipation, and urinary incontinence**.

Evaluation
Findings on general examination may include **scoliosis, stunted leg growth, or foot deformity** (*pes cavus*), **pigmentation, tufts of hair,** or a **deep dermal sinus**

over the **lower spine**. On neurologic examination, **spastic leg weakness, hyper-reflexia,** and **extensor plantar responses** are present.

Treatment

Surgery is required to release the cord.

Syringomyelia

Etiology

Syringomyelia is a **cavity within the spinal cord,** usually resulting from a congenital neural tube malformation. This condition most commonly occurs in the cervical and lumbar spinal cord segments.

Clinical Features

Syringomyelia often presents in adolescence or later with **progressive weakness and sensory loss**. Motor examination results depend on the **location of the lesion**. **Cervical lesions** show flaccid paralysis and hyporeflexia of the arms with spasticity and hyperreflexia in the legs; **lumbar lesions** present with flaccid paralysis of the legs with hyporeflexia, fasciculations, and muscle atrophy. Interruption of the **crossing spinothalamic fibers** in the central cord produces a "cape distribution" of pain and temperature sensation loss with relative sparing of light touch and proprioception.

Evaluation

The diagnostic test of choice is an **MRI**.

Treatment

Symptomatic congenital cord malformations are treated **surgically**.

Familial Spastic Paraparesis

Etiology

Familial spastic paraparesis is an **inherited progressive spastic paraparesis**. The genetics are complex, with autosomal dominant transmission seen in 70% of patients, but autosomal recessive transmission and X-linked recessive transmission are also reported. The mean age of onset in childhood type I familial spastic paraparesis is 11 to 16 years.

Clinical Features

Toe walking and slowly progressive gait disturbance are typical. A third of patients present with **urinary symptoms**. On examination, **spasticity** is out of proportion to weakness. **Hyperreflexia** involves all four extremities, and **ankle clonus** may be present. A third of patients have **pes cavus deformity**. The autosomal recessive form can also be associated with ataxia, sensory neuropathy, and pseudobulbar palsy.

Evaluation

Genetic testing for familial spastic paraparesis is of limited clinical utility at present. **Exclusion** of other, treatable disorders is critical. **MRI** of the spine can be useful to rule out structural disorders (e.g., vascular malformation, tumor, syringomyelia) or demyelination. **Vitamin B$_{12}$, vitamin E, and very-long-chain fatty acid levels** should be obtained. Eliciting a **family history** of similarly affected individuals is critical.

Treatment
No specific treatment is available.

Spastic Diplegia
Etiology
In this form of cerebral palsy, **all four extremities** are involved to some degree; however, the lower extremities are affected much more significantly than the upper extremities.

Clinical Features
In early infancy (<4 months of age), muscle tone is usually normal or hypotonic. Between 4 months and 1 year of age, there is an **insidious onset of lower extremity spasticity,** often associated with delay in sitting, crawling, and walking. **Toe walking** is common. On examination, there is **spasticity and hyperreflexia,** involving the legs more than the arms. **Scissoring** of the legs, ankle clonus, and extensor plantar responses are common.

Evaluation
Historical information suggesting premature birth or possible perinatal injury could be significant. **Brain MRI** may demonstrate evidence of periventricular leukomalacia or other evidence of perinatal injury.

Treatment
Supportive therapy often includes **physical and occupational therapy, bracing,** and, if needed, **botulinum toxin injections or surgical release** for treatment of contractures.

EVALUATION OF PARAPLEGIA
Patient History
The history should include the following information:

- Timing of onset of symptoms (acute, subacute, or chronic)
- Trauma
- Fever
- Back pain
- Changes in sensation—if so, in what distribution?
- Bowel and bladder dysfunction
- Visual problems—past or present
- Previous weakness, numbness, or other neurologic symptoms
- Family history of leg weakness

Physical Examination
The following should be sought on physical examination:

- **General examination**—evidence of head, neck, or back trauma; scoliosis; stunted leg growth; foot deformity (pes cavus); or pigmentation, tufts of hair, or a deep dermal sinus over the lower spine.
- **Cranial nerve examination**—look for papillitis (associated with transverse myelitis in Devic disease); eye movement abnormalities (associated with transverse myelitis secondary to MS); Horner syndrome (associated with cervical

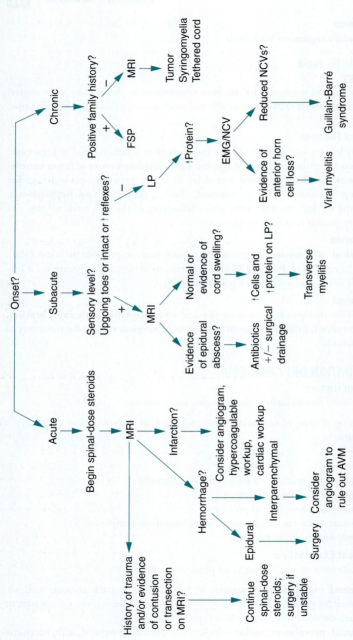

FIGURE 58-1 Evaluation of a patient with paraplegia. *AVM*, arteriovenous malformations; *EMG*, electromyogram; *FSP*, familial spastic paraparesis; *LP*, lumbar puncture; *MRI*, magnetic resonance imaging; *NCVs*, nerve conduction velocities; ↑, increased.

cord trauma); facial diplegia and decreased gag reflex (associated with Guillain–Barré syndrome).
- **Motor strength, tone, and reflexes in arms and legs**—weak, flaccid leg muscles and absent reflexes (associated with acute cord processes and Guillain–Barré syndrome); spasticity, hyperreflexia, and extensor plantar responses (associated with chronic spinal cord processes).
- **Sensation to all sensory modalities**—a sensory level (associated with spinal cord problems); mild distal sensory changes (associated with Guillain–Barré syndrome).
- **Autonomic disturbances**—associated with cord processes (usually found below the level of the lesion) or Guillain–Barré syndrome.

Laboratory Studies and Diagnostic Modalities

The usual workup for a patient with paraplegic symptoms includes an **MRI,** an **electromyogram, nerve conduction velocity studies,** and an **LP**. Several timing factors may cause false-negative results (e.g., CSF protein levels and nerve conduction studies may be normal for up to 1 week in patients with Guillain–Barré syndrome; MRI may not demonstrate cord swelling or signal changes in the first 24 hours in patients with transverse myelitis or cord infarction).

TREATMENT OF ACUTE PARAPLEGIA

If there is any suspicion of cord trauma, the **neck should be stabilized** and spinal-dose **steroids** should be administered. **DVT prophylaxis with sequential compression stockings** is essential. **Subcutaneous heparin,** 5,000 U twice a day, or low-molecular-weight heparin may be added in patients at particularly high risk of DVT but only after hemorrhage is ruled out. Urinary retention is common, so an **indwelling bladder** (Foley) **catheter** should be placed or intermittent bladder catheterizations should be performed. **Histamine blockers** should be administered to prevent gastritis. Autonomic instability may be a problem, so careful monitoring of heart rate and **blood pressure** are essential.

APPROACH TO THE PATIENT

A structured approach to evaluation of a patient with paraplegia is presented in Figure 58-1.

Suggested Readings

de Bot STT, van de Warrenburg BPC, Kremer HPH, et al. Hereditary spastic paraplegia in children. *Neurology.* 2010;75:e75–e79.

Dias MS. Traumatic brain and spinal cord injury. *Pediatr Clin N Am.* 2004;51:271–303.

Hughes RAC, Wijdicks EFM, Barohn R, et al. Practice parameter: immunotherapy for Guillain–Barré syndrome. *Neurology.* 2003;61:736–740.

Pidcock FS, Krishnan C, Crawford TO, et al. Acute transverse myelitis in childhood. *Neurology.* 2007;68:1474–1480.

Renoux C, Vukusic S, Mikaeloff Y, et al. Natural history of multiple sclerosis with childhood onset. *N Engl J Med.* 2007;356:2603–2613.

Sladky JT. Guillain–Barré syndrome in children. *J Child Neurol.* 2004;19:191–200.

Transverse Myelitis Consortium Working Group. Proposed diagnostic criteria and nosology of acute transverse myelitis. *Neurology.* 2002;59:499–505.

Pelvic Pain

INTRODUCTION

Knowledge regarding the location of organs in the female pelvic region and how they may cause discomfort is key to the evaluation of pelvic pain in female patients. There may be distinct causes of pelvic pain depending on the timing and onset of pain. **Acute pelvic pain** is intense with a sudden and sharp onset of short duration. **Chronic pelvic pain** has been present for >6 months and is severe enough to cause functional disability.

DIFFERENTIAL DIAGNOSIS LIST

Acute Pelvic Pain

- Obstetric—ectopic pregnancy, abortion (threatened, missed, or incomplete), and labor
- Gynecologic—endometriosis, adenomyosis, dysmenorrhea, mittelschmerz, pelvic adhesions, ovarian/adnexal torsion, stable/ruptured ovarian cyst, and obstructive Müllerian tract anomaly
- Infectious—endometritis, pelvic inflammatory disease (PID), and tubo-ovarian abscess
- Gastrointestinal—gastroenteritis, appendicitis, Meckel diverticulitis, pancreatitis, inflammatory bowel disease, constipation, volvulus, intestinal obstruction, irritable bowel syndrome, mesenteric adenitis, and regional enteritis
- Genitourinary—cystitis, radiation cystitis, urinary tract infection, pyelonephritis, and ureteral/renal lithiasis
- Musculoskeletal—hernia, back pain, pelvic bone and joint infection, slipped femoral epiphysis, and muscular strain/sprain
- Others—falls, accidents, and sexual abuse

Chronic Pelvic Pain

- Obstetric—pregnancy
- Gynecologic—obstructive Müllerian tract anomaly, cervical stenosis, ovarian tumor, pelvic adhesions, and endometriosis
- Gastrointestinal—hernia, inflammatory bowel disease, irritable bowel syndrome, midgut malrotation, lactose malabsorption, and chronic constipation
- Genitourinary—ureteropelvic junction obstruction, detrusor instability, pelvic kidney, and cystitis
- Musculoskeletal—scoliosis, kyphosis, fibromyalgia, and abdominal wall trigger points
- Neurologic—neurofibromatosis and nerve entrapment syndrome
- Psychological—abuse and emotional stress

DIFFERENTIAL DIAGNOSIS DISCUSSION
Ectopic Pregnancy
Etiology

An ectopic pregnancy is one in which a **fertilized ovum implants itself outside the uterine cavity (most often in the fallopian tube)** as a result of **delayed passage** of the fertilized ovum into the uterine cavity. **Abdominal, cornual, cervical, and ovarian ectopic pregnancies** can also occur. Delayed passage of the fertilized ovum into the uterine cavity usually results from a **condition that interferes with tubal structure or function** (e.g., chronic salpingitis, pelvic adhesive disease, tubal surgery, congenital abnormalities of the fallopian tube).

Clinical Features

The **classic triad of symptoms** consists of **abdominal pain, history of amenorrhea, and new vaginal bleeding,** which is present in about 50% of patients. The abdominal pain may develop **suddenly or gradually**. In **unruptured ectopic pregnancies,** the pain tends to be **unilateral, colicky, and localized** to the involved adnexa. In case of a **rupture,** the pain becomes **diffuse and intense**. **Referred shoulder pain** may occur in the presence of hemoperitoneum. **Dizziness and syncope** are the result of anemia and hypotension.

Evaluation

- **Vital signs.** Vital signs are often within the normal limits. However, with excessive pain and/or blood loss, the patient may be tachycardic. If there has already been significant blood loss, patient may also be hypotensive.
- **Abdominal examination.** Localized tenderness may be revealed in the lower quadrant. With rupture and intra-abdominal bleeding, rebound tenderness and guarding may be elicited. On pelvic examination, the cervix and uterus may be soft and tender from the effects of pregnancy hormones. Adnexal fullness or a discrete, tender mass may be noted in some patients.
- **Complete blood count (CBC).** The hemoglobin and hematocrit values may be low in patients with acute or gradual intraperitoneal hemorrhage; in the absence of bleeding, they are usually normal.
- **Type and screen.** Rh status is assessed in case blood replacement is necessary, and Rh-negative patients who may need Rhogam are identified.
- **A pregnancy test.** A quantitative beta human chorionic gonadotropin (beta-hCG) should be drawn.
- **Vaginal ultrasonography** can detect an intrauterine gestational sac as early as 4 weeks of gestation when the quantitative β-hCG is 1,500 to 2,000 mIU/mL. However, distinguishing between an intrauterine gestational sac and endometrial fluid, sometimes referred to as a pseudosac, can be difficult. A pseudosac can form when an ectopic pregnancy causes changes within the uterus. Therefore, the clinician performing the ultrasound should identify other markers of an intra- or extrauterine pregnancy (i.e., double decidual sign). In addition, the ultrasound may show an adnexal mass or complex free fluid in the pelvis. An adnexal mass seen on ultrasound further substantiates the diagnosis of an ectopic pregnancy. Free fluid in the cul-de-sac seen

on ultrasound suggests hemoperitoneum and the necessity of early surgical intervention.

 HINT: A quantitative β-hCG >2,000 mIU/mL and an empty uterus by vaginal ultrasound is presumptive evidence of an ectopic pregnancy.

Treatment

Surgical diagnosis and treatment via **laparoscopy or laparotomy** is almost always indicated to manage an ectopic pregnancy with a tubal mass ≥3.5 cm. Medical treatment with **methotrexate** can be considered when an intrauterine pregnancy is absent, no adnexal mass is present, or the mass is <3.5 cm in the setting of a positive β-hCG. **Early gynecology consultation** is highly recommended.

Dysmenorrhea

Etiology

- Primary dysmenorrhea is **painful menstruation with no demonstrable cause**. Patients with primary dysmenorrhea have a greater endometrial production of prostaglandins, which cause uterine contractions, uterine ischemia, and pelvic pain.
- **Secondary dysmenorrhea** results from various pathologic conditions (e.g., endometriosis, salpingitis, or congenital Müllerian anomalies).

Clinical Features

Symptoms of **primary dysmenorrhea** usually begin 1 to 2 years after menarche when ovulatory cycles are established. The pain is described as **crampy, lower abdominal pain,** starting within **several hours of the onset of menses**. The pain usually lasts for **2 to 3 days**. Associated symptoms include **headache, nausea, vomiting, diarrhea, and backache**. The symptoms of **secondary dysmenorrhea** are **similar** to those of primary dysmenorrhea, although they develop years after menarche.

Evaluation

In patients with **primary dysmenorrhea,** the **physical examination is normal**. Findings in **secondary dysmenorrhea** are related to the **underlying cause**. A **CBC and screening tests for *Neisseria gonorrhoeae* and *Chlamydia trachomatis*** are obtained to evaluate for possible infection. A **pregnancy test** is obtained to rule out pregnancy. **Pelvic ultrasonography** is useful for delineating the internal pelvic anatomy and evaluation of adnexal pathology. **Magnetic resonance imaging (MRI)** is helpful in the diagnosis of Müllerian abnormalities.

Treatment

If the pelvic examination is normal, treatment is aimed at **symptomatic relief**. **Nonsteroidal anti-inflammatory drugs (NSAIDs)** should be initiated 1 day prior to expected menses and continued for 2 to 3 days. If dysmenorrhea persists, a trial of **combination oral contraceptives (COCs)** may be initiated. **COCs** may also be used continuously to decrease the number of withdrawal bleeds. While irregular spotting may occur with this method, number of bleeding days and symptoms of dysmenorrhea often decrease. **Depot medroxyprogesterone acetate (DMPA),** commonly known as Depo-Provera®, may also improve symptoms in the setting of primary dysmenorrhea. Furthermore, Implanon®, a single subdermal rod impregnated with etonogestrel, has been shown to improve dysmenorrhea due to specific causes of pelvic pain (i.e., endometriosis); thus, Implanon® could be used in this setting. When the pain is refractory to all medical therapy, a **diagnostic laparoscopy** is warranted to evaluate for pelvic pathology, such as endometriosis, adhesions, or ovarian cysts.

Adnexal Torsion

Etiology

Adnexal torsion is the **twisting of a fallopian tube or both the fallopian tube and the ovary on its pedicle**. This may result in **vascular occlusion, ischemia, and tissue death**. Usually, a normal tube or ovary does not "twist" without **predisposing factors** (e.g., ovarian cysts, tumors, tubal neoplasm, parovarian cysts, or pregnancy). The risk of ovarian torsion is greatest if there is an ovarian cyst >5 cm.

Clinical Features

Abdominal pain may develop **suddenly or gradually**. It is usually **paroxysmal and intermittent**. It tends to be **unilateral and localized** to the involved adnexa. If ischemia occurs, the **pain worsens and becomes persistent**. Associated symptoms include **nausea, vomiting, anorexia, and a sense of fullness in the lower abdomen**.

Evaluation

The patient usually appears in **acute distress** and may present with **mild tachycardia** and a **slight elevation of temperature**. The abdominal examination may reveal **tenderness in the iliac fossa**. With increasing ischemia and peritoneal irritation, **guarding, rebound tenderness, and decreased bowel sounds** may be noted. On pelvic examination, a **tender adnexal mass** may be noted.

The white blood cell count is normal or slightly elevated as a marker of an inflammatory process or stress response. Urinalysis is normal. **Pelvic ultrasonography** reveals an **adnexal mass** and Doppler flow may or may not be present, depending if twisting is intermittent.

Treatment

Evidence of an acute surgical abdomen warrants **laparoscopy** and possibly **exploratory laparotomy**. A conservative approach is paramount and every effort should be made to preserve the adnexa. Recent studies have shown that necrotic-appearing ovaries may still be viable and functional. Despite theoretical concerns, studies have not demonstrated an increase in thromboembolic events after untwisting the adnexa.

Ovarian Cysts

Etiology

During puberty, secretion of gonadotropin-releasing hormone from the hypothalamus resumes and **levels of the gonadotropins** (follicle-stimulating hormone and luteinizing hormone) **rise**. The surge in gonadotropins usually is **not cyclical** in adolescents, as it is in adults. The **constant stimulus of gonadotropins on the ovaries results in multiple follicles or cysts** that may range from a few millimeters to 8 cm. Pain is caused by follicular distention, rupture, hemorrhage, ovarian torsion, or peritoneal irritation after rupture.

Clinical Features
Most follicular cysts are **asymptomatic**. **Large follicular cysts** may cause a **vague, constant, dull sensation, or a heaviness in the pelvis**. **Extreme distention with rupture or torsion of the cyst and ovary** may result in **acute, severe pelvic pain**.

Evaluation
Tender, slightly enlarged ovaries may be appreciated. Rarely, a large cystic ovary is identified. A **CBC** is obtained to **rule out rupture and internal hemorrhage**. A **pregnancy test** is ordered to rule out pregnancy. **Pelvic ultrasound** may reveal ovarian cysts or fluid in the cul-de-sac.

Treatment
For **mildly symptomatic** patients, **reassurance** may be all that is necessary. The cyst should be observed using **serial ultrasounds,** typically at 3-month intervals, to monitor for resolution. Most follicular cysts resolve before the first repeat ultrasound; however, it is not uncommon to require several months for cyst resolution. **NSAIDs** may be prescribed for pain management, and **oral contraceptives** to suppress the new cyst formation. **Laparoscopy** is indicated in the presence of a ruptured hemorrhagic cyst accompanied by severe anemia, ovarian torsion, or a persistent cyst, particularly those at risk for torsion.

Congenital Obstructive Müllerian Malformations
Etiology
The differentiation and development of the urogenital system in the embryo and fetus is complex. Developmental errors may occur along this sequential process, resulting in distinctive structural abnormalities. Obstructive Müllerian malformations include **imperforate hymen, transverse vaginal septum, and various types of uterine anomalies**.

Clinical Features
Often obstructive Müllerian abnormalities are **asymptomatic** and not diagnosed **until an adolescent girl presents with primary amenorrhea and recurrent pelvic pain**. The obstruction, leading to **increasing collection of menstrual fluid,** causes **distention of the uterus and vagina** and results in **monthly cyclic pain**.

Evaluation
A **genital or rectal examination** is essential whenever a child complains of pelvic or abdominal symptoms. A **pediatric otoscope or vaginal speculum** (Huffman "virginal," pediatric regular, and pediatric narrow) may be used to visualize the vagina and cervix. The child can be examined in either the **lithotomy or knee-chest position**. An **imperforate hymen** is diagnosed by **simple inspection**. In **infants and children, the hymen** may be **bulging and distended by mucus**.

In **adolescents, menstrual blood fills the vagina**. The **transverse vaginal septum** may be **complete or incomplete** and is recognized on vaginoscopy. Uterine anomalies are more difficult to detect unless an abnormally shaped uterus or pelvic mass is noted on examination.

 HINT: Prior to puberty, rectal examination is often the best method for the evaluation of upper genital tract.

Laboratory studies are nondiagnostic. **Abdominopelvic MRI** is the most useful in the detection of uterine anomalies. Because the embryonic differentiation and development of the urologic system occurs around the same time as that of the genital system, **errors in development of the urologic system** must be sought using **intravenous pyelography**.

Treatment
An imperforate hymen is **opened surgically**. **In infants,** the hymenal membrane is tented and excised centrally with scissors. **In postmenarchal patients,** a portion of the membrane should be excised. In complete transverse vaginal septum, a simple incision is made to allow the egress of secretions in premenarchal patients. The **definitive surgical treatment,** which involves excision of the vaginal septal membrane with a surrounding ring of dense connective tissue, should be **delayed until after puberty** because technical difficulties may be encountered if the surgery is performed on immature structures. **Anomalies of the uterus** (e.g., a blind rudimentary uterine horn) **should not be resected until the patient is postmenarchal**.

Endometriosis
Etiology
Endometriosis is the presence of **endometrial tissue outside of the uterus**. Theories of pathogenesis include retrograde menstruation, direct implantation, coelomic metaplasia, and lymphatic and hematogenous spread. A polygenic multifactorial mode of inheritance has also been demonstrated. The risk of endometriosis is seven times greater if a first-degree relative is affected. The major distinction between endometriosis in adolescents and adults is its **association with congenital anomalies of the reproductive tract in the pubertal patient**. Premenarchal patients are not affected by this disease because the **onset of menses must precede the development of endometriosis**.

Clinical Features
Characteristically, the pelvic pain is described as **cramping in the pelvic or sacral region** that is **aggravated during menstruation**. The pain may also be **intermittent, chronic, and not related to the menstrual cycle**.

Evaluation
Examination under anesthesia may be necessary for an adequate pelvic examination **in the virginal adolescent**. A search for **anomalies of the hymen, vagina,**

cervix, uterus, and adnexa is mandatory. In **older patients,** the finding of **pain on palpation of the adnexa** (i.e., the ovary and fallopian tube), **in the cul-de-sac, or along the uterosacral ligaments** suggests the possibility of endometriosis. Occasionally, **enlargement of the ovary, fixation of the pelvic organs as a result of adhesions,** or decreased mobility of pelvic organs on bimanual exam may be noted.

Screening tests (either endocervical or urine based) for *N. gonorrhoeae* and *C. trachomatis* are obtained to rule out the possibility of pelvic infection. A **pregnancy test** is obtained to rule out pregnancy.

Pelvic ultrasonography is useful when examination is difficult, and indicated when a palpable pelvic mass is noted. **MRI** is helpful in delineating the pelvic anatomy and establishing the diagnosis of congenital Müllerian anomalies. **Diagnostic laparoscopy with visualization and biopsy** of endometrial implants is essential to confirm the diagnosis.

Treatment

NSAIDs remain the first line of medical therapy for pain control; **narcotics** are reserved for severe cases. If pain persists, **COCs** may be prescribed in a continuous fashion to suppress ovulation and promote endometrial atrophy. Alternatively, Depo-Provera® (DMPA) or Implanon® may be administered. DMPA may temporarily cause some decrease in bone mineral density, but most women return to baseline after discontinuation. When medical therapy fails, **laparoscopy** is indicated to **fulgurate, laser vaporize, or excise** endometrial implants and **perform lysis of adhesions**.

Pelvic Inflammatory Disease

Pelvic inflammatory disease is discussed in Chapter 70, "Sexually Transmitted Diseases."

Constipation

Constipation is discussed in Chapter 22, "Constipation."

EVALUATION OF PELVIC PAIN

There are various causes of acute and chronic pelvic pain (Tables 59-1 and 59-2). The most important tool for making the correct diagnosis is a **detailed history,** physical examination, and laboratory and radiographic evaluation. The following information should be sought:

Patient History

- Medical, surgical, sexual, gynecologic history; including method of contraception in postmenarchal patients.
- Psychosocial history (to assess the possibility of stress, substance abuse, or sexual or physical abuse).
- Pain history (mnemonic: **OLD CAARTS**):
  - **O**nset: When and how did the pain start? Did it change over time?
  - **L**ocation: Localize specifically. Can you put a finger on it?

TABLE 59-1 Age-Related Prevalence of Principal Laparoscopic Findings in 121 Adolescent Females 11 to 17 Years Old with Acute Pelvic Pain (The Children's Hospital, Boston, 1980–1986)

Diagnosis	Number of Patients		
	Age 11–13	Age 14–15	Age 16–17
Ovarian cyst	12 (50%)	16 (35%)	19 (37%)
Acute pelvic inflammatory disease	4 (17%)	7 (16%)	10 (19%)
Adnexal torsion	0 (0%)	7 (16%)	2 (4%)
Endometriosis	0 (0%)	2 (4%)	4 (7%)
Ectopic pregnancy	0 (0%)	3 (7%)	1 (2%)
Appendicitis	3 (13%)	4 (9%)	6 (12%)
No pathology	5 (20%)	6 (13%)	10 (19%)
Total	24 (20%)	45 (37%)	52 (43%)

Adapted from Goldstein DP. Acute and chronic pelvic pain. *Pediatr Clin N Am*. 1989;36(3):576.

- **D**uration: How long does it last?
- **C**haracteristics: Cramping, aching, stabbing, burning, tingling, and itching?
- **A**lleviating/**A**ggravating factors: What makes it better (medication, stress reduction, heat/ice, position change) or worse (specific activity, stress, menstrual cycle)?
- **A**ssociated symptoms: Gynecologic—dyspareunia, dysmenorrhea, abnormal bleeding, discharge, and infertility. Gastrointestinal—constipation, diarrhea, bloating, gas, and rectal bleeding. Genitourinary—frequency, dysuria, urgency, and incontinence.
- **R**adiation: Does it move to other areas?

TABLE 59-2 Age-Related Incidence of Laparoscopic Findings in 129 Adolescent Females 11 to 21 Years Old with Chronic Pelvic Pain (The Children's Hospital, Boston, 1980–1983)

Diagnosis	Number of Patients				
	Age 11–13	Age 14–15	Age 16–17	Age 18–19	Age 20–21
Endometriosis	2 (12%)	9 (28%)	21 (40%)	17 (45%)	7 (54%)
Postoperative adhesions	1 (6%)	4 (13%)	7 (13%)	5 (13%)	2 (15%)
Serositis	5 (29%)	4 (13%)	0 (0%)	2 (5%)	0 (0%)
Ovarian cyst	2 (12%)	2 (6%)	3 (5%)	2 (5%)	0 (8%)
Uterine malformation	1 (6%)	0 (0%)	1 (2%)	0 (0%)	1 (0%)
Others	0 (0%)	1 (3%)	2 (4%)	1 (3%)	0 (0%)
No pathology	6 (35%)	12 (37%)	19 (36%)	11 (29%)	3 (23%)

Adapted from Goldstein DP. Acute and chronic pelvic pain. *Pediatr Clin N Am*. 1989;36(3):580.

- **T**emporal: What time of day? Relation to menstrual cycle and activities of daily living?
- **S**everity: Scale of 0 to 10.

Physical Examination

The following should be sought on physical examination:

- Abnormal vital signs
- Structural abnormalities
- The reproduction of pain on palpation of specific abdominopelvic structures
- Signs of peritonitis (guarding, rigidity, rebound tenderness)

Laboratory Studies

In the patient with a suspected acute abdomen, the following laboratory studies should be considered:

- CBC with differential
- Blood electrolytes
- Blood type and screen
- Pregnancy test (β-hCG)
- Urinalysis
- Urine culture
- Testing for *N. gonorrhoeae* and *C. trachomatis*

Radiographic Studies

- Pelvic ultrasound
- Abdominal/pelvic computed tomography scan or MRI (if indicated)

Suggested Readings

Carrico CW, Fenton LZ, Taylor GA, et al. Impact of sonography on the diagnosis and treatment of acute lower abdominal pain in children and young adults. *Am J Roentgenol.* 1999;172(2):513–516.

Goldstein DP. Acute and chronic pelvic pain. *Pediatr Clin N Am.* 1989;365:573–580.

Harel Z, Johnson CC, Gold MA, et al. Recovery of bone mineral density in adolescents following the use of depot medroxyprogesterone acetate contraceptive injections. *Contraception.* 2010;81(4):281–291.

Khoiny FE. Pelvic inflammatory disease in the adolescent. *J Pediatr Health Care.* 1989;3(5):230–236.

Laufer MR, Goitein L, Bush M, et al. Prevalence of endometriosis in adolescent girls with chronic pelvic pain not responding to conventional therapy. *J Pediatr Adolesc Gynecol.* 1997;10:199–202.

Propst AM, Laufer MR. Endometriosis in adolescents: incidence, diagnosis, and treatment. *J Reprod Med.* 1999;44:751–758.

Sanfilippo JS. Dysmenorrhea in adolescents. *Female Patient.* 1993;18:29–33.

Seeber BE, Barnhart KT. Suspected ectopic pregnancy. *Obstet Gynecol.* 2006;107(2):399–413.

Vercellini P, Fedele L, Arcaini L, et al. Laparoscopy in the diagnosis of chronic pelvic pain in adolescent women. *J Reprod Med.* 1989;34(10):827–830.

Pleural Effusions

INTRODUCTION

A pleural effusion is an **accumulation of fluid between the parietal and visceral pleura**. Normally, fluid is produced by the capillaries of the parietal pleura and absorbed by the capillaries of the visceral pleura; only a trivial amount of fluid is left within the pleural space. The Starling relationship governs the net flow of fluid at each capillary bed:

$$F = k[(\boldsymbol{P}_{cap} - \boldsymbol{P}_{pl})] - \sigma(P_{cap} - P_{pl})]$$

where

F is the rate of fluid movement
$\boldsymbol{P}$ is the hydrostatic pressure
P is the oncotic pressure
k is the filtration coefficient
σ is the osmotic reflection coefficient for protein

A larger difference between capillary and pleural hydrostatic pressure, or a smaller difference between capillary and pleural oncotic pressure, results in a larger amount of fluid left in the pleural space. Lymphatic drainage normally removes excess fluid from the pleural space. Accumulation of a pleural effusion may result from **increased capillary hydrostatic pressure, decreased hydrostatic pressure in the pleural space, decreased capillary oncotic pressure, capillary leak, lymphatic obstruction, movement of fluid from the peritoneal space,** or a combination of these factors.

Pleural effusions are classified according to their etiology as **transudative or exudative**. Pleural fluid analysis can often distinguish a transudate from an exudate and serves as the first step in the differential diagnosis.

- **Transudative effusions** are usually secondary to increased capillary hydrostatic pressure or decreased capillary oncotic pressure. The most common etiology of a transudative effusion is congestive heart failure.
- **Exudative effusions** are typically seen in diseases that injure the capillary membrane, result in increased capillary permeability, or impair lymphatic drainage. A broad differential diagnosis is implied by an exudative effusion and may require more extensive workup.

DIFFERENTIAL DIAGNOSIS LIST

Transudative Effusion
- **Cardiac**
  - Congestive heart failure
  - Increased pulmonary arterial pressure
  - Superior vena caval obstruction
  - Constrictive pericarditis
- **Pulmonary**
  - Acute atelectasis
- **Hepatic**
  - Cirrhosis
  - Hypoalbuminemia
- **Renal**
  - Peritoneal dialysis
  - Nephrotic syndrome
- **Iatrogenic**
  - Extravasation from subclavian or jugular central venous lines into the pleural space
- **Endocrine**
  - Hypothyroidism

Exudative Effusions
- **Infectious**
  - Bacterial infection (Most common—*Streptococcus pneumoniae, Staphylococcus aureus*)
  - Viral infection (Most common—*Adenovirus*)
  - Mycoplasma infection
  - Fungal infection
  - Parasitic infection
- **Neoplastic**
  - Hematologic neoplasm
  - Cervical teratoma
  - Pleural mesothelioma
  - Pheochromocytoma
- Wilms tumor
- Metastatic sarcoma—Ewing sarcoma, rhabdomyosarcoma, and clear cell sarcoma
- Squamous cell carcinoma
- Bronchogenic carcinoma
- **Gastrointestinal Disease**
  - Esophageal rupture
  - Sub-diaphragmatic abscess
  - Pancreatic pseudocyst
  - Acute pancreatitis
  - Intrahepatic abscess
- **Pulmonary Disease**
  - Pulmonary embolism
  - Acute respiratory distress syndrome
  - Chronic atelectasis
  - Hemothorax
- **Collagen Vascular Disease**
  - Rheumatologic—rheumatoid arthritis, systemic lupus erythematosus, sarcoidosis, and Wegener granulomatosis
  - Sjögren syndrome
- **Lymphatic**
  - Traumatic chylothorax
  - Obstruction of lymphatic drainage
  - Congenital lymphangiectasis
  - Noonan syndrome
  - Lymphedema
- **Iatrogenic**
  - Radiation therapy
  - Surgery
  - Esophageal sclerotherapy
  - Extravasation from subclavian or jugular central venous lines

DIFFERENTIAL DIAGNOSIS DISCUSSION
If the etiology of the effusion is unclear, the distinction should be made between a transudate and an exudate by thoracentesis and pleural fluid analysis.

Transudative Effusions

Transudative effusions usually **resolve with treatment of the underlying disease process**.

Exudative Effusions: Infectious Causes
Parapneumonic Effusions

A parapneumonic effusion is any effusion that occurs in the **presence of pneumonia, lung abscess, or bronchiectasis**. Between 50% and 70% of the pleural effusions in hospitalized children are parapneumonic.

Bacterial Infections

The most common bacterial causes of parapneumonic pleural effusions and empyema are *Staphylococcus aureus, Streptococcus pneumoniae, and Streptococcus pyogenes. Streptococcus pneumoniae* is becoming less common now that the conjugated vaccine is given to all immunized children. *Haemophilus influenza* type B was a major cause of infection in the preimmunization era. Oral anaerobes can be causal in neurologically impaired children. Gram-negative rods are seen in neonates and chronically ventilated children.

A minority of bacterial parapneumonic effusions progress to an **empyema,** leading to **deposition of fibrin** in the pleural space and loculation of the effusion. Loculation of the effusion makes clearance of infection difficult and ultimately results in the development of a fibroblast "peel" on the visceral and parietal pleural surfaces. Parapneumonic effusions are classified as **uncomplicated,** those that will resolve with systemic antibiotic therapy alone, and **complicated,** those that require drainage for resolution. Pleural fluid analysis can be helpful in predicting the parapneumonic effusions that are likely to be complicated.

Viral Infections

Pleural effusions occur in 10% to 15% of patients with viral lower respiratory tract infections. **Adenoviral infection** is the most common cause of virus-related effusions. Effusions rarely occur with influenza, cytomegalovirus, herpes simplex virus, Epstein–Barr virus, or hepatitis virus infections. An effusion usually **resolves spontaneously** within a few weeks.

Other Causes

Table 60-1 lists the frequency of various causes of a pleural effusion in two hospital-based series.

APPROACH TO THE PATIENT WITH PLEURAL EFFUSION
Physical Examination

The clinical findings in a patient with a pleural effusion vary, depending on the size and cause of the effusion. With small effusions, patients may be asymptomatic or have a cough, chest pain, fever, or a combination of the three. Patients with moderate effusions may develop shallow, rapid respirations as the lung becomes compressed. With large effusions, cyanosis may be seen as intrapulmonary

TABLE 60-1	Causes of Pleural Effusions in Hospitalized Children	
	Alkrinawi and Chernick[a] n = 127	**Hardie et al.[b] n = 210**
Cause	**Number (%)**	**Number (%)**
Parapneumonic	64 (51%)	143 (68%)
Congenital heart disease	22 (17%)	23 (11%)
Malignancy	13 (10%)	10 (5%)
Renal	11 (9%)	
Liver failure		7 (3%)
Trauma	9 (7%)	
Sickle cell disease		7 (3%)
Ruptured appendix		6 (3%)
Miscellaneous	8 (6%)	14 (7%)

[a]Alkrinawi S, Chernick V. Pleural fluid in hospitalized pediatric patients. *Clin Pediatr.* 1993;35:5–9.
[b]Hardie W, BoKulic R, Garcia VF, et al. Pneumococcal pleural empyemas in children. *Clin Infect Dis.* 1996;22:1057–1063.

shunting occurs. Examination of the chest reveals decreased breath sounds and dullness to percussion on the affected side. If the lung is compressed by the effusion, egophony ("E to A" changes) may also be noted.

Diagnostic Modalities

In chest radiographs, pleural fluid is best seen on an upright postero-anterior and lateral films or a decubitus film. A supine film may show only a hazy lung field. With small effusions, only blunting of the costophrenic angle may be seen. As fluid accumulates, the hemithorax begins to opacify. On a lateral decubitus film, as little as 50 mL fluid can be seen. If the opacity does not layer out, a loculated effusion, empyema, or lobar consolidation should be considered. An ultrasound or computed tomography scan may be useful in distinguishing consolidation from effusion and identifying loculations within the fluid.

Laboratory Studies

Thoracentesis and Pleural Fluid Analysis

Thoracentesis should be performed if the cause of the effusion is unclear, to determine the need for drainage in a parapneumonic effusion, or if the pleural effusion is causing respiratory distress with impairment of oxygenation and/or ventilation. If the **effusion is small or loculated, ultrasound or computed tomography–guided thoracentesis** may be necessary.

Classification of Transudates Versus Exudates

Pleural fluid should be sent for analysis of pH, lactate dehydrogenase (LDH), and total protein with concurrent determination of serum LDH and total protein. If there is a concern for a chylothorax, the fluid should be sent for a white blood cell

TABLE 60-2	Other Pleural Fluid Studies That May Be Helpful in the Differential Diagnosis of an Exudate
Test	**Comments**
White blood cell count and differential	Lymphocyte predominance in neoplastic processes, tuberculosis, chylothorax, or certain fungal infections Segmented neutrophil predominance in bacterial infections, connective tissue disease, pancreatitis, or pulmonary infarction Eosinophil count may be elevated in patients with bacterial infections, a neoplastic process, or a connective tissue disease
Red blood cell count	Red blood cell count >100,000/mm^3: consider trauma, neoplasia, or pulmonary infarction
Microbiologic studies • Gram stain and fluid culture for aerobes and anaerobes • Acid-fast bacillus smear and culture • Viral culture • Fungal culture	Consider the clinical context
Cytology	May reveal malignant cells
Rheumatoid factor, lupus erythematosus preparation, and antinuclear antibody levels	Useful if a collagen vascular disorder is suspected
Amylase	Elevated in pancreatitis or esophageal rupture
Triglycerides	>110 mg/dL in chylothorax
Cholesterol	May be markedly elevated in certain inflammatory conditions, especially tuberculosis and rheumatoid arthritis

count with differentiation. Light's criteria define an effusion as an exudate if it fulfills at least one of the following criteria. In adult studies, this definition is 98% sensitive and 83% specific for an exudate.

- Pleural fluid protein-to-serum protein ratio >0.5
- Pleural fluid LDH >200 IU/L
- Pleural fluid-to-serum LDH ratio >0.6

Table 60-2 lists other studies that may be helpful in the differential diagnosis of an exudate.

Unexplained exudates require further workup beyond the scope of this chapter.

TREATMENT OF PLEURAL EFFUSION

In all cases, the underlying disease-stimulating effusion formation should be treated. The patient's respiratory status should be monitored closely. If the effusion significantly compromises the patient's respiratory status, **therapeutic thoracentesis or chest tube placement** is indicated. Rarely, **pleurodesis with a sclerotic agent** (e.g., talc or tetracycline) is used to fibrose the two pleural linings to prevent fluid from accumulating. **The management of parapneumonic effusions has attracted much attention because of the risk of empyema, and variations in the management approach exist.**

An uncomplicated parapneumonic effusion is defined as one that will resolve only with systemic antibiotic therapy.

A complicated parapneumonic effusion requires chest tube or surgical drainage for resolution.

A chest ultrasound should be obtained to evaluate for loculation. Diagnostic thoracentesis may be helpful. A pleural fluid pH <7.0, glucose >40 mg/dL, or LDH >1,000 UI/L predicts a complicated effusion and is an indication for tube drainage. In addition, a positive Gram stain or culture is an indication for tube drainage. Importantly, *British Thoracic Society Guidelines* do not rely on biochemical parameters but recommend tube drainage of any significant pleural effusion associated with infection. Fibrinolytics, **video-assisted thoracoscopic debridement, or open drainage** is used for patients with loculated effusions or for those who do not respond to tube drainage. Some authors advocate earlier, more universal use of fibrinolytics or video-assisted thoracoscopic debridement in complicated parapneumonic effusion, but this approach remains controversial. **Surgical decortication** has been used in the organized stage of empyema.

Suggested Readings

Gene CL, Curtis A, Deslauriers J, et al. Medical and surgical treatment of parapneumonic effusions: an evidence based guideline. *Chest.* 2000;118:1158–1171.

Jahani IA, Fakhoury K. Management and prognosis of parapneumonic effusion and empyema in children. www.uptodate.com, Accessed November 28, 2007.

Montgomery M, Sigalet D. Air and liquid in the pleural space. In: Chernick V, Boat TF, eds. *Kendig's Disorders of the Respiratory Tract in Children.* 7th ed. Philadelphia, PA: WB Saunders; 2006:368–387.

Wong CL, Holroyd-Leduc J, Straus SE. Does this patient have a pleural effusion? *JAMA.* 2009;301(3):309–317.

Precocious Puberty

INTRODUCTION
Normal Pubertal Development
Girls

In girls, **puberty** usually begins at 10.5 to 11 years with a range of **9 to 11 years**. **Breast development (thelarche)** is usually the **first sign** of normal sexual development; however, in a small number of girls, pubic hair development may precede breast development by 6 months. **Pubic hair development (adrenarche)** usually **follows thelarche** by 6 months and **axillary hair** 12 to 18 months later. The **growth spurt occurs early** in pubertal development in girls at a mean age of 11.5 years (between Tanner stages 2 to 3; see Chapter 2, "The Physical Examination," Table 2-6). **Menses (menarche)** begin 18 to 24 months after thelarche and become ovulatory in most girls within 18 months. Puberty is completed within 1.5 to 6 years. Pubertal growth in girls contributes 25 cm to overall height.

Breast development and cornification of the vaginal mucosa are controlled primarily by **ovarian estrogens,** which are influenced by follicle-stimulating hormone (FSH). Pubic and axillary hair growth is stimulated primarily by **adrenal androgens,** although there may also be an ovarian contribution.

Boys

In boys, puberty usually begins at 11.5 to 12 years with a range of **10 to 14 years**. **Testicular enlargement** occurs first, followed by the **development of pubic hair** ~6 months later. **Phallic enlargement** usually begins 12 months after testicular size begins to increase. The pubertal **growth spurt** in boys occurs between Tanner stages 3 and 4, with progression of male pubertal development occurring over 2 to 4.5 years (see Chapter 2, "The Physical Examination," Table 2-5). The average growth during puberty is 28 cm. Onset of **spermatogenesis** occurs early in puberty with the mean age of conscious ejaculation of 13.5 years (range 12.5 to 15.5 years).

The virilizing changes seen at puberty are mainly the result of **testosterone secretion** from the testes. Growth of the penis and pubic hair are stimulated primarily by **testicular androgens;** however, **adrenal androgens** also contribute. Luteinizing hormone (LH) stimulates Leydig cell production of testosterone, whereas FSH supports spermatogenesis. It is now clear that peripheral **conversion of testosterone to estrogen** is important in bone growth and maturation in males.

Precocious Puberty

Precocious puberty is defined as the development of secondary sexual characteristics at <6 years of age in African-American girls and at <7 years of age in white American girls, and at <9 years of age in boys regardless of race. These age limits in girls are based on a large study completed in 1997 within the Pediatric Research in the Office Setting network. This recommendation has been somewhat controversial because Tanner staging of breast development was done visually and not by palpation. With increasing obesity in the pediatric population, it has been argued that their data may have been skewed because of the inability to distinguish fat from true breast tissue by inspection only. Two recently published longitudinal studies have confirmed these data (see Suggested Readings). Many experts still recommend evaluation, including magnetic resonance imaging (MRI) of the head, in girls with premature onset of puberty at >6 years of age if the tempo of pubertal progression is unusually rapid, bone age is advanced by >2 years of age, or predicted height is <150 cm; or if neurologic signs or symptoms are detected. Precocious puberty is classified as either **central (gonadotropin-dependent)** precocious puberty (CPP), which is caused by an elevation of FSH and LH, or **peripheral (gonadotropin-independent)** precocious puberty (PPP), which is caused by an elevation of sex steroids.

 DIFFERENTIAL DIAGNOSIS LIST

Central (Gonadotropin-Dependent) Precocious Puberty (CPP)

- **Infectious Causes**
  - Brain abscess
  - Meningitis—viral or bacterial
  - Encephalitis
  - Granulomatous disease
  - Tuberculosis, sarcoidosis, or histiocytosis
- **Toxic Causes**
  - Chronic exogenous androgen or estrogen exposure (initially presenting as PPP)
- **Brain Tumor**
  - Glioma
  - Astrocytoma
  - Ependymoma
  - Hypothalamic hamartoma
- **Brain Injury**
  - Head trauma
  - Brain surgery
  - Cranial irradiation
  - Hemorrhage and stroke

- **Congenital Causes**
  - Central nervous system (CNS) malformation
  - Suprasellar cyst
  - Hydrocephalus
  - Idiopathic precocious puberty
  - Constitutional precocious puberty

Peripheral (Gonadotropin-Independent) Precocious Puberty (PPP)

- **Toxic Causes**
  - Exogenous estrogens—face creams, breast-enlarging creams, contraceptive pill, and vaginal creams
  - Excess ingestion of phytoestrogens in soy products
  - Exogenous androgens—transdermal testosterone gel and anabolic steroid abuse

- **Neoplastic Causes**
  - **Boys**
    - Human chorionic gonadotropin (hCG)-secreting tumors—brain and liver choriocarcinomas
    - Leydig cell tumor
    - Virilizing adrenal tumor
  - **Girls**
    - Ovarian tumors
    - Adrenal tumors

- **Congenital Causes**
  - Congenital adrenal hyperplasia (CAH)
  - Familial gonadotropin-independent Leydig cell maturation—testotoxicosis
  - McCune–Albright syndrome
  - Ovarian follicular cysts

DIFFERENTIAL DIAGNOSIS DISCUSSION
Central (Gonadotropin-Dependent) Precocious Puberty
Etiology

Central precocious puberty, or true precocious puberty, refers to sexual precocity **secondary to elevations in the gonadotropins (FSH and LH)**. CPP arises from early activation of the hypothalamic–pituitary–gonadal axis. CPP is investigated five times more often in girls than in boys.

In most cases of CPP, especially in girls, **no cause is identified** (idiopathic precocious puberty). The younger the onset, the more likely an etiological factor will be found. Other cases involve various forms of **CNS pathology,** including malformations and benign or malignant tumors. **Hamartomas of the tuber cinereum** are the CNS tumors most frequently identified as causing precocious puberty. These tumors contain ectopic gonadotropin-releasing hormone (GnRH) neurosecretory cells. The pulsatile release of GnRH from these cells stimulates the pituitary gland. These hamartomas may be associated with gelastic (involving emotional features) seizures. CPP has also developed after **cranial irradiation therapy** for CNS tumors and after **head trauma**. Children with malformations of the CNS, such as septo-optic dysplasia and hydrocephalus, also have an increased incidence of precocious puberty.

Clinical Features

As with children progressing through normal puberty, the first physiologic change is an increase in the amplitude and frequency of hypothalamic GnRH pulses. This causes **increased FSH and LH secretion** from the pituitary gland, **maturation of the gonads, and increased release of sex steroids**.

Evaluation

Boys have pubertal FSH and LH levels, a pubertal response to GnRH, and a pubertal value of **testosterone**. **Girls** have pubertal FSH and LH levels, a pubertal response to GnRH, and a pubertal value of **estradiol** (see Tables 61-1 and 61-2). The diagnosis of **CPP in boys is almost always serious** and necessitates a search for a **CNS tumor**. Unfortunately, GnRH, which was considered the gold standard stimulation test for diagnosis of CPP, is no longer available. Alternative methods of diagnosis include stimulation tests using nafarelin or leuprolide, ultrasound evidence of ovarian and uterine enlargement, and ultrasensitive assays for LH and estradiol.

TABLE 61-1	Normal Ranges for Gonadotropin and Sex Steroid Levels: Females			
	LH (mIU/mL)	FSH (mIU/mL)	Estradiol (ng/dL)	Testosterone (ng/dL)
0–1 yr	0.02–7.0	0.24–14.2	0.5–5.0	<10
Prepubertal	0.02–0.3	1.0–4.2	<1.5	<3–10
Tanner 2	0.02–4.7	1.0–10.8	1.0–2.4	7.0–28
Tanner 3	0.10–12.0	1.5–12.8	0.7–6.0	15–35
Tanner 4	0.4–11.7	1.5–11.7	2.1–8.5	13–32
Tanner 5	0.4–11.7	1.0–9.2	3.4–17.0	20–38
Adult	—	—	—	10–55
Follicular phase	2.0–9.0	1.8–11.2	3.0–10.0	—
Midcycle	18.0–49	6.0–35.0	—	—
Luteal phase	2.0–11.0	1.8–11.2	7.0–30.0	…

FSH, follicle-stimulating hormone; *LH,* luteinizing hormone.

Treatment

CNS tumors associated with CPP are rarely completely resectable because of their proximity to vital structures. Therefore, a **joint medical and surgical approach** is required. Usually a **biopsy** is performed and treatment is determined based on the results.

Hamartomas of the tuber cinereum are benign tumors of the hypothalamus that are usually asymptomatic, except for causing precocious puberty and gelastic seizures. Surgical treatment is not indicated for these hamartomas; treatment is directed at **medically halting the puberty**.

The treatment of choice for CPP is a **synthetic GnRH agonist,** which, when administered chronically, suppresses gonadotropin secretion and gonadal steroid

TABLE 61-2	Normal Ranges for Gonadotropin and Sex Steroid Levels: Males			
	LH (mIU/mL)	FSH (mIU/mL)	Estradiol (ng/dL)	Testosterone (ng/dL)
0–1 yr	0.02–7.0	0.16–4.1	1.0–3.2	<10
Prepubertal	0.02–0.3	0.26–3.0	<1.5	<3–10
Tanner 2	0.2–4.9	1.8–3.2	0.5–1.6	18–150
Tanner 3	0.2–5.0	1.2–5.8	0.5–2.5	100–320
Tanner 4	0.4–7.0	2.0–9.2	1.0–3.6	200–620
Tanner 5	0.4–7.0	2.6–11.0	1.0–3.6	350–970
Adult	1.5–9.0	2.0–9.2	0.8–3.5	350–1030

FSH, follicle-stimulating hormone; *LH,* luteinizing hormone.

output. Several different forms of GnRH analogs are available, including long-acting forms that can be administered monthly. In 2007, a subdermal implant containing histrelin was approved for treatment of CPP after a multicenter study. The implant needs to be replaced annually and is as effective as the monthly injections of GnRH analogs.

Peripheral (Gonadotropin-Independent) Precocious Puberty
Etiology
The secondary sexual development in PPP results from circulating sex steroids that originate independently of gonadotropin stimulation. Possible sources of sex steroids are the following:

- The **gonads** (e.g., ovarian cysts, ovarian tumors, testicular tumors)
- The **adrenal glands** (e.g., CAH, adrenal tumors)
- **Exogenous administration** in the form of estrogen creams, birth control pills, or anabolic steroids

Isosexual precocity occurs when the hormonal changes are consistent with gender (e.g., excess estrogens in a female), and **heterosexual precocity** occurs when the hormonal changes are of the opposite gender (e.g., adrenal carcinoma-producing androgens in a female).

PPP may develop in boys via **autonomous secretion of sex steroids** or as a result of **hCG secretion,** which stimulates testosterone secretion from the Leydig cells. **Autonomous androgen secretion** can result from adrenal 21-hydroxylase deficiency or 11-β-hydroxylase deficiency, adrenal carcinomas, interstitial cell tumors of the testes, or premature Leydig cell maturation. **Tumors that secrete hCG** include hepatomas; hepatoblastomas; teratomas; chorioepitheliomas of the gonads, mediastinum, retroperitoneum, or pineal gland; and germinomas of the pineal gland.

PPP can develop in girls from **ovarian or adrenal estrogen secretion** or from **exogenous estrogen**. Follicular ovarian cysts, granulosa cell tumors, gonadoblastomas, lipoid tumors, and ovarian carcinomas can all secrete estrogen.

Importantly, certain forms of PPP, such as poorly controlled CAH, can eventually activate the hypothalamic–pituitary–gonadal axis and, therefore, initiate true precocious puberty via central mechanisms.

Clinical Features
The hypothalamic–pituitary–gonadal axis has not been activated and, therefore, the sexual characteristics that are manifested are limited to those stimulated by the elevated sex steroid level (e.g., breast development following estrogen production). Adrenal tumors can produce excessive androgens or estrogens, resulting in **virilization or feminization**. Ovarian abnormalities can also produce both androgens and estrogens. The classical features of PPP in boys are **development of the penis without testicular enlargement**.

Evaluation
If sex steroid levels are elevated but gonadotropin levels are decreased, the diagnosis is likely PPP. LH cross-reacts with hCG on some radioimmunoassays; therefore, **measurement of hCG** along with **LH, FSH, and testosterone** should be

done to rule out an hCG-secreting tumor in boys. An **ultrasound evaluation** of the pelvis should be performed if ovarian pathology is suspected.

Treatment

Treatment of PPP is dictated by the cause. In the case of steroid-producing tumors, **surgery, chemotherapy,** or both may be indicated. PPP has been treated with **ketoconazole** (steroidogenesis inhibitor), **tamoxifen,** and a combination of **spironolactone** (androgen receptor inhibitor) **and testolactone and anastrozole** (aromatase inhibitors).

Premature Adrenarche
Etiology

Premature adrenarche, the **isolated appearance of sexual hair** at <6 or 7 years of age in girls and at 9 years of age in boys, is the most common cause of premature pubic hair development. Premature adrenarche, which is more common in girls, is a **benign condition** that appears to be secondary to premature increased secretion of adrenal androgens or increased end-organ sensitivity, or both.

Clinical Features

Affected children may have only pubic hair, or they may also have **axillary hair, acne, perspiration, and body odor**. There is no premature growth spurt. Girls do not have associated clitoromegaly. **Repeat observation** is the most important evaluation and diagnostic tool.

Evaluation

The need for laboratory studies is dictated by the **degree of concern** raised by the results of complete and repeated examinations and by the **bone age**. Premature adrenarche is usually slowly progressive. Dehydroepiandrosterone sulfate levels are modestly elevated in patients with premature adrenarche. Plasma levels of gonadotropin and gonadal steroids are normal. Measurements of 17-α-hydroxyprogesterone, androstenedione, and testosterone are indicated to differentiate premature adrenarche from true precocious puberty (in boys) and from adrenal tumors or adrenal hyperplasia (in boys and girls). The bone age is often mildly advanced, but not significantly. Beware of the patient with **rapidly progressive pubic hair development and normal bone age**. This may suggest an aggressive androgen-producing tumor.

Treatment

Because of no other long-term sequelae except progression into central puberty, **observation** is the only necessary treatment. However, there is data that links premature adrenarche with later development of hyperandrogenic states such as polycystic ovarian syndrome. Therefore, it is important to follow these girls into the later stages of puberty to monitor for the development of irregular menses, hirsutism, and acne.

Premature Thelarche
Etiology

Premature thelarche refers to **isolated breast development,** which usually appears in the first 3 years of life. It is felt to be secondary to episodic formation of ovarian cysts or increased sensitivity of the breasts to estradiol.

Clinical Features

Affected children have **unilateral or bilateral** premature breast development. There are **no other signs of estrogen effect** or precocious puberty (e.g., vaginal cornification, pubic hair, or growth spurt).

Evaluation

As with premature adrenarche, **regular examinations** for several months should precede any laboratory or radiologic evaluations. **Plasma levels of FSH, LH, and estradiol** should be obtained if significant progression or signs of other estrogen effects develop with repeat observations. Gonadotropin levels, estradiol levels, and bone age are usually normal. **Continued observation** is necessary because this may be the first sign of CPP or PPP.

Treatment

Because of no long-term sequelae, **observation** is the only necessary treatment.

EVALUATION OF PRECOCIOUS PUBERTY

Patient History

The following information should be sought:

- History of accelerated growth
- Behavioral changes
- CNS infections or trauma
- Use of steroid medications

Family History of Precocious Puberty

> **HINT:** Ask specifically about the presence of estrogen- or testosterone-containing preparations in the house.

Physical Examination

- Breast, genital, and sexual hair development should be carefully assessed and Tanner staged.
- Special measuring devices such as testicular volume beads (Prader orchidometer) may be useful.
- Skin should be examined for acne, oiliness, and hirsutism (signs of androgen secretion), and also for café-au-lait spots (McCune–Albright syndrome).
- Funduscopic and neurologic evaluations should be performed to investigate the possibility of intracranial lesions.

Laboratory Studies

Initial laboratory and radiologic evaluations should be guided by the history and physical examination findings. In general, **blood work** should include determination of LH, FSH, estradiol, testosterone, and adrenal steroid levels. If these initial studies are abnormal or equivocal, **provocative testing with synthetic GnRH or leuprolide** may be indicated. Normal pubertal children and children with true precocious puberty have a mature LH response to exogenous GnRH administration. Normal ranges for gonadotropin and sex steroid levels are presented in Table 61-1 (girls) and Table 61-2 (boys). β-hCG should be measured in boys with signs of puberty. Thyroid function tests should also be drawn as hypothyroidism can be associated with CPP.

Imaging Studies

The **bone age** should be determined. If indicated, **ultrasound of the ovaries and adrenal glands** should be performed. The need for additional studies, such as an **MRI scan** of the head to investigate the cranial cavity and pituitary fossa, is dictated by the results of these initial studies.

> **HINT:** Small cysts on the ovaries are not uncommon in girls who have no clinical evidence of puberty.

APPROACH TO THE PATIENT

Treatment options for precocious puberty are dictated by the cause. However, while the inciting cause of the precocious pubertal development is being sought and treated, the physician must also focus on the **long-term consequences of the physical changes** that are occurring. **Short stature** is the most obvious result of early pubertal development. The advanced skeletal maturity associated with some forms of precocious puberty results in a child who initially is taller and stronger than his or her peers but who, ultimately, if the disorder is untreated, loses years of growth potential as a result of fusion of the epiphyseal growth plates.

Suggested Readings

Biro FM, Galvez MP, Greenspan LC, et al. Pubertal assessment method and baseline characteristics in a mixed longitudinal study of girls. *Pediatrics.* 2010;126(3):e580–590.

Cesario SK, Hughes LA. Precocious puberty: a comprehensive review of literature. *J Obstet Gynecol Neonatal Nurs.* 2007;36(3):263–274.

Eugster EA, Clark W, Kletter GB, et al. Efficacy and safety of histrelin subdermal implant in children with central precocious puberty: a multicenter trial. *J Clin Endocrinol Metab.* 2007;92(5):1697–1704.

Haddad N, Eugster E. An update on the treatment of precocious puberty in McCune-Albright syndrome and testotoxicosis. *J Pediatr Endocrinol Metab.* 2007;20(6):653–661.

Kaplowitz P. Precocious puberty: update on secular trends, definitions, diagnosis, and treatment. *Adv Pediatr.* 2004;51:37–62.

Muir A. Precocious puberty. *Pediatr Rev.* 2006;27(10):373–381.

Nathan BM, Palmert MR. Regulation and disorders of pubertal timing. *Endocrinol Metab Clin N Am.* 2005;34:617–664.

Susman EJ, Houts RM, Steinberg L, et al. Longitudinal development of secondary sexual characteristics in girls and boys between ages 9½ and 15½ years. *Arch Pediatr Adolesc Med.* 2010;164(2):166–173.

Proteinuria

INTRODUCTION

Proteinuria, the presence of excessive protein in the urine, is a **common finding in school-age children**. As many as 10% of children test positive for proteinuria (1+ **on urine dipstick**) at some time (Table 62-1). The prevalence of proteinuria increases with age and **peaks during adolescence**. Although most proteinuria is transient or intermittent, it is the most **common laboratory finding indicative of renal disease**. The challenge is to differentiate proteinuria caused by renal disease from that associated with benign conditions. Normal urinary protein excretion in adults is <150 mg/day, whereas in children it is <4 mg/m^2/hour (Table 62-2).

DETECTION OF PROTEINURIA
Qualitative

The **dipstick measures the concentration of protein in urine**. It is impregnated with tetrabromophenol blue, which changes color in the presence of albumin when the pH is in the normal range. A urine sample is considered positive for protein if it measures 1+ when the specific gravity of urine is <1.015 or 2+ when the specific gravity is >1.015. A child is said to have persistent proteinuria if the dipstick is **positive for protein** on **two of three random urine samples** collected at least a week apart.

Although not as convenient as dipstick analysis, a reagent called **sulfosalicylic acid detects all forms of proteinuria**. False-positive results by this method may result from radiographic contrast material, penicillins, cephalosporins, sulfonamides, and high uric acid concentrations.

 HINT: The following can cause false-positive results on dipstick analysis: alkaline urine (pH >7.0), prolonged immersion, placing the strip directly in the urine stream, cleansing of the urethral orifice with quaternary ammonium compounds prior to collecting the sample, pyuria, and bacteriuria. False-negative results can occur when the urine is too dilute (i.e., the specific gravity is <1.005) or when the patient excretes abnormal amounts of proteins other than albumin.

Quantitative

A timed urine collection for protein quantitation is essential to establish the degree of proteinuria. A **24-hour urine collection** can be done by asking the child to void

TABLE 62-1	Qualitative Evaluation of Proteinuria by Dipstick
Grade	**Protein Concentration (mg/dL)**
Trace	10–20
1+	30
2+	100
3+	300
4+	1,000–2,000

as soon as he wakes up and discarding the specimen; then every void should be collected for the next 24 hours including the first void the next morning. In clinical practice, it is difficult to obtain timed urine collections in children. A **random urine specimen** can be analyzed for protein and creatinine concentration, and the ratio of the urine protein (in milligrams) to urine creatinine (in milligrams) can be used as a measure of 24-hour urine protein. The normal ratio of urine protein to urine creatinine in children >2 years is <0.2 and in children <2 years is <0.5.

Microalbuminuria

It is recommended that children with diabetes of more than 5 years' duration have their urine checked for microalbuminuria to monitor for signs of chronic kidney disease. First-morning collections are optimal to avoid a confounding effect of postural proteinuria. A value of <30 mg albumin per gram of creatinine is normal. A level between 30 and 300 mg/g creatinine is consistent with microalbuminuria and a level >300 mg/g indicates clinical proteinuria. Both microalbuminuria and clinical proteinuria necessitate further evaluation by a nephrologist because they may signal early diabetic nephropathy.

DIFFERENTIAL DIAGNOSIS LIST

Transient Proteinuria
- Fever
- Dehydration
- Exercise
- Cold exposure
- Congestive heart failure
- Seizures
- Epinephrine administration

Isolated Proteinuria
- Orthostatic proteinuria
- Persistent asymptomatic isolated proteinuria (PAIP)

Glomerular Disease
- Minimal change nephrotic syndrome (MCNS)
- Focal segmental glomerulosclerosis (FSGS)
- Postinfectious glomerulonephritis
- Membranoproliferative glomerulonephritis
- Membranous nephropathy
- Immunoglobulin A nephropathy
- Henoch–Schönlein purpura
- Hemolytic uremic syndrome
- Hereditary nephritis

- Systemic lupus erythematosus
- Diabetes mellitus
- Sickle cell disease
- Human immunodeficiency virus (HIV)-associated nephropathy

Tubulointerstitial Disease
- Reflux nephropathy
- Pyelonephritis
- Interstitial nephritis

- Fanconi syndrome—cystinosis, tyrosinemia, and Lowe syndrome
- Toxins—drugs (aminoglycosides, penicillins, heavy metals)
- Ischemic tubular injury
- Renal hypoplasia or dysplasia
- Polycystic kidney disease

DIFFERENTIAL DIAGNOSIS DISCUSSION
Transient Proteinuria
Transient proteinuria is **unrelated to renal disease** and resolves when the inciting factor disappears. It is rarely >2+ on the dipstick. **Febrile proteinuria** usually appears with the onset of fever and resolves by 10 to 14 days. Proteinuria that occurs **after exercise** usually abates 48 hours after cessation of exercise. Transient proteinuria seen with fever, exercise, and congestive heart failure is caused by hemodynamic alterations in glomerular blood flow.

Orthostatic Proteinuria
Etiology and Incidence
Orthostatic proteinuria is abnormal protein excretion that **occurs only when the patient is in an upright position**. Although the exact mechanism is unclear, orthostatic proteinuria is most likely the result of excessive glomerular filtration of protein. Orthostatic proteinuria is the most common form, accounting for **60% of all proteinuria in children**. The prevalence is even higher among **teenagers, especially girls**. Orthostatic proteinuria is an incidental finding, and there are no specific clinical features.

Evaluation
The diagnosis of orthostatic proteinuria can be made if urinary protein excretion is abnormal in samples obtained while the patient is upright but normal in samples obtained when the patient is recumbent. Total protein excretion should be <1 g/day. In some patients, orthostatic proteinuria is reproducible; in others, it is intermittent. There are three approaches to evaluating orthostatic proteinuria:

Dipstick analysis of first-morning (recumbent) and daytime (upright) random urine samples. Negative or trace protein in the first-morning sample with >1+ protein in the daytime urine sample is suggestive of orthostatic proteinuria.

Quantitative evaluation of proteinuria in a split collection. Urine samples may be collected at timed intervals while recumbent, as well as while ambulating, and evaluated quantitatively for protein excretion (see Table 62-2). The timed urine samples should be collected by asking the child to void and discard the urine just before going to bed. Collect the void into a container marked "recumbent"

TABLE 62-2	Quantitative Evaluation of Proteinuria by Timed 24-hr Urine Collection
Normal	<4 mg/m^2/hr
Abnormal	$4–40$ mg/m^2/hr
Nephrotic range	>40 mg/m^2/hr

immediately on arising. Then collect all the urine during the day including the specimen voided just before going to bed in a separate container labeled "ambulatory." With orthostatic proteinuria, the amount of protein in the ambulatory collection should be 2 to 4 times that of the recumbent collection.

Calculation of the urine protein-to-urine creatinine ratio. The urine protein-to-urine creatinine ratio is calculated on first-morning and upright random urine samples.

The prognosis for orthostatic proteinuria is thought to be very good.

Persistent Asymptomatic Isolated Proteinuria
Etiology
Persistent asymptomatic isolated proteinuria is defined as proteinuria **detected persistently for 3 months in >80% of the urine specimens taken,** including recumbent samples, in an **otherwise healthy child.** The prevalence in school-age children is 6%. It is usually <2 g/day and is never associated with edema. Numerous studies have revealed that children with PAIP have normal histology or mild nonspecific glomerular abnormalities. Other studies have reported divergent results with a significant number of patients having glomerular abnormalities such as focal sclerosis. Children with PIAP form a heterogeneous group, and in the absence of large prospective studies, the prognosis of PAIP should be viewed with caution.

Nephrotic Syndrome
Nephrotic syndrome is defined by the presence of proteinuria, edema, hypercholesterolemia, and hypoalbuminemia.

Etiology
Nephrotic syndrome can be **primary or secondary** (part of a systemic disease, such as systemic lupus erythematosus). Glomerular diseases that can cause primary nephrotic syndrome include MCNS (77%), FSGS (8%), membranoproliferative glomerulonephritis (7%), and membranous nephropathy (2%).

Clinical Features
Edema is the cardinal finding in nephrotic syndrome. One of the most common manifestations is periorbital edema on awakening, which is sometimes mistaken for an allergic reaction. The **edema increases over time,** and the child may develop ascites, pleural effusion, and labial or scrotal edema.

Clinical features that favor a diagnosis of MCNS are **male gender,** age **<6 years** at onset of disease, **absence of hypertension,** and absence of impaired renal function. There may be microscopic hematuria in up to 30% of patients with MCNS.

Evaluation

Evaluation should include a **urinalysis,** a **serum albumin level,** blood chemistries including **serum creatinine,** and a **serum cholesterol level**. Nephrotic syndrome is characterized by proteinuria >40 mg/m²/hour, a serum albumin level typically <2.5 g/dL, and hypercholesterolemia, with total cholesterol >200 mg/dL.

A biopsy is indicated for patients who:

- Are <1 year or >12 years
- Have atypical features such as hematuria with red blood cell casts, severe hypertension, and strong family history of nephrotic syndrome
- Fail to achieve remission with 4- to 6-week course of prednisone (steroid resistance)

Treatment

More than 80% of patients with nephrotic syndrome and ~95% of children with MCNS respond favorably to **corticosteroid therapy**. Corticosteroids are generally started with a dose of 2 mg/kg/day (to a maximum dose of 80 mg/day), administered in two divided doses for 4 to 8 weeks. Remission is defined as urine dipstick negative/trace or urine protein:creatinine ratio <0.2 for 3 consecutive days. Patients who achieve remission within 4 to 8 weeks of steroid therapy are considered steroid-sensitive. If the patient achieves remission, then steroids are tapered over 4 to 8 weeks. The taper should be gradual enough to reduce the rate of relapse, without causing side effects (e.g., growth retardation).

Approximately 80% of children who initially respond to prednisone **relapse,** which is defined as urine dipstick >1+ or urine protein:creatinine ratio >2 for 3 consecutive days. Patients who relapse during a steroid taper or within 2 weeks of discontinuation of steroid therapy are considered steroid-dependent. Patients who fail to achieve remission with 4 weeks of daily steroids or who achieve an initial remission then no longer respond to steroids are considered steroid-resistant. Patients who are steroid-resistant or those with frequent relapses (more than two relapses in 6 months or more than three relapses per year) are candidates for additional **immunosuppressive medications,** such as intravenous steroids, cyclophosphamide, cyclosporine, or tacrolimus.

 HINT: Most children with MCNS have fewer relapses as they grow older and generally do well.

Proteinuria Caused by Structural Abnormalities

Damage to the glomerulus or tubules can cause proteinuria. Proteinuria from glomerular insult can be in the nephrotic range (Table 62-2), whereas proteinuria from tubular injury rarely exceeds 1 g/day.

EVALUATION OF PROTEINURIA

Once abnormal proteinuria is found and confirmed, a stepwise workup can be initiated.

Phase I Workup

The initial workup of proteinuria should begin with a complete history and physical examination. The physician should elicit history of **recent infections** (streptococcal, impetigo), **urinary tract infections, oliguria/hematuria, and family history** of renal disease. The physical examination should be focused on looking for **hypertension** (glomerulonephritis), **edema** (nephrotic syndrome), **rash/arthritis** (vasculitis), and **short stature** (chronic kidney disease). Laboratory investigations in this phase should include a **urine dipstick** (ambulatory and recumbent), a **urinalysis** including microscopic examination, and a **urine protein-to-creatinine ratio**.

Phase II Workup

If the patient is edematous, laboratory workup should include serum albumin, serum chemistries including serum creatinine, and total cholesterol to confirm nephrotic syndrome. Additional laboratory studies to look for secondary causes of nephrotic syndrome should be obtained based on the history and physical examination; these include complement levels, ANA, hepatitis B/C, and HIV. A PPD is typically placed prior to initiating steroid therapy. For patients without nephrotic syndrome, a urine protein/creatinine ratio (preferably on a first morning sample) or a **24-hour urinary protein level** should be obtained.

A **renal ultrasound** should be performed to look for abnormalities of size and structure in the kidney.

Phase III Workup

If the initial workup suggests the presence of an underlying renal disease, a **referral to a pediatric nephrologist** should be made. A referral should be made in the following situations:

- Persistent fixed (i.e., nonorthostatic) proteinuria
- Family history of glomerulonephritis
- Systemic complaints (e.g., fever, rash, arthralgias)
- Hypertension
- Edema
- Cutaneous vasculitis or purpura
- Hematuria
- Abnormal renal function
- Abnormal ultrasound
- Increased parental anxiety

The nephrologist may perform a renal biopsy to define the etiology of proteinuria in some of these situations.

Most cases of proteinuria in children can be managed by a primary care physician at times in consultation with a pediatric nephrologist. **Long-term follow-up** is important because prognosis in some of the conditions is not well defined.

APPROACH TO THE PATIENT

An algorithm for the approach to a patient with proteinuria is presented in Figure 62.1.

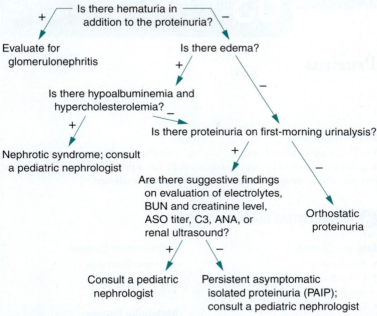

FIGURE 62-1   Approach to the patient with proteinuria. *ANA*, antinuclear antibody; *ASO*, antistreptolysin-O; *BUN*, Blood urea nitrogen.

Suggested Readings

Bergstein JM. A practical approach to proteinuria. *Pediatr Nephrol.* 1999;13:697–700.

Ettenger RB. The evaluation of the child with proteinuria. *Pediatr Ann.* 1994;23(9):486–494.

Gipson DS, Massengill SF, Yao L, et al. Management of childhood onset nephrotic syndrome. *Pediatrics.* 2009;124(2):747–757.

Hogg RJ, Portman RJ, Milliner D, et al. Evaluation and management of proteinuria and nephrotic syndrome in children: recommendations from a pediatric nephrology panel established at the National Kidney Foundation Conference on Proteinuria, Albuminuria, Risk, Assessment, Detection and Elimination (PARADE). *Pediatrics.* 2000;105:1242–1249.

Roy S. Proteinuria. *Pediatr Ann* 25(5):277–278, 281–282, 1996.

Yoshikawa N, Kitagawa K, Ohta K, et al. Asymptomatic constant isolated proteinuria in children. *J Pediatr.* 1991;119(3):375–379.

Pruritus

INTRODUCTION

Pruritus, simply defined, means "itching." Pruritus that is **persistent and severe** requires further investigation. Pruritus usually has a primary **dermatologic** cause but may also be **drug induced** or caused by **systemic disease**.

 DIFFERENTIAL DIAGNOSIS LIST

Allergic Causes
- Anaphylaxis
- Contact dermatitis and allergen mediated
- Drug eruptions

Congenital Causes
- Erythropoietic protoporphyria
- Hemochromatosis
- Neurofibromatosis
- Urticaria pigmentosa

Hematologic Causes
- Hypereosinophilic syndrome
- Iron deficiency anemia
- Polycythemia

Infectious Causes
- Hookworms
- Parvovirus
- Pediculosis
- Pinworms
- Ringworm
- Scabies
- Trichinosis
- Varicella

Inflammatory Causes
- Atopic dermatitis
- Lichen planus
- Psoriasis

Metabolic Causes
- Diabetes mellitus
- Hypercalcemia
- Hyperparathyroidism
- Hypothyroidism or hyperthyroidism

Neoplastic Causes
- Carcinoid syndrome
- Hepatobiliary tumors
- Hodgkin's disease
- Leukemia
- Non-Hodgkins Lymphoma

Neurologic and Psychiatric Causes
- Delusional parasitosis
- Postherpetic pruritus

Rheumatologic Causes
- Dermatomyositis
- Sarcoidosis

- Sjögren syndrome
- Systemic lupus erythematosus

Traumatic Causes
- Coelenterata (jellyfish) envenomation
- Insect bites
- Contact dermatitis and irritant mediated
- Overbathing, dry heat, and harsh detergents
- Ultraviolet or chemical burns

Miscellaneous Causes
- Cholestasis
- Opiates
- Pityriasis rosea
- Pregnancy
- Seborrheic dermatitis
- Uremia
- Xerosis (dry skin)

DIFFERENTIAL DIAGNOSIS DISCUSSION

Any skin condition comprising exudation, lichenification, and pruritus falls under the broad category of eczema. Two common forms of eczema, atopic dermatitis and contact dermatitis, are first discussed, followed by other common causes of pruritus.

Atopic Dermatitis
Etiology
Although, it is one of the **most common causes of pruritus** in children, this condition is **poorly understood**. Characterized by **inflammatory hyperreactivity,** the disease is currently believed to be caused by aberrancies in T-cell function, with immunoglobulin E overproduction and cell-mediated immune dysfunction in the skin.

Clinical Features and Evaluation
Most children with atopic dermatitis have a **family history of atopic disease** (asthma, allergic rhinitis, or atopic dermatitis), and may later develop these conditions. The rash usually appears in susceptible patients during the first year of life, and starts on the cheeks and extensor surfaces of the extremities. As the child ages, the distribution changes to involve the **flexor creases of the elbows and knees** as well as the wrists, ankles, and trunk. The diaper area and nose are usually spared. The eruption consists of **erythematous, poorly demarcated patches, and initially is exudative, later forming crusts**. There may be **associated papules or vesicles**. With the **scratching** that ensues, the lesions become **thickened or lichenified** and may develop a **surface scale**. **Pigmentation changes** are common complications. Atopic dermatitis has a **chronic, recurrent, or recalcitrant nature**.

 HINT: It may be difficult to differentiate seborrheic dermatitis from atopic dermatitis in infants. Classically, seborrheic dermatitis appears in the first 2 months of life, whereas atopic dermatitis may appear later. The scale of seborrhea is yellow and greasy and is often seen behind the ears and in the diaper area. The diagnosis of atopic dermatitis may be delayed until repeated outbreaks occur.

HINT: For an eczematous rash in the diaper area that is refractory to topical therapy, think about zinc deficiency. Zinc deficiency may be inherited (acrodermatitis enteropathica) or nutritional. Diarrhea and failure to thrive are often present.

Treatment

Treatment focuses on **moisturizing the skin, avoiding overdrying, and eliminating possible irritants**. Children should **bathe no more than 3 times per week and apply a moisturizer at least twice a day**. A **topical steroid,** such as 1% or 2.5% hydrocortisone ointment, is used initially to control flares. Unresponsive or severe cases may require treatment with more potent steroids or pimecrolimus (Elidel) or tacrolimus (Protopic), which inhibit cytokines. The patient with severe atopic dermatitis is at a risk for **secondary skin infections** with staphylococci, herpes simplex virus (eczema herpeticum), and varicella zoster infection.

Contact Dermatitis
Etiology

Contact dermatitis can be mediated by irritants or allergens.

Primary irritant dermatitis is a direct response of the skin to an irritant. The most common irritants are soaps, bubble baths (a common cause of severe vaginal pruritus in prepubertal girls), saliva, urine, feces, perspiration, citrus juice, chemicals, and wool. Irritant diaper dermatitis is common in infants, and is differentiated from fungal diaper dermatitis by its sparing of the inguinal folds.

- **Allergic contact dermatitis** requires reexposure to an allergen and is characterized by a delayed hypersensitivity reaction. The most common allergens implicated include poison ivy, poison oak, and poison sumac (rhus dermatitis) (Figure 63-1); jewelry (nickel); cosmetics (causing eyelid involvement) and nail polish; topical medications; shoe materials (rubber, dyes); and clothing materials (elastic or latex compounds).

Clinical Features and Evaluation

In either case, the **rash is the key to diagnosis,** being **most prominent in the areas of direct approximation to the trigger**. It may appear as erythematous papules, patches, vesicles, or bullae.

Treatment

The cornerstone of treatment is **removal of the offending agent**. A short course of **topical steroids** may help speed recovery. Severe contact dermatitis due to poison ivy may require a 2-week course of oral steroids including a taper to prevent rebound dermatitis. **Failure to respond** to these measures **indicates possible misdiagnosis**.

Scabies
Etiology

Scabies is caused by an **infestation with the mite** *Sarcoptes scabiei.* The mites burrow into the stratum corneum and deposit eggs and feces, which cause the intense itching.

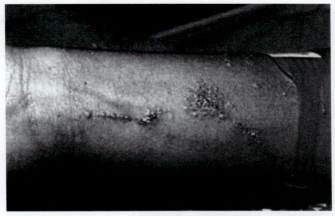

FIGURE 63-1 Rhus dermatitis (poison ivy), an example of allergic contact dermatitis.
(Reprinted with permission from Avery ME, First LR. *Pediatric Medicine.* 2nd ed. Baltimore: Williams & Wilkins; 1994.)

Clinical Features and Evaluation

Lesions may be **papules, pustules, or vesicles** (Figure 63-2). Fewer than 15% of patients have the classic S-shaped burrows. The **rash distribution on infants** (neck, face, scalp, axilla, and genitalia) **differs from that of older children** (wrists, axilla, **interdigital webs,** intragluteal web, and belt line). Scabies is a clinical diagnosis, though skin scrapings from an unscratched burrow in immersion oil under 10× magnification should reveal the female mite, her eggs, and her feces.

Treatment

Permethrin 5% cream is applied to the **entire body** and left on **for 12 hours**. This treatment may be repeated every 2 weeks, if necessary. Because the **infestation is highly contagious,** household contacts should also be treated. **Bedding and clothing** may harbor the mites and should be **laundered;** the dryer heat kills the remaining mites.

Bedbugs
Etiology

The **bedbug (*Cimex lectularius*)** has reemerged as a cause of pruritus. The **insect is 5 mm long with a brown body** that turns mahogany red after feeding. It emerges during the **night**. The insect attaches itself to the skin and injects an enzyme, anticoagulant, and vasodilator. Following feeding, it returns to **dark crevices of mattresses, furniture, wallpapers, and suitcases**. Unlike mosquitoes, **bedbugs are not known to transmit diseases**.

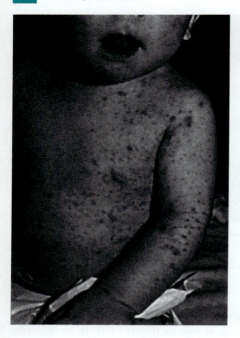

FIGURE 63-2 **Erythematous papules, pustules, vesicles, and crusted lesions of scabies.** (Reprinted with permission from Avery ME, First LR. *Pediatric Medicine.* 2nd ed. Baltimore: Williams & Wilkins; 1994.)

Clinical Features and Evaluation

Most patients present with pruritic **macules that become papular, erythematous, and indurated**. The lesions may be in linear groups ("breakfast, lunch, and dinner"). **Bullous lesions, wheals, and anaphylactoid reactions** are also reported. Younger patients may develop **papular urticaria**. When healed, the lesions may be hypopigmented. History and physical examination should suggest the diagnosis, with **small dark brown stains on the bedding** as a clue. **Recent travel** may precede the infestation. A **careful search of the bedroom,** including turning the mattress over, may reveal the culprit.

Treatment

Local care of the lesions, with twice-daily cleansing and application of topical antibiotic ointment is usually all that is necessary. **Eradication** of the insect from the home usually requires an **exterminator and may be difficult** because of the multiple stages of insect larvae.

Varicella
Etiology

Varicella is caused by **primary infection with varicella zoster virus,** usually from droplet contact with a primarily infected individual. It is contagious from 1 or 2 days before the outbreak of lesions until all of the lesions are crusted over. Varicella vaccine is now a component of the routine immunization schedule, and the incidence of varicella has decreased substantially since universal immunization began in 1995. Children who have received the vaccine may exhibit milder or atypical symptoms.

Clinical Features and Evaluation

The rash of primary varicella infection is characterized by a **progression of lesions from erythematous macules, to papules, to fluid-filled vesicles, and to crusted lesions**. Crops of lesions appear on the **face, trunk, and scalp,** with minimal involvement of the distal extremities. The **mucous membranes** can be involved with superficial ulcerations appearing on the oral mucosae. Classically, lesions in various stages of evolution are simultaneously present. **Fever and malaise** may accompany the rash. Herpes zoster ("shingles") occurs due to reactivation of latent virus in the dorsal root ganglia and presents as grouped vesicles occurring in a dermatomal distribution.

Treatment

Treatment is **supportive,** including attempts to **alleviate the itching**. **Antiviral agents** (e.g., acyclovir) are effective only in shortening the course of illness, **if given within 24 hours** of the onset of lesions. Immunization with varicella vaccine is recommended for contacts without evidence of immunity, ideally within 72 hours (but up to 120 hours) after exposure. Varicella immunoglobulin (VariZIG) should be administered to immunocompromised patients within 96 hours after exposure. Aspirin use in patients with varicella is associated with Reye syndrome and is contraindicated.

 HINT: Immunocompromised hosts and neonates are at risk for disseminated disease and warrant special precautions, intravenous acyclovir therapy, and consultation with infectious disease specialists. Newborns are especially at a high risk of infection if the mother develops lesions within 5 days prior to delivery or 2 days after the delivery.

 HINT: Toxic shock syndrome secondary to *Streptococcus pyogenes* (Group A Strep) is a possible complication of varicella infection. Toxic shock syndrome is characterized by fever, hypotension, erythroderma, and dysfunction in three organ systems.

Xerosis
Etiology

Xerosis refers to **dryness of the skin** and may be the diagnosis of exclusion in common pruritus. Children of any age may be affected.

Clinical Features and Evaluation

The rash often has a **fine, flaky, white, and diffuse scale,** which may be **excoriated from scratching**. The **lower legs** are commonly involved. The **hands** may also be afflicted in older children, especially when exposed to frequent washing of hands or dishes. The condition is **made worse by dry heat, frequent bathing in hot water, and wool fabrics**.

Treatment

Treatment with **emollients and cessation of causative behaviors** are effective.

Drug Reaction

Etiology

Many medications can cause pruritus, either by **drug-induced intrahepatic cholestasis** (from erythromycin, oral contraceptives, anabolic steroids, phenothiazines) or **mast cell degranulation** (from opioids, aspirin, penicillin).

Clinical Features and Evaluation

In addition to pruritus, the rash of a drug reaction can be diverse, ranging from papules to target lesions (Stevens Johnson syndrome) to urticaria (see below).

Treatment

Treatment of most drug reactions is supportive. If clinically feasible, a **trial period** during which the **patient is off medication** should be attempted. Relief of pruritus should occur **within several days if it is histamine mediated** but can take **several weeks to resolve if it is caused by cholestasis**. Pruritus associated with opioids without associated urticaria or systemic symptoms is a side effect of the medication, not an allergy, and can be prevented by giving antihistamines prior to subsequent doses.

Urticaria

Etiology

This classic pruritic rash, also known as hives, is caused by the release of histamine and other vasoactive mediators into the dermis. Urticaria may be acute or chronic. Acute urticaria is most often due to an **immediate hypersensitivity reaction,** but may also be due to other types of hypersensitivity reaction. The most common triggers are **foods** (nuts, berries, shellfish, dairy products), **drug reactions, environmental triggers, viral infections, and *Mycoplasma pneumoniae*.** Intravenous injection of **radiopaque contrast material or blood products** may cause **severe reactions**. Less commonly, the trigger may be **cold, heat, tactile stimuli, or sunlight**. Chronic urticaria is defined by hives that last for more than 6 weeks, and may be caused by autoimmune or other systemic disease.

Clinical Features and Evaluation

Diagnosis is made clinically. The classic appearance of urticaria is a **rash of erythematous raised, often evanescent, wheals** scattered over the body. Laboratory workup to evaluate for autoimmune disease or malignancy should be considered in patients with chronic urticaria.

Treatment

If signs of anaphylaxis are present (wheezing, stridor, gastrointestinal symptoms, hypotension), **intramuscular injection of epinephrine should be administered**

emergently. Systemic steroids are also given for anaphylaxis. **Antihistamines** are commonly prescribed for urticaria of any cause to help alleviate itching. Attempts should be made to **identify and remove the trigger,** although often none can be found.

> **HINT:** Up to 20% of patients with anaphylaxis will not have urticaria, pruritus, or angioedema. Suspect anaphylaxis in patients with respiratory and gastrointestinal symptoms, or hypotension, after exposure to a possible or known allergen.

EVALUATION OF PRURITUS
Patient History
Key components are the duration of symptoms and the presence of rash, fever, or other systemic symptoms. Answers to the following questions should be sought:

- Are there any new or unusual exposures?
- What is the patient's medication history?
- Are any household contacts also suffering from similar symptoms?
- What is the patient's past medical history, including renal and hepatic disorders, atopic disease, psychiatric disorders, and autoimmune diseases?

Physical Examination
Physical examination findings that may point to the diagnosis include wheezing, oral lesions, organomegaly, and any abnormal skin findings. The pattern of distribution should be noted.

Laboratory Studies and Diagnostic Modalities
Appropriate laboratory studies and diagnostic modalities are indicated by the history and physical examination, and may include the following:

- Complete blood count
- Blood urea nitrogen and creatinine levels
- Liver function tests
- β-human chorionic gonadotropin level
- Chest radiograph
- Skin biopsy
- Microscopic examination of skin scrapings

TREATMENT OF PRURITUS
If **urticaria** is present, the patient should be **urgently assessed for signs of anaphylaxis** as discussed earlier. Treatment is otherwise dictated by the underlying cause.

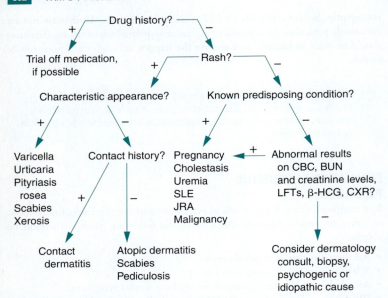

FIGURE 63-3 **Evaluation of a patient with pruritus.** If the diagnosis remains elusive, refer the patient to a dermatologist. *β-hCG,* β-human chorionic gonadotropin; *BUN,* blood urea nitrogen; *CBC,* complete blood count; *CXR,* chest radiograph; *JRA,* juvenile rheumatoid arthritis; *LFTs,* liver function tests; *SLE,* systemic lupus erythematosus.

APPROACH TO THE PATIENT

An approach to the evaluation of the patient is presented in Figure 63-3.

Suggested Readings

Angel TA, Nigro J, Levy ML. Infestations in the pediatric patient. *Pediatr Dermatol.* 2000;47(4):921–935.

Boguniewicz M. Atopic dermatitis: beyond the itch that rashes. *Immunol Allergy Clin N Am.* 2005;25(2):333–351.

Frieden IJ, Resnick SD. Childhood exanthems: old and new. *Pediatr Clin N Am.* 1991;38(4):859–887.

Hurwitz S. *Clinical Pediatric Dermatology: A Textbook of Skin Disorders of Childhood and Adolescence.* 2nd ed. Philadelphia, PA: WB Saunders; 1993.

Wolf R, Orion E, Marcos B, et al. Life-threatening acute adverse cutaneous drug reactions. *Clin Dermatol.* 2005;23(2):171–181.

CHAPTER **64**

Leslie Castelo-Soccio
Kara Shah

Rashes

Rash is a common reason for children to be brought for evaluation by a health-care provider. The examination of the rash can provide key clues to the diagnosis. Rashes can be categorized by type and by accompanying symptoms to organize the differential diagnosis.

 DIFFERENTIAL DIAGNOSIS LIST

Rash Accompanied by a Fever

- **Bacterial Causes**
  - Scarlet fever
  - Staphylococcal scalded skin syndrome
  - Toxic shock syndrome
  - Acute meningococcemia
  - Rocky Mountain spotted fever
- **Viral Causes**
  - Herpes simplex
  - Varicella
  - Roseola infantum
  - Erythema infectiosum
  - Enteroviruses
  - Measles
  - Rubella
  - Lyme disease
- **Miscellaneous**
  - Juvenile idiopathic arthritis
  - Kawasaki disease

Rash in a Neonate

- Erythema toxicum neonatorum
- Transient neonatal pustular melanosis
- Miliaria
- Infantile seborrheic dermatitis
- Candidiasis
- Neonatal acne
- Acropustulosis of infancy

Eczematous Dermatitis

- Atopic dermatitis
- Contact dermatitis
- Nummular dermatitis
- Asteatotic eczema
- Id reaction

Papulosquamous Disease

- Psoriasis
- Lichen planus
- Seborrheic dermatitis
- Tinea (dermatophyte) infections
- Tinea versicolor
- Pityriasis rosea
- Secondary syphilis
- Pityriasis lichenoides et varioliformis acuta
- Acrodermatitis enteropathica
- Exfoliative dermatitis

Vesiculobullous Disease

- Herpes simplex
- Herpes zoster
- Varicella
- *Rhus* dermatitis (poison ivy)
- Contact dermatitis
- Insect bite or papular urticaria
- Urticaria pigmentosa

Annular Erythema

- Lyme disease
- Erythema multiforme (EM)

Papular Eruptions
- Scabies
- Papular acrodermatitis of childhood (Gianotti–Crosti syndrome)
- Papular urticaria
- Molluscum contagiosum
- Warts

DIFFERENTIAL DIAGNOSIS DISCUSSION
Scarlet Fever
Etiology
Scarlet fever is caused by **group A β-hemolytic** *Streptococcus*.

Clinical Features
Illness begins with **fever and pharyngitis** followed by **enanthem and exanthem** in 24 to 48 hours.

The face appears flushed, except for circumoral pallor. The tongue initially has a white coating (**white strawberry tongue**) that fades by the fourth day, revealing a very erythematous tongue with prominent papillae (**red strawberry tongue**). Cervical and submandibular lymphadenopathies are noted.

The rash appears as a **diffuse erythema; small fine papules give it a **sandpaper-like** quality. The rash begins on the neck and spreads rapidly to the trunk and extremities. It is accentuated in the intertriginous areas (i.e., the axillae and antecubital, inguinal, and popliteal creases), and the palms and soles are spared. The rash resolves in 4 to 5 days with **fine peeling** of the skin. Peeling begins on the face, spreading to the trunk and extremities. On the hands and feet, peeling in large sheets may occur.

> **HINT:** Petechiae may occur on the soft palate and uvula or in streaks in the intertriginous areas (Pastia lines).

Evaluation
Diagnosis is by **culture or rapid test of a pharyngeal swab. Antistreptolysin-O titers or antideoxyribonuclease B titers** may also be used to indicate recent infection. Complete blood count commonly reveals leukocytosis. Urinalysis and liver function test may reveal changes associated with complications of scarlet fever.

Treatment
Treatment of choice is with **penicillin, amoxicillin, or a first-generation cephalosporin. Erythromycin** can be used in penicillin-allergic patients.

Staphylococcal Scalded Skin Syndrome
Etiology
Staphylococcal scalded skin syndrome is caused by two **epidermolytic toxins, epidermolytic toxins A and B,** which are produced by some strains of *Staphylococcus aureus*. These toxins cause intraepidermal splitting through the granular layer by specific cleavage of **desmoglein 1,** a cadherin protein that mediates cell-to-cell adhesion of keratinocytes.

Clinical Features
Staphylococcal scalded skin syndrome typically occurs in children younger than **5 years**. The illness begins with **fever and/or irritability** after an episode of

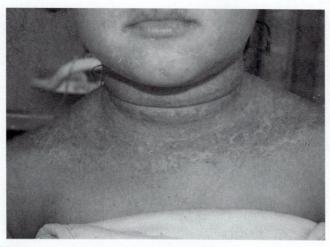

FIGURE 64-1 Crusted superficial erosions favoring intertriginous sites in staphylococcal scalded skin syndrome.

conjunctivitis, rhinitis, or an upper respiratory tract infection. The skin initially becomes **erythematous and tender.** The eruption usually begins around the **nose and mouth and spreads to the trunk.** The rash is most **prominent in the flexures** and can involve the hands and feet. After 1 to 2 days, the **skin develops bullae** and begins **peeling in sheets.** After 2 days, the involved **skin surfaces become crusted** and then begin to **develop scaling,** which lasts up to 5 days (Figure 64-1).

Evaluation

Staphylococcus aureus can sometimes be isolated by **bacterial culture of the nose, nasopharynx, throat, conjunctiva, or perianal area.**

 HINT: Periocular and perioral crusting in association with tender erythema and blisters and/or superficial erosions that favor intertriginous areas (the neck, axillae, groin, and perineum), is characteristic of this disease.

Treatment

Treatment is with a **penicillinase-resistant antibiotic,** such as **nafcillin or oxacillin** (parenteral) or **dicloxacillin or amoxicillin-clavulanate** (oral). **Clindamycin** reduces the bacterial production of the toxin and is increasingly used because of concern about methicillin-resistant *Staphylococcus aureus.*

Toxic Shock Syndrome
Etiology

Toxic shock syndrome (TSS) is a multisystem disease caused by **exotoxin-producing strains** of either *S. aureus* (TSS) or **Streptococcus pyogenes** (STSS). These exotoxins—toxic shock syndrome toxin-1 in the case of *S. aureus* and most commonly

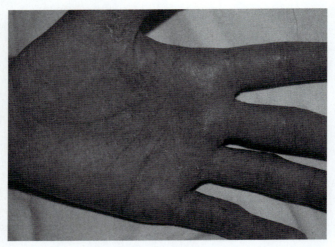

FIGURE 64-2 Desquamation of the palms in toxic shock syndrome.

streptococcal pyrogenic exotoxin-A in the case of *S. pyogenes*—function as superantigens and stimulate the release of massive amounts of proinflammatory cytokines, including tumor necrosis factor-alpha and interleukin-1. Although **classic TSS** is seen in association with **menstruation,** nonmenstrual TSS is now more common. **STSS** is usually seen as a complication of a **wound infection**.

Clinical Features

The association of **fever, rash, and hypotension** is the hallmark of TSS. Involvement of other organ systems may present as **myalgias, acute renal failure, encephalopathy, disseminated intravascular coagulopathy, diarrhea, metabolic acidosis, and/or hepatitis**. The rash may appear **morbilliform** (resembling measles) or as **confluent erythema** (erythroderma). Involvement of the **palms and soles** is common, and late **desquamation** of these areas is a key feature (Figure 64-2). A **strawberry tongue** is also characteristic.

> **HINT:** The presence of fever, hypotension, and an erythematous rash in combination with dysfunction of at least three organ systems is diagnostic of TSS.

Evaluation

Blood cultures should be sent, although they are not always positive. In TSS only about 5%–15% of cultures are positive and in STSS about 50% are positive. Culture of any **cutaneous wounds** should also be performed. Evaluation for systemic involvement should include complete blood counts, serum chemistries, liver function tests, urinalysis, creatine kinase, and coagulation studies. Other diagnostic tests that may be helpful when indicated include electrocardiogram, echocardiography, and chest radiography. Skin biopsy is rarely needed.

Treatment

Appropriate antibiotic therapy should be promptly initiated. Use of an agent that is effective against both *S. aureus* and *S. pyogenes* is required if the causative agent is unknown. Initial choices include use of **oxacillin or vancomycin.** Addition of **clindamycin** is recommended as an adjunct to decrease toxin production.

Meningococcemia
Etiology

Meningococcemia is caused by ***Neisseria meningitidis.*** Asymptomatic nasopharyngeal carriage occurs and transmission occurs via respiratory droplets.

Clinical Evaluation

The illness begins with symptoms of a **mild upper respiratory tract infection,** followed by **fever, malaise, headache,** and the development of a **petechial eruption** on the skin and mucous membranes. In addition, patients can have **erythematous macules, papules, and urticarial lesions**. In severe cases, the purpura can involve **large areas that eventually necrose**.

Many patients develop meningitis, disseminated intravascular coagulation, and hypotension.

 HINT: Always think of meningococcemia when a patient presents with fever and petechiae.

Evaluation

Cultures of blood and cerebrospinal fluid are indicated. The organism can sometimes be recovered from a small petechial lesion if a **biopsy of the lesion** is performed and cultured. A **Gram stain** of a scraping of a petechial lesion may reveal organisms.

Treatment

Initial treatment is with a **broad-spectrum antibiotic;** once the diagnosis is confirmed, the patient can be treated with **penicillin, ceftriaxone, or cefotaxime**.

Rocky Mountain Spotted Fever
Etiology

Rocky Mountain spotted fever is caused by ***Rickettsia rickettsii,*** which is transmitted by **ticks**. Humans are accidental hosts.

Clinical Features

After a prodrome characterized by headache, malaise, photophobia, and joint and muscle pain, the patient develops a fever followed by a rash on the fourth day.

The rash begins on the **wrists and ankles** as small erythematous macules that eventually become petechial or purpuric. The rash then spreads to the trunk and within 2 days is generalized, with involvement of the palms and soles.

Other findings may include **generalized edema** (especially affecting the periorbital area in children), **severe muscle tenderness, photophobia, and hyponatremia**.

 HINT: Consider Rocky Mountain spotted fever in any patient with fever and a petechial eruption involving the palms and soles.

Evaluation

Diagnosis is with the detection of **rickettsial-specific antibodies**. Indirect immunofluorescence antibody, enzyme immunoassay, and indirect hemagglutination are the most sensitive and specific diagnostic tests. Direct immunofluorescence of a skin lesion biopsy specimen and serum polymerase chain reaction (PCR) are useful for confirming a clinical diagnosis. Owing to poor sensitivity and specificity, the Weil–Felix assay is no longer used.

Treatment

The treatment of choice for all patients is a **tetracycline derivative**.

Herpes Simplex Virus

Herpes simplex virus is discussed in Chapter 70, "Sexually Transmitted Diseases."

Varicella (Chickenpox)

Varicella is discussed in Chapter 63, "Pruritus."

Roseola Infantum
Etiology

Roseola is caused by **human herpes virus-6** infection. Transmission occurs through saliva.

Clinical Features

Usually seen in infants, roseola classically presents with **3 days of high fever,** followed by rapid defervescence. **Febrile seizures** are common. After the fever abates, a **diffuse, faint, blanchable, erythematous reticulated rash** appears. It lasts for several days. An **enanthem** characterized by erythematous macules on the soft palate and uvula may also develop.

Evaluation

The diagnosis is usually made clinically, although serology and/or serum PCR for human herpes virus-6 DNA may be performed if the diagnosis is unclear.

Treatment

The disease is self-limiting.

Erythema Infectiosum
Etiology

Erythema infectiosum is caused by infection with parvovirus B19. Transmission occurs via respiratory droplets. Clinical signs and symptoms are probably the result of immune complexes in the skin and joints rather than from the virus itself.

Clinical Features

Erythema infectiosum is seen predominantly in **school-age children**. Prodromal symptoms such as **fever, pharyngitis, malaise, or coryza** may occur, followed by the development of the classic **"slapped cheek" erythema**. A **lacy, reticulated, erythematous exanthem** then develops most commonly on the extremities. It may wax and wane over several weeks. Older children and adults may complain of **arthralgias or arthritis**.

Evaluation

The diagnosis is usually made clinically. Serologic tests and serum PCR for parvovirus B19 DNA may be performed if the diagnosis is unclear.

Treatment

The disease is self-limiting. Patients with sickle cell or other hemolytic disease may require treatment for anemia due to decreased red cell production associated with parvovirus infection.

Enterovirus

Etiology

Several human enteroviruses are capable of causing disease with cutaneous manifestations. **Coxsackievirus A 1–10, 16, and 22** are common causes of **herpangina**. **Coxsackievirus B16** is the most common cause of **hand-foot-mouth disease**. Other enteroviruses including echoviruses may cause pustular, morbilliform, vesicular, or papular exanthems.

Clinical Features

Prodromal symptoms such as fever, malaise, headache, pharyngitis, or diarrhea may be present. Herpangina presents with small gray-white vesicles and erosions with an erythematous ring on the uvula, soft palate, and tonsils. Hand-foot-mouth disease presents with similar vesicles and erosions that favor the hard palate, buccal mucosa, tongue, and gingiva. Small oval vesicles with an erythematous ring are seen on the lateral aspects of the hands and feet, as well as on the palms and soles. Papules and vesicles may also be seen on the buttocks. Many patients with herpangina or hand-foot-mouth disease have significant oral pain and decreased oral intake; young infants are at risk for dehydration.

Evaluation

The diagnosis is usually made clinically.

Treatment

Enterovirus infections are self-limiting. Intravenous hydration and analgesics may be required in severe cases.

Juvenile Idiopathic Arthritis

Juvenile idiopathic arthritis is discussed in Chapter 47, "Joint Pain."

Kawasaki Disease

Etiology

The cause of Kawasaki disease is **unknown**.

Clinical Features

The patient must present with five of the following six criteria to make the diagnosis of typical Kawasaki disease. Atypical cases of Kawasaki disease are increasingly recognized and an approach to these cases has been summarized in recent practice guidelines (see Suggested Readings):

- Fever >5 days
- Bilateral nonpurulent conjunctivitis
- Erythema and crusting of the lips
- Edema or erythema of the palms and soles with subsequent desquamation
- Rash
- Cervical adenopathy

The **rash** can have many different forms, including **generalized erythema, scarlatiniform lesions, EM, and pustular lesions**. The **lips** are usually **bright red** with some **crusting,** and the patient may have a **strawberry tongue**.

> **HINT:** An important cutaneous finding is that of fine desquamation of the perineal area early in the course of the disease.

Evaluation

Thrombocytosis is present by the second week of illness. Sterile pyuria, hyponatremia, hypoalbuminemia, elevated erythrocyte sedimentation rate, anemia, and leukocytosis may be seen. An **echocardiogram** should be performed to look for coronary artery aneurysmal dilation.

Treatment

Treatment is with **intravenous gamma globulin and aspirin**.

Erythema Toxicum Neonatorum
Etiology and Clinical Features

The cause of erythema toxicum neonatorum is **unknown**. Affected infants appear healthy. The rash develops **within 3 to 4 days of birth** and is characterized by **erythematous macules and patches, some with a central papule or pustule**. The rash may occur **anywhere on the body except in the palms and soles**. There may be **few or several hundred lesions**.

Clinical Evaluation

A **smear** of a pustule reveals **clusters of eosinophils;** Gram staining is negative for bacteria. As many as 15% of patients have **peripheral eosinophilia**.

Treatment

No treatment is needed. The eruption generally resolves by the time the patient reaches 2 weeks of age.

Transient Neonatal Pustular Melanosis
Etiology and Clinical Features

The cause of transient neonatal pustular melanosis is **unknown**. This condition is more commonly seen in **African-American infants** and is characterized by **pustules,** vesicles, and hyperpigmented macules that are **present at birth**. Pustules **rupture,** leaving a **fine white collarette of scale**. The eruption **resolves within several days,** most of the time **leaving pigmented macules**. The eruption can appear **anywhere on the body, including the palms and soles**. A **smear** of the pustules shows neutrophils.

Evaluation and Treatment
Gram stain, a Tzanck preparation, and potassium hydroxide preparation are negative for infection. **No treatment** is needed.

Miliaria
An **eruption,** characterized by **small nonfollicular, erythematous papules,** is caused by **sweat retention in eccrine ducts**. The rash is most commonly seen in the **intertriginous or flexor regions** of the body but can appear anywhere. There is no evidence of infection. Treatment entails **avoidance of excessive heat, humidity, and friction**.

Infantile Seborrheic Dermatitis
Etiology
The cause is **unknown** but may be related to **maternal hormonal stimulation**.

Clinical Features
The eruption often begins during the **first 12 weeks of life** with **scaling of the scalp,** sometimes associated with **erythema ("cradle cap");** the eruption generally **clears by 1 year of age**. The eruption is characterized by **greasy yellow scales** associated with **patches of erythema, fissuring, and occasional oozing** on the **scalp, face, ears, trunk, and intertriginous areas**.

Treatment
Parents should be advised to **gently loosen the scale with a soft comb or brush**. Application of **baby oil** to the scalp prior to shampooing may be helpful. A **low-potency topical corticosteroid** (i.e., hydrocortisone) may be applied to acutely inflamed areas.

Candidiasis
Etiology
Cutaneous candidiasis is common in neonates and infants. It is most commonly caused by infection with the yeast *Candida albicans,* although other *Candida* species are also implicated. Transmission usually occurs during or after delivery. Congenital candidiasis, which results from antepartum infection, is rare.

Clinical Features
The presence of **superficial erythematous papules and pustules,** often with a **collarette of scaling,** is seen. Involvement of the **diaper area** and other **intertriginous areas such as the neck** is common. Congenital candidiasis may present with more diffuse erythema and pustules.

Evaluation
The diagnosis is usually clinical. **Microscopic examination of a potassium hydroxide preparation** of a skin scraping may demonstrate **budding yeast**. A **fungal culture** can be performed if the diagnosis is unclear.

Treatment

Use of a topical antifungal cream or ointment such as nystatin or clotrimazole is effective. Affected areas should be kept dry, and frequent diaper changes should be performed.

Neonatal Acne

The cause is **unknown,** but the condition is probably related to **stimulation of sebaceous glands** by the maternal and infant **androgens**. Neonatal acne is **more commonly seen in boys** and is reported in as many as 20% of newborns. **Closed comedones (whiteheads)** are most common, but **open comedones, inflammatory papules, and pustules** may also be noted. **No treatment** is necessary for most patients; patients with **moderate to severe cases** should be **referred to a pediatric dermatologist**.

Atopic Dermatitis and Contact Dermatitis

Atopic dermatitis and contact dermatitis are discussed in Chapter 63, "Pruritus."

Nummular Dermatitis

The cause of nummular dermatitis is **unknown,** although it tends to be a manifestation of **dry skin and ichthyosis**. The **rash** is characterized by **coin-shaped lesions** with **vesicles, papules, erythema, and scaling that enlarge by confluence** or peripheral extension. Lesions are treated with **mid-potency topical steroids**.

> **HINT:** Nummular dermatitis lesions may be confused with impetigo or tinea corporis.

Id Reaction

Etiology

An id reaction is a **reactive inflammatory dermatitis** that develops in response to a primary infection, often a **cutaneous dermatophyte (tinea) or bacterial infection,** or an eczematous dermatitis such as a **contact dermatitis**.

Clinical Features

Patients present with an **acute, pruritic rash** characterized by a **symmetric eruption of multiple, small papules and/or vesicles** (Figure 64-3). Sites of predilection include the **face, ears, and extremities,** although any area may be involved.

Evaluation

The diagnosis is usually made clinically. Patients should be examined for evidence of an associated dermatophyte infection such as tinea corporis or tinea capitis, impetigo, or contact dermatitis.

Treatment

Most patients respond to treatment of the underlying infection or eczematous dermatitis. The use of **topical corticosteroids and systemic antihistamines** may afford symptomatic relief.

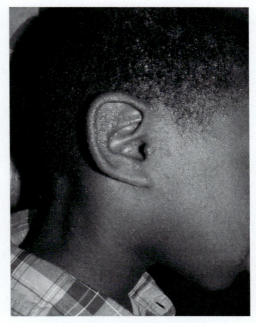

FIGURE 64-3   Id reaction in tinea capitis.

Psoriasis
Etiology
The cause is **unknown,** although some evidence indicates a **genetic** component. An **immune defect** may be a primary or secondary factor.

Clinical Features
Psoriasis is characterized by erythematous plaques with silvery scale located symmetrically on the elbows, knees, extensor surfaces of the wrist, genitalia, and scalp. Children may present with guttate (teardrop-like) plaques on the trunk (Figure 64-4). Patients can also present with large plaques, pustular plaques, or as an erythroderma, whereby most of the body's skin is erythematous and scaling. Nail changes include pitting on some or all of the fingers and onycholysis (i.e., separation of the nail plate from the nail bed).

Evaluation
Psoriasis is a **clinical diagnosis,** but if there is doubt, a **skin biopsy** may be beneficial.

Treatment
Mid-potency topical steroids, topical retinoids, topical calcipotriene (a vitamin D derivative), tar preparations, and antiseborrheic shampoos are useful. Patients with

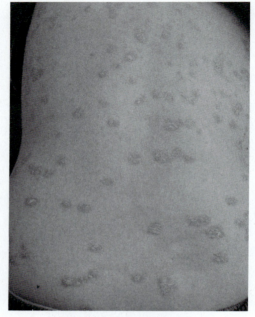

FIGURE 64-4 Guttate psoriasis.

severe cases may require ultraviolet light therapy or systemic medication. Referral to a pediatric dermatologist is recommended for all patients with psoriasis, except those with very mild cases.

 HINT: Guttate psoriasis may be triggered by an antecedent Group A α-hemolytic *Streptococcus* infection.

Lichen Planus
Etiology and Clinical Features
Lichen planus is a dermatologic disorder with lesions characterized by the **"five Ps"—pruritic, polygonal, purple, planar, and papules**—located on the **flexor surfaces, genitalia, mucous membranes, scalp, and nails** (Figure 64-5). The cause is **unknown**. The disease can eventually lead to **scarring of the scalp and nails**.

Evaluation
A **skin biopsy** confirms the diagnosis when the clinical lesions do not conform to the classic description.

Treatment
Initial treatment is with **mid- to high-strength topical steroids**. Some patients may require oral corticosteroids or phototherapy; these patients are best managed by a dermatologist.

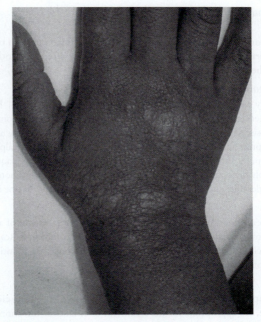

FIGURE 64-5 Polygonal, pruritus, and purple papules of lichen planus.

Seborrheic Dermatitis

Etiology

The cause is **unknown,** although there appears to be a relation to the yeast *Pityrosporum ovale*. In addition, there may be a **hormonal component** because it usually appears in neonates or after the onset of puberty.

Clinical Features

Typically, scalp scaling is present and may be associated with erythema and pruritus. In addition, erythematous patches with greasy scaling may be present behind the ears, on the forehead and eyebrows, and in the nasolabial folds. The eruption can occasionally be seen in the presternal area, axillae, and inguinal folds.

> **HINT:** Seborrheic dermatitis is usually not seen in patients between 1 year of age and puberty. In patients in this age group, one must always think of the possibility of dermatophyte (tinea) infections.

Treatment

Treatment entails frequent shampooing with an antidandruff shampoo and the application of low-potency topical steroids.

Tinea (Dermatophyte) Infections
Etiology
Tinea infections are caused by superficial cutaneous infection with one of many species of **dermatophyte molds**. They may be transmitted from other persons, animals, or the environment.

Clinical Features
Infection may involve the body (tinea corporis), face (tinea facie), hands (tinea manuum), feet (tinea pedis), groin (tinea cruris), scalp (tinea capitis), or nails (onychomycosis). Cutaneous involvement usually presents with pruritus and scaly erythematous papules and annular plaques. Tinea capitis may present as scalp scaling, erythematous papules and pustules, hair loss, or painful, boggy, scaling plaques (kerion). Cervical lymphadenopathy may be prominent in tinea capitis. Onychomycosis presents with brittle, thickened, discolored nails. One or several nails may be involved.

Evaluation
Microscopic examination of a **potassium hydroxide preparation** of a skin scraping may demonstrate **fungal hyphae**. **Fungal culture** from skin or scalp scrapings or from nail clippings are the diagnostic test of choice and can identify the causative species of mold.

Treatment
A variety of topical antifungal agents, such as **clotrimazole, naftifine, ciclopirox, or ketoconazole,** are appropriate for the treatment of cutaneous infection. Treatment of tinea capitis requires the use of a systemic antifungal, usually **griseofulvin**. Adjuvant therapy with antifungal shampoo, such as ketoconazole, ciclopirox, or selenium sulfide, is recommended to decrease the shedding of spores. Treatment of onychomycosis also requires the use of a systemic antifungal agent such as **terbinafine**.

Tinea Versicolor
Etiology and Clinical Features
Tinea versicolor is caused by superficial infection with the mold *Malassezia furfur*.

Tinea versicolor presents with **hypopigmented or hyperpigmented round, oval, coalescent macules** with **slight superficial scale** on the chest, back, abdomen, or proximal extremities. It is usually asymptomatic.

Evaluation
The diagnosis is usually made clinically. **Microscopic examination of a potassium hydroxide preparation** of a skin scraping may demonstrate **fungal spores and hyphae** with a characteristic **"spaghetti and meatballs"** appearance.

Treatment
Intermittent use of a topical antifungal shampoo or cream such as **ketoconazole** or **selenium sulfide** is usually effective.

Pityriasis Rosea
Etiology and Clinical Features
Pityriasis rosea is an **acute, self-limited eruption**. The cause is **unknown**. Most cases start with a **single, large, oval, scaling plaque** known as a **herald patch**.

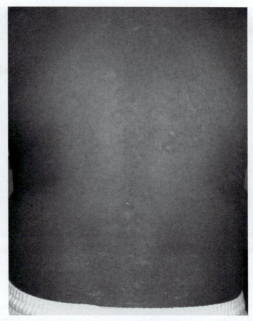

FIGURE 64-6 Oval scaling macules arranged along skin tension lines in pityriasis rosea.

Within 1 week of the initial lesion, crops of **small, pink, finely scaled plaques** develop on the **trunk** (Figure 64-6). These lesions have a tendency to follow **skin cleavage lines,** creating a **"Christmas tree" pattern**. The rash usually **spares the face, except in children,** in whom facial involvement is common. The eruption may be associated with **moderate pruritus**.

> **HINT:** The eruption of secondary syphilis can mimic pityriasis rosea and should be considered in sexually active adolescents.

Treatment
Topical steroids and oral antihistamines can help alleviate the itching.

Lyme Disease
Etiology
Lyme disease is a tick-borne illness caused by the spirochete ***Borrelia burgdorferi***. It is most commonly seen in the northeastern United States.

Clinical Features
The most characteristic finding is the presence of an **expanding annular patch of erythema with central clearing** (erythema chronicum migrans) at the site of the

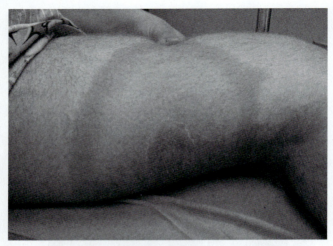

FIGURE 64-7   Annular patch of erythema with central clearing (erythema chronicum migrans) in Lyme disease.

tick bite (Figure 64-7). Early symptoms may include **fever, myalgias, arthralgias, headache, and fatigue**. Late manifestations include arthritis, carditis, and neurologic abnormalities such as aseptic meningitis and Bell palsy.

Evaluation
Serologic testing of acute and convalescent sera is helpful. Skin biopsy is rarely needed.

Treatment
The treatment of choice for early Lyme disease in children above 8 years is **doxycycline**. In younger children, use of **amoxicillin** is appropriate.

Erythema Multiforme
Etiology
Erythema multiforme is a reactive, inflammatory dermatosis. It usually occurs in response to an antecedent infection, although medications may also trigger the reaction. The most common cause is a **herpes simplex virus infection,** although other viruses as well as bacteria and fungi are reported to cause EM. Recurrent episodes are often associated with herpes simplex virus infection.

Clinical Features
The characteristic rash is the **target lesion,** which is characterized by a central area of **dusky erythema, surrounded by a ring of pallor (edema) and a peripheral ring of erythema** (Figure 64-8). Common sites of involvement are the **palms and extremities,** although any area may be involved. Some patients complain of pruritus or burning. Mucous membrane involvement of the lips or oropharynx

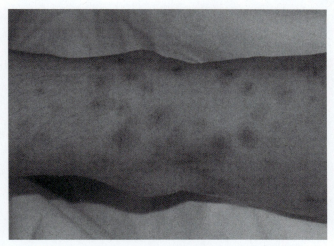

FIGURE 64-8 Classic acral "target lesions" of erythema multiforme.

may be seen but is generally mild. Associated symptoms are generally mild and may include **fever, fatigue, or pharyngitis**. Stevens–Johnson syndrome is a more severe form of this entity with mucosal involvement.

> **HINT:** EM may be confused with annular forms of urticaria, which presents with transient pruritic annular and polycyclic plaque characterized by erythematous lesions with central clearing.

Evaluation
The diagnosis is usually made clinically. Skin biopsy is rarely needed.

Treatment
The use of **topical steroids and systemic antihistamines** may be helpful. Systemic steroids may be required for more extensive cases. Analgesics, emollients, and oral hygiene may be required for painful oral lesions. The condition is self-limited.

Scabies
Scabies is discussed in Chapter 63, "Pruritus."

Papular Acrodermatitis of Childhood (Gianotti–Crosti Syndrome)
Etiology
Papular acrodermatitis of childhood is associated with many viruses, most commonly **Epstein–Barr virus** in the United States. In Europe, there is a strong association of this disease with nonicteric hepatitis B virus infection.

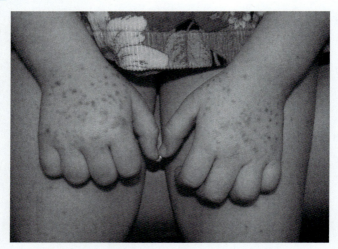

FIGURE 64-9 Acrally located papular rash of Gianotti–Crosti syndrome.

Clinical Features

The patient presents with **skin-colored to erythematous flat-topped papules** that are found on the **face, extremities, and buttocks,** with the trunk usually spared (Figure 64-9). **Pruritus** is sometimes associated with the eruption. **Hepatomegaly and lymphadenopathy** are occasionally present.

Evaluation and Treatment

Liver function tests may be abnormal in those patients with hepatomegaly. Usually, there is no need for any laboratory tests because the diagnosis can be made clinically and the eruption is **benign and self-limiting,** usually **resolving in 3 to 6 weeks**.

Papular Urticaria

Etiology and Clinical Features

Papular urticaria, caused by a **hypersensitivity reaction to insect bites,** is characterized by **intensely pruritic wheals** (5 to 10 mm in diameter) **and papules** that contain a **central punctum**. Many times, the central punctum cannot be seen secondary to excoriation. Mosquitoes, fleas, and bedbugs are the most common exposures.

Lesions can be seen on any part of the body but are typically observed on exposed areas such as **the extremities, head, neck, and shoulders**. The eruption can **persist for months** and lesions can become **secondarily infected**. Extremely sensitive patients can develop **bullous lesions**. Fully resolved lesions tend to develop **temporary hyperpigmentation**.

 HINT: Always consider an insect bite reaction when a patient presents with grouped urticarial papules that occur only on exposed areas.

Evaluation

The history and physical examination are diagnostic.

Treatment

In patients with prolonged episodes, it is important to **identify the arthropod exposure**. Pets should be **treated for infestations**. An exterminator may need to inspect the home. Secondarily infected lesions should be treated with the appropriate topical or systemic **antibiotics**.

Molluscum Contagiosum

Etiology

Molluscum contagiosum is caused by cutaneous infection with the molluscum virus, a poxvirus. It may be spread by close physical contact, sharing of swimming pools or fomites such as towels, and autoinoculation.

Clinical Features

Infection is most commonly seen in school-age children. From a few to several dozen **small pearly, umbilicated papules** develop. These papules may occur anywhere on the body, but involvement of the face is common. Lesions are usually asymptomatic. During the resolution of individual lesions, an intense inflammatory reaction with surrounding erythema may develop. The condition is self-limited and generally resolves over 9 to 15 months.

Evaluation

The diagnosis is made clinically.

Treatment

Since the infection is self-limited, no treatment is required. When treatment is considered, therapeutic options include topical application of **cantharidin,** a blistering agent; **cryotherapy; curettage; and topical retinoids**.

EVALUATION OF RASH

Patient History

Details regarding the **associated symptoms** such as fever, pharyngitis, and malaise should be elicited. It is important to ascertain **how the rash has evolved** and if any **topical or systemic treatment** has been rendered. A **complete drug and immunization history** should be obtained.

Physical Examination

Important features include the **morphology** of the eruption and its **distribution**. A complete examination of the **skin, hair, nails, and mucous membranes** should be performed.

TREATMENT OF RASH

Table 64-1 summarizes commonly used topical corticosteroids but is not all inclusive. In general, the use of class 1 and 2 topical steroids is best avoided in children.

TABLE 64-1	Topical Corticosteroids		
Class	**Generic Name**	**Brand Name**	**Formulation**
1. Highest potency	Clobetasol propionate 0.05%	Temovate	Cream, ointment
	Betamethasone dipropionate 0.05%	Diprolene	Cream, ointment
	Diflorasone diacetate 0.05%	Psorcon	Ointment
2. High potency	Fluocinonide 0.05%	Lidex	Cream, ointment, gel
	Desoximetasone 0.25%	Topicort	Cream, ointment
3. Mid-to-high potency	Triamcinolone acetonide 0.5%	Aristocort	Cream, ointment
	Mometasone furoate 0.1%	Elocon	Cream, ointment
	Betamethasone valerate 0.1%	Valisone	Ointment
4. Mid potency	Triamcinolone acetonide 0.1%	Aristocort	Ointment
	Mometasone furoate 0.1%	Kenalog	Ointment
	Fluocinolone acetonide 0.025%	Elocon	Cream
	Desoximetasone 0.05%	Topicort LP	Cream
5. Low-to-mid potency	Alclometasone dipropionate 0.05%	Aclovate	Cream, ointment
	Betamethasone valerate 0.1%	Valisone	Cream, lotion
	Fluocinolone acetonide 0.025%	Synalar	Cream
	Hydrocortisone valerate 0.2%	Westcort	Cream, ointment
6. Low potency	Triamcinolone acetonide 0.025%	Aristocort	Cream
	Desonide 0.05%	DesOwen	Cream
	Fluocinolone acetonide 0.01%	Synalar	Cream, lotion
7. Lowest potency	Hydrocortisone 1% Hydrocortisone 2.5%	Numerous over-the-counter preparations	Cream, ointment

Suggested Readings

Dyer JA. Childhood viral exanthems. *Pediatr Ann.* 1997;36(1):21–29.

Folster-Holst R, Kreth HW. Viral exanthems in childhood (infectious exanthems): Part 1: classic exanthems. *J Deutschen Dermatologischen Gesselschaft.* 2009;7(4):309–316.

Folster-Holst R, Kreth HW. Viral exanthems in childhood (infectious exanthems): Part 2: other viral exanthems. *J Deutschen Dermatologischen Gesselschaft.* 2009;7(5):414–418.

Gable EK, Liu G, Morrell DS. Pediatric exanthems. *Prim Care.* 2000;27(2):353–369.

Nelson JS, Stone MS. Update on selected viral exanthems. *Curr Opin Pediatr.* 2000;12(4):359–364.

Newburger JW, Takahashi M, Gerber MA, et al. Diagnosis, treatment, and long-term management of Kawasaki disease. American Heart Association Scientific Statement. *Circulation.* 2004;110:2747–2771. Available at: http://www.circ.ahajournals.org/cgi/content/full/110/17/ 2747.

Wagner A. Distinguishing vesicular and pustular disorders in the neonate. *Curr Opin Pediatr.* 1997;9(4): 396–405.

Red Eye

INTRODUCTION

Red eye may refer to **erythema of the ocular adnexa, conjunctiva, sclera, or cornea, or inflammation of deeper structures**.

DIFFERENTIAL DIAGNOSIS LIST

Ocular Adnexa

- **Infectious Causes**
  - Hordeolum and chalazion
  - Dacryocystitis
  - Molluscum contagiosum
  - Blepharitis
  - Phthiriasis (louse)
  - Frontal sinus infection or other sinusitis
  - Periostitis of orbital bones
  - Orbital cellulitis, periorbital cellulitis
  - Dental abscess
- **Neoplastic Causes**
  - Neuroblastoma
  - Leukemia
  - Neurofibroma
- **Traumatic Causes**
  - Insect bites
  - Basilar skull fracture
  - Trauma to eyelid or nose
- **Miscellaneous Causes**
  - Frequent eye rubbing
  - Cavernous sinus thrombosis
  - Prolonged crying
  - Contact dermatitis
  - Seborrhea

Conjunctiva

- **Infectious Causes**
  - Bacteria
  - Viruses
  - Fungi
  - Protozoans
  - Helminths—onchocerciasis (river blindness)
- **Toxic Causes**
  - Atropine, scopolamine
  - Irritants—makeup, smoke, smog, chemicals, contact lenses, caterpillar hair, wind, ultraviolet light, tobacco
- **Neoplastic Causes**
  - Orbital tumors—retinoblastoma
- **Traumatic Causes**
  - Foreign body
  - Entropion, ectropion
  - Child abuse
  - Blunt or penetrating trauma
  - Traumatic glaucoma
  - Subconjunctival hemorrhage
- **Immunologic Causes**
  - Allergic/inflammatory conjunctivitis
  - Keratoconjunctivitis sicca and other dry eye disorders

- Nasal inflammation
- Sjögren syndrome and other collagen vascular diseases
- Kawasaki syndrome
- Stevens–Johnson syndrome
- Inflammatory bowel disease
- Juvenile rheumatoid arthritis
- Graves disease
- **Miscellaneous Causes**
  - Bone marrow transplant
  - Ectodermal dysplasia
  - Subconjunctival hemorrhage (secondary to severe cough, bacteremia, blood dyscrasia, or vomiting)

Cornea
- **Infectious Causes**
  - Keratitis
  - Syphilis

- **Traumatic Causes**
  - Contact lenses
  - Corneal ulcer
  - Corneal abrasion
  - Chemical irritant

Uveal Tract
- Iridocyclitis
- Reiter syndrome

Sclera
- Episcleritis
- Scleritis
- Collagen vascular disease

Pupil
- Hyphema
- Globe
- Glaucoma

DIFFERENTIAL DIAGNOSIS DISCUSSION
Neonatal Conjunctivitis
Etiology

Neonatal conjunctivitis is most often **secondary to infection or chemical irritation**.

- **Infection.** Causes of infectious conjunctivitis in the neonates include sexually transmitted and nonsexually transmitted organisms. Sexually transmitted agents, in order of decreasing frequency, are *Chlamydia trachomatis, Neisseria gonorrhoeae,* and herpes simplex virus (HSV), usually type 2. *Staphylococcus aureus* is the most common nonsexually transmitted infectious pathogen. Other bacterial causes include enteric Gram-negative rods.
- **Chemical irritation.** Silver nitrate is the most common cause of neonatal chemical conjunctivitis, although other antibiotics used for prophylaxis can also cause conjunctivitis.

Clinical Features

Conjunctivitis that presents in the **first 24 hours of life** is most likely **secondary to chemical irritation,** unless there was prolonged rupture of membranes before delivery.

- **Gonococcal conjunctivitis,** which presents 2 to 6 days after birth, is an acute to hyperacute infection that causes edema of the eyelids and conjunctiva (chemosis), local pain, and a copious purulent discharge. Swelling and discharge can be so extensive that the orbit is difficult to view. Often there is a palpable preauricular node, a finding otherwise uncommon in bacterial conjunctivitis.
- **Chlamydial conjunctivitis** has a slightly later onset than gonococcal conjunctivitis but can be symptomatic as early as 4 to 5 days after birth. Modest purulent

drainage and mild-to-moderate inflammation are seen. As with gonococcal conjunctivitis, the preauricular lymph node may be tender.
- **Herpes simplex conjunctivitis** is associated with clusters of vesicles on the face, eyelids, and mucous membranes.

> **HINT:** Chlamydial conjunctivitis, in general, is markedly less acute and impressive than gonococcal conjunctivitis.

> **HINT:** Chlamydial pneumonitis occurs in as many as a one-third of infants with chlamydial conjunctivitis, although it presents later, typically at 3 to 16 weeks of age.

Evaluation

Bacterial culture, including **chocolate agar or Thayer–Martin plates and Gram stain of the purulent material,** should be obtained. In up to 95% of cases of gonococcal conjunctivitis, Gram-negative intracellular diplococci are identified by Gram stain.

Chlamydia **culture** should be obtained on **conjunctival scrapings** (not purulent material) using **a Dacron-tipped swab.** Nucleic acid amplification techniques can be used to identify both the organisms in laboratories with these testing capabilities. In patients with suspected herpes simplex conjunctivitis, conjunctival scrapings reveal mononuclear cells and giant multinucleated epithelial cells.

Treatment
- **Chlamydial conjunctivitis.** Hospitalization is not necessary. Treatment consists of 14 days of oral erythromycin combined with topical erythromycin.
- **Gonococcal conjunctivitis.** Hospitalization and consultation with an ophthalmologist are required. The eye should be irrigated every 1 to 2 hours to reduce bacterial load and local irritation. Improperly treated gonococcal conjunctivitis can quickly damage vision. Intravenous therapy for 7 days is indicated for disseminated infection, and up to 14 days for meningitis; one dose is adequate for isolated conjunctivitis. Cefotaxime or ceftriaxone are appropriate until sensitivities are known; **use ceftriaxone with caution in patients with hyperbilirubinemia.**
- **Herpes simplex conjunctivitis.** Patients must be followed by an ophthalmologist to minimize the chances of permanent scarring and damage to vision.

Infectious Conjunctivitis (Outside the Neonatal Period)
Etiology

The most common bacterial cause of conjunctivitis is *S. aureus,* which affects all age groups. *Haemophilus influenzae* and *Streptococcus pneumoniae* are common causes of conjunctivitis in **young children. Adolescents** can also present with **gonococcal** conjunctivitis **secondary to sexual contact.**

Epidemic keratoconjunctivitis, the name given to rapidly spreading viral conjunctivitis, most often occurs secondary to adenoviral infection. **HSV, types 1 and 2, and varicella-zoster virus** are more serious causes of viral conjunctivitis; these organisms are associated with **corneal destruction** (keratitis) and **loss of vision**. Herpes simplex keratitis is the most common infectious cause of corneal blindness in developed countries.

Protozoal infections, specifically *Acanthamoeba,* are seen almost **exclusively in contact lens wearers**.

 HINT: Contact lens wearers are more susceptible to virulent Gram-negative infections and unusual fungal infections of the conjunctiva.

Clinical Features

The clinical signs and symptoms of **bacterial** conjunctivitis include **tearing, purulent discharge, conjunctival hyperemia, and foreign body sensation** (Table 65-1). The **eyelids** are often **crusted closed** on arising in the **morning**. *H. influenzae* and *S. pneumoniae* conjunctival infections are often associated with **subconjunctival hemorrhage**. Infection is often **bilateral**.

The physical findings of **nonherpetic viral** conjunctivitis include a **serous or lightly purulent discharge, minimal-to-moderate eyelid swelling, a unilateral or bilateral presentation, and occasional systemic symptoms** (e.g., malaise, fever, or sore throat). **Profuse tearing** is often present. Viral conjunctivitis is much more likely than bacterial infection to be associated with **tender preauricular adenopathy**.

 HINT: Clinical features cannot definitively distinguish between bacterial and viral etiologies; patients with no or watery discharge, no glued eye in the morning, age 6 years or older, and who present in April through November have been shown to have a high likelihood of viral etiology.

 HINT: Subconjunctival hemorrhage may point to adenoviral conjunctivitis.

In patients with **herpetic viral** conjunctivitis, the **initial HSV infection** is clinically **indistinguishable from other causes of viral conjunctivitis,** with the exception that it is almost always **unilateral**. Herpetic recurrences are unilateral in 96% of patients, are often **corneal** (keratitis), and produce the classic **dendritic lesion of the cornea best seen with fluorescein**.

Evaluation

Culture is necessary only **if an unusual or serious pathogen** is suspected. Although recovery of the offending organism is difficult once antibiotic therapy has been initiated, cultures are also recommended in case of **treatment failure**. Culture recovery of HSV is successful in only 70% of patients with herpetic conjunctivitis.

TABLE 65-1	Differentiation of Conjunctivitis (Outside the Neonatal Period)			
Clinical Findings	**Viral**	**Bacterial**	**Chlamydial**	**Allergic**
Itching	Minimal	Minimal	Minimal	Severe
Hyperemia	Generalized	Generalized	Generalized	Generalized
Tearing	Profuse	Moderate	Moderate	Moderate
Exudation	Minimal	Profuse	Profuse	Minimal
Preauricular node	Common	Uncommon[a]	Inclusion conjunct	None
Sore throat/fever	Occasionally	Occasionally	Never	Never

[a]Except in gonococcal conjunctivitis.
PMNs, polymorphonuclear cells.
Modified with permission from Schwab I, Dawson C. Conjunctiva. In: Vaughan D, Ashbury T, Riordan-Eva P, eds. *General Ophthalmology.* 14th ed. Norwalk, CT: Appleton & Lange; 1995:98.

Treatment

Viral and bacterial conjunctivitis are **self-resolving** illnesses **except for herpes simplex** conjunctivitis and conjunctivitis caused by **varicella-zoster virus**. Since it is **impossible clinically to differentiate viral and bacterial** conjunctivitis with certainty, **nonherpetic viral** conjunctivitis is **treated in the same fashion as bacterial** conjunctivitis. Watchful waiting can be used; if treatment is preferred, instillation of **antibiotic drops and periodic removal of eye discharge with warm wet washcloth is recommended**. Improvement usually occurs within 3 to 4 days. Without treatment, both bacterial and viral conjunctivitis usually resolve within 5 days, although treatment for bacterial conjunctivitis has been shown to speed clinical recovery. In the event of **treatment failure,** a **second antibiotic** with a significantly **different spectrum** from the first antibiotic should be prescribed.

Any child who presents with red eye with a **prior history of herpetic conjunctivitis** should be assumed to have **recurrent herpes infection** and must be **referred to an ophthalmologist urgently. Steroid use** in all types of conjunctivitis is best **left to an ophthalmologist** because **serious harm** can result **if steroids** are inadvertently **prescribed for a patient with herpetic conjunctivitis**.

Allergic Conjunctivitis

Etiology

Common environmental allergens (e.g., animal dander, dust, molds, grass, pollens) can cause allergic conjunctivitis. **Antibiotic drops and facial creams or lotions** are also implicated.

Clinical Features

The hallmark of allergic conjunctivitis is **pruritus**. Symptoms include significant **erythema and swelling of the eyelids,** most often in a **bilateral** distribution. These symptoms can be confused with those of periorbital or orbital cellulitis; however, a **lack of tenderness and** the **absence of systemic symptoms** make cellulitis unlikely. **Conjunctival hyperemia** is **diffuse**. **Discharge** is **moderate** in volume, and **clear**. Adenopathy is not found.

The **onset of symptoms** can be **abrupt,** after acute exposure to the offending agent, or **chronic,** with repeated or continuous exposure. Symptoms may show a **seasonal variation,** commonly **worsening in the spring. Rhinitis and other allergic symptoms** may also be present.

Treatment

Treatment depends on the age of the child and on the subjective symptoms. **Erythema alone does not warrant intervention. Cold compresses** are effective for short-term relief of pruritus. **Topical vasoconstrictors and antihistamines** are the first-line medications if treatment is undertaken. If the treatment is unsuccessful, **topical steroids** may be required. **Systemic antihistamines and nasal steroids** often provide relief.

Chalazia and Hordeola

Etiology

A chalazion is a **chronic inflammatory lipogranuloma of the meibomian gland** resulting from obstruction of the gland duct. **Secondary infection** is common. An infected chalazion is sometimes referred to as an **internal hordeolum**.

An **external hordeolum (stye)** is a **purulent,** usually **staphylococcal, infection of the follicle of an eyelash** or its associated **sebaceous or sweat gland**.

Clinical Features and Evaluation

Uninfected chalazia are characterized by **gradual, painless swelling** in the body of the **eyelid.** Chalazia that become **secondarily infected** usually **point and drain on the inside of the eyelid** (the conjunctival side).

Hordeola present with **swelling, induration, and purulent drainage** at or near the margin of the eyelid. Hordeola tend to **point and drain outward**. Hordeola often occur in **groups,** following the spread of infection from one follicle to another.

Both chalazia and hordeola may be **unilateral or bilateral**. The child with either a hordeolum or an infected chalazion is **afebrile and appears otherwise well**.

Treatment

Small, uninfected chalazia may **resolve spontaneously. Large chalazia** must be **surgically removed. Infected** chalazia require **medical management**.

Hordeola and infected chalazia are treated identically. **Warm to hot compresses** should be applied to the affected eye for **20 minutes, four times per day,** to encourage spontaneous drainage of the purulent collections. Some advocate daily **cleaning of the lid margins, using baby shampoo and water on a washcloth** rubbed on the lid margin with the eyes held shut. **Topical antibiotic ointment or drops** should be instilled daily. Attention to **general hygiene** keeps recurrences to a minimum.

Corneal Abrasion

Etiology

Corneal abrasions result from **traumatic removal of part of the corneal epithelium**.

Clinical Features

The signs and symptoms seen with corneal abrasion often mimic those of infectious conjunctivitis—**diffuse injection of the conjunctiva, watery discharge, pain,** and, often, **decreased visual acuity**. The main difference is found in the history—**trauma,** even if apparently minor, **immediately precedes the onset of symptoms** in patients with corneal abrasion.

Evaluation

Patients presenting with **red eye** and any **history of trauma** should have a **fluorescein examination of the eye** to rule out an abrasion. The eye should be carefully examined to **exclude** the possibility of a **retained foreign body** or a **deeper injury**. This includes performing a **maneuver to flip the upper lid and inspect the inner surface**. If the **pain** persists for **>24 hours** after the initial trauma, the patient should be referred to **an ophthalmologist**.

Treatment

The primary goal of treatment is to **prevent further injury. Foreign bodies** should be **removed by irrigation** with sterile saline solution. If this is ineffective, an **ophthalmologist** should be **consulted** for removal. Many authors recommend **topical antibiotic eyedrops**. For large abrasions or those involving the visual axis, the eye should be **examined daily** until fully healed.

 HINT: Topical anesthetics should never be given to a patient for repeated home instillation after corneal injury. Their use delays healing, masks damage, and can lead to permanent corneal scarring.

Orbital and Periorbital Cellulitis

Etiology

Periorbital cellulitis refers to **infection of the tissues anterior to the globe**. Infection occurs either via **hematogenous spread or local trauma**. In the past, hematogenously spread disease was most often caused by *H. influenzae*, but *S. pneumoniae* and other organisms are becoming more prevalent as a result of the success of the universal *H. influenzae* type B vaccination. In patients with a **history of local trauma**, *S. aureus* and *Streptococcus* are the most common pathogens.

Orbital cellulitis most commonly results from **direct spread of infection from the sinuses**. The infectious process in orbital cellulitis involves the **retrobulbar tissues**, including the **ocular muscles, orbital fat, and bone**.

Clinical Features

Periorbital cellulitis is a unilateral disease that presents with **significant swelling, induration, tenderness, and erythema of the eyelids** and a variable amount of **purulent discharge. Fever** is common.

Orbital cellulitis presents with a clinical picture **similar to** that of **periorbital** cellulitis. In addition, orbital cellulitis is characterized by a **decreased range of motion of ocular muscles, proptosis, changes in vision, and papilledema**. Other potential risk factors for invasive disease include previous antibiotic therapy, older age (3 years or older), and edema beyond the eyelid.

Evaluation

Children with periorbital or orbital cellulitis may be **bacteremic, and blood cultures** should be considered in highly febrile patients. **Computed tomography** should be used whenever **orbital** cellulitis is considered.

Treatment

Hospitalization and the intravenous administration of antibiotics are indicated for patients with orbital cellulitis. Medications such as **ampicillin–sulbactam, oxacillin, and ceftriaxone** are appropriate antibiotic choices, although coverage for methicillin-resistant *S. aureus* should also be considered. **Surgical drainage** may be required. Patients with periorbital cellulitis often require hospitalization, but outpatient therapy can be considered if they are older (generally >2 years), afebrile, well appearing, and have close follow-up with their primary care physician. Antibiotics like **amoxicillin–clavulanic acid and cefuroxime axetil** are appropriate choices.

Patients with **orbital** cellulitis should be seen by an **ophthalmologist** because orbital cellulitis carries **a significant risk for damage to the visual axis**—specifically, **optic neuritis with atrophy**. **Significant extraocular complications** are also associated with orbital cellulitis, including **cavernous sinus thrombosis, meningitis, and brain abscess**.

Suggested Readings

Block SL, Hedrick J, Tyler R, et al. Increasing bacterial resistance in pediatric acute conjunctivitis (1997–1998). *Antimicrob Agents Chemother.* 2000;44(6):1650–1654.

King RA. Common ocular signs and symptoms in childhood. *Pediatr Clin North Am.* 1993;40:753–766.

Leibowitz HM. The red eye. *N Engl J Med.* 2000;343(5):345–351.

Limberg M. A review of bacterial keratitis and bacterial conjunctivitis. *Am J Ophthalmol.* 1991;112:2S–9S.

Meltzer JA, Kunkov S, Crain EF. Identifying children at low risk for bacterial conjunctivitis. *Arch Pediatr Adolesc Med.* 2010;164(3):263–267.

Rose P. Management strategies for acute infective conjunctivitis in primary care: a systematic review. *Expert Opin Pharmacother.* 2007;8(12):1903–1921.

Roy FH. *Ocular Differential Diagnosis.* 6th ed. Baltimore, MA: Williams & Wilkins; 1996.

Rudloe TF, Harper MB, Prabhu SP, et al. Acute periorbital infections: who needs emergent imaging? *Pediatrics.* 2010;125(4):e719–e726.

Respiratory Distress

INTRODUCTION

Respiratory distress is defined by **increased work of breathing** that can lead to respiratory failure, a state of inadequate oxygenation and/or ventilation. Symptoms and signs may include cough, tachypnea, retractions, grunting, stridor, wheezing, shortness of breath, chest tightness, chest pain, and altered mental status in later stages.

 DIFFERENTIAL DIAGNOSIS LIST

Infectious Causes
- Peritonsillar abscess
- Retropharyngeal abscess
- Epiglottitis
- Croup (viral laryngotracheobronchitis)
- Bacterial tracheitis
- Bronchiolitis
- Meningitis
- Pertussis
- Pneumonia

Structural Lesions
- Laryngeal lesions/masses
- Laryngomalacia
- Vocal cord paralysis
- Subglottic stenosis
- Tracheomalacia
- Bronchomalacia
- Lobar emphysema
- Bronchogenic cyst
- Vascular ring and other aberrant vessels
- Mediastinal or other intrathoracic mass (cystic hygroma, teratoma, cystic adenomatoid malformation, neuroblastoma, diaphragmatic hernia, or eventration)

Toxic Causes
- Carbon monoxide poisoning
- Heavy metal poisoning
- Methemoglobinemia
- Organophosphate poisoning

Neoplastic Causes
- Hemangioma
- Papilloma
- Brainstem tumor

Traumatic Causes
- Foreign body aspiration
- Aspiration caused by gastroesophageal reflux disease
- Near drowning
- Pneumothorax

Metabolic or Genetic Causes
- Cystic fibrosis
- Hypocalcemic tetany
- Immune deficiency
- Metabolic acidosis

Psychosocial Causes
- Psychogenic hyperventilation

Neuromuscular Disorders
- Respiratory muscle weakness, myopathy
- Duchenne muscular dystrophy
- Spinal muscle atrophy
- Prune belly syndrome
- Werdnig–Hoffmann disease

Miscellaneous Causes
- Anaphylaxis
- Asthma

- Atelectasis
- Cardiac disease (congestive heart failure, tamponade, myocarditis)
- Central nervous system (increased intracranial pressure)
- Pleural disease (effusion, empyema)
- Pulmonary hemorrhage
- Pulmonary edema
- Pulmonary embolism
- Sickle cell crisis—acute chest syndrome
- Vocal cord dysfunction

DIFFERENTIAL DIAGNOSIS DISCUSSION
Infectious Causes

Infections causing respiratory distress may be **bacterial or viral** and may **affect any part of the respiratory tract**. Some infections are more common in different age groups, aiding in the diagnosis. In addition to the earlier-mentioned symptoms of respiratory distress, the patient may have **congestion or rhinitis** or a variety of constitutional symptoms such as **fever, malaise, poor appetite, or body aches**. The causative agent may be identified by cultures of the nasopharynx, pharynx, or sputum.

Epiglottitis
Etiology

Infection of the epiglottis is most commonly caused by *Haemophilus influenzae* type B and results in **rapid swelling and airway compromise,** creating a **medical emergency**. Fortunately, near universal use of the *H. influenzae* type B vaccine has dramatically reduced the incidence of this disease in children. Other pathogens that may cause epiglottitis include Streptococci, Staphylococci, and *Candida albicans.*

Clinical Features

Epiglottitis is most common in children **between the ages of 3 and 6** years who have not been vaccinated against *H. influenzae* type B. Symptoms develop over several hours, which include **high fever, dysphagia, drooling, inspiratory stridor, and holding the head in an upright "sniffing" position,** with the neck extended and the jaw protruding.

Evaluation

When the history is suggestive, **the child should not be excessively disturbed**. Attempts to visualize the pharynx directly may result in **complete occlusion** of the airway and **respiratory arrest**. Vaccination status of a patient with suspected epiglottitis must be assessed, although a positive history of vaccination does not rule out the possibility of epiglottitis. A **lateral neck radiograph** should not be attempted until a secure airway is established if the diagnosis is strongly suspected. A **characteristic "thumbprint" epiglottis** (the epiglottis is swollen) is diagnostic. A blood culture drawn after an airway is established may help determine the causative bacteria.

Treatment

The **most experienced staff** available should **establish an artificial airway under controlled circumstances,** preferably by an otolaryngologist or anesthesiologist in an operating room. When intubation of the trachea cannot be accomplished, **tracheostomy** is indicated. **Broad-spectrum antibiotics** are then administered **intravenously**.

Croup (Viral Laryngotracheobronchitis)

Etiology

Most cases of croup are caused by **parainfluenza virus types 1 and 3,** although other pathogens have been described. **Inflammation of the larynx, trachea, and bronchi** results in increased airway resistance and obstruction. Rarely is airway obstruction so severe that cardiopulmonary arrest ensues.

Clinical Features

Patients are usually in the typical age range of **6 months to 6 years**. The presence of symptoms in the first few months of life should prompt evaluation for congenital anomalies. Patients with mild cases may demonstrate a **bark-like cough, nasal congestion, and fever**. Typically, a mild cough with intermittent stridor **progresses to continuous stridor, especially at night**. Many patients improve after exposure to cool night air.

Evaluation

On physical examination, **critical airway narrowing** is denoted by severe retractions, inspiratory stridor, and decreased air entry. In patients with severe airway obstruction, **cyanosis and fatigue** may be noted. **Cyanosis, tachycardia, and mental status changes** may accompany hypoxia. **Lateral and anteroposterior neck radiographs** can help differentiate croup from epiglottitis, although radiographs should not be required in typical presentations. A characteristic **"steeple sign"** is often seen in the subglottic airway in croup, and the epiglottis is normal.

Treatment

An **artificial airway** should be established for patients with impending respiratory failure. Therapeutic strategies include the following:

- **Humidified oxygen.** Cool, humidified oxygen is often provided for patients with mild-to-moderate cases of croup, although this practice is not clearly supported in randomized clinical trials.
- **Steroids.** A single dose of oral dexamethasone is helpful in reducing respiratory symptoms even in mild cases with symptomatic relief within 4 to 6 hours.
- **Racemic epinephrine.** Patients with severe cases may temporarily benefit from the inhalation of racemic epinephrine. These patients may need to be hospitalized

to observe for rebound effects, which may occur within 1 to 4 hours after the administration of racemic epinephrine.
* **Intravenous fluids.** Fluids are helpful in maintaining adequate hydration in patients with severe tachypnea.
* **Antibiotics.** Unless a secondary bacterial infection is suspected, antibiotics are not indicated.

Bronchiolitis

Etiology
Viruses (e.g., respiratory syncytial virus [RSV], human metapneumovirus, parainfluenza viruses, and adenoviruses) infect the **lining of the small airways (bronchioles),** resulting in **mucosal edema and intraluminal accumulation of mucus and cellular debris.** Infants **less than 2 years** are predominantly affected because the small caliber of their airways predisposes them to the development of increased airway resistance with even mild airway narrowing.

Clinical Features
A **prodrome of nasal congestion and coryza** lasting several days is usual. **Fever and anorexia** may be present, particularly in young infants with severe nasal congestion who may have difficulty feeding. Often, another family member has a mild upper respiratory tract infection. **Respiratory distress** usually **develops gradually** and is characterized by a worsening cough and wheezing. Typically, the **symptoms are worse at night, especially days 3 to 5 of illness.**

Evaluation
On physical examination, infants may be **tachypneic,** with a respiratory rate of 60 to 80 breaths/minute. The **expiratory phase is usually prolonged, and diffuse wheezing, crackles, and rhonchi** are often present. **Breath sounds** may be diminished in severe cases. **Severe retractions and the use of accessory muscles** are common. Lung hyperinflation and depression of the diaphragm may result in a **palpable liver and spleen.** Clinicians should diagnose bronchiolitis and assess disease severity on the basis of history and physical examination. Clinicians **should not** routinely order laboratory and radiologic studies for diagnosis unless there is concern for another disease entity. A **chest radiograph,** when obtained, may show hyperinflation, peribronchial thickening, and, in many patients, subsegmental atelectasis. The diagnosis of bronchiolitis is a clinical one, although **nasopharyngeal swab** or washing for RSV may help support the diagnosis in some cases.

Treatment
Supportive care entails administration of **humidified oxygen for oxygen saturation less than 90%,** and frequent **nasal suctioning** is often very helpful. **Intravenous or nasogastric fluids** are useful in maintaining hydration in the presence of tachypnea and decreased oral intake. The use of nebulized medications has been studied extensively, with inconclusive and variable results. A trial of **nebulized albuterol may be administered although** it is not effective in most cases. **Nebulized racemic epinephrine** has been shown to be beneficial in some studies. Systemic

corticosteroids also show variable results in clinical trials, although they are not currently recommended for routine use. **Hypertonic normal saline** may improve symptom scores. **Sedatives should not be used,** and antibiotics are generally not helpful. In infants with a severe course, or those with underlying cardiac or pulmonary disease, **ribavirin** may have a role in treating bronchiolitis caused by RSV.

> **HINT:** Neonates and infants with a history of premature birth (with or without associated lung disease) or chronic heart or lung disease are at greater risk for apnea and poor outcome. A monoclonal antibody (Palivizumab), given in monthly intramuscular injections through the typical RSV season, is available for patients who meet high-risk criteria.

Pertussis

Etiology

The classic causative organism is *Bordetella pertussis,* but *Bordetella parapertussis* and adenovirus infection can also cause pertussis, which is characterized by **necrosis** and desquamation of the superficial epithelium of the pharynx. Infants **less than 2 months** of age are most at risk, even if immunized. Adolescents and adults are often first affected because of waning immunity, and the diagnosis should be entertained in a younger child if an adult contact has a prolonged coughing illness.

Clinical Features

- A **catarrhal stage,** consisting of symptoms of an upper respiratory tract infection, lasts 1 to 2 weeks.
- A **paroxysmal stage** follows and is characterized by a distinctive, repeated, staccato cough that occurs during a single expiration, often emptying the lungs of all their vital capacity. In the following inspiration, a "whoop" sound is produced as the edematous, narrowed glottis oscillates between the open and the closed position, causing the column of inspired air to vibrate. Whoops are not always present; rather some patients demonstrate posttussive emesis at the end of a paroxysm. Patients are usually well between paroxysmal attacks. With repeated coughing, facial redness or cyanosis and neck vein distension may occur. Petechiae of the head and neck and conjunctival hemorrhages may develop after severe coughing. Infants may develop respiratory distress, apnea, or both.
- During the **convalescent stage,** the frequency of paroxysms gradually decreases, although the cough often persists for several months (called the "100-day cough"). Habitual (or psychogenic) coughing may result in a few patients.

Evaluation

During the early paroxysmal phase, a **complete blood cell count may** reveal lymphocytosis. **Chest radiographs** may show perihilar infiltrates and subsegmental atelectasis. **Fluorescent antibody staining or polymerase chain reaction** can be performed on nasopharyngeal swabs to detect *B. pertussis.* A positive culture can also confirm the diagnosis. Many states require notification to the department of health, and contacts may warrant prophylaxis.

Treatment

Although **erythromycin estolate** can help reduce the spread of infection, it does not shorten the disease once it progresses to the paroxysmal phase. Alternative therapy with clarithromycin or azithromycin may be effective and is more likely to be tolerated based on frequency of dosing, duration of therapy, and side effects. Supportive care consists of maintaining adequate **hydration,** administering **supplemental oxygen** for patients with respiratory distress, and **suctioning nasal secretions** in infants. **Inhaled bronchodilators** may help reduce coughing paroxysms. Cough suppressants are generally neither helpful nor recommended in young children, although they may sometimes be considered at bedtime in older patients with significant sleep disruption.

Structural Lesions

Structural lesions may occur at any point along the respiratory system and may cause respiratory symptoms any time from the early neonatal period onward. The symptoms may worsen in the face of an intercurrent acute respiratory illness such as a viral infection or asthma exacerbation. Treatment for lesions may involve **observation, medical therapy, or surgical intervention**.

Laryngomalacia, Tracheomalacia, and Bronchomalacia

Etiology

Weakened or softened underlying cartilaginous and/or muscular infrastructure of the airway results in **collapse of the airway and luminal narrowing**. The process may be **primary or secondary,** often caused by insults such as prolonged mechanical ventilation in the premature newborn or recurrent aspiration from gastroesophageal reflux disease.

Clinical Features

The patient may demonstrate **stridor if the lesion is extrathoracic or wheezing if the lesion is intrathoracic**. The wheeze is often homophonous and vibratory. The symptoms may be accentuated during crying or agitation or during an intercurrent acute respiratory illness.

Evaluation

The history and physical examination are often highly suggestive of the diagnosis. Confirmation requires visualization by **endoscopy**. Radiography, with lateral neck radiographs and/or airway fluoroscopy, is less helpful, although anterior and lateral chest films should be performed to evaluate for other causes of respiratory symptoms.

Treatment

Since airway collapsibility improves with increasing age, malacia usually **resolves spontaneously by 15 to 18 months of age**. Some children with tracheomalacia continue to have a characteristic loud or barky "smoker's" cough well into school age. Intercurrent acute illnesses should be managed accordingly, and causative diseases, such as reflux, should be treated appropriately. In severe cases, **positive airway pressure** (either noninvasively or invasively through a tracheostomy) or **surgical procedures** may be needed. Poor feeding, poor growth, cyanotic spells or recurrent apparent life-threatening events, or failure to follow a typical course of spontaneous improvement and resolution should all prompt further evaluation and intervention.

Traumatic Causes

Foreign Bodies

Etiology

Foreign bodies may be **inhaled into the airway,** or they may get **caught in the esophagus** and externally compress the trachea. Foreign body aspiration is more common in toddlers and infants, who tend to put objects in their mouths. Parents may recall the exact time of the start of symptoms, and the symptoms often start suddenly without a prodrome of infection symptoms.

Clinical Features

If the object is in the esophagus, **drooling, dysphagia, and anorexia** may accompany **respiratory distress**. Respiratory symptoms may be **acute or chronic,** with a history of **chronic cough** unresponsive to other treatments.

Evaluation

A **monophonic wheeze or absent breath sounds on one side** may be noted on chest examination.

- **Chest and neck radiographs** with lateral views may be helpful in identifying the location of an object. **Inspiratory and expiratory lateral decubitus films** may denote an area of hyperinflation. Fluoroscopy may be used to show abnormal inflation or deflation in real time. Retained foreign bodies, if small and not obstructing the larger airways, may result in chronic infection with persistent opacification on plain films and later bronchiectasis.
- **Arterial blood gas analysis** (to establish the adequacy of gas exchange) is indicated when the patient is in severe distress.

Treatment

- If the child is calm with good air exchange, removal of the foreign body should take place under controlled circumstances because manipulation may change the position of the object, inducing more severe obstruction.
- **If the child is in significant distress, chest thrusts (for age <1 year) or abdominal thrusts (for >1 year)** may be performed as per the standard technique for cardiopulmonary resuscitation. **Emergency tracheostomy** may be necessary.

Aspiration Caused by Gastroesophageal Reflux Disease

Etiology

Gastroesophageal reflux disease (GERD) may cause respiratory symptoms from **large bolus aspiration, recurrent microaspiration, or reflex laryngospasm or bronchospasm**. Patients with underlying neurologic disorders are at an increased risk of aspiration, although GERD may be found in children of all ages in the absence of other predisposing conditions.

Clinical Features

Patients may or may not have a history of overt reflux with vomiting followed by coughing or choking. Some patients may simply have recurrent cough (especially at night), frequent stomachaches, heartburn or chest pain, globus, or sour burps. With aspiration pneumonitis, symptoms of significant respiratory distress and hypoxemia, as well as fever, may develop.

Evaluation

GERD is often clinically diagnosed by symptom recognition and trial of GERD therapy. Diagnostic procedures include **radionucleotide scan** (milk scan), **pH probe, and impedance pH testing**. To ensure the absence of an anatomic abnormality causing the reflux, an **upper gastrointestinal series** is often performed prior to the initiation of therapy. After aspiration, a **chest radiograph** may show a consolidation in the affected area.

Treatment

Aspiration pneumonitis requires **antibiotic therapy,** usually intravenous antibiotics until fever and significant respiratory symptoms have resolved. GERD is usually treated with feeding precautions (liquid volume limitation, positioning) as well as **an H_2 blocker or proton pump inhibitor,** sometimes in combination with a **prokinetic agent.** In severe reflux that does not respond to medical therapy, **surgical treatment** (fundoplication) may be necessary.

Pneumothorax
Etiology

Trauma to the chest, foreign body aspiration (with a ball-valve effect), **severe underlying pulmonary disease, or idiopathic bulla formation** may result in the entry of air into the potential space between the parietal and visceral pleurae, impairing the ability of the chest wall to inflate the lung parenchyma adequately on the affected side. Patients with **asthma, cystic fibrosis, and connective tissue diseases** (e.g., Marfan syndrome) may be at an **increased risk of pneumothorax**. Often, the precipitating event is a **Valsalva maneuver,** which causes a transient elevation of intrathoracic pressure. Other risk factors include **commercial air travel** in pressurized cabins and **scuba diving**.

Tension pneumothorax (a life-threatening event that results from the rapid filling of the pleural space by gas under pressure) can **distort the vascular flow** via compression and **cause rapid death**. Patients undergoing positive-pressure mechanical ventilation are at risk for tension pneumothorax.

Clinical Features

Symptoms are usually **abrupt in onset** and consist of **pleuritic chest pain, cough, cyanosis, tachypnea, and hypoxemia**. Shoulder pain may be a more subtle presenting symptom. The degree of distress is related to the size of the pneumothorax, usually described as a percentage of the thoracic volume on the affected side. Small pneumothoraces may be asymptomatic.

Evaluation

A **history** of trauma, underlying lung disease, or past pneumothoraces from bullae should be explored. **Chest examination** demonstrates **decreased breath sounds** on the affected side and **tympany** to percussion. **Heart tones may be shifted** toward the affected side (as a result of lung collapse) or away from the affected side (in patients with tension pneumothorax). **Transillumination of the chest** is helpful in demonstrating pneumothorax in young infants. **Chest radiographs** should be done in the expiratory phase to accentuate areas of hyperlucency. **Arterial blood gas analysis** may help establish the degree of ventilatory compromise. Chest computed tomography (CT) may be performed to evaluate for the presence of bullae, especially in spontaneous pneumothorax.

Treatment

Tension pneumothorax is a **medical emergency**. **Thoracentesis** should be attempted by placing a needle at the second anterior intercostal space at the midclavicular line. Care must be taken not to puncture the underlying lung. For large pneumothoraces, **tube thoracostomy** may be necessary to drain the air until the visceral pleura can repair itself. Occasionally, in patients with recurrent pneumothoraces, **sclerosing the pleura by chemical or physical means** to the internal chest wall is necessary to allow the lung to remain reexpanded. **Supplemental oxygen** should be given to hypoxemic patients. Inhalation of **100% oxygen can displace the nitrogen** in the gas that forms the pneumothorax, although this practice is not supported in research trials. Since oxygen is more readily absorbed by the body, displacement of nitrogen with oxygen can hasten resolution of the pneumothorax. A history of pneumothorax may result in delayed airplane travel and is considered a contraindication to scuba diving.

Neuromuscular Disorders
Etiology
Respiratory muscle weakness accompanies skeletal muscle weakness, and this weakness results in failure of the respiratory pump that functions in ventilation. Patients with neuromuscular diseases also may have a **weak cough** resulting in impaired airway clearance, potentially causing recurrent infections or atelectasis. Progressive muscular disease may result in the development of chronic respiratory insufficiency and failure. In the face of an acute respiratory illness, these patients are at risk for significant respiratory decompensation and acute respiratory failure.

Clinical Features
The patient may demonstrate **shallow, rapid respiratory pattern and a weak cough**. Worsening chronic respiratory failure may result in **morning headaches** and **poor sleep quality**. Hypoxemia and respiratory distress may accompany an acute illness.

Evaluation
Pulmonary function testing, including spirometry, lung volumes, and maximal respiratory pressures, should be measured on a regular basis to follow the patient's trend. **End tidal carbon dioxide level** may indicate worsening ventilatory failure. **Overnight polysomnography** is used to evaluate sleep pattern, respiratory events, and oxygenation and ventilation during sleep.

Treatment

Aggressive airway clearance and assisted coughing, on a regular basis as well as during an acute illness, are the mainstays of therapy. **Early recognition** of impending chronic respiratory failure should be followed by early **initiation of nocturnal noninvasive ventilation**. Some patients progress to needing 24-hour support, which warrants consideration for invasive chronic mechanical ventilation via **tracheostomy**.

Miscellaneous Causes

Asthma

The triggers for asthma are discussed in Chapter 23, "Cough." This discussion focuses on asthma as a cause of respiratory distress and impending respiratory failure.

Clinical Features

Important differential diagnoses include **anaphylaxis and foreign body aspiration**. A thorough patient history should be taken, including the **duration, frequency, and severity of attacks;** the **medications** the patient uses acutely and chronically, as well as those used during this particular exacerbation; **peak flows** (if the patient keeps a log); and the **family history**. On physical examination, the **expiratory phase is prolonged**. **Breath sounds are often tubular or decreased** at the bases. **Heterophonous wheezing** is usually appreciated diffusely, but it may be absent when air exchange is severely affected.

Evaluation

Pulse oximetry is useful for determining oxygenation status. **Spirometry** may be helpful in patients with mild-to-moderate symptoms but should not be performed in the presence of significant distress. In severe status asthmaticus, an **arterial blood gas** may be obtained to assess oxygenation and carbon dioxide elimination. Table 66-1 lists the normal values. A **pulsus paradoxus** may be observed when the patient is in extremis.

> **HINT:** A near-normal carbon dioxide tension in the presence of significant tachypnea heralds impending respiratory failure. Decision to mechanically ventilate is based on progressive hypercapnia and hypoxemia, hemodynamic instability, and altered mental status, but not carbon dioxide level.

Treatment

- **Oxygen** should be administered to all patients with evidence of hypoxemia.
- **Bronchodilators.** Patients with mild symptoms may improve with the inhalation of a β-agonist, such as albuterol. The continuous use of nebulized albuterol (administered at a rate of 10 to 40 mg/hour) in severely affected patients with impending respiratory failure is often necessary. Care must be taken to monitor for hypokalemia, a side effect of high-dose albuterol therapy. Subcutaneous or intravenous bronchodilators, such as terbutaline, may also be considered in severe cases.

TABLE 66-1	Normal Blood Gas Values from the Children's Hospital of Philadelphia Blood Gas Laboratory	
Parameter	**Age of Patient**	**Normal Value**
pH	1 day	7.29–7.45
	3–24 months	7.34–7.46
	>7 years	7.37–7.41
PCO$_2$	1 day	27–40 mm Hg
	3–24 months	26–42 mm Hg
	>7 years	34–40 mm Hg
PO$_2$	1 day	37–97 mm Hg
	3–24 months	88–103 mm Hg
	>7 years	88–103 mm Hg
Base excess	1 day	.8–(–2)
	3–24 months	–7–0
	>7 years	–4–12
HCO$_3$	1 day	19 mmol/L
	3–24 months	16/24 mmol/L
	>7 years	22–27 mmol/L
O$_2$ saturation	—	94%–99%
Venous pH	—	7.32–7.42
Venous CO$_2$	—	25–47 mm Hg
Venous O$_2$	—	25–47 mm Hg

CO_2, carbon dioxide; HCO_3, bicarbonate; O_2, oxygen; PCO_2, carbon dioxide tension; PO_2, oxygen tension.

- **Anticholinergics.** Administration of multiple doses (2 to 3 doses) of ipratropium bromide in conjunction with bronchodilators is recommended in the early treatment of moderate-to-severe asthma exacerbations.
- **Steroids.** Prompt administration of oral or intravenous steroids (usually prednisone or methylprednisolone sodium succinate, 1 to 2 mg/kg/day) is vitally important in the management of an asthma exacerbation to treat the inflammation.
- **Fluids.** Patients with severe symptoms may benefit from intravenous fluids as the patients are often dehydrated from the underlying viral illness or from increased fluid loss caused by the work of breathing.
- **Magnesium.** Intravenous magnesium has been shown to improve pulmonary function in severe exacerbations.

Atelectasis
Etiology
Partial or complete collapse of normally aerated pulmonary parenchyma can result from an **intraluminal obstruction, extrinsic compression of the airway, or decreased respiratory muscle strength**. Loss of gas-exchanging regions of the lung may lead to **ventilation-perfusion mismatching and respiratory distress**.

Atelectasis is common in **postoperative patients** with impaired respiratory drive or muscle strength, **patients with infection or bronchospasm** leading to airway plugging, and **patients with alterations in the normal airway structure** as a result of congenital lesions, bronchopulmonary dysplasia, or recurrent aspiration.

Evaluation

Breath sounds may be decreased in the affected area. Anteroposterior and lateral **chest radiographs** help delineate the affected region. Volume loss results in the displacement of fissures or hemidiaphragm toward the area of atelectasis.

Treatment

Definitive treatment entails eliminating the pathologic process that is responsible for the atelectasis. **Chest physiotherapy and postural drainage** combined with **bronchodilator therapy** can help reexpand atelectatic areas. In refractory cases, **bronchoscopy** may help remove a particularly tenacious mucus plug. **Supplemental oxygen** is indicated for patients with hypoxemia. In the postoperative period, **early incentive spirometry, early ambulation, and good pain control** are helpful in preventing atelectasis.

Vocal Cord Dysfunction

Etiology

Vocal cord dysfunction (VCD) is a paradoxical closure of the vocal cords (of unclear etiology) during periods of high-flow breathing (such as exercise or hyperventilation). It is often misdiagnosed as asthma, but it is unresponsive to typical bronchodilator therapy or even long-term controller therapy with inhaled corticosteroids. Although most often seen in competitive athletes and high-performing individuals, it often develops as a somatic manifestation of **psychosocial stress** in preadolescents and adolescents.

Clinical Features

The **associated cough and respiratory distress are real** and are the result of paradoxical vocal cord movement. Stridor or difficulty in inspiration may be noted, especially during sporting events or stressful activities. Sour taste or heartburn, caused by GERD, may also be noted before or at the same time as the respiratory difficulty.

Evaluation

Consideration should be made in the patient diagnosed with asthma who does not respond to appropriate asthma therapy, especially if the patient has a competitive, high-achieving, or anxious temperament. An attempt should be made to **identify significant psychosocial stressors** in the patient's life. Sometimes sports and exercise are withheld by parents and/or coaches until a diagnosis is confirmed. On physical examination, **wheezing is absent** or a monophonic inspiratory wheeze is heard on auscultation of the neck. **Flow-volume loops** performed as a part of pulmonary function testing may show **flattening of the inspiratory curve. Exercise testing** may reproduce symptoms or demonstrate flattening of the inspiratory loop, often without reduction in spirometry flows seen with exercise-induced asthma.

Flexible laryngoscopy can sometimes identify paradoxical vocal cord movement.

Treatment

Vocal cord muscle relaxation exercises, taught by an experienced speech pathologist, are often very effective. **Psychological counseling and/or biofeedback** may be appropriate if symptoms persist. Many patients with VCD also have true **asthma;** for these patients, appropriate asthma therapy is indicated. A protocol often is provided for the patient to use for relief of symptoms in cases where both VCD and asthma exist. With therapy, the patient should be able to continue or resume sports and other activities that triggered the symptoms.

APPROACH TO THE PATIENT

The physician should consider typical and common illnesses for the patient's age and underlying medical conditions. A focused history should be taken, with special attention to onset of symptoms, presence of prodromal symptoms of infection, course and duration of symptoms, and response to therapies tried. A detailed history may be postponed in the case of severe respiratory distress, so that emergency life support measures may be performed. On physical examination, one may note **tachypnea (Table 66-2 lists normal values), tachycardia, decreased oxyhemoglobin saturation, positioning with the neck hyperextended, cyanosis, nasal flaring, retractions or accessory muscle use, grunting, wheezing, or stridor.** Helpful diagnostic studies include **arterial blood gas, radiographic studies** (chest radiograph, chest CT scan, upper airway films, fluoroscopy, barium swallow, bronchogram, pulmonary arteriogram, ventilation perfusion scan), **endoscopy, and pulmonary function testing.** Some procedures may need to be delayed in severe distress. The underlying cause of respiratory distress should be sought and treated, if possible. In some cases, supportive care is the only recommended option for treatment. Hallmarks of therapy include **maintaining airway patency, oxygenation, and circulation,** first and foremost. Continuing care may involve a variety of medical treatments including **bronchodilators, anti-inflammatories, airway clearance, antimicrobials, analgesia,** and invasive or noninvasive **mechanical ventilation.** Surgical procedures, such as **airway endoscopy, thoracentesis or lung biopsy,** may be necessary for diagnosis or treatment. Untreated respiratory distress may advance to respiratory failure, in which oxygenation and ventilation are impaired.

TABLE 66-2	Definition of Tachypnea by Age
Age	**Breaths per min**
<2 mo	>60
2–12 mo	>50
1–5 yr	>40
>5 yr	>20

Suggested Readings

American Academy of Pediatrics Subcommittee on Diagnosis and Management of Bronchiolitis. Diagnosis and management of bronchiolitis. *Pediatrics.* 2006;118(4):1774–1793.

Bent J. Pediatric laryngotracheal obstruction: current perspectives on stridor. *Laryngoscope.* 2006;116(7): 1059–1070.

Corneli HM, Zorc JJ, Majahan P, et al. A multicenter, randomized, controlled trial of dexamethasone for bronchiolitis. *N Engl J Med.* 2007;357(4):331–339.

Lichenstein R, Suggs AH, Campbell J. Pediatric pneumonia. *Emerg Med Clin North Am.* 2003;21(2):437–451.

National Asthma Education and Prevention Program: Expert Panel Report 3. NIH Publication No. 08–4051. Bethesda, MD. Available at: www.nhlbi.nih.gov/guidelines/asthma. Accessed July 1, 2011.

Panitch HB. Respiratory issues in the management of children with neuromuscular disease. *Respir Care.* 2006;51(8):885–893; discussion 894–895.

Rafei K, Lichenstein R. Airway infectious disease emergencies. *Pediatr Clin North Am.* 2006;53(2):215–242.

Sanchez I, Navarro H, Mendez M, et al. Clinical characteristics of children with tracheobronchial anomalies. *Pediatr Pulmonol.* 2003;35(4):288–291.

Werner HA. Status asthmaticus in children: a review. *Chest.* 2001;119(6):1913–1929.

Scrotal Pain, Acute

INTRODUCTION

When evaluating a patient with acute scrotal pain, **testicular torsion** should be considered **the diagnosis until proven otherwise**. Testicular torsion is the **only condition in the differential diagnosis of acute scrotum that absolutely requires emergent surgical intervention**. This complaint must be **evaluated in an emergency setting;** telephone consultation for such symptoms is dangerous because valuable time may be wasted, leading to testicular loss. One in every 4,000 males less than 25 years of age will develop testicular torsion. The incidence is bimodal, although testicular torsion can occur at any age. A peak incidence is seen in the first few days of life and again at puberty. Between 16% and 42% of boys and young adults presenting with acute scrotal pain to a hospital emergency department prove to have testicular torsion. This represents a **surgical emergency** because **irreversible ischemic injury can occur after 4 hours, and testicular viability decreases significantly beyond 6 hours from the onset of pain**. Therefore, patients presenting with this complaint must be given high priority in an acute-care setting.

DIFFERENTIAL DIAGNOSIS OF ACUTE/SUBACUTE SCROTUM

Anatomic
- Testicular torsion
- Torsion of the appendix testis
- Torsion of the appendix epididymis
- Inguinal hernia
- Hydrocele

Inflammatory
- Epididymitis
- Epididymo-orchitis
- Trauma
- Insect bite

- Inflammatory vasculitis (Henoch–Schönlein purpura)
- Idiopathic scrotal edema

Others
- Dermatologic lesions
- Varicocele
- Tumor
- Ureteral colic (referred pain)
- Nonurogenital pathology (e.g., musculoskeletal)

DIFFERENTIAL DIAGNOSIS
Common Causes

Testicular torsion, torsion of the testicular appendices, and epididymitis account for approximately 95% of all acute scrotum cases. In one study, almost 70% of all cases of acute scrotal pain were classified as either a testicular torsion or torsion of the appendix testis.

Testicular Torsion

Testicular torsion results from a **complete twist of the testis on its vascular pedicle**. The **resulting ischemia** produces **pain** that can be **constant or colicky**. The **sudden onset of pain** is often accompanied by **nausea and vomiting**. The testis in question **is pulled up high in the scrotum** (secondary to the twists in the spermatic cord). In majority of the cases, **no cremasteric reflex** can be elicited. Since the cremasteric reflex is not always present, especially in older males, **absence of a cremasteric reflex does not invoke a diagnosis of testicular torsion**.

Testicular torsion may be extravaginal or intravaginal. Extravaginal torsion occurs almost exclusively in neonates and accounts for approximately 10% of testicular torsion. It results from twisting of the tunica vaginalis and testis before complete descent into the scrotum and fusion of the tunica to the scrotal wall. The majority of testicular torsion cases are intravaginal in which the testis rotates freely within the tunica vaginalis. This occurs due to a **congenital anatomic malpositioning of the testis,** termed the **bell-clapper deformity**. A normal testis and its blood supply are attached to the tunica vaginalis posteriorly. However, with the bell-clapper deformity, **no such posterior attachment exists to anchor the testis** and prevent it from twisting completely around the spermatic cord. Establishing this **diagnosis early is crucial,** for the situation presents a **surgical emergency;** the longer the delay in diagnosis, the lower the chances for testicular salvage.

Torsion of the Testicular Appendices

Torsion of the testicular appendices results when these tiny vestigial remnants twist around their base and become ischemic. The typical presentation is characterized by a **gradual onset of pain,** and patients often note significant **scrotal swelling** and **erythema** secondary to a **reactive hydrocele**. The appetite is unaffected, and nausea and vomiting are rare. It is often possible to elicit a **strong cremasteric reflex,** which greatly aids in distinguishing this condition from torsion of the testis. If the patient presents early on, **point tenderness** is noted **on the upper outer pole**. Some patients have a "**blue-dot sign**" on the scrotum. Once the diagnosis is established, treatment consists of **nonsteroidal anti-inflammatories and rest**. Over a 1-week period, 90% to 95% of these patients improve with no need for further treatment. In about 5% to 10% of cases, the **appendix torses intermittently, and surgical excision of the appendix testis** is warranted.

Epididymitis

This diagnosis is **extremely rare in the prepubertal boy**. A true bacterial epididymitis in a prepubertal boy is usually secondary to a structural anomaly of the genitourinary tract. In the adolescent male, the usual causes of bacterial epididymitis are **chlamydia and gonorrhea.** However, at times the adolescent male may present with a **normal urinalysis and a tender, inflamed epididymis.** Often these patients present **following a period of heavy physical exertion** such as weight lifting. It is believed that **reflux of sterile urine via the prostatic ducts under pressure** sets up **inflammation** within the epididymis. Regardless of etiology, the diagnosis of epididymitis is established by the history and physical findings. The **onset of pain is slow,** and the **appetite is preserved.** A history of **urethral discharge and/ or dysuria** may be noted. The physical examination demonstrates a **nontender testis** with a **large and very tender epididymis palpable posteriorly.** If a bacterial process is suspected, appropriate therapy with antibiotics should be prescribed. Noninfectious epididymitis should be treated with scrotal support, limited physical activity, and nonsteroidal anti-inflammatory medications until symptoms improve.

Hernia/Hydrocele

Patients may present with an incarcerated hernia that produces **significant pain.** The hernia sac represents an extension of the peritoneal cavity, which can cause pain when suddenly entrapped. The findings of an **enlarged scrotum** that transilluminates in conjunction with a **thickened inguinal bulge** provide evidence for a **patent processus vaginalis.** This allows for **peritoneal fluid to roll down and pool within the scrotum.** The **testis is not tender** in this setting. On occasion, the patent processus vaginalis expands from a **small tunnel** that only allows for **passage of fluid to a much larger diameter** that enables **bowel or omentum to herniate** into the sac. Presence of bowel or omentum produces a **thicker spermatic cord.** On occasion, the bowel or omentum becomes **inflamed,** causing pain and becoming more difficult to reduce. At this point, **surgical consultation** is required.

EVALUATION OF ACUTE SCROTAL PAIN

Despite technological advances in Doppler sonography, the vast majority of patients presenting with scrotal pain may be accurately diagnosed with a **complete history and physical examination,** especially when patients present early in the course of their symptoms (Figure 67-1). **After 8 to 12 hours of inflammation,** it becomes much more difficult to distinguish the individual scrotal contents, and it is in this setting that **Doppler sonography** becomes especially useful. Table 67-1 summarizes the diagnostic features for acute scrotal pain.

History

The history provides valuable clues to the cause of acute scrotal pain. Answers to the following specific questions should be sought:

- Has the patient ever experienced pain like this before? Often patients with torsion have had several episodes of intermittent torsion preceding the current presentation.
- Was the onset sharp and acute or slow and gradual? Patients with testicular torsion may be able to note the time of day when the pain began. In some instances, the pain awakens the patient from sleep.
- Does the patient have nausea, vomiting, or anorexia? The presence of these symptoms has a positive predictive value up to 98% with testicular torsion. In

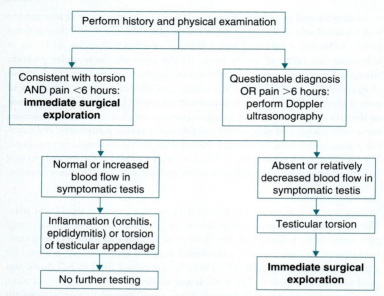

FIGURE 67-1 **Evaluation of acute scrotal pain.** Algorithmic approach to the evaluation of the patient with acute scrotal pain. (Adapted from Ringdahl E, Teague L. Testicular torsion. *Am Fam Physician.* 2006;74(10):1739–1743).

TABLE 67-1	Diagnostic Features of Acute Scrotal Pain			
	Testicular Torsion	**Torsed Appendix**	**Epididymitis**	**Hernia/ Hydrocele**
History				
Sudden onset	+	+/−	−	+/−
Nausea/vomiting	+	−	−	−
Altered gait	−	+	−	−
Prior episodes	+	−	+/−	+
Physical examination				
High-riding	+	−	−	−
Transilluminates	−	+/−	−	+
Cremasteric reflex	−	+	+	+/−
Laboratory				
Urine dipstick	−	−	+/−	−
Radiology				
Doppler flow	−	+	+	+
Radionuclide perfusion	−	+	+	+

contrast, boys presenting with epididymitis or a torsed testicular appendix often have an appetite.

Physical Examination

Observation of the patient provides useful clues. The patient who is in **obvious pain and writhing** at times has a higher **likelihood of having testicular torsion**. In contrast, the **patient with a torsed testicular appendix** prefers to **lie still**. The **appearance of the scrotum** is also helpful. The scrotal skin should be palpated for edema, fluid collections, tenderness, and crepitus. A testis that is **high-riding** or has a **horizontal lie** favors **testicular torsion**. The torsed testis may have a shorter spermatic cord because of the twisting that has produced the ischemia. A major component of the physical examination is the eliciting of the **cremasteric reflexes**. A brisk stroking of the inner thigh should result in a rise in the testis that is prominent (at least 2 cm). Such a brisk cremasteric reflex **is not seen in cases of testicular torsion** in which the twisted cord precludes such movement. Absence of the ipsilateral cremasteric reflex is 92% sensitive and 94% specific for testicular torsion.

> ♡ **HINT:** A high-riding testis and absent cremasteric reflex are strong signs
> ⚲ suggesting the presence of testicular torsion.

An effort should be made to **distinguish pain within the testis from pain in the epididymis or an inflamed testicular appendix**. With a **gentle touch,** it is often possible to isolate the **localized point tenderness** associated with an early torsed appendix, usually located on the **upper outer pole**.

Findings on the remainder of the genitourinary exam may lend clues to the diagnosis as well. The penis should be examined for masses or discharge. Fullness in the groin may suggest an inguinal hernia, and inguinal lymphadenopathy may indicate an inflammatory or infectious process.

Finally, note that **manual detorsion of a torsed testis** can be **temporarily therapeutic**. The spermatic cord rotates in the medial direction in 67% of testicular torsion cases. Gently turning the testis in a lateral direction while stabilizing the spermatic cord may result in detorsion. The motion should not be forced if the patient is suffering significant pain, as the remaining 33% of patients will have torsion in the lateral direction and only medial rotation will detorse the testis. If successful, the spermatic cord will lengthen and the testis will sit in a normal position in the scrotum. Once the testis is detorsed, the **relief of pain is instantaneous**. If access to the operating room or surgical subspecialist is limited, however, manual detorsion can be a valuable maneuver. This is not a substitute for scrotal exploration and bilateral testicular fixation since retorsion or residual torsion can still put the testis at risk.

Laboratory Studies

A **urinalysis** should be performed to assist in the workup of acute scrotum, **regardless of age**. Results demonstrating greater than 10 WBC/HPF or 10 RBC/HPF suggest epididymitis but do not confirm the diagnosis. If the patient is sexually active, urethral cultures should be sent for **gonorrhea and chlamydia** screening.

Imaging Studies

Scrotal pain lasting **for more than 12 hours** is often associated with **significant inflammation and edema** that renders the physical examination less accurate. The **exquisite point tenderness** seen with a torsed appendix testis **becomes less prominent as a reactive hydrocele forms,** and the **tunica vaginalis and tunica albuginea become inflamed**. When the diagnosis is unclear, radiographic imaging can help differentiate testicular torsion from other causes of acute scrotum.

Color Doppler ultrasound has become the gold standard for imaging the acute scrotum. This noninvasive test is readily available and provides a quick answer to whether or not blood flow is present within the testis itself. Color Doppler sonography is 86% sensitive, 100% specific, and 97% accurate in diagnosing ischemia in the acute scrotum. The role of **nuclear scintigraphy** has faded because limited accessibility to the isotope, elevated cost, and increased duration of the study make this a less efficient method of assessing testicular blood flow when time is of the essence.

Surgery

When in doubt regarding the diagnosis of testicular torsion, it is prudent to perform **exploratory surgery**. It is **never wrong to operate and establish an exact diagnosis** of the acute scrotum by ruling out torsion. **If clinical findings alone suggest testicular torsion, then immediate surgical exploration is warranted,** and radiologic studies are not indicated. Although Doppler sonography has decreased negative exploratory surgery, the study is not perfect. **Testes may torse and detorse** to a point **allowing for arterial inflow at the time of actual study**. The best way to establish the diagnosis is by examining the patient at the time of symptom occurrence. Occasionally, physicians are asked to assess the patient who has pain of short duration without classic symptoms. This patient may have **intermittent torsion** and could benefit from elective orchiopexies. Such patients should still be **referred for urologic evaluation** and are advised to **keep a diary** of such episodes, noting their **frequency, degree of pain, and duration**.

Suggested Readings

Barada JH, Weingarten JL, Cromie WJ. Testicular salvage and age-related delay in the presentation of testicular torsion. *J Urol.* 1989;142:746–747.

Cattolica EV. Preoperative manual detorsion of the torsed spermatic cord. *J Urol.* 1985;133:803–804.

Ciftci AO, Senocak ME, Tanyel FC, et al. Clinical predictors for differential diagnosis of acute scrotum. *Eur J Pediatr Surg.* 2004;14:333.

Cronan KM, Zderic SA. Manual detorsion of the testes. In: Henretig FM, King C, eds. *Textbook of Pediatric Emergency Procedures.* Baltimore, MA: Williams & Wilkins; 1991:1003–1006.

Jefferson RH, Perez LM, Joseph DB. Critical analysis of the clinical presentation of acute scrotum: a 9-year experience at a single institution. *J Urol.* 1997;158:1198–1200.

Kadish HA, Bolte RG. A retrospective review of pediatric patients with epididymitis, testicular torsion, and torsion of testicular appendages. *Pediatrics.* 1998;102:73–76.

Kass EJ, Lundak B. The acute scrotum. *Pediatr Clin North Am.* 1997;44(5):1251–1266.

Lewis AG, Bukowski TP, Jarvis PD, et al. Evaluation of acute scrotum in the emergency department. *J Pediatr Surg.* 1995;30(2):277–282.

Sessions AE, Rabinowitz R, Hulbert WC, et al. Testicular torsion: direction, degree, duration and disinformation. *J Urol.* 2003;169:663.

Siegel A, Snyder H, Duckett JW. Related epididymitis in infants and boys: underlying urogenital anomalies and efficacy of imaging modalities. *J Urol.* 1987;133:1100–1103.

Wein AJ, Kavoussi LR, Novick AC, et al., eds. *Campbell-Walsh Urology.* 9th ed. Philadelphia, PA: Elsevier Saunders; 2007.

CHAPTER 68

Katherine S. Taub
Nicholas S. Abend

Seizures

INTRODUCTION

A seizure is an episode characterized by altered behavior, consciousness, movement, sensation, or autonomic function due to hypersynchronous excessive firing of a network of neurons. The differential diagnosis of seizures is listed in Table 68-1. **Generalized** seizures rapidly engage bilaterally distributed networks. **Focal** seizures begin in one portion of the brain with symptoms related to that region's function. Prior classification systems separated focal seizures into simple partial seizures (remain restricted to a region without affected alertness), complex partial seizures (spread to involve adjacent regions such that consciousness is affected), and secondarily generalized seizures (spread widely to involve the entire cortex). In the most recent International League Against Epilepsy (ILAE) classification, the terms simple and complex are replaced with the more descriptive phrases "without impairment of consciousness or awareness" and "with impairment of consciousness or awareness," respectively, and can also be designated as "evolving to a bilateral, convulsive seizure."

Seizures may occur in an individual with an underlying tendency to have recurrent seizures (**epilepsy**) or may be secondary to an ongoing process that primarily or secondarily affects the brain (**acute symptomatic seizures**). The initial evaluation of a patient with a seizure must focus on identifying and treating any underlying condition that may be causing seizures. Prolonged or multiple recurrent seizures without return to baseline mental status are called **status epilepticus**. Types of seizures are listed in Table 68-2.

Epilepsy is defined by recurrent unprovoked seizures. In more detail, the ILAE defines epilepsy as a disorder of the brain characterized by an enduring predisposition to generate epileptic seizures and by the neurobiologic, cognitive, psychological, and social consequences of this condition. Epilepsy may be classified based on the underlying etiology as **genetic, structural-metabolic, and unknown**. **Genetic** refers to epilepsy caused by a known or presumed genetic defect. The genetic mutation may be known, such as a mutation in a sodium ion channel (e.g., SCN1A mutation) or may be suspected due to a family history of seizures. **Structural-metabolic** includes epilepsy related to an underlying structural or metabolic etiology. Structural defects include cortical malformations (e.g., dysplasias, tubers) or acquired defects such as strokes or trauma. **Unknown** indicates that the etiology of the epilepsy is not known and may be related to an undiagnosed genetic defect or an unrecognized disorder. In some patients, the clinical history, age, seizure type, and electroencephalographic (EEG) findings can be grouped into an epilepsy

TABLE 68-1	Nonseizure Etiologies of Transient Neurological Events

Neurological
- Stroke/transient ischemic attack
- Migraine headache
- Movement disorders
- Reflex movements

Cardiac
- Vasovagal syncope (which may be followed by a seizure in syncopal convulsion)
- Arrhythmia
- Hypotension

Endocrine/metabolic
- Hypoglycemia
- Hyponatremia

Sleep disorders
- Hypnic jerks
- Benign sleep myoclonus
- Parasomnias
- Narcolepsy/cataplexy

Psychological
- Nonepileptic psychogenic seizures (pseudoseizures)—conversion disorder

Others
- Breath holding
- Masturbation
- Gastroesophageal reflux
- Behavior
- Apparent life-threatening events

TABLE 68-2	Classification of Epileptic Seizures by ILAE 2010 Terminology

Generalized
Tonic–clonic

Absence
- Typical absence
- Atypical absence
- Absence with special features (myoclonic absence, eyelid myoclonia)

Myoclonic
- Myoclonic
- Myoclonic atonic
- Myoclonic tonic

Clonic

Tonic

Atonic

Focal seizures
- With impairment of awareness or consciousness
- Without impairment of awareness or consciousness
- Evolving to bilateral convulsive seizure

Unknown
- Epileptic spasms (including infantile spasms)

syndrome that can guide management and suggest prognosis. Common pediatric epilepsy syndromes are listed in Table 68-3 and described in the following.

> **HINT:** Consider acute symptomatic etiologies when evaluating a patient with a first seizure. Epilepsy (unprovoked seizures) is a diagnosis of exclusion.

DIFFERENTIAL DIAGNOSIS LIST

Neurological Etiologies

Neurovascular
- Ischemic stroke
- Sinovenous thrombosis
- Intracerebral hemorrhage
- Subarachnoid hemorrhage
- Arteriovenous malformation
- Hyperperfusion syndrome

Tumor
- Primary
- Metastatic

Infection
- Meningitis
- Encephalitis
- Abscess
- Cat-scratch disease
- Tick-borne disorders

Inflammatory
- Acute disseminated encephalomy-
  elitis
- Vasculitis
- Lupus cerebritis
- Rasmussen

Trauma
- Contusion
- Epidural hematoma
- Subdural hematoma
- Subarachnoid hemorrhage
- Depressed skull fracture

Neurosurgery

Inherited
- Neurodegenerative disorders

Congenital and Intrauterine
- Brain malformations
- Neonatal hypoxic ischemic injury
- Congenital infections

Primary Epilepsy

Systemic Etiologies

Hypoxia-ischemia

Drug Toxicity
- Amphetamines
- Cocaine
- Phencyclidine
- Local anesthetics
- Antipsychotics
- Antidepressants
- Immunosuppressants
- Antibiotics

Drug Withdrawal
- Benzodiazepines
- Barbiturates
- Opiods
- Alcohol

Febrile Infection (not involving the central nervous system [CNS])

Metabolic Abnormalities
- Hypoglycemia
- Hyponatremia
- Hypophosphatemia
- Renal dysfunction
- Hepatic dysfunction

Metabolic Disorders
- Urea cycle disorders
- Aminoacidopathies
- Organic acidurias
- Mitochondrial encephalopathies
- Storage diseases
- Vitamin B_6 (pyridoxine) deficiency
- Folinic acid–responsive seizures
- Nonketotic hyperglycinemia

TABLE 68-3	**International League Against Epilepsy Classification of Electroclinical Syndromes and Other Epilepsies**

Neonatal period
- Benign familial neonatal epilepsy (BFNE)
- Early myoclonic encephalopathy (EME)
- Ohtahara syndrome

Infancy
- Epilepsy of infancy with migrating focal seizures
- West syndrome
- Myoclonic epilepsy of infancy (MEI)
- Benign infantile epilepsy
- Benign familial infantile epilepsy
- Dravet syndrome (severe myoclonic epilepsy of infancy)
- Myoclonic encephalopathy in nonprogressive disorders

Childhood
- Febrile seizures plus (FS+)
- Panayiotopoulos syndrome (early onset benign childhood occipital epilepsy)
- Epilepsy with myoclonic atonic seizures
- Benign epilepsy with centrotemporal spikes (BECTS, Rolandic epilepsy)
- Autosomal dominant nocturnal frontal lobe epilepsy (ADFNLE)
- Late onset childhood occipital epilepsy (Gastaut syndrome)
- Epilepsy with myoclonic absences
- Lennox–Gastaut syndrome
- Landau–Kleffner syndrome (LKS)
- Epileptic encephalopathy with continuous spike-and-waves during sleep (CSWS)
- Childhood absence epilepsy (CAE)

Adolescence–adult
- Juvenile absence epilepsy (JAE)
- Juvenile myoclonic epilepsy (JME)
- Epilepsy with generalized tonic–clonic seizures alone
- Progressive myoclonic epilepsies (PME)
  - Lafora body disease
  - Unverricht–Lundborg syndrome (Baltic myoclonus)
  - Neuronal ceroid lipofuscinosis
  - Myoclonic epilepsy with ragged red fibers (MERRF)
  - Sialidoses
- Autosomal dominant epilepsy with auditory features (ADEAF)
- Reflex epilepsies
  - Photosensitive occipital lobe epilepsy
  - Primary reading epilepsy
  - Startle epilepsy

Distinctive constellations
- Mesial temporal lobe epilepsy with hippocampal sclerosis
- Rasmussen syndrome
- Gelastic seizures with hypothalamic hamartoma
- Hemiconvulsion-hemiplegia-epilepsy

TABLE 68-3	International League Against Epilepsy Classification of Electroclinical Syndromes and Other Epilepsies (*Cont.*)

Epilepsies attributed to and organized by structural-metabolic causes
- Malformations of cortical development (e.g., hemimegalencephaly, heterotopias)
- Neurocutaneous syndromes
- Tumor
- Infection
- Trauma
- Angioma
- Perinatal insults
- Stroke

Conditions with epileptic seizures that are traditionally not diagnosed as a form of epilepsy
- Benign neonatal seizures (BNS)
- FS

DIFFERENTIAL DIAGNOSIS DISCUSSION

Benign Epilepsy with Centro-Temporal Spikes (Rolandic Epilepsy)

Onset is typically between 2 and 13 years, with most between 5 and 10 years. It most often presents with predominantly nocturnal seizures that include salivation, clonic mouth movements, and gurgling sounds. Daytime seizures are less common and generally consist of speech arrest and face/arm clonic movements with preserved consciousness. These children have **normal cognitive function** and a normal neurological examination. EEG demonstrates **sharp waves** in one or both central-temporal regions. Antiepileptic drug treatment is considered optional, and it is usually easy to control seizures if treatment is initiated. The syndrome is often outgrown by adolescence.

Juvenile Myoclonic Epilepsy

Juvenile myoclonic epilepsy generally starts in the early teenage years. It is characterized by myoclonic seizures seen **soon after awakening** with involvement of the upper extremities. These are often initially considered morning clumsiness. Patients later usually come to medical attention after their first generalized tonic–clonic seizure. These adolescents have normal cognitive function and neurological examinations. EEG may be entirely normal in the waking state, but typically shows irregular fast spike and wave pattern during sleep, and is occasionally precipitated by photic stimulation. Seizures may be exacerbated by sleep deprivation, stress, and alcohol consumption. While seizures are usually easily treated, they often recur if treatment is discontinued, so individuals may require lifelong therapy.

Childhood Absence Epilepsy

The typical onset is between 4 and 10 years, with a peak at 5 to 7 years. Most children have normal cognitive function and neurological examination, although associated behavioral impairments (e.g., attention deficit hyperactivity disorder) are overly represented. Seizures are brief (4 to 10 seconds), with frequent (>10/day) arrests of activity with loss of awareness. They may occur hundreds of times per day, (often far more often than recognized by caregivers), and thus may interfere with learning. Seizures may be elicited on examination by having the child **hyper-ventilate**. EEG demonstrates 3 Hz generalized spike and waves discharges provoked by hyperventilation. Seizures are usually easily treated and often remit by adolescence. Refractory absence epilepsy may prompt consideration of GLUT-1 deficiency which may be treated with the ketogenic diet.

Juvenile Absence Epilepsy

This is very similar to childhood absence epilepsy, but has a later onset at 10 to 17 years with a peak at 12 to 14 years. Normal cognitive function and neurological examination are usually present. EEG demonstrates generalized spike-wave discharges at 3.5 to 4.5 Hz. Seizures are much less frequent, often less than a few per week, and also brought out by fatigue and hyperventilation. They are also usually easily treated but often recur if treatment is discontinued, so lifelong therapy may be required. Some develop generalized tonic–clonic seizures.

West Syndrome

This is an age-related epileptic encephalopathy with typical onset between 4 and 12 months. Only one-third are neurologically and developmentally normal before onset (idiopathic), while two-thirds have preexisting abnormalities (symptomatic). West syndrome is defined by the triad of **infantile spasms,** mental retardation, and **hypsarrhythmia** on EEG. Infantile spasms describe the seizure type that can be flexor or extensor (also referred to as jackknife seizure or "salaam" attacks). They tend to occur at sleep-wake transition and often occur in clusters. The EEG pattern is hypsarrhythmic (irregular, high amplitude, disorganized, multifocal spikes, and slow waves). Etiologies vary widely from neonatal hypoxic ischemic injury or infection to brain malformations, tuberous sclerosis, and Down syndrome. Evaluation for etiology generally includes magnetic resonance imaging (MRI) and sometimes genetic and metabolic testing. Treatment is usually adrenocorticotropic hormone as a daily intramuscular injection or high-dose oral steroids; it is important to rule out infections before initiating treatment and monitor closely for side effects. Vigabatrin may be especially useful in patients with tuberous sclerosis. Typical antiepileptic drugs (AEDs [especially topiramate]) may be appropriate with structural etiology. About half progress to Lennox–Gastaut syndrome. Only about 10% have good outcome, mostly those in the idiopathic group.

Lennox–Gastaut Syndrome

This syndrome is a triad of diffuse slow spikes-waves on EEG, mental retardation, and multiple types of often refractory generalized seizures. Onset is usually 2 to 8 years. It can appear *de novo* or evolve from West syndrome. Common seizure types include atypical absence, tonic, and atonic seizures. Remission is rare, and severe cognitive impairment is common.

Landau–Kleffner Syndrome

Insidious onset of aphasia at 3 to 8 years (typically progressive verbal auditory agnosia) may mimic autistic regression. Most have seizures preceding or with the onset of language problems, although epilepsy is generally mild with seizures that are easy to control. EEG demonstrates bilateral temporal or parieto-occipital spikes and spike-waves that are dramatically activated during slow-wave sleep (called *electrical status epilepticus of sleep,* if a substantial portion of the record contains epileptiform discharges). While EEG abnormalities may be controlled by medication and in some children is linked to language improvement, the language disorder may be more difficult to treat and persists in half of affected children.

Febrile Seizures

This is the most common cause of seizures in children, occurring in 2% to 4% of children between 6 months and 5 years. Simple febrile seizures (FS) are seizures that occur associated with fever in children without an underlying neurologic disorder; they are generalized, last less than 15 minutes, and there is only one seizure in 24 hours. With simple FS, there is up to a 50% recurrence, but only a 2% to 3% risk of epilepsy. There is no effect on development or cognition. Complex FS are those which are focal, last longer than 15 minutes, and recurrent in 24 hours. If all three characteristics are present, then there is a 50% risk of epilepsy. Research is ongoing, but at this time it is unclear whether prolonged FS cause mesial temporal sclerosis. MRI should be performed if there are focal features.

Diagnostic evaluation begins with the identification and treatment of the source of fever. Common etiologies include otitis media, upper respiratory infection, viral syndrome, pneumonia, urinary tract infection, gastroenteritis, varicella, and bronchiolitis. Since seizure can be the initial manifestation of CNS infection, one should consider lumbar puncture (LP) in an infant less than 12 to 18 months of age in whom it may be difficult to rule out CNS infection by clinical exam, or if an older patient remains lethargic, irritable, or does not return to baseline. Neuroimaging and EEG are generally not required if the seizure was simple. Antipyretics have not been shown to be effective in preventing the recurrence of FS, which often occur at the onset of fever. Rectal diazepam (Diastat) may be prescribed for patients with prolonged FS.

Neonatal Seizures

Seizures in the first weeks of life are usually subtle rather than well-localized partial or symmetric, generalized tonic–clonic seizures. Typically, they show lip-smacking, eye deviation, focal motor, autonomic variability, or myoclonus. Most neonatal seizures are response to injury from an identifiable cause (60% hypoxic-ischemic injury, 20% intracerebral hemorrhage or infarction, 5% to 10% infections, and 5% to 10% other disorders including metabolic disease). In the first 3 days of life, one should primarily consider hypoxic-ischemic encephalopathy, intracranial hemorrhage, metabolic abnormalities, pyridoxine dependency, nonketotic hyperglycinemia, local anesthetic intoxication, sepsis, and meningoencephalitis. After 3 days of life, one needs to consider as more likely metabolic disease, brain malformations, "fifth day fits" (healthy term infant with seizures on about day 5 of life which resolve by about 2 weeks and carry a good prognosis), benign (nonepileptic) neonatal sleep myoclonus, and familial neonatal seizures (autosomal dominant, seizures often persisting for 1 to 6 months with a good prognosis). Prognosis depends on underlying etiology.

Specific Disorders to Consider

- Pyridoxine sensitive seizures may respond to pyridoxine (vitamin B_6) or pyridoxal phosphate administration.
- GLUT-1 deficiency (low cerebrospinal fluid [CSF] glucose <40% of the serum glucose) may be treated with the ketogenic diet.

Routine evaluation includes blood sugar, electrolytes, arterial blood gas, ammonia, drug screen, LP, computed tomography (CT)/MRI, blood and CSF cultures, EEG, and pyridoxine trial. Neonatal seizures may be electrographic-only, referring to seizures detectable with EEG monitoring but without any clinical manifestations, especially after treatment with anticonvulsants; so prolonged EEG monitoring may be indicated for some neonates. Additional evaluation, if indicated, may include plasma amino acids, urinary organic acids, very long chain fatty acids, lysosomal enzymes, CSF, as well as blood lactate/pyruvate and CSF glycine. If these studies are negative, then genetic testing should be considered.

Initial treatment is generally **phenobarbital** (20 mg/kg IV), which can be repeated if needed to achieve serum levels of 20 to 40 µg/mL. Persistent seizures can be treated with phenytoin (20 mg/kg IV); additional doses are administered if needed to achieve serum levels of 15 to 20 µg/mL. Other anticonvulsants including topiramate and levetiracetam are often utilized although dosing and efficacy data are not available. If seizures are completely controlled for 1 to 2 weeks, and the underlying acute etiology is stable or resolved, it is reasonable to discontinue AEDs.

 HINT: There is almost always an underlying cause for neonatal seizures. It is essential to identify and treat the underlying etiology, in addition to managing seizures.

Posttraumatic Seizures

Seizures can occur as an acute consequence of blunt or penetrating head trauma or as a delayed posttraumatic consequence.

- Impact seizures occur within an hour of head trauma and may or may not be associated with associated brain injury. They are the least likely type of trauma-related seizure to persist.
- Early posttraumatic seizures occur within 1 week of the injury and are associated with cerebral edema; epidural, subdural, and intracerebral hematomas; and traumatic subarachnoid hemorrhages. Neuroimaging is indicated. These are not associated with future epilepsy.
- Late posttraumatic seizures (after 1 week) are considered to be remote symptomatic seizures and recurrent spells should be treated.

EVALUATION OF A PATIENT WITH A FIRST SEIZURE

Seizures should initially be considered acute symptomatic seizures to avoid missing treatable causes. Unprovoked recurrent seizures (e.g., epilepsy) can only be diagnosed after symptomatic etiologies are considered and ruled out. All children should undergo a detailed history and physical examination. Useful history questions regarding seizures are listed in Table 68-4. They should have blood glucose and electrolyte evaluation if they do not quickly return to baseline alertness and neurological status, or if they develop recurrent seizures. A CT scan should be performed emergently in children with risk factors including head trauma, seizure >15 minutes, focal postictal deficits (Todd paralysis), persistently altered level of consciousness, sickle cell disease, bleeding disorders, malignancy, and human immunodeficiency virus infection. MRI is more sensitive than CT in detecting abnormalities related to seizures, and thus is preferred to CT when nonurgent imaging is required. Nonurgent MRI should be considered if the child is <1 year old, has focal seizures, has focal neurological examination signs, or has other motor/cognitive deficits. ILAE guidelines recommend imaging when "localization-related epilepsy is known or suspected, when the epilepsy classification is in doubt, or when an epilepsy syndrome with remote symptomatic cause is suspected," and describe that, "MRI is preferred to CT because of its superior resolution, versatility, and

---

TABLE 68-4	**History Taking in a Patient with Seizure**

Patient history
- Birth history
- History of febrile seizures
- Neurological problems
- Developmental problems
- Psychiatric problems
- Medication use

Related to suspected seizure event
- Precipitating factors

Factors lowering seizure threshold (sleep deprivation, alcohol, systemic infection, fever)
- Preceding symptoms
- Duration of symptoms
- Motor and sensory symptoms
- Level of awareness and responsiveness
- Injury
- Incontinence
- Breathing or skin color changes
- Duration of event
- Duration and description of time after the event

Related to the pattern of events
- Frequency of events
- Stereotyped quality or variable

Family history

Social history: Household medications/toxins

lack of radiation." CNS infection must be ruled out with a LP if infection is suspected. A toxicology screen should be performed if ingestion is possible. Neonates and infants can present with seizures as the initial manifestation of CNS infections, so absence of fever or clear encephalopathy should not preclude LP in these young children if infection is suspected. If the child has returned to baseline and the history is not suggestive of an underlying disorder or focality, then laboratory testing, LP, and urgent neuroimaging are generally not indicated.

Immediate EEG is indicated for persistently altered mental status or movements of unclear etiology to evaluate for subclinical seizures or confirm that movements are epileptic in nature. Otherwise, emergent EEG is not needed since soon after a seizure, the EEG is likely to show nonspecific slowing. An EEG can generally be performed nonurgently to help determine the seizure type and identify any underlying epilepsy syndrome.

MANAGEMENT OF SEIZURES
Antiepileptic Drugs

When seizures are provoked by an acute condition, it is essential to treat the underlying condition, but AEDs may not be indicated. AEDs may be utilized for several weeks or months when recurrent seizures complicate an acute condition or if additional seizures might threaten the neurological status (as in posttraumatic seizures) further increasing intracranial pressure.

If a first seizure is unprovoked, only 40% of children will have a second seizure, and thus AEDs are not generally initiated after a first unprovoked seizure. After a second unprovoked seizure, about 60% to 70% of children will have a third seizure, and thus AEDs are often initiated. Decisions regarding initiating AED therapy also take into account the child's age, an identifiable epilepsy syndrome, EEG findings, and the duration between subsequent seizures.

Commonly used antiepileptic drugs are summarized in Table 68-5. Medication choices are based on epilepsy classification, seizure frequency, efficacy data, possible adverse reactions, titration schedule, dosing schedule, and the availability of pediatric-friendly formulations (liquids, sprinkle capsules).

Diastat® (preloaded syringe of rectal diazepam) is approved for use in children with repetitive seizures. There is evidence that it is also effective in terminating prolonged seizures. It is generally administered for cluster seizures or if a seizure persists for >5 minutes. Not every child with a seizure needs rectal diazepam, but it should be considered in children with a history of prolonged seizures or who live far from medical attention.

Other Treatment Modalities
- Ketogenic diet: This employs a high fat, low carbohydrate regimen. Common adverse events to consider include hypoglycemia and nephrolithiasis. If intravenous fluids are required, they should be dextrose-free.
- Vagal nerve stimulator: This surgically implanted device can be set to cycle continuously, but also can be programmed to provide a higher current over a longer

TABLE 68-5	Antiepileptic Medications		
AED	**Indications**	**Advantages**	**Side Effects**
Carbamazepine (Tegretol, Carbatrol)	Focal epilepsy Initial mono- therapy	Possible mood stabilization Available as suspension and sprinkles	Hepatic enzyme induction rash and hypersensitivity reactions Idiosyncratic leukopenia and aplastic anemia Long-term use: osteoporosis
Ethosuximide (Zarontin)	Absence epilepsy	Available as suspension	Idiosyncratic rash and leuko- penia
Felbamate (Felbatol)	Broad spec- trum Intractable epilepsy	Available as suspension	Idiosyncratic aplastic anemia and hepatic failure Frequent blood tests and consent form
Gabapentin (Neurontin)	Focal epilepsy	Neuropathic pain Available as suspension	Prolonged use: weight gain
Lacosamide (Vimpat)	Partial epi- lepsy Adjunctive therapy >17 yr old	IV formulation No weight gain <15% protein bound	Dizziness Headache Nausea Diplopia Prolongs PR interval
Lamotrigine (Lamictal)	Broad spec- trum	Possible mood stabilization Available as a chew tablet	Slow titration Rash and hypersensitivity reactions Valproate coadministration increases lamictal levels Rash (especially with rapid titration)
Levetiracetam (Keppra)	Broad spec- trum	IV formulation Available as suspension	May exacerbate behavior problems
Oxcarbazepine (Trileptal)	Focal epilepsy Initial mono- therapy	Available as suspension	Rash and hypersensitivity reactions Hyponatremia
Phenobarbital	Focal epilepsy Initial mono- therapy (but no longer used as first line in children)	IV formulation Quick load and bolus Available as suspension	Cognitive concerns Hepatic enzyme induction Rash and hypersensitivity reactions Rapid administration may cause hypotension and reduced respiratory rate Long-term use: osteoporosis
Phenytoin (Dilantin)	Focal epilepsy Initial mono- therapy (but no longer used as first line in children)	IV formulation Quick load and bolus Available as suspension	Hepatic enzyme induction Rash and hypersensitivity reactions Unpredictable pharmacokinetics May cause cardiac arrhythmias Long-term use: gingival hyper- plasia Long-term use: osteoporosis

(continued)

TABLE 68-5	Antiepileptic Medications (*Cont.*)		
AED	**Indications**	**Advantages**	**Side Effects**
Rufinamide (Banzel)	Seizures associated with Lennox–Gastaut syndrome >4 yr old		QT shortening Headache Dizziness Somnolence Nausea
Topiramate (Topamax)	Broad spectrum Initial monotherapy	Migraine and tic prevention No weight gain Available as sprinkle	Word finding difficulty Weight loss Nephrolithiasis Hypohydrosis (overheating) Metabolic acidosis Acute angle closure glaucoma
Valproate (Depakote, Depakene)	Broad spectrum	IV formulation Available as suspension and sprinkles	Hepatic enzyme inhibition Idiosyncratic pancreatitis and hepatic failure (especially in young children, polypharmacy, metabolic disease) Dose related thrombocytopenia Long-term use: weight gain, hair loss, tremor, menstrual irregularities Highly teratogenic
Vigabatrin	Partial epilepsy Infantile spasms (drug of choice for tuberous sclerosis patients with infantile spasms)		Asymptomatic MRI changes in the basal ganglia, thalamus, brainstem, and dentate nucleus Progressive, permanent, bilateral concentric visual field constriction Fever (19%–29% of infants)
Zonisamide (Zonegran)	Broad spectrum	No weight gain	Weight loss Nephrolithiasis Hypohydrosis (overheating) Metabolic acidosis

time course upon a magnet swipe that can be used to abort seizures. It must be turned off prior to MRI scans.

- Epilepsy surgery: Options include resective surgery, standard lobectomy, tailored cortical resections, and rarely hemispherectomy. Other options are corpus callosotomy and multiple subpial transections. Outcomes are best for lesional epilepsy with concordant EEG and imaging findings. Children with focal epilepsy who have continued seizures despite adequate trials of two to three anticonvulsants should be referred to an epilepsy surgery program for evaluation.

Discontinuing Antiepileptic Drugs

One should consider an attempt to discontinue AEDs once the child is seizure-free for 2 years, since more than half will continue to do well without medication. Predictors of successful discontinuation include 2 years of seizure freedom, normal EEG, normal examination, and a single seizure type.

Epilepsy Patient with Increased Seizure Frequency

When seizures suddenly increase in frequency or severity, one must consider epilepsy exacerbation, but more frequently worsening is caused by missed medication doses, recent growth leading to lower AED levels, and exacerbation due to intercurrent infection (with or without fever). On occasion, one must consider acute symptomatic etiologies since children with preexisting epilepsy can also develop additional CNS disorders such as infection. If a bridge medication is needed for acute exacerbation (e.g., during an intercurrent infection), consider administering a long-acting benzodiazepine such as clorazepate or clonazepam, for several days.

Epilepsy Comorbidities

While much of epilepsy management focuses on seizure control, identification and management of comorbidities is important and may have a substantial impact on quality of life. Common comorbidities include depression, anxiety, learning disabilities, attention-deficit hyperactivity disorder, and headaches. Some studies of patients with even well-controlled seizures report high rates of unplanned pregnancy, academic underachievement, and unemployment, suggesting that attention to these psychosocial issues is necessary.

STATUS EPILEPTICUS

Status epilepticus is a life-threatening emergency characterized by prolonged or recurrent seizures without return to baseline mental status. The older definition of status is 30 minutes of persistent seizure activity (or 30 minutes of recurrent seizures without full recovery of consciousness). However, given the evidence that most seizures stop spontaneously within 5 minutes, prolonged seizures become harder to terminate, and prolonged seizures are associated with worse outcome, treatment for status is now typically initiated at **5 to 10 minutes**. Status epilepticus may be convulsive or nonconvulsive (requiring EEG for detection). In patients with preexisting epilepsy, common etiologies include poor compliance with medication, recent medication changes, benzodiazepine or barbiturate withdrawal, or exacerbation by intercurrent infection. Acute symptomatic etiologies predominate in first attacks of status epilepticus. One must consider meningoencephalitis, stroke, intracranial hemorrhage, acute head injury, cerebral neoplasm, demyelinating disorders, metabolic disorders, and medication/drug overdose. Evaluation and treatment must focus on terminating the seizure and treating the underlying condition. Particular attention to traditional resuscitation issues (the ABCs) is important as abnormalities may worsen or cause secondary brain injury. A status epilepticus guideline is presented in Table 68-6.

TABLE 68-6	Status Epilepticus Protocol
Stage	**Management**
Impending SE **< 5 min**	Out-of-hospital Consider buccal midazolam or rectal diazepam Benzodiazepines Lorazepam 0.1 mg/kg IV (max 5 mg) over 1 min Diazepam 0.2 mg/kg IV (max 10 mg) over 1 min Allow 5 min to determine whether seizure terminates Give oxygen. Stabilize airway, respiration, and hemodynamics as needed Obtain IV access. Check bedside glucose. Begin EKG monitoring

Established SE **5–10 min**	Repeat benzodiazepine administration
	Administer fosphenytoin 20 mg/kg phenytoin equivalents IV at 2 mg/kg/min
	    (max 150 mg/min)
	(or phenytoin 20 mg/kg IV at 1 mg/kg/min [max 50 mg/min])
	OR
	If <1 yr, consider phenobarbital (20 mg/kg IV); if <2 yr, consider pyridoxine
	    100 mg IV push
	If hypoglycemic administer bolus of 2 mL/kg 50% glucose, consider thiamine
	    100 mg IV first
	Testing:
	Bedside glucose CBC cultures
	BMP, Mg, Phos LFT toxicology (serum, urine)
	AED levels PT, PTT
	Head CT
	Draw phenytoin/phenobarbital level (10 min after infusion)
	Support airway, respiration, hemodynamics as needed. Continuous vital
	    sign and EKG monitoring
	Consult neurology service

Initial refractory SE	If seizure continues 10 min after receiving a benzodiazepine and an additional anticonvulsant, then patient has refractory SE regardless of time elapsed Third-line medications to consider: • Phenobarbital 30 mg/kg IV at 2 mg/kg/min (max rate 60 mg/min) Carefully monitor and prepare to support ventilation and blood pressure • Phenytoin 20 mg/kg IV at 1 mg/kg/min (max 50 mg/mL) Carefully monitor EKG • Levetiracetam 40 mg/kg IV at 5 mg/kg/min (max 3 g) • Valproate 20 mg/kg at 5 mg/kg/min Contraindicated if liver or metabolic disease

Later refractory SE	Admit to PICU. Prepare to secure airway, mechanically ventilate, and obtain
	    central venous access and continuous hemodynamic monitoring through
	    arterial line
	Once clinical seizure terminates will likely need EEG monitoring to assess
	    for subclinical seizures

Coma induction	If seizure continues then initiate coma with midazolam 0.2 mg/kg bolus
	    (max 10 mg) over 2 min and then initiate infusion at 0.1 mg/kg/hr. If clini-
	    cal seizures persist 5 min after initial midazolam bolus, then administer
	    additional midazolam bolus of 0.2 mg/kg bolus. Continue infusion. Titrate
	    up as needed to terminate seizures and generally to achieve a burst
	    suppression pattern on EEG
	If seizure persists at maximum midazolam (generally 2 mg/kg/hr) or mid-
	    azolam infusion is not tolerated, then consider transition to pentobarbital
	    or isoflurane

HINT: Status epilepticus is an emergency that requires rapid and aggressive treatment.

Suggested Readings

Abend NS, Gutierrez-Colina AM, Dlugos DJ. Medical treatment of pediatric status epilepticus. *Semin Pediatr Neurol.* 2010;17:169–175.

Berg AT, Berkovic SF, Brodie MJ, et al. Revised terminology and concepts for organization of seizures and epilepsies: Report of the ILAE Commission on Classification and Terminology, 2005–2009. *Epilepsia.* 2010;51(4):676–685.

Gaillard WD, Chiron C, Cross J, et al. Guidelines for imaging infants and children with recent-onset epilepsy. *Epilepsia.* 2009;50(9):2147–2153.

Hirtz D, Berg A, Bettis S, et al. Practice parameter: treatment of the child with a first unprovoked seizure. *Neurology.* 2003;60:166–175.

Subcommittee on Febrile Seizures. Clinical Practice Guideline—neurodiagnostic evaluation of the child with a simple febrile seizure. *Pediatrics.* 2011;127(2):389–394.

Waruiru C, Appleton R. Febrile seizures: an update. *Arch Dis Child.* 2004;89:751–756.

Sexual Abuse

INTRODUCTION

Child sexual abuse is defined as the involvement of children in sexual activities that they cannot understand, are not developmentally prepared for, cannot give informed consent to, and that violate societal taboos. "Sexual abuse" is a general term that includes a broad range of activities, including **noncontact activities** (e.g., pornography, either in its production or in its viewing; inappropriate observation of the child while dressing, toileting, or bathing; and perpetrator exhibitionism directed at the child) and **contact activities**. Sexual abuse **frequently occurs over time** as the perpetrator gains the trust of the child, and it can progress from noncontact to contact forms of abuse.

 DIFFERENTIAL DIAGNOSIS LIST

Child sexual abuse can have various presenting signs and symptoms. The following are physical signs associated with sexual abuse and the differential diagnosis for each.

Vaginal or Penile Discharge
Infectious Causes
- Sexually transmitted infections (STIs)—*Neisseria gonorrhoeae, Chlamydia trachomatis, Trichomonas vaginalis*
- *Group A Streptococcus*
- *Haemophilus influenzae*
- *Staphylococcus aureus*
- *Corynebacterium diphtheriae*
- *Mycoplasma hominis*
- *Gardnerella vaginalis*
- *Shigella*

Anatomic Causes
- Ectopic ureter
- Rectovaginal fistula
- Draining pelvic abscess

Traumatic Causes
- Foreign body
- Chemical irritation (e.g., bubble bath)
- Tight, nonporous clothing

Miscellaneous Causes
- Nonspecific vulvovaginitis
- Leukorrhea
- Lipschutz ulcerations

Genital Bleeding
Infectious Causes
- Urinary tract infection with gross hematuria
- Vaginitis

Anatomic Causes
- Vaginal polyp
- Urethral prolapse
- Vulvar hemangioma

Traumatic Causes
- Straddle injuries (usually anterior lacerations)
- Impaling (penetrating) injuries
- Foreign body (e.g., toilet paper, small toys)

Dermatologic Causes
- Lichen sclerosus et atrophicus (girls)
- Balanitis xerotica obliterans (boys)

Endocrinologic Causes
- Neonatal estrogen withdrawal
- Precocious puberty

Neoplastic Causes
- Sarcoma botryoides
- Vaginal rhabdomyosarcoma
- Estrogen-producing tumors

Genital Inflammation or Pruritus
Infectious Causes
- Nonspecific vulvovaginitis
- STIs—*N. gonorrhoeae, C. trachomatis, T. vaginalis*
- Pinworms
- Scabies
- Vaginal candidiasis
- Group A streptococcal perianal cellulitis

Traumatic Causes
- Poor hygiene
- Poorly ventilated or tight underwear
- Chemical irritation
- "Sandbox" vaginitis

Dermatologic Causes
- Atopic dermatitis
- Contact dermatitis
- Seborrhea
- Diaper dermatitis
- Psoriasis
- Lichen sclerosus et atrophicus (girls)
- Balanitis xerotica obliterans (boys)

Systemic Causes
- Urticaria
- Crohn disease

- Kawasaki syndrome
- Stevens–Johnson syndrome

Bruising
Infectious Causes
- Purpura fulminans
- Disseminated intravascular coagulation

Traumatic Causes
- Straddle injuries
- Accidental penetrating injuries

Dermatologic Causes
- Lichen sclerosus et atrophicus (girls)
- Balanitis xerotica obliterans (boys)
- Erythema multiforme
- Mongolian spots
- Vascular nevi

Hematologic Causes
- Idiopathic thrombocytopenic purpura
- Leukemia
- Vitamin K deficiency
- Coagulopathies
- Disseminated intravascular coagulation

Metabolic Causes
- Ehlers–Danlos syndrome
- Osteogenesis imperfecta

Autoimmune Causes
- Henoch–Schönlein purpura
- Vasculitis

Anatomic Variations
Acquired
- Labial agglutination
- Hair thread tourniquet syndrome
- Phimosis
- Paraphimosis
- Urethral prolapse

Congenital
- Septate hymen
- Cribriform hymen

- Microperforate hymen
- Imperforate hymen
- Urethral caruncles
- Vestibular bands
- Median raphe
- Ectopic ureterocele

DIFFERENTIAL DIAGNOSIS DISCUSSION

A few diagnoses are commonly mistaken for sexual abuse and deserve comment.

Lichen Sclerosus et Atrophicus
Etiology
Lichen sclerosus et atrophicus, a **dermatologic condition,** generally affects **prepubertal and postmenopausal women** and is characterized by **thin, atrophic vulvar skin that is easily injured**. The atrophic skin typically involves the labia majora, perineum, and perianal area in an hourglass configuration. The hymen is not usually involved.

Clinical Features and Evaluation
Leukoplakia and hemorrhagic bullae may develop. Children often present with **pruritus and vaginal bleeding after minimal trauma**. The diagnosis is usually made clinically, although biopsy is sometimes required.

Treatment
Treatment is usually **symptomatic, with attention to hygiene. Hydrocortisone** can be used to relieve irritation and pruritus.

Straddle Injuries
Etiology
Straddle injuries, common injuries to the genitalia of both boys and girls, result from the **crushing of the genital tissues between the bony pelvis and a solid structure** (e.g., a bicycle bar or the arm of a chair).

The term "straddle injury" is also used to describe **accidental penetrating trauma to the genitals**. These injuries can occur in any area of the genitalia and in girls can potentially lead to injury of the hymen. Accidental penetrating injuries to the genitals are far less common than nonpenetrating straddle injuries and should be accompanied by a history that confirms an impaling injury.

Clinical Features
In girls, most nonpenetrating straddle injuries cause **ecchymosis and/or lacerations of the anterior vulva,** often involving the labia minora. Because of its posterior location and recessed position, the hymen is not typically involved. **In boys,** straddle injuries commonly cause **scrotal and penile lacerations or ecchymoses**. These injuries **heal quickly** and usually no treatment is needed other than **sitz baths**. Some lacerations or impaling injuries require **surgical repair,** with the patient under general anesthesia.

Vulvovaginitis
Etiology
There are many causes of vulvovaginitis in children, many of which do not relate to sexual abuse. In **adolescent females,** most cases of vulvovaginitis are caused

by a **specific infectious organism**. The most common type of vulvovaginitis in **prepubertal children,** however, is **nonspecific vulvovaginitis,** which results from a combination of **anatomic, physiologic, and hygienic factors**. Vulvovaginitis may also result from **sexual abuse,** either as a result of mechanical trauma and irritation or from STIs.

Clinical Features

The **discharge** associated with nonspecific vulvovaginitis is **generally chronic, intermittent, scant to moderate,** and may or may not be seen in the introitus during the examination.

Evaluation

The laboratory evaluation of a genital discharge in a child can include **testing for *N. gonorrhoeae*, *C. trachomatis*, and *T. vaginalis*, a general vaginal culture, antigen testing for *T. vaginalis* and "clue cells"** (vaginal epithelial cells with adherent bacteria), a **Gram stain** of the discharge, and a **potassium hydroxide preparation** for *Candida*. A **whiff test** is done by mixing a sample of the **vaginal discharge** with a **small amount of potassium hydroxide;** an **amine-like odor** is present in **bacterial vaginosis** as well as in **trichomoniasis. Nucleic amplification tests that identify *N. gonorrhoeae* and *C. trachomatis* are quickly replacing cultures for the identification of gonorrhea and Chlamydia infections.**

Treatment

The treatment of **nonspecific vulvovaginitis** is aimed at **modifying hygiene practices** (e.g., wiping front to back after a bowel movement; wearing loose-fitting clothing and white cotton underwear). The treatment of vulvovaginitis caused by STIs and other infectious pathogens is detailed in Chapter 70, "Sexually Transmitted Diseases."

EVALUATION OF CHILD SEXUAL ABUSE

Discovery of sexual abuse is usually by one of the following mechanisms:

- The child discloses abuse
- A third party discovers the abuse (e.g., a sibling walks in the room during an assault)
- The child presents with physical injuries
- The child develops an STI

Many sexually abused children **do not have physical injuries at the time of an examination,** either because the child did not sustain physical injury during the abuse or the injuries have healed. The evaluation of a patient in whom sexual abuse is suspected, therefore, requires **careful attention to the history, physical examination, and laboratory specimen collection** and must include **meticulous documentation** of both historical and physical findings.

Patient History

Complaints may be related to physical injuries or STIs, but, more commonly, the signs and symptoms of sexual abuse are nonspecific and are **manifestations of the**

psychological stress associated with the abuse. These include **nonspecific behavioral complaints** (e.g., hypersexualized behaviors, phobias, sleep disturbances, poor school performance, runaway behaviors, truancy, aggressive behavior, symptoms and signs of depression) as well as **nonspecific physical complaints** (e.g., enuresis—secondary, day or night; encopresis; headaches; abdominal, genital, and/or rectal pain; dysuria; vaginitis; genital erythema; vaginal or penile discharge; genital and/or rectal bleeding; pregnancy). Information related to both physical and behavioral symptoms of abuse should be explored.

In most cases, the diagnosis of child sexual abuse depends on the **history obtained from the child**. Ideally, the **interview** of the child is **conducted by a professional** who is familiar with the dynamics of sexual abuse, knowledgeable about child development, and comfortable speaking to children about these issues. **Joint interviews** (with a representative from Child Protective Services and a law enforcement official) are **recommended,** although in the medical setting, this is often not possible. The child should be **interviewed with the parents absent,** because some children are hesitant to talk with a parent present and others may be overly coached by anxious parents.

The child should be asked **nonleading questions,** although specific questions to clarify statements are necessary of course. It is best to start the interview with an **open-ended question** such as "Can you tell me why you were brought here today"? The interviewer should ask **developmentally appropriate questions**. For example, a young child's sense of dates and time is best approximated by references to seasons, holidays, and other important events in the child's life. Statements made by the child should be **recorded verbatim** in the medical record, if possible.

It is important to try and elicit the following information:

- Identity of the alleged perpetrator and his or her relationship to the child
- The time of the last contact
- The reason why the child chose to disclose the incident at this time
- The frequency of abuse (one time vs. chronic)
- The specific types of sexual contact included in the abuse
- History of perpetrator ejaculation
- Whether threats were made to the child by the alleged perpetrator
- Whether prior official reports of the abuse have been made

Physical Examination

The type of examination performed depends on the age of the child. **Adolescent girls or children with suspected intravaginal injury** may require a **full pelvic examination,** whereas **most children** usually require only **careful inspection of the vulva**. Common positions used for examination of children include the supine, frog-leg position with labial traction (young girls), lithotomy position (adolescent girls), knee-chest position, and lateral decubitus position.

Few physical findings are pathognomonic of sexual abuse. Many genital findings are nonspecific, but with a history may support the diagnosis of sexual abuse. **Definitive findings** of sexual abuse include the **finding of semen or sperm**. In **pregnant patients and those with STIs** or injuries **without a history of sexual**

activity, sexual abuse is a very likely possibility. Further investigation is warranted for patients with **suspicious injuries or anatomic variants** (e.g., posterior angular concavities or transections of the hymen). **Less serious vaginal problems** (e.g., infections, adhesions) are **common in children** and do not independently suggest sexual abuse. Perianal erythema or hyperpigmentation are examples of nonspecific changes.

The decision to complete a **"rape kit"** is **determined by clinical presentation**. Recent research suggests that forensic evidence collection for prepubertal children can be limited to those who present for medical evaluation **within 24 hours of the last assault** or those who have **injury or bleeding** on examination. Adolescents who present within 72 hours (or up to 5 days in some recommendations) require forensic collections. Local crime laboratories have different protocols for collection of evidence. In general, the following evidence may be collected:

- **Victim's clothing.** Clothing provides the highest yield of forensic evidence in child sexual assault and should be vigorously sought. The clothing the child was wearing at the time of the assault is collected by having the child undress while standing on a sterile sheet and placing all items into a clean paper bag. (Plastic bags should not be used because they may be airtight; the buildup of heat and moisture can degrade evidence.) Police should be notified of unwashed clothing at home that might provide forensic evidence.
- **Swabs for semen, sperm, acid phosphatase, P30 analysis, and DNA analysis.** Moist secretions should be collected from the oral cavity (e.g., the pharynx, gum line), vagina, and rectum with a swab and allowed to air-dry before packaging. Swabs may also be collected from areas of the body that appear to have dried secretions, either by scraping a dry sample into a paper envelope or using a swab slightly moistened with sterile water, which is then allowed to air-dry.
- **Fingernail scrapings for foreign debris** should be placed into a paper envelope.
- **Pubic hair collection.** Collect combed pubic hairs into a paper envelope.
- **Foreign debris.** Any suspicious foreign debris found on the victim should be placed in a paper envelope.
- **Victim identification samples.** Collect a saliva sample and a blood sample from the victim to be used for identification of secretor status of the patient or for later DNA analysis.

Laboratory Studies

Laboratory evaluation is not universally required. When indicated, recommended tests to screen for STIs include the following:

- Culture or nucleic acid amplification tests (NAATs) of the cervix, vagina, or urethra; rectum; and pharynx for *N. gonorrhoeae*
- NAAT or culture of the cervix/vagina/urethra and rectum for *C. trachomatis*
- Wet preparation of vaginal secretions for *T. vaginalis*
- Culture of lesions for herpes simplex virus
- Serology for syphilis

- Serology for HIV, based on the prevalence of infection and suspected risk (should be repeated 3 and 6 months after last assault; obtain written consent)
- Gram stain and general culture of any vaginal, urethral, or anal discharge
- Nucleic acid amplification techniques are now approved for use in adolescent and adult women for STI screening, although appropriate confirmation is required for positive screening tests

Documentation

A **detailed medical record** is imperative to ensure that the best interests of the child are served. A well-documented medical evaluation in the medical record can serve as the basis for future discussion of the case. The physician should not rely on memory alone to reconstruct what occurred. The following hints are offered as a quick reference:

Do:

- Describe findings simply.
- Be aware of the child's developmental status.
- Use the child's words, defining the child's language if necessary.
- Ask nonleading questions.
- Record questions asked and specific answers given.
- Use diagrams and photographs to supplement the written record.

Do not:

- Use leading questions, if at all possible.
- Use the terms "virginal" or "intact hymen," because these terms are imprecise and can be problematic during the legal investigation of the case.
- State conclusions in absolute terms; rather, describe findings and comment if they are consistent with expectations based on information known at that time.

TREATMENT OF CHILD SEXUAL ABUSE

Medical treatment is guided by the **specific injuries or infections**. Hospitalization of sexually abused children is rarely required and, in general, is limited to children with severe genital trauma or systemic manifestations of STIs. Victims of sexual abuse, nonoffending parents, and perpetrators may all benefit from **therapy,** and referrals for patients should be made.

APPROACH TO THE PATIENT

All cases of suspected sexual abuse must be reported to law enforcement, Child Protective Services (for abuse committed by a caretaker or household member), **or both**. Each state has laws that define child sexual abuse, and physicians should be aware of the laws operating in their state of practice. Individual institutions often have policies or guidelines regarding the evaluation of abuse, and some hospitals have a multidisciplinary team with expertise in recognizing and evaluating child abuse. Physicians who report suspected abuse "in good faith" are given immunity should a suit be brought against a physician for "false reports." **Parents should be informed of the need to report** before doing so.

Suggested Readings

Adams JA, Harper K, Knudson S, et al. Examination findings in legally confirmed child sexual abuse: it's normal to be normal. *Pediatrics.* 1994;94:310–317.

American Academy of Pediatrics Committee on Child Abuse and Neglect. The evaluation of sexual behaviors in children. *Pediatrics.* 2009;124:992–998.

American Academy of Pediatrics Committee on Child Abuse and Neglect. The evaluation of sexual abuse in children. *Pediatrics.* 2005;116:506–512.

American Academy of Pediatrics Committee on Adolescence. Care of the adolescent sexual assault victim. *Pediatrics.* 2008;122:462–470.

Berenson AB, Chacko MR, Wiemann CM, et al. A case-control study of anatomic changes resulting from sexual abuse. *Am J Obstet Gynecol.* 2000;182:820–834.

Christian CW, Lavelle JM, De Jong AR, et al. Forensic evidence findings in prepubertal victims of sexual assault. *Pediatrics.* 2000;106:100–104.

Heger AH, Tiscon L, Guerra L, et al. Appearance of the genitalia in girls selected for nonabuse: review of hymenal morphology and nonspecific findings. *J Pediatr Adolesc Gynecol.* 2002;15:27–35.

Kellogg ND, Menard SW, Santos A. Genital anatomy in pregnant adolescents: "normal" does not mean "nothing happened." *Pediatrics.* 2004;113(1 Pt 1):e67–e69.

CHAPTER 70

Lisa K. Tuchman
Amy L. Weiss

Sexually Transmitted Diseases

INTRODUCTION

Among all age groups, adolescents and young adults are at the highest risk of being diagnosed with a sexually transmitted disease (STD) due to a combination of factors, including risk-taking behaviors, increased biologic susceptibility, and barriers to accessing appropriate reproductive health care services. Although young people between the ages of 15 and 24 years comprise a quarter of the sexually experienced population, they account for up to a half of newly acquired STDs. In 2009, women aged 15 to 19 years had the highest rates of Chlamydia, gonorrhea, and HPV infection compared to all other age groups.

While often asymptomatic, the clinical presentation of most STDs in adolescents can be highly variable. Females may present with **vaginal discharge, abnormal vaginal bleeding, vaginal itching, dysuria, or pain** (lower abdominal, right upper quadrant, or rectal). **Males** may present with **urethral discharge, dysuria, testicular pain or swelling, or rectal pain**. Presentation can also include rash, pharyngitis, arthralgia or arthritis, and inguinal adenopathy.

Clinicians should **educate adolescents about the transmission of STDs and the importance of protecting oneself**. **Primary prevention** includes helping guide the development of healthy sexual behaviors and providing accurate sexual and reproductive health information, as well as access to reproductive health resources. Providers should remember that adolescents with chronic conditions engage in intimate relationships like their healthy peers and are also at risk for acquiring STDs. Adolescents across the United States, with limited exceptions, can consent to the confidential diagnosis and treatment of STDs, and medical care for STDs can be provided to adolescents without parental consent or knowledge. Providers should inform adolescents of their right to confidentiality and should comply with state laws and policies to ensure the confidentiality of STD-related services for adolescents.

Appropriate treatment of both the patient and the partner is essential.

DIFFERENTIAL DIAGNOSIS LIST

Bacterial Infection

- Chancroid (*Haemophilus ducreyi*)
- Gonorrhea (*Neisseria gonorrhoeae*)
- Granuloma inguinale (*Calymmato-bacterium granulomatis*)
- Lymphogranuloma venereum (*Chlamydia trachomatis*)
- Shigella species
- Syphilis or condyloma latum (*Treponema pallidum*)

- Ureaplasma urealyticum
- Bacterial vaginosis (*Gardnerella vaginalis*)

Parasitic Infection
- Pubic lice (*Phthirus pubis*)
- Scabies (*Sarcoptes scabiei*)

Protozoal Infection
- *Trichomonas vaginalis*
- *Entamoeba histolytica*
- Giardiasis (*Giardia lamblia*)

Viral Infection
- Cytomegalovirus infection
- Hepatitis A, B, or C
- Herpes simplex virus (HSV) infection
- HIV
- HPV (genital warts, condyloma acuminatum)
- Molluscum contagiosum

DIFFERENTIAL DIAGNOSIS DISCUSSION
Selected Diseases That Cause Genital Lesions
Syphilis
Etiology
Syphilis is caused by the spirochete *T. pallidum.*

Clinical Features
- **Primary syphilis** is characterized by a painless ulcer or chancre at the site of inoculation.
- **Among children and adolescents, secondary syphilis is most common,** typically presenting with a maculopapular rash involving the palms and soles. Other symptoms include mucocutaneous lesions (condyloma lata) and systemic symptoms (e.g., adenopathy, fever, pharyngitis, malaise).
- **Tertiary syphilis** includes aortitis, neurologic dysfunction, and gummatous lesions of the bone, kidney, and liver.
- **Latent syphilis** describes disease in patients who have no symptoms of infection. Early latent syphilis refers to infection within the past year. Late latent syphilis and syphilis of unknown duration make up the remainder of this category.
- Men who have sex with men (MSM) accounted for 62% of all primary and secondary syphilis cases in the United States in 2009. Rates of coinfection of syphilis and HIV in MSM varied across the United States in 2009, with a median of 44.4% (30%–74%).

Evaluation
The diagnosis of syphilis is generally made by using a **nonspecific** (nontreponemal) **antibody test** such as the **venereal disease research laboratory (VDRL) test** and the **rapid plasma reagent test**. The specific tests for treponemal antibody, fluorescent treponemal antibody, absorbed (FTA-ABS), or the *T. pallidum* particle agglutination (TP-PA) test, remain positive for life; therefore, they do not denote activity. Nontreponemal tests can be quantified by **testing serial dilutions of serum. Quantification is important** because the appearance of clinical lesions correlates with a rise in titers. These titers diminish with appropriate treatment and can be used to follow response to therapy.

> **HINT:** FTA-ABS or TP-PA helps differentiate infections from diseases such as lupus that produce a false-positive VDRL. However, these tests are positive in Lyme disease, which does not have a positive VDRL.

- *T. pallidum* cannot be cultured in artificial media but **darkfield examination and direct fluorescent antibody tests** of lesion exudate or tissue are definitive ways to diagnose syphilis.

Treatment
Parenteral penicillin G is the treatment of choice for all stages of syphilis (see Table 70-1 for details).

Treatment may be complicated by an acute febrile syndrome known as the Jarisch–Herxheimer reaction. This reaction resolves within 24 hours.

The expected serologic response to treatment is a minimum fourfold decrease in nontreponemal test titers within 6 months.

Herpes Genitalis
Etiology
Most recurrent cases of herpes genitalis result from **herpes simplex virus-type 2 (HSV-2),** although up to 50% of primary cases of genital herpes are caused by **HSV-1,** the type more commonly associated with stomatitis. These viruses account for up to 90% of all ulcerative lesions of the genitalia and are highly contagious; as many as 90% of women exposed to infected men develop genital herpes. Transmission can occur in patients who are asymptomatic and often unaware that they are infected, but are still shedding virus and therefore contagious.

Clinical Features
Primary infection is characterized by **single or multiple vesicles** that may appear anywhere on the genitalia. These vesicles **spontaneously rupture to form shallow ulcers,** which are exquisitely **painful** but **resolve spontaneously** without scarring. Some cases of primary genital herpes are severe enough to require **hospitalization**. Mild to severe **systemic symptoms** may accompany the genital lesions. The mean duration of the initial episode of HSV is 12 days.

Recurrent infections, which occur in some patients, are less painful and of shorter duration, lasting 4 to 5 days.

Evaluation
Viral culture allows detection of the virus in 1 to 3 days. New vesicles are unroofed and scraped for inoculation of viral media. The yield of culture diminishes over time. **Direct fluorescent antibody tests** are available and are rapid and highly sensitive. Serologic testing is available but is of limited value in the management of the patient.

Treatment
- **Management of a first episode** of genital herpes includes antiviral therapy and counseling regarding the natural history of genital herpes with particular emphasis on potential recurrent episodes, asymptomatic viral shedding, sexual

TABLE 70-1 Selected Sexually Transmitted Diseases

Etiology	Disease	Diagnostic Tests	Treatment
Treponema pallidum	Syphilis[a]	Darkfield microscopy or direct fluorescent antibody Serology Nontreponemal (VDRL, RPR) Treponemal (TP-PA, FTA-ABS)	
	Primary: chancre Secondary: rash adenopathy, fever		Benzathine penicillin G, 2.4 million U IM × 1 Benzathine penicillin G, 2.4 million U IM × 1
	Tertiary: cardiac, gummatous Neurosyphilis Early latent Late latent or latent of unknown duration		Benzathine penicillin G, 2.4 million U IM weekly × 3 doses Aqueous penicillin G, 18–24 million U daily for 10–14 d Benzathine penicillin G, 2.4 million U × 1 Benzathine penicillin G, 2.4 million U IM weekly × 3 doses
Herpes simplex	Herpes[b]	Culture virus Rapid fluorescent antibody test	
	Primary: painful genital mucosal lesions and mild systemic symptoms		Acyclovir, 400 mg PO three times daily or 200 mg PO 5 times daily for 7–10 d Famciclovir, 250 mg PO three times daily for 7–10 d Valacyclovir, 1 g PO twice daily for 7–10 d
	Secondary: less severe recurrence		Acyclovir, 400 mg PO three times daily or 800 mg PO twice daily for 5 d or 800 mg PO 3 times daily for 2 d Famciclovir, 125 mg PO twice daily for 5 d or 1 g PO twice daily for 1 d or 500 mg PO once, followed by 250 mg twice daily for 2 d Valacyclovir, 500 mg PO twice daily for 3 d or 1 g PO once daily for 5 d

(continued)

TABLE 70-1	Selected Sexually Transmitted Diseases (*Cont.*)		
Etiology	Disease	Diagnostic Tests	Treatment
Trichomonas vaginalis	Trichomoniasis: vaginal discharge, dysuria, and local irritation	Wet mount Culture	Metronidazole, 2 g PO × 1, or Tinidazole, 2 g orally in a single dose
Human papilloma virus	Condyloma acuminata (genital warts)[c]	Visual inspection	Patient applied: Podofilox, 0.5% solution or gel. Apply twice daily for 3 d then 4 d off up to four cycles Imiquimod, 5% cream. Apply three times weekly up to 16 wk Wash off after 6–10 hr Sinecatechins, 15% ointment. Apply three times daily for up to 16 wk Provider administered: Cryotherapy. Every 1–2 wk Podophyllin resin, 10%–25%. Apply weekly. Wash off in 1–4 hr Trichloroacetic acid (TCA) or bichloracetic acid (BCA), 80%–90% Apply weekly Surgical removal
Chlamydia trachomatis	Uncomplicated cervicitis Urethritis Epididymitis Proctitis	NAAT (urethral, cervical, urine) Culture	Azithromycin, 1 g PO × 1, or Doxycycline, 100 mg PO twice daily for 7 d In pregnant women: Azithromycin, 1 g PO × 1, or Amoxicillin, 500 mg PO 3 times daily for 7 d
	Neonatal conjunctivitis or pneumonia		Neonatal: Erythromycin, 50 mg/kg/d, in four divided doses for 14 d

Neisseria gonor-rhoeae	Uncomplicated cervicitis	NAAT (urethral, cervical, urine)	Ceftriaxone, 250 mg IM, × 1 or Cefixime,[d] 400 mg PO × 1 or Single-dose injectable cephalosporin regimens plus Azithromycin 1 g orally in a single dose or Doxycycline 100 mg a day for 7 d Quinolones[e] are no longer recommended as first-line therapy because of increasing resistance and should only be used in culture-proven quinolone sensitive strains
	Urethritis Pharyngitis Epididymitis Proctitis	Culture Gram stain (urethral discharge)	
		Conjunctivitis Disseminated disease	Ceftriaxone, 1 g IM × 1; consider eye lavage with saline Ceftriaxone,[f] 1 g IV every 24 hr

FTA-ABS, fluorescent treponemal antibody, absorbed (test); *IM*, intramuscularly; *IV*, intravenously; *NAAT*, nucleic acid amplification test; TP-PA, *Treponema pallidum* particle agglutination; *PO*, orally; *VDRL*, Venereal Disease Research Laboratory (test).

[a]All doses listed for adolescents and adults. Doses for children and alternative regimens for persons with penicillin allergies can be found in Centers for Disease Control and Prevention. Sexually transmitted diseases treatment guidelines 2010. *MMWR Recomm Rep.* 2010;59(RR-12):1–110.

[b]Regimens for suppressive therapy for recurrent genital herpes can be found in Centers for Disease Control and Prevention. Sexually transmitted disease treatment guidelines 2010. *MMWR Recomm Rep.* 2010;59(RR-12):1–110.

[c]Exact regimens for the treatment of external genital warts and future inflammation in treatment of cervical warts can be found in Centers for Disease Control and Prevention. Sexually transmitted diseases treatment guidelines 2010. *MMWR Recomm Rep.* 2010;59(RR-12):1–110.

[d]The tablet form of cefixime is currently not available in the United States.

[e]Fluoroquinolones have not been recommended for patients younger than 18 years because of possible damage to articular cartilage. Because of the lack of data, the CDC recommends any adult regimen for patients ≥45 kg.

[f]See the 2010 CDC STD guidelines for other treatment options for disseminated gonorrhea. The parenteral regimens can be switched to oral regimens for 7 days after 24 to 48 hr of improvement.

transmission, risk for neonatal infection for women of childbearing age, and risk reduction. Acyclovir, famciclovir, and valacyclovir can all be used (see Table 70-1 for details). Analgesics as well as local care (e.g., sitz baths, barrier creams) may offer some relief. Herpes proctitis or herpes in the setting of immune dysfunction (e.g., HIV/AIDS, status post bone marrow transplant) may require higher doses of antiviral medication.

- **For recurrent disease,** acyclovir, famciclovir, or valacyclovir have been effective in decreasing severity and length of infection but are most beneficial if initiated within 1 day of the onset of lesions (see Table 70-1 for details). In patients who have frequent recurrences (at least six per year), the physician may want to consider suppressive oral therapy, which requires continuous treatment with antiviral agents.

Human Papilloma Virus

Etiology

There are more than **40 types of HPV** that can infect the genital tract. Although most HPV infections are asymptomatic, types 6 and 11 are implicated in 90% of **visible genital warts** and types 16, 18, 31, 33, and 35 have been strongly **associated with cervical dysplasia**. The virus is **transmitted by direct contact**. The incubation period can be as long as 20 months. **In children, the presence of genital warts** can be secondary to **vertical transmission at birth or sexual abuse**.

A quadrivalent HPV vaccine, for strains 6, 11, 16, and 18, was licensed in the United States in June, 2006, and a bivalent HPV vaccine, against types 16 and 18, was licensed in October, 2009. The current recommendation is that young women aged 9 to 26 years receive either vaccine, while young men aged 9 to 26 years receive the quadrivalent vaccine. It is unclear what effect these vaccines will have on future prevalence rates of various types of HPV.

Clinical Features

Warts can be **asymptomatic or symptomatic** and are found in a variety of locations, including the uterine cervix, vagina, urethra, anus, and extragenital areas (conjunctival, nasal, oral, laryngeal). Depending on the location and size of the warts, they can be **painful, friable, and pruritic**.

Evaluation and Screening

Identification of the characteristic lesion is diagnostic. Application of **3% acetic acid** produces a **classic acetowhite appearance**. Depending on the location and appearance, condyloma acuminatum can be confused with urethral prolapse, syphilis, vulvar tumors, and sarcoma botryoides.

Current recommendations are that adolescents do not start undergoing cervical cytology, either conventional or liquid-based Pap testing, until the age of 21 years, unless they are infected with HIV or have another form of immunocompromise. HPV testing is similarly not recommended in adolescents.

Treatment

The primary goal of treating genital warts is the **removal of symptomatic or visible warts**. Treatment often induces wart-free periods but does not necessarily decrease infectivity. There is no known effect of treatment on the subsequent development of cervical cancer. Without treatment, genital warts can resolve spontaneously, remain unchanged, or increase in both size and number.

Because none of the available treatments is superior, treatment should be guided by the preference of the patient and the experience of the health care provider. Medical and surgical treatments are available. Treatments include patient-applied therapies (e.g., podofilox and imiquimod) and provider-administered therapies (e.g., cryotherapy, podophyllin resin, trichloroacetic acid, interferon, and surgery). Warts on moist surfaces respond better to topical treatment. The treatment modality should be changed if a patient does not have significant improvement after three provider-administered treatments. Recurrences are most common in the first 3 months after treatment.

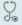
HINT: The HPV vaccines are prophylactic immunizations and only protect against strains of HPV to which one has not been exposed prior to receiving the vaccination; there are no therapeutic benefits if someone has already been infected with a particular stain of HPV.

Selected Diseases That Cause Mucopurulent Discharge
Chlamydia Trachomatis
Etiology

C. trachomatis is a Gram-negative, intracellular organism. It is the most commonly reported notifiable disease in the United States.

Clinical Features

In females, *C. trachomatis* can cause **cervicitis, urethritis, or pelvic inflammatory disease (PID)**. Although the majority of **females** are asymptomatic or mildly symptomatic (vaginal discharge, dysuria, dyspareunia, urinary frequency), serious sequelae include **PID, ectopic pregnancy, and potential tubal scarring leading to fertility difficulties**.

Like females, chlamydia infection is often asymptomatic in males but can result in urethritis, epididymitis, proctitis, or prostatitis. Clinical signs of epididymitis are pain and swelling of the epididymis; for prostatitis, the patient has pain in the testicles and scrotum; for proctitis, the patient complains of rectal pain on defecation or of tenesmus.

Reiter syndrome (conjunctivitis, dermatitis, urethritis, and arthritis) or reactive arthritis can occur in males and females.

Evaluation

In symptomatic females, genitourinary examination is essential. Nucleic acid amplification tests (NAATs) are highly sensitive and specific permitting collection of less invasive specimens for testing. Urine or swabs from the endocervical or vaginal canal can be used. The cervix can appear normal or be friable with the presence of mucopurulent discharge. Cervical cultures range in sensitivity from 50% to 85% and should be used if NAAT testing available to the provider is unreliable in the presence of gross blood, if the sample is being obtained in a prepubertal girl, or in case of specimen collection in medicolegal cases.

In males, urine or urethral swab can be sent for chlamydia NAAT.

The Centers for Disease Control and Prevention (CDC) does not recommend that a chlamydia test be performed for a "test of cure" after completing treatment, unless there are persistent symptoms or suspicion of reinfection. Testing with NAAT that is done <3 weeks after completion of therapy may give false-positive results because of detection of nonviable organisms.

Because of high reinfection rates secondary to partners not being treated and the increased risk of PID with repeat infection, adolescents with chlamydia infections should be rescreened 3 to 4 months after treatment.

Treatment

Most recommended regimens include either **azithromycin or doxycycline**. In the past, given high coinfection rates with gonococcal infection, presumptive treatment for chlamydia and gonorrhea was universally recommended. Given the high sensitivity of NAATs, patients with a positive chlamydia and a negative gonorrhea NAAT result need only be treated for chlamydia. If a non-NAAT assay is performed or gonorrhea infection is not ruled out, presumptive treatment for coinfection is appropriate. Empirical treatment is indicated for patients who may not return for test results. See Table 70-1 for treatment regimens.

Partners with sexual contact within 60 days preceding symptoms or diagnosis should be evaluated, tested, and treated. Patients should abstain from sexual intercourse until 1 week after they and their partners have completed treatment.

Gonorrhea

Etiology

Gonorrhea is caused by a Gram-negative diplococcus, *N. gonorrhoeae*. In the United States, ~600,000 new infections occur each year. Because gonococcal **infections in women** are often asymptomatic and **can lead to PID, tubal scarring, and subsequent tubal infertility or ectopic pregnancy,** screening is of utmost importance in women younger than 25 years.

Clinical Features

In **premenarchal females,** the **vagina** is the primary site of infection, whereas in **postmenarchal females** the organism can cause **endocervicitis, urethritis, bartholinitis, perihepatitis, or upper genital tract disease**. Common presentations include vaginal discharge, dysuria, labial swelling and tenderness, abnormal vaginal bleeding, or abdominal pain. Only about 50% of women with gonorrhea are symptomatic.

In **males,** *N. gonorrhoeae* infection can cause **urethritis, prostatitis, or epididymitis**.

In both **males and females,** infection in **extragenital sites** includes **pharyngitis, conjunctivitis, or disseminated infection** presenting as meningitis, septic arthritis, osteomyelitis, or septic shock. Gonococcal endocarditis and pericarditis have been described, though are rare. **Adolescents** commonly have **migratory arthritis or tenosynovitis**. The two patterns of arthritis are the **arthritis-dermatitis syndrome**

and monoarticular arthritis. The arthritis-dermatitis syndrome, characterized by fever, chills, and arthritis or tenosynovitis, is accompanied by skin lesions that affect ~50% of patients. The lesions are usually small, tender papules or pustules on the distal extremities. The remainder of patients with gonococcal arthritis have a mono-articular arthritis affecting, in order of frequency, the knees, elbows, ankles, wrists, and small joints of the hands and feet.

Evaluation

Culture and Gram stain have been the mainstays of diagnosis for gonorrhea in symptomatic patients, but **NAATs** are now available for detection of genital *N. gonorrhoeae* infection. Diagnosis of the gonococcal infection depends on the location and circumstances of the infection.

- **In males, a Gram stain of the urethral exudates** (revealing typical Gram-negative intracellular diplococci) is sufficient for the diagnosis of gonorrhea, but, in the absence of urethral exudate, cultures or preferably NAAT specimens from urine or **anterior urethra** swab should be obtained to rule out a gonorrheal infection.
- **In female patients depending on available NAAT assays, the presence of blood** may necessitate testing with cultures from the endocervix. Otherwise, NAAT can be used. Endocervical Gram stain is not helpful in females.
- **In patients with gonococcal arthritis-dermatitis syndrome, blood cultures** may be positive.
- **In patients with gonococcal monoarticular arthritis, joint fluid culture** may be positive; blood cultures are usually negative.

Treatment

Given the **high coinfection rates of *N. gonorrhoeae* with *C. trachomatis*,** patients who are treated empirically for gonococcal infection are also routinely treated with a regimen effective against uncomplicated genital *C. trachomatis* infection. The most recent recommendations from the Centers for Disease Control and Prevention recommend treatment for both organisms even if testing for *C. trachomatis* is negative.

Pelvic Inflammatory Disease

Etiology

The term PID refers to a spectrum of infections of the **upper female genital tract** including endometritis, salpingitis, tubo-ovarian abscess, and pelvic peritonitis. Although *C. trachomatis and N. gonorrhoeae* are the most important causative organisms of PID, it should be managed as a **polymicrobial infection** of microorganisms that are part of the **vaginal flora** (e.g., anaerobes, *G. vaginalis, H. influenzae,* enteric Gram-negative rods, and *Streptococcus agalactiae*) as well as other organisms (e.g., *M. hominis, Mycobacterium genitalium, U. urealyticum*).

Risk factors for PID include age (highest rate in 15- to 19-year-olds), increased number of sexual partners, previous history of PID, sexual partner with an STD, and socioeconomic factors such as drug use, youth with behavioral and emotional problems, and disadvantaged youth.

Clinical Features

The wide variety of signs and symptoms plus many asymptomatic patients make the **diagnosis of PID difficult**. PID is more likely to present during the first half of the menstrual cycle. **Bilateral lower abdominal pain** is the most common presenting symptom. Other associated symptoms include abnormal vaginal discharge, abnormal uterine bleeding, dysuria, dyspareunia, nausea, vomiting, and fever. Because of this presentation, **other common causes of lower abdominal pain** (e.g., ectopic pregnancy, ovarian torsion, acute appendicitis, urinary tract infection, functional pain) **must be considered and ruled out**.

Evaluation

Given the potential for **devastating sequelae if left untreated,** the diagnosis of PID should be **considered in any female of childbearing age who has pelvic pain**. As noted earlier, history can be very helpful and information should be obtained regarding past episodes of PID (increased risk for recurrent PID) and date of last menstrual cycle. Because visualization of the pelvic structures for inflammation by laparoscope (the golden standard) is almost never practical, the diagnosis is made on clinical evidence. Most women with PID have pelvic tenderness in addition to either mucopurulent discharge or evidence of white blood cells in saline preparation of vaginal fluid. Table 70-2 reviews the criteria for the diagnosis of acute PID.

Important laboratory testing includes a **pregnancy test** (to rule out pregnancy or complications of pregnancy), **complete blood cell count (CBC) with differential, erythrocyte sedimentation rate (ESR), C-reactive protein (CRP), NAAT** (or cultures) for *N. gonorrhoeae and C. trachomatis*, **urinalysis, and urine culture**. **Blood cultures** should be obtained in ill-appearing patients. **Pelvic ultrasonography (with Doppler if ovarian torsion is suspected)** should be considered in all adolescents with the diagnosis of PID because a tubo-ovarian abscess (TOA) may not be noted on the examination, and physical examination and laboratory findings are not sensitive or specific for the diagnosis of TOA. **Ultrasonography** can also help rule out acute appendicitis and torsion. **Transvaginal sonography**

TABLE 70-2	Criteria for the Diagnosis of Acute PID

Minimum criteria (initiate empirical treatment if present and no other causes)
Uterine OR adnexal tenderness OR
Cervical motion tenderness

Additional criteria to support a diagnosis of pelvic inflammatory disease
Abnormal cervical or vaginal mucopurulent discharge
Presence of white blood cells on saline microscopy of vaginal secretions
Elevated erythrocyte sedimentation rate
Elevated C-reactive protein
Laboratory documentation of cervical infection with *Neisseria gonorrhoeae or Chlamydia trachomatis*
Oral temperature >101°F (38.3°C)

may show thickened fluid-filled tubes with or without free pelvic fluid or tubo-ovarian complex in cases of PID. **Laparoscopy** is only indicated when the diagnosis of PID is uncertain or for patients with a diagnosis of PID who have recurrent abdominal pain.

Treatment

Because even mild disease can result in long-term sequelae, clinicians should have a **low threshold for making the diagnosis** and initiating treatment.

PID treatment regimens must provide empirical **broad-spectrum coverage** of likely pathogens. Coverage should include *N. gonorrhoeae, C. trachomatis,* anaerobes, Gram-negative facultative bacteria, and streptococci. Table 70-3 reviews appropriate antibiotic regimens for the treatment of PID.

The CDC recommends considering **hospitalization when the diagnosis is unclear, the possibility of surgical emergencies** (e.g., appendicitis, ectopic pregnancy) **cannot be excluded, the patient is pregnant, the patient has a TOA,** the patient has severe illness (severe nausea and vomiting or high fever), or there is **intolerance or failure of an outpatient regimen** (after 72 hours). Because there are no data to suggest that either adolescent women or women with HIV infection benefit

TABLE 70-3	Regimens for the Treatment of Pelvic Inflammatory Disease in Adolescents

Outpatient Regimens
Ceftriaxone, 250 mg IM once
or
Cefoxitin, 2 g IM once WITH probenecid, 1 g PO once
or
Other parenteral third-generation cephalosporin (e.g., ceftizoxime or cefotaxime)
plus
Doxycycline, 100 mg PO twice daily for 14 d, WITH or WITHOUT metronidazole, 500 mg orally twice daily for 14 d

Inpatient Regimens
Regimen A
Cefoxitin, 2 g IV every 6 hr
or
Cefotetan, 2 g IV every 12 hr
plus
Doxycycline, 100 mg orally or IV every 12 hr
Regimen B
Clindamycin, 900 mg IV every 8 hr
plus
Gentamicin, 2 mg/kg IV loading dose, followed by a maintenance dose of 1.5 mg/kg every 8 hr

Parenteral therapy can be discontinued 24 hr after clinical improvement with continuation of PO doxycycline 100 mg twice daily or clindamycin 450 mg PO four times daily (preferred when tubo-ovarian abscess is present) to complete a 14-d course.
IM, intramuscularly; *IV,* intravenously; *PO,* orally.
Adapted from Centers for Disease Control and Prevention. Sexually transmitted diseases treatment guidelines 2010. *MMWR Recomm Rep.* 2010;59(RR-12):1–110. Published by the United States Centers for Disease Control and Prevention.

from hospitalization for PID treatment, clinical judgment and an assessment of the patient's compliance is recommended based on the previously described considerations. All patients treated as outpatients should be reevaluated within 72 hours to ensure clinical improvement.

EVALUATION OF SEXUALLY TRANSMITTED DISEASES

Patient History

Important questions to ask include:

- Are there any common symptoms consistent with infection (e.g., presence of abnormal vaginal discharge or bleeding, dysuria, abdominal pain, genital lesions)?
- Is there testicular pain or swelling?
- What type of birth control method is used?
- Is the person currently trying to get pregnant?
- Is there a previous history of STDs or known exposure to an infected partner?
- What was the first day of the last menstrual period?
- Is there a history of pregnancy or abortion?
- When was the last pelvic examination done?

Physical Examination

In all patients, when there is concern about an STD, the **external genitalia** must be examined. In sexually active adolescent females, the **internal genitalia** should be examined by bimanual examination; using a speculum is indicated if cervical cultures need to be collected. In males, the **penis, testes, scrotum, and rectum** should be examined. Vaginal or meatal discharge, skin lesions, lacerations, contusions, epididymal or testicular tenderness, or inguinal adenopathy should be noted.

 HINT: Avoid using lubricant for speculum insertion because the lubricant may interfere with cultures and/or NAAT. Instead, rinse the speculum with warm water before inserting.

Laboratory Studies

- **Cultures or NAAT** should be performed on samples from the endocervical canal, vagina, or urine (for females) and from the urethra or urine (for males) if chlamydia or gonorrhea is suspected.
- **Wet mount.** In females, a wet mount should be done if trichomonas is suspected. Some centers may have access to rapid trichomonas polymerase chain reaction testing, which is preferred over direct visualization due to higher sensitivity.
- Gram stain of a vaginal specimen should be done if vaginal candidiasis or bacterial vaginosis is suspected, and to assess for white blood cells.
- **Gram stain** of urethral discharge can be useful in diagnosing gonococcal urethritis in males.

- **Blood tests.** In females with suspected upper genital tract disease, a complete blood cell count and erythrocyte sedimentation rate or C-reactive protein should be considered.
- **Urinalysis.** In males, a urinalysis should be performed. A leukocyte esterase test in men has a good negative predictive value (97%) for *C. trachomatis.*

TREATMENT OF SEXUALLY TRANSMITTED DISEASES
Females
Empirical therapy for gonorrhea and chlamydia should be instituted **for patients with a mucopurulent cervical or vaginal discharge** while awaiting results of cultures or NAAT. Additionally, empirical therapy is warranted **if the partner** (or perpetrator, in the case of suspected sexual abuse) **has been diagnosed** with an STD. In most other patients, treatment can be deferred until the results of testing are available, provided appropriate follow-up is feasible.

Males
Empirical therapy for gonorrhea and chlamydia should be **considered in males with a urethral discharge**. In patients with dysuria or an abnormal urinalysis, further workup for STD is warranted prior to treatment.

SCREENING, PROPHYLAXIS, AND PREVENTION OF SEXUALLY TRANSMITTED DISEASES
The consideration of an STD in a sexually active adolescent or young adult serves as an important opportunity to **initiate STD screening, prophylaxis,** and a discussion about **prevention**.

Screening
All patients diagnosed with an STD should be **screened for syphilis and offered HIV antibody testing**. The CDC recommends routine opt-out screening for HIV among adults aged 13 to 64 years presenting to health-care settings without the need of a separate written consent.

Yearly screening for chlamydia and gonorrhea by culture or NAAT should be considered for all sexually active males and females. For females with a history of an STD, more frequent screening (every 3 to 4 months) is indicated.

The most current recommendation is that adolescents with intact immune systems begin cervical cytology screening, with either conventional or liquid-based Pap test, at the age of 21 years, regardless of the age of onset of sexual activity. Infection with HPV is extremely common and nearly always self-resolving in this population. The rate of cervical cancer in women younger than 21 years is exceedingly low, and screening does not appear to prevent cervical cancer in this age group. HPV testing is also not recommended in adolescents or young adults. Cervical cytology, either conventional or liquid-based Pap test, **should not be obtained** in the presence of an STD. Routine cervical cytology testing should be deferred until symptoms of vaginitis/cervicitis resolve. Although there are no formal guidelines recommending anal cytology screening, some providers perform these tests on MSMs and individuals with HIV. An anal cytology test is performed by inserting a Dacron swab into the anus until it hits the rectal wall, then withdrawing while using a spiral motion and applying lateral pressure. The same cytology techniques used for cervical specimens, conventional or liquid-based Pap tests, can be applied for anal cytology.

Prophylaxis

- **Hepatitis B.** Effective prophylaxis for hepatitis B can be accomplished with the hepatitis B vaccine. The vaccine should be considered in all sexually active individuals without hepatitis B disease or prior vaccination.
- **HIV.** There is no consensus on the use of antiretroviral medications for HIV-negative patients with sexual exposure to an HIV-infected or suspected HIV-infected individual. In certain settings, however, postexposure prophylaxis may be considered for reducing the risk of HIV transmission.
- **HPV.** The quadrivalent HPV vaccine confers prophylactic protection against the high-risk strains 16 and 18 and those most commonly associated with genital warts, strains 6 and 11. The vaccine is recommended for all females and males aged 9 to 26 years, regardless of sexual activity status. The bivalent HPV vaccine protects against strains 16 and 18, and is recommended in girls and women aged 9 to 26 years.
- **Hepatitis A (HAV).** Vaccination is important to prevent fecal-oral transmission during sexual contact, with the majority of cases reported in MSMs.

Prevention

Information regarding major STDs should be **provided to all adolescents and individuals diagnosed with an STD**.

Education on the correct use and efficacy of condoms in preventing pregnancy and STDs should be given to all patients, male and female, diagnosed with an STD or engaging in sexual activity. The **limitations of condoms should also be stated,** namely, that they may not prevent many cases of HPV, HAV, and some cases of HSV. Providers should advocate for dual contraception.

Treatment of partners of patients with chlamydia, gonorrhea, syphilis, and trichomonas is an effective means of preventing symptomatic disease in the partner. It also minimizes the risk of reinfection in the patient and future infection of other sexual partners. Understanding the complex developmental and biologic issues that contribute to adolescents' risk for STDs is an important first step in providing sexual and reproductive health care for this population.

Suggested Readings

Berlan ED, Holland-Hall C. Sexually transmitted infections in adolescents: advances in epidemiology, screening, and diagnosis. *Adolesc Med State Art Rev.* 2010;21(2):332–346.

Catallozzi M, Rudy BJ. Lesbian, gay, bisexual, transgendered, and questioning youth: the importance of sensitive and confidential sexual history in identifying the risk and implementing treatment for sexually transmitted infections. *Adolesc Med.* 2004;15:353–367.

Centers for Disease Control and Prevention. Quadrivalent human papilloma virus vaccine. Recommendations of the Advisory Committee of Immunization Practice (ACIP). *MMWR Recomm Rep.* 2007;56(RR-2):1–24.

Centers for Disease Control and Prevention. Sexually transmitted diseases treatment guidelines 2010. *MMWR Recomm Rep.* 2010;59(RR-12);1–110. See: www.cdc.gov/std/treatment/2010/

English A, Ford CA. The HIPAA Privacy Rule and adolescents: legal question and clinical challenges. *Perspect Sex Reprod Health.* 2004;36:80–86.

Ford CA, English A, Sigman G. Confidential health care for adolescents: position paper of the Society for Adolescent Medicine. *J Adolesc Health.* 2004;35:160–167.

Neinstein LS. Sexually transmitted diseases. In: Neinstein LS, ed. *Adolescent Health Care: A Practical Guide.* 5th ed. Philadelphia, PA: Lippincott, Williams, & Wilkins; 2008.

Schnee DM. Pelvic inflammatory disease. *J Pediatr Adolesc Gynecol.* 2009;22(6):387–389.

Straub DM. Sexually transmitted diseases in adolescents. *Adv Pediatr.* 2009;56(1):87–106.

Tarr MR, Gilliam ML. Sexually transmitted infections in adolescent women. *Clin Obstet Gynecol.* 2008;51(2):306–318.

The American College of Obstetricians and Gynecologists, Committee on Adolescent Health Care. Cervical cancer in adolescents: Screening, evaluation, and management. *Obstet Gynecol.* 2010;116(2):469–472.

Tramont EC. *Treponema pallidum* (syphilis). In: Mandell GL, Bennett JE, Dolin R, eds. *Principles and Practice of Infectious Diseases.* 7th ed. New York, NY: Churchill Livingstone; 2010:3035–3054.

CHAPTER 71

Dorit Koren
Adda Grimberg

Short Stature

INTRODUCTION

Linear growth is an integral part of childhood development. Human growth generally occurs in a predictable pattern:

- Rapid growth of intrauterine life—how much the fetus grows is primarily determined by maternal health and nutrition.
- Less rapid growth of infancy—genetic factors gradually come into play and eventually outweigh the intrauterine conditions that initially determined fetal size; in practice, this means that infants often cross growth percentiles (channelize) to a percentile more in line with their genetic potential, whether tall or short. Growth gradually slows such that average rates of growth are 25 cm over first year of life and 10 cm over second year of life.
- Slow, relatively constant rate of growth of early-to-mid childhood: from ages 2 to beginning of puberty: 4 to 6 cm/year.
- Growth acceleration of mid-puberty—also known as the pubertal "growth spurt"—occurs early in puberty in girls (Tanner stages 3 to 4) and later in puberty in boys (Tanner stages 4 to 5). Average peak pubertal growth velocity: 9 cm/year in females and 10.3 cm/year in males. (This difference in growth velocity and, the fact that puberty [and hence, growth plate fusion] occurs later in boys than in girls, underlies the average 13 cm difference between the 50th percentile height for men and women.)
- Cessation of growth with epiphyseal (growth plate) fusion.

Deviations from this pattern may represent a number of different possibilities, including the benign variants of normal growth to abnormal patterns with a wide differential diagnosis ranging from an underlying genetic abnormality, psychosocial or nutritional deprivation, endocrine abnormalities, or systemic illness. Early detection of any such deviations, with diagnosis and treatment of underlying illness (if any), is essential to maximizing potential adult height. Thus, interval growth should be accurately assessed at each child care visit, and any deviations from standard growth patterns should be evaluated. It is crucial to differentiate between normal variants of growth and abnormal patterns—that is, between a healthy petite child and a child with an underlying systemic illness and/or other abnormality of growth.

HINT: The more a child's growth pattern deviates from the usual pattern, the greater the chances of an underlying abnormality.

Definition of Important Terms

- **Short stature:** Because height is a continuous variable, the definition of "short" involves a selected cutoff; a height that is more than 2 standard deviations (SD) below the mean for age and sex is the most commonly accepted threshold. It is important to recall that, given the nature of bell curves and SDs, ~ 2% of the population (including a number of healthy children) will obligatorily be classified as short by definition. Thus, **short stature may or may not be pathological**. It is important to take the child's height and growth velocity in the context of the overall picture, including the variables discussed below.
- **Height/growth velocity:** The annualized rate of linear growth.
- **Growth failure:** A height velocity that is less than expected for a child's age, sex, genetic potential (as determined by parental heights—see below), and stage of puberty; alternately defined as the crossing downward of two or more major height percentiles (beyond 2 years of age) and/or dropping below the third height percentile.

 HINT: Growth failure is by definition pathological.

- **Chronological age:** Age since birth.
- **Bone/skeletal age:** The stage of bone development or maturation as assessed by radiography.

Assessment of Growth
Length/Stature

Measurement of length/stature must be accurate and reproducible in order to correctly assess the degree of interval growth. Children <2 years should be measured supine, children >3 years should be measured standing, and children between ages 2 and 3 years can be measured either way, depending on the child's ability to stand erect for the time it takes to be measured. **Recumbent lengths should be recorded on the length (ages from birth to 36 months) chart and standing heights on the height (ages 2 to 20 years) chart, as they will differ slightly.** Recumbent length is best measured with the child's head against an inflexible board in the Frankfurt plane (wherein the long axis of the trunk is perpendicular to the line formed by connecting the inferior margin of the eyes to the top of the external auditory meatus), legs fully extended, and the feet placed perpendicularly against a movable footboard. To measure height, a stadiometer fixed to the wall is most accurate. The child's feet are placed together in parallel to each other, and the child's heels, buttocks, thoracic spine, and back of head should all be up against the stadiometer's vertical axis. The child should be standing fully erect, heels touching the ground, and the head must be in the Frankfurt plane (see above).

Growth Charts

Evaluation of a child's current height and overall growth pattern occurs within the context of standards typical for the population. Most general pediatric and pediatric endocrine offices use the Centers for Disease Control (CDC) growth charts—percentile curves that illustrate the distribution, in U.S. children, of length or height, weight, head circumference (for ages from birth to 36 months), and body mass index (BMI = weight (kg)/height (m)^2 for ages 2 to 20 years). The data used to construct the 2000 growth curves came from the National Health and Nutrition Examination Survey. The CDC growth curves were derived from cross-sectional population surveys, rather than longitudinal surveys that follow the same children over a course of years to determine their growth rates over time. Therefore, an individual's growth pattern may differ somewhat from the standardized pattern, especially during periods of rapid growth (infancy and the pubertal growth spurt).

In April 2006, the World Health Organization (WHO) released new international growth charts for children aged 0 to 59 months. Similar to the 2000 CDC growth charts, these charts describe weight for age, length (or stature) for age, weight for length (or stature), and body mass index for age, but the methodology for the infant growth charts differed. The growth of infants aged 0 to 24 months was tracked longitudinally, although the growth data on older children (up to 71 months of age) was obtained cross-sectionally; thus, the WHO charts for infants aged 0 to 24 months are in fact true growth standards, describing the linear growth of healthy children under optimal conditions. In September 2010, the CDC recommended that clinicians in the United States use the 2006 WHO growth charts, rather than the 2000 CDC growth charts, for tracking linear growth of children aged 0 to 24 months.

WHO charts are available online at www.who.int/childgrowth/standards/en.

 HINT: Use a growth chart based on the appropriate reference population (ethnicity, age and if applicable, genetic syndrome).

Parental Heights

Because genetics play a large role in determining both the rate of maturation and the eventual adult height, it is important to consider the heights of the biological mother and father in order to place the child's current stature and predicted height in proper context. A significant deviation from the familial growth pattern should raise suspicion of possible pathological processes.

Body Proportions

Several conditions underlying growth abnormalities cause disproportionate growth (e.g., extremities more shortened than trunk in SHOX insufficiency, skeletal dysplasias, and chondrodysplasias). Thus, measurement of the following body proportions can aid the diagnosis of the underlying defect:

- Occipitofrontal head circumference
- Lower body segment: distance from top of pubic symphysis to the floor

- Upper body segment: distance from top of head to top of symphysis pubis
- Arm span: distance between the tips of the middle digits with both arms fully extended

Published standards exist for each of these measurements relative to the child's age.

Skeletal Maturation (Skeletal or Bone Age)

The determination of bone age is predicated on the fact that ossification centers appear and progress in a predictable sequence in most children, so that a radiograph may be compared to a standard. **The bone age, or skeletal age, is the only quantitative determination of somatic maturation; thus, it mirrors the tempo of growth and maturation and gives an indication of the remaining growth potential.** Once the child is beyond infancy, an anteroposterior (AP) radiograph of the left hand and wrist is taken and compared to published standards (Greulich–Pyle or Tanner–Whitehouse method); knee films can be used at ages when hand/wrist films are not yet informative. Factors that impact the rate of skeletal maturation include genetic predisposition, thyroid hormone, growth hormone (GH), insulin-like growth factor (IGF)-1, glucocorticoids, and estrogens (in children of both sexes). Once a bone age is assigned, this value, in combination with the child's present height, is entered into one of several commonly used algorithms (Bayley–Pinneau, Roche–Wainer–Thissen, or Khamis–Roche method) to generate an adult height prediction. However, as demonstrated in a study published in *Pediatrics* in October 2010, a fair amount of variability exists between the predicted heights generated by these various methods. Thus, such predictions may be less reliable than was previously believed to be the case.

 HINT: It is critical to evaluate the child's present height in the greater context of the parents' heights, the historical pattern of linear growth and weight gain, the presence or absence of abnormalities on history or physical examination, and the degree of skeletal maturation. These all help assess whether the growth pattern is pathological or a variant of normal.

 DIFFERENTIAL DIAGNOSIS LIST

Normal Variants

- Familial (genetic) short stature (excluding genetic problems inherited in an autosomal dominant fashion, which can also cause short stature in successive family generations)
- Constitutional delay of growth and puberty

Intrauterine Growth Retardation (IUGR)

Metabolic or Genetic Causes

Bone Disorders

Osteochondrodysplasias: Genetic abnormalities of cartilage and/or bone. Examples:
- Achondroplasia and hypochondroplasia

- Achondrogenesis
- Mesomelic dysplasias
- Epiphyseal and metaphyseal dysplasias
- Osteogenesis imperfecta

Chromosomal Abnormalities:

- Trisomy 21
- Turner syndrome
- Trisomies 8, 13, 18
- 18q deletion

Other Genetic Conditions

- Deletions of *SHOX* gene region of X (or Y) chromosome
- Polymorphism—Chromosome 1q12, 2q36, 6q24, 12q11
- Russell–Silver syndrome
- Prader–Willi syndrome
- Noonan syndrome
- Others: Cornelia de Lange syndrome, insulin receptor gene mutations (leprechaunism, or "Donovan" syndrome), Rubinstein–Taybi syndrome, Aarskog syndrome, Bloom syndrome, Cockayne syndrome, progeria, Seckel syndrome)

Inborn Errors of Metabolism

- Glycogen storage diseases
- Galactosemia
- Mucopolysaccharidoses
- Glycoproteinoses
- Mucolipidoses

Malnutrition

- Protein-calorie (kwashiorkor)
- Generalized (marasmus)
- Anorexia nervosa
- Bulimia nervosa
- Nutritional dwarfing and failure to thrive
- Micronutrient deficiencies (especially iron and zinc)

Psychosocial (Deprivation) Dwarfism
Iatrogenic

- Chronic glucocorticoid exposure (e.g., in severe asthma, inflammatory conditions)
- Stimulant medications for attention deficit and hyperactivity disorder

Chronic Systemic Diseases
Renal Disease

- Fanconi syndrome
- Renal Tubular acidosis
- Uremia/chronic renal failure

Heart Disease

- Congenital (especially cyanotic)
- Congestive heart failure

Malabsorption

- Celiac disease
- Inflammatory bowel disease (IBD)
- Short gut syndrome

Liver Disease

- Chronic liver disease and/or liver failure

Lung Disease

- Cystic fibrosis

Hematologic

- Profound anemia
- Thalassemia (especially if transfusion dependent)
- Hemosiderosis

Oncologic

- Primary malignancy
- Secondary to chemotherapy
- Secondary to irradiation

Collagen Vascular Diseases
Infectious

- Acquired immunodeficiency syndrome (AIDS) or human

immunodeficiency virus (HIV) infection (untreated)

- Tuberculosis
- Intestinal parasites

Endocrine Disorders

- Diabetes mellitus (DM) (Mauriac syndrome)
- Glucocorticoid excess (Cushing syndrome)
- Hypothyroidism
- Growth hormone deficiency (GHD)
- Primary IGF deficiency
  - GH insensitivity (Laron Dwarfism)
  - Post-GH receptor defects
- Pseudohypoparathyroidism
- Rickets
- Pituitary and/or hypothalamic dysfunction:
  - Structural abnormalities:
    - Associated with other midline defects (e.g., holoprosencephaly, septo-optic dysplasia)
    - Isolated hypothalamic/ pituitary malformation/s (e.g., empty sella syndrome, ectopic neurohypophysis)
  - Trauma—generalized brain trauma or trauma specific to hypothalamus, pituitary stalk, or anterior pituitary
- Surgical resection of pituitary and/or pituitary stalk
- Inflammation of pituitary and/or hypothalamus
- Brain and/or hypothalamic tumors (e.g., germinomas, gliomas)
- Pituitary tumors (e.g., cranio-pharyngiomas, histiocytosis X)
- Irradiation of brain and/or hypothalamus
- Genetic causes:
  - Idiopathic GHD
  - Growth hormone releasing hormone (GHRH) receptor mutation
  - Isolated: *GH1 and GH2* mutations, *CSHP1* mutation, *CSH1 and CSH2* mutations, idiopathic
  - GH secretagogue receptor mutation
  - Multiple pituitary hormone deficiencies: *HESX1* mutation, *PROP1* mutation, *POU1F1* mutation

DIFFERENTIAL DIAGNOSIS DISCUSSION

A comprehensive discussion of all the causes of short stature is beyond the scope of this chapter. The following is a focused review of a select number of normal variants and abnormal causes of short stature (see section on "Differential Diagnosis List").

Familial Short Stature

Familial short stature (FSS) is a height that, while representing the lower end of the population norm, is nonetheless in keeping with the child's genetic potential. **This is usually a normal variant.** However, some causes of abnormal short stature such as GH gene deletions can be inherited in a dominant fashion, so even if there is a family history of short stature, taking a careful history, including heights and pubertal timing of parents, siblings and extended family members, and performing a focused physical examination remain important.

Clinical Features

Both parents' heights are usually in the lower height percentiles, often below the 10th. The child's pattern of growth is **consistent** with that of his/her parents (and often siblings, too). The child's growth velocity is usually normal, so that the growth curve is low, but parallel to the normal lines. The predicted adult height is in keeping with midparental target height. In the absence of a family history of delayed puberty, the timing of puberty is usually average.

Evaluation

The past medical history, review of systems, and physical examination are typically unremarkable, with no abnormalities of body proportions in either the patient or the parents. As skeletal growth is not delayed, the bone age should be within the normal range. Laboratory workup, including growth factors and a chemistry panel, should be within the normal range. Abnormalities of history, physical examination, or laboratory studies should prompt the investigator to look for other causes of short stature.

Treatment

The child and family should be reassured that **this is not a disease,** that the child will likely enter puberty within the same average time frame as his or her peers, and that the child's height will likely be in keeping with the family trend. **As this is not a disease, treatment is not indicated.**

Constitutional Growth Delay

(Also known as constitutional delay of growth and puberty or constitutional delay of growth and maturation)

Delayed puberty is defined as the absence of secondary sexual characteristics by an age that is delayed by more than 2 to 2.5 S.D. beyond the mean for the population: the absence of thelarche in girls over 12 years of age, of signs of puberty in boys over 13 years of age, or of menarche in girls over 16 years of age (primary amenorrhea). Constitutional delay of growth and puberty (CDGP) represents the late end of the spectrum of pubertal development. Children with CDGP enter puberty later than most of their peers. Thus, the pubertal growth spurt is also delayed, and these children continue to grow at the prepubertal rate of 4 to 6 cm/year while their peers' height velocity increases, resulting in a gap between the heights of children with CDGP and the heights of age-matched peers—**a transient relative short stature**.

Clinical Features

These children usually have a normal birth length, begin to cross height percentiles early in life, and settle in the lower percentiles by the age of 2 years. Between the ages of 2 years and the onset of puberty in their peers, the children's height velocity usually places them along the lower margins of the growth curve (around or sometimes below the 5th to 10th percentile). Then, as their peers begin the pubertal growth spurt and the growth curve slope increases, the children with CDGP commonly fall further below the fifth percentile. They enter puberty spontaneously at a later-than-usual age and eventually attain an adult height within the normal range, although this height can fall short of the predicted adult height. There is often a family history of maternal and/or paternal relatives with similarly delayed puberty. CDGP can sometimes occur together with FSS, leading to pronounced short stature.

Evaluation

History, review of systems, and physical examination are usually normal except for short stature and the delayed pubertal status relative to age norms. **Taking a detailed history and thoroughly reviewing the child's growth curve are essential steps to establishing this diagnosis;** an isolated point on the growth curve at the time of the visit is insufficient. The differential diagnosis for CDGP includes Kallman syndrome and partial gonadotropin deficiency; lack of anosmia can exclude the former, but only time can help distinguish between CDGP and the latter. **Bone age is significantly delayed, enough so that the predicted adult height should be normal.** Any abnormalities on physical examination or laboratory workup should suggest another diagnosis.

Treatment

After a thorough evaluation has excluded other causes of delayed puberty/abnormal growth, it is reasonable to reassure the child and family and monitor growth expectantly, given that spontaneous entry into puberty and attainment of a typical adult height are anticipated. However, because delayed puberty and consequent short stature in adolescence can have a significant psychosocial impact, it is also reasonable to offer a short course of low-dose androgens (for boys) or estrogen (for girls) to jump-start puberty. Low-dose, short-term courses are used to avoid acceleration of skeletal maturation and thus impairment of adult height from decreased time to grow. **This intervention only causes the child to enter puberty earlier—it does not increase the adult height.** There are no data indicating that GH therapy increases adult height in patients with CDGP.

HINT: FSS versus CDGP:
- FSS: Average timing of puberty, low predicted adult height, normal bone age.
- CDGP: Delayed timing of puberty, predicted adult height in the normal range, delayed bone age.
- Sometimes the two can occur simultaneously.

Intrauterine Growth Retardation/Small for Gestational Age

IUGR has been defined as birth weight and/or length >2 SD below the mean for gestational age. Small for gestational age (SGA) has been defined as birth weight <2,500 g at a gestational age of 37 weeks or above or length below the third percentile for gestational age. Affected infants are a diverse group, as there are a variety of maternal, placental, environmental, and intrinsic fetal causes that can lead to IUGR/SGA, including:

- Maternal causes: malnutrition, hypertension or pre-eclampsia, uterine malformations
- Placental abnormalities: two-vessel cord, vascular insufficiency or infarction, abnormal implantation
- Genetic disorders: Russell–Silver syndrome, Cornelia de Lange syndrome, others
- Congenital infections: rubella, varicella

- Intrauterine exposure to medications, drugs, or toxins: amphetamines, cocaine, nicotine, alcohol, propranolol, methotrexate
- IGF deficiency or resistance

Clinical Features

Most infants experience sufficient catch-up growth (i.e., an accelerated rate of weight gain and linear growth above the upper statistical limit for the child's age following a period of growth failure) in the first few years of life to place them on the normal height curve. However, a subset (10% to 25% in various studies) does not and remains below the fifth percentile throughout life. Children with IUGR who experience catch-up growth and, more importantly, accelerated weight gain are at higher risk of childhood obesity than children who were appropriate for gestational age at birth. Children whose IUGR is due to a genetic abnormality (such as Russell–Silver syndrome) continue to have poor postnatal growth, a condition that has been termed "primordial dwarfism."

Evaluation

The evaluation of a child with IUGR should begin with a careful history and physical examination. If the history or physical examination findings are suggestive of an intrinsic abnormality, the appropriate evaluation should be obtained (e.g., chromosomal analysis and/or referral to a geneticist to evaluate for a possible syndrome). If the limbs are disproportionate, skeletal radiographs should be obtained.

Treatment

GH was shown to improve final height prognosis in two large multicenter studies of short children who were born SGA and to improve adult height in another recent study of prepubertal children who were born SGA. Yet another study of GH administration, this one in young children (ages 2 to 5 years) who were born SGA with continuing short stature, showed a significant increase in growth velocity in response to GH therapy without significant acceleration of bone age or side effects. Some caution in the interpretation of studies of GH in SGA children is indicated, however, for the following reasons:

- The group of SGA children is quite heterogeneous; there are a number of causes of SGA, and not all respond equally well to GH.
- Since GH is one of the counterregulatory hormones, GH therapy can increase insulin resistance—a particular concern in children born SGA, who have been shown to be at greater risk for developing obesity and insulin resistance later in childhood than children born appropriate for gestational age.

Each individual child should be carefully evaluated to see whether he or she is a candidate for GH therapy, and the risks and benefits should be clearly explained to the family.

Osteochondrodysplasias

The osteochondrodysplasias are a diverse group of disorders whose common denominator is genetic abnormalities of cartilage and/or bone.

Clinical Features

Over 100 different conditions falling under this heading have been identified, each defined by specific skeletal and nonskeletal abnormalities and by radiographic features. The three broad groups are as follows:

- Defects of tubular and flat bones and/or axial skeleton (e.g., achondroplasia)
- Disorganized development of cartilaginous and fibrous components of the skeleton
- Idiopathic osteolyses

Nearly all children with a skeletal dysplasia grow slowly. If not, their growth is usually *disproportionate*—the **ratio of upper-to-lower (U:L) body segment growth is abnormal,** resulting in short limbs and/or trunks, and disproportionate rates of growth between limb segments (rhizomelic, mesomelic, or acromelic) are also frequently seen.

Evaluation

A careful family history should be obtained, as the osteochondrodysplasias are hereditary (e.g., classical achondroplasia is an autosomal dominant disorder). However, many cases represent *de novo* mutations, so the absence of a family history does not rule out the possibility. A careful measurement of body proportions should be taken. Clinical and radiographical evaluation can determine what is primarily involved: long bones, vertebrae, and/or skull; and epiphyses, metaphyses, or diaphyses.

Treatment

GH therapy has been studied in several skeletal dysplasias. A few studies of GH in children with achondroplasia and hypochondroplasia showed an increase in height velocity (from 3.8 to 6.6 cm/year in one study in the first year, with a slight slowing of height velocity in subsequent years). A worsening of the disproportion between limb and trunk lengths in response to GH therapy was inconsistently seen.

Turner Syndrome

Turner syndrome, a disorder in females associated with the partial or complete absence of one X chromosome, is a relatively common condition, with a prevalence of 50/100,000 liveborn girls based on widespread genetic screening or 32/100,000 liveborn girls based upon clinical postnatal diagnosis. This discrepancy suggests the possibility of mild or even normal phenotype in girls with Turner syndrome. Short stature is the most common phenotypic manifestation of Turner syndrome in children and adults. The *SHOX* (short stature, homeobox-containing) gene encodes a transcription factor that is expressed in the growth plate and helps regulate chondrocyte differentiation and proliferation. The *SHOX* gene is located in the pseudoautosomal region (PAR) 1 on the distal end of the X and Y chromosomes (Xp22.3 and Yp11.3). Genes in the pseudoautosomal regions do not undergo X inactivation, so healthy 46,XX and 46,XY individuals express two copies of these genes. Patients with Turner syndrome are missing part or all of the second X chromosome, and (in most cases) thus have only 1 functional copy of the

SHOX gene, a condition termed "*SHOX* haploinsufficiency." This haploinsufficiency appears to underlie the 20-cm average difference in height between women with Turner syndrome and other women of the same ethnic group.

Clinical Features

Turner syndrome may be recognized in infancy due to characteristic webbed neck (formed following the resolution of cystic hygromas) and/or lymphedema of the extremities. Beyond infancy, the two most common features are short stature and sexual infantilism. Aside from short stature, other skeletal abnormalities may be seen, including relatively large hands and feet, a wide body, a short neck, cubitus valgus, genu valgum, and shortened fourth metacarpals. Madelung's deformity of the wrist (bilateral bowing of the radius with a dorsal subluxation of the distal ulna) is occasionally seen. Girls with Turner syndrome are at higher risk for developmental dysplasia of the hip in infancy and scoliosis during later childhood.

Other physical examination findings may include: ptosis, strabismus, low-set or deformed ears, micrognathia, high-arched palate, dental abnormalities, low posterior hairline, shield chest, and hypoplastic areolae. Girls with Turner syndrome are at risk for a number of associated abnormalities of multiple organ systems (Table 71-1).

Evaluation

A careful physical examination may reveal some phenotypic features of Turner syndrome. However, not all girls with Turner syndrome will manifest the classic

---

TABLE 71-1	**Complications of Turner Syndrome**

- Cardiac (seen in ~1/3 of all patients with Turner syndrome)
  - Coarctation of the aorta (~10%)
  - Bicuspid aortic valve (increased incidence of this in patients with residual neck webbing at birth)
  - Aortic stenosis
  - Partial anomalous pulmonary venous connection
  - Conduction and repolarization anomalies (e.g., prolonged QT)
  - **Increased risk of developing progressive aortic root dilatation and, eventually, a dissecting aortic aneurysm**—careful monitoring throughout life is warranted
- Renal and urinary tract
  - Duplicated or cleft renal pelvis
  - Horseshoe kidney
  - Abnormal renal position or alignment
  - **Increased risk of recurrent urinary tract infections**
- Reproductive tract
  - Underdeveloped uterus, oviducts
  - Streak gonads

Although most women with Turner syndrome are infertile, up to 10% of women with Turner syndrome will undergo some spontaneous pubertal development, and 2–5% will be able to become spontaneously pregnant.

- Sensorineural hearing loss
- Conductive hearing loss from recurrent otitis media during early childhood
- Autoimmune diseases: Thyroiditis, celiac disease, Crohn disease

phenotype, so the diagnosis should be considered in any female with unexplained short stature, and a standard karyotype should be sent (chromosomal analysis of 30 peripheral lymphocytes) to evaluate for possible mosaicism. Given the number of possible associated systemic problems, a comprehensive evaluation should be performed, including but not limited to:

- Echocardiogram at diagnosis to evaluate for cardiac anomalies; monitoring cardiac magnetic resonance imaging (MRI) throughout life, to look for abnormalities of the aortic arch and descending aorta. (Turner syndrome is associated with a higher mortality risk due to aortic dissection.)
- Renal and pelvic ultrasound to evaluate the kidneys and pelvocaliceal collecting system as well as the reproductive tract.
- Auditory evaluation at diagnosis and every 1 to 5 years thereafter to look for possible sensorineural hearing loss.

Treatment

GH therapy is standard of care in pediatrics to increase adult height in patients with Turner syndrome. **It is recommended that GH therapy be initiated as soon as growth failure is detected.** If pubertal development does not begin spontaneously, exogenous estrogen therapy should be initiated with the goal of reflecting as much as possible the process of normal puberty. If GH treatment is started young enough, sufficient growth is attained during the prepubertal years such that estrogen therapy need not be delayed.

Abnormalities of the GH/IGF Axis
Background

Human GH is produced in and secreted by the somatotrophs of the anterior pituitary. Its secretion is regulated by GHRH and somatostatin, which respectively stimulate and inhibit its release. Another hormone which may be involved in the regulation of GH release is ghrelin, a GH secretagogue produced in the stomach (primarily) and in the hypothalamus. Synthetic ghrelin analog administration causes an immediate and massive GH release; however, it is less clear what the physiologic role in regulating GH release may be. IGF-1 and free fatty acids inhibit GH secretion at the level of the pituitary and hypothalamus.

Many, though not all, of GH's actions are mediated through the IGF peptides, in accordance with the somatomedin hypothesis. IGF-1 (aka somatomedin-C), the primary IGF in humans, circulates in the bloodstream bound to IGF-binding proteins (especially IGFBP-3). IGF-1 then binds to IGF receptors, leading to activation of second messenger systems and multiple downstream effects, including insulin-like activity in extra-skeletal tissue, promotion of incorporation of sulfate into cartilage, and stimulation of DNA synthesis. Other players in the growth system include insulin and IGF-2, which along with IGF-1 are the main mediators of fetal growth; androgens and estrogens, which induce the pubertal growth spurt and (estrogens only—in both sexes) epiphyseal fusion; and thyroid hormone, which has a permissive effect on GH secretion and exerts direct action on the growth plates.

GH Deficiency and Related Conditions

Dysfunction may appear at a number of levels of the GH/IGF axis, including the following:

1. Hypothalamic and higher centers
   - Congenital hypothalamic malformations
   - GHRH receptor mutations
   - Trauma or inflammation of the brain and/or hypothalamus
   - Central nervous system and/or hypothalamic tumors
   - Irradiation of brain and/or hypothalamus; chemotherapy
   - GH neurosecretory dysfunction
2. Pituitary
   - Absence of pituitary (empty sella syndrome) or other structural defects
   - Pituitary tumors (e.g., craniopharyngioma)
   - Hypophysitis
   - Genetic abnormalities of GH production or secretion (e.g., *PROP1 or POU1F1* mutations, production of a bioinactive GH)
   - Pituitary trauma
   - Idiopathic GHD
3. GH Insensitivity (Laron syndrome): due to GH receptor defect—high GH levels, but low IGF-1 levels and, often, low GHBP levels
4. Postreceptor signaling defects (primary IGF-1 deficiency): e.g., mutations in STAT5b

A study of U.S. children with short stature found an incidence of GHD of 1/3,500 children.

Factors that should raise suspicion for GHD include the following:

- (Infants): a history of prolonged jaundice, hypoglycemia, microphallus, or traumatic delivery
- Craniofacial midline abnormalities (e.g., septo-optic dysplasia, holoprosencephaly, central maxillary incisor)
- Consanguinity or family history of similar presentations
- History of a suprasellar tumor (e.g., craniopharyngioma)
- History of cranial irradiation, head trauma or central nervous system infection/infarction

Clinical Features

Since insulin plays a major role in intrauterine growth, infants with congenital isolated GHD tend to have normal length and weight at birth. They may have a history of prolonged neonatal jaundice, microphallus, or hypoglycemia. Postnatal growth is overtly abnormal; in severe cases, growth failure is seen within the first months, and in less severe cases, poor linear growth manifests later. Other features of congenital GHD overlap with those of acquired GHD, and include the following:

- Relatively normal skeletal proportions that correlate better with bone age than with chronological age
- Increased adiposity (especially truncal) with poor lean body mass gain

- Growth deceleration and/or growth failure
- Standing height significantly below normal for the population and parental target height
- Delayed dentition
- Delayed average age of pubertal onset
- Depressed midfacial development, prominent forehead

Diagnosis of GHD

A child suspected of having GHD should be referred to a pediatric endocrinologist for diagnostic evaluation. Due to the circadian rhythm of GH secretion, there is no one single test that can definitively diagnose GHD, so the workup involves a combination of different studies, including growth factors and provocative GH testing. Once the diagnosis of GHD has been established, **the child's ability to secrete other pituitary hormones must be evaluated (i.e., thyroid, adrenal, and, if age-appropriate, gonadal function); there is an increased risk of mortality in patients with GHD due to underrecognized and undertreated central adrenal insufficiency (CRI).** Brain MRI with and without contrast, with special cuts of the pituitary and hypothalamus (which must be specifically requested), should be performed to evaluate for an intracranial tumor or structural abnormality as cause of the GHD.

Recombinant Human GH and IGF-1 Treatment

GH and IGF-1 replacement therapy should be managed by pediatric endocrinologists. Doses and preparations vary. Recombinant human GH (rhGH) is administered as a nightly subcutaneous injection. Those who care for patients on rhGH or rhIGF-1 therapy should be aware of the potential side effects (see Table 71-2 for more details).

Current Non-GHD Indications Approved by the FDA for GH Therapy

- Chronic renal insufficiency
- Turner syndrome
- AIDS wasting syndrome
- Prader–Willi syndrome

TABLE 71-2	Possible Side Effects of rhGH and rhIGF-1 Therapy

Possible Adverse Effects of rhGH Therapy
- Pseudotumor cerebri (increased intracranial pressure)
- Slipped capital femoral epiphysis
- Increased insulin resistance
- Increased size and number of nevi (but no increased risk of malignancy)
- Transient gynecomastia
- Increased severity of scoliosis

Possible Adverse Effects of rhIGF-1 Therapy
- Adenoidal hypertrophy
- Hypoglycemia

Malignancy: current evidence supports a permissive role, but not a causal role, for both GH and IGF-I in cancer development

- SGA/IUGR
- Idiopathic short stature
- *SHOX* haploinsufficiency
- Noonan syndrome

Chronic Systemic Illness

Many chronic illnesses are associated with short stature. The general mechanisms by which chronic illnesses lead to poor growth include:

- Anorexia/poor appetite/poor intake
- Malabsorption of nutrients
- Chronic acidosis
- Anemia
- Chronic hypoxemia
- Increased energy requirements
- Medical therapy for the condition (e.g., glucocorticoids)

   Some general categories of chronic illnesses associated with poor growth:

- Malabsorptive disorders: inadequate calorie or protein absorption leading to growth failure. In other words, dropping height and/or weight percentiles, even with a normal history, review of systems, and physical examination, can be the first sign of a serious systemic illness, for example, celiac disease, IBD, and cystic fibrosis.

> **HINT:** Abnormal growth can predate other disease manifestations.

- Chronic Renal Insufficiency (CRI): Metabolic acidosis, loss of electrolytes essential to growth, protein-wasting, decreased caloric intake, chronic anemia, deficiency of 1,25-dihydroxy vitamin D3, and cardiac dysfunction can all play a role in the growth failure associated with CRI. Examples: Fanconi syndrome and renal tubular acidosis. GH has been demonstrated to accelerate growth in children with chronic renal failure prior to renal transplantation, which is an FDA-approved indication for GH therapy.
- Cardiovascular disease: Congestive heart failure and cyanotic heart diseases can both be associated with growth failure, due to a combination of increased energy demands and chronic hypoxemia. Sometimes they occur in the context of dysmorphic syndromes.
- Pulmonary disease: Chronic hypoxemia is associated with poor growth. The classical example is cystic fibrosis. Severe asthma can also be associated with growth failure; however, the chronic systemic glucocorticoids these children require also play a role in the growth failure.
- Chronic anemias: Can contribute to poor growth for a number of reasons:
  - Poor oxygen delivery to tissues
  - Increased cardiac work to maintain cardiac output

- Higher energy needs due to increased hematopoiesis
- In transfusion-dependent conditions such as thalassemias or severe sickle cell disease: The metabolic consequences of iron overload from chronic transfusion
- Chronic inflammation and infection: Poor growth in these conditions may be mediated in part by the inflammatory mediators; for example, IL-6 has been shown to mediate a decrease in serum IGF-1 levels. Examples: AIDS and tuberculosis (the two top chronic illnesses causing growth failure worldwide), intestinal parasites (e.g., hookworms). Growth failure can be the initial presentation of HIV infection in children.
- DM: Chronically poorly controlled DM can lead to growth failure in association with hepatomegaly due to excessive glycogen deposition. This condition is termed Mauriac syndrome. Insulin inhibits the transcription of IGF-binding protein-1 (IGFBP-1) in the liver. In the setting of insulin deficiency, IGFBP-1 synthesis increases, decreasing the bioavailability of serum IGF-1.
- Inborn errors of lipid, protein, or carbohydrate metabolism.

Clinical Features
In many children with short stature caused by chronic illness, the weight tends to be depressed to a greater extent than the height, or there is a lag between the onset of weight deceleration and subsequent height deceleration. Bone age is usually delayed and approximates the height age.

Evaluation
A careful history and examination of the growth curve are important. The typical pattern is a period of normal growth followed by growth deceleration or even cessation, suggesting the onset of illness. Past medical history may reveal a previously diagnosed chronic illness, and review of systems may reveal features suggestive of certain illnesses (e.g., hematochezia and chronic abdominal pain in IBD). However, it is important to remember that growth failure can be the presenting sign of a chronic illness such as celiac disease or IBD; thus, even in the absence of concerning findings in the medical history or physical examination, the clinician should always consider and evaluate for chronic illnesses in children presenting for short stature evaluation.

Laboratory studies that screen for chronic illness include complete blood cell count with differential, erythrocyte sedimentation rate, C-reactive protein, serum biochemistry profile (including creatinine and hepatic enzymes), serum albumin level, celiac autoimmunity, and urinalysis. These preliminary screens may suggest the pathway for future diagnostic tests or procedures, such as endoscopy, small bowel biopsy, or renal biopsy.

Treatment
Once the underlying condition is treated, catch-up growth often occurs. If the underlying disease is treated late or incompletely, a permanent height deficit may ensue.

Poor Nutrition
Optimal linear growth requires optimal nutrition. Globally, malnutrition is the most common cause of poor growth. Malnutrition affects the GH/IGF system.

Total calorie and/or protein–calorie malnutrition cause decreased hepatic production of IGF-1. The lower IGF-1 levels provide decreased IGF-1-mediated negative feedback to the hypothalamus and pituitary, which can lead to increased GH production and secretion, and thus higher than normal basal and stimulated serum GH levels.

Causes of malnutrition include social/societal (e.g., poverty, child neglect, societal upheaval), psychological (e.g., anorexia nervosa), self-imposed severe dietary restrictions (e.g., fear of hypercholesterolemia), chronic illness, malformations of the oropharynx (e.g., Pierre Robin sequence, cleft lip, or palate), abnormal oral-motor function (e.g., pervasive developmental delay or severe cerebral palsy), or certain medications (e.g., stimulants for treatment of attention deficit hyperactivity disorder or chemotherapeutic agents). Isolated nutrient deficiencies, such as zinc, iron, and vitamin D (deficiency of which leads to rickets), can also cause short stature.

Clinical Features
Poor weight gain generally precedes the decrease and eventual failure of linear growth. The bone age is often delayed. With more advanced cases of malnutrition, signs of wasting may be seen on examination. Pubertal delay may be seen.

Evaluation
Taking a detailed dietary history is essential to establishing this diagnosis. A 3-day diet log is a useful tool. Everything the child eats and drinks should be quantified and recorded. This record can be analyzed for intake of total calories, macronutrients, and micronutrients (i.e., vitamins and minerals, including vitamin D, calcium, iron, and zinc). Parental dietary recall is not sufficient, as it is often inaccurate, although a 24-hour diet recall may shed some light during an initial clinic visit. Physical examination should look for the above-mentioned pubertal delay, evidence of malnutrition, and signs of systemic illness. Laboratory evaluations should include all those involved in the evaluation for chronic illness (see previous section.)

Treatment
The treatment is **nutritional restitution**. Children unable to consume sufficient calories by mouth can be fed either enterally (via nasogastric or gastrostomy tube) or parenterally (partial or total parenteral nutrition). Chronically malnourished children provided with sufficient calories can experience catch-up growth.

 HINT: The treatment of poor growth due to inadequate nutrition is assuring adequate caloric intake. GH is NOT helpful in treating undergrowth due to undernutrition.

Hypothyroidism
Growth failure is one of the most common and significant aspects of congenital and acquired hypothyroidism in children. Because of the significant cognitive consequences of hypothyroidism in the first 3 years of life, newborn screening

programs have been implemented to allow early diagnosis and treatment before any phenotypic manifestation. Thus, growth failure associated with hypothyroidism generally occurs now in the context of acquired hypothyroidism, which is most commonly due to autoimmune Hashimoto (chronic lymphocytic) thyroiditis or iodine deficiency. Growth retardation due to acquired hypothyroidism can take several years to clearly manifest, though once clinically significant, it tends to be severe and progressive.

Clinical Features
Children with undiagnosed or untreated congenital hypothyroidism experience profound growth failure, delayed fontanelle closure in infancy, and mental retardation (cretinism). Fortunately, most of these children are diagnosed by newborn screening and adequately treated, so this condition is now uncommon. Children with acquired hypothyroidism over time experience poor linear growth in the setting of increased weight gain. They have immature body proportions, with an increased upper to lower (U:L) body segment ratio, delayed dentition, and a profoundly delayed bone age. Puberty is often delayed, but precocious puberty can be seen as well.

Evaluation
Primary hypothyroidism is diagnosed by an elevated thyroid stimulating hormone level; total thyroxine (T4) level is normal in compensated hypothyroidism and low in uncompensated hypothyroidism. Autoimmune thyroiditis is confirmed by the presence of antithyroglobulin and/or antithyroid peroxidase antibodies. Secondary and tertiary hypothyroidism (of pituitary and hypothalamic etiologies, respectively) most often occurs with other pituitary hormone deficiencies and is best screened for with a free T4 level.

Treatment
The treatment of hypothyroidism is daily replacement with levothyroxine. Thyroid hormone replacement is associated with rapid catch-up growth.

EVALUATION OF SHORT STATURE
Patient History
A careful history can uncover risk factors for short stature and signs or symptoms of underlying conditions or illnesses.

1. Pregnancy history—specific points of inquiry:
   - Exposure to medications, drugs (e.g., alcohol, tobacco), or toxins
   - Maternal illnesses or pregnancy complications, especially infections or hypertension
   - History of any perinatal complications (e.g., traumatic delivery, perinatal asphyxia)
   - Birth weight and length (to see whether child was born SGA)
2. Growth curve
   - Annualized growth velocity, and any changes therein
   - Changes in height percentile

3. Dietary history
4. Past medical history
   - History of chronic/systemic illnesses or frequent hospitalizations (e.g., cystic fibrosis, IBD, or anemias requiring transfusion)
   - Medication history (e.g., history of systemic glucocorticoid therapy)
   - History of pediatric cancer and its treatment
5. Review of systems
   - Symptoms suggestive of underlying illness (e.g., chronic diarrhea or abdominal pain, headache or visual disturbances, shortness of breath or lower extremity swelling, etc.)
   - Behavior problems or changes in school performance
   - Timing of pubertal onset and progression, if relevant (look for pubertal delay)
6. Family history:
   - Document heights of parents and other relatives (siblings, grandparents, aunts, and uncles)
   - Determine whether anyone in the family had a pattern of late growth and/or delayed puberty
   - Calculate midparental height
   - Girls: (mother's height in cm + father's height in cm − 13)/2
   - Boys: (mother's height in cm + 13 + father's height in cm)/2
7. Social history: any suspicion of abuse or of a neglectful environment

Physical Eamination
- Measure and plot current and prior height and weight accurately; calculate height-to-weight ratio in younger children and BMI in older children to see whether height or weight are disproportionately affected.
- General physical examination—look for signs of underlying genetic abnormalities (e.g., dysmorphic features), midline defects suggestive of possible hypothalamic or pituitary malformations (e.g., central maxillary incisor), or of systemic illness (e.g., aphthous ulcers, truncal adiposity, rachitic rosary).
- Dental examination—dental maturation correlates well with skeletal maturation, so delayed dentition can be a clue to delayed bone age.
- Tanner staging—look for pubertal delay (e.g., CDGP, Turner syndrome).
- Upper body segment to lower body segment ratio (normal ratio: 1.7 at birth, 1.3 at 3 years of age, and 1.0 at 7 years of age).
  - Abnormal ratio—possible rickets or skeletal dysplasia.
- Arm span—less than the height before age 8 years, equal to the height at ages 8 to 12 years, and greater than the height above age 12 years.
- Examine for scoliosis.

Laboratory Studies
- Complete blood count with differential—look for anemia or other abnormalities
- Erythrocyte sedimentation rate and C-reactive protein—elevated in inflammatory conditions

- Serum electrolytes, blood urea nitrogen and creatinine levels, calcium, phosphate, and alkaline phosphatase levels—screen for renal dysfunction and calcium homeostasis
- Total protein, albumin, prealbumin, and transaminase levels in evaluation of potential synthetic defects, inflammation/injury, and cholestasis
- Tissue transglutaminase and antiendomyseal IgA to exclude celiac disease
- Thyroid stimulating hormone and total T4 levels
- IGF-1 and IGFBP-3 levels—screen for GHD and malnutrition
- Urinalysis
- Karyotype for females to evaluate for Turner syndrome

Depending on the clinical diagnosis, other studies may be indicated, such as 25-hydroxy-vitamin D level to evaluate for vitamin D-deficiency rickets, sweat chloride analysis to exclude cystic fibrosis, tine testing or PPD to screen for tuberculosis, HIV testing, or screening for *SHOX* gene deletion or mutation.

Imaging Studies
- Bone age determination
  - AP left hand and wrist radiograph
  - AP and lateral knee radiographs, in children under the age of 2 years
- Skeletal survey, if indicated (suspected skeletal dysplasia)
- MRI of brain with pituitary cuts, if indicated (e.g., if neurological symptoms or hypopituitarism)

PSYCHOSOCIAL RAMIFICATIONS OF SHORT STATURE

Many patient families seek evaluation and treatment of short stature to avoid the discrimination against shorter individuals, a phenomenon termed heightism. Although there is general agreement that short stature is associated with psychosocial stressors, whether they significantly impact the psychosocial function of the short individual remains controversial. The results of studies of the social function of children with short stature vary depending on the study population; children from a sample referred for medical evaluation of short stature are more likely to demonstrate problems than a population-based sample. The psychosocial, anthropological, historical, and biological aspects of short stature are comprehensively reviewed in the book by Stephen Hall (see section on "Suggested Readings"). Social pressures for tallness seem to affect males more than females in U.S. society. This has led to a referral bias for short stature evaluations. However, because growth failure can be the only presenting sign of an underlying health problem, the evaluation of short stature should be given equal attention for both girls and boys. The primary job of the evaluating physician is to distinguish healthy variants from pathological growth.

APPROACH TO THE PATIENT WITH SHORT STATURE

Short stature is a relatively common complaint in the pediatric patient and is one of the most common reasons for referral to a pediatric endocrinologist. A careful history, including family history, can uncover the cause in many cases. The growth curve must be evaluated to determine patterns of growth and whether height and weight are affected equally. Other key components of the evaluation include a detailed dietary history to evaluate for malnutrition, a thorough physical examination (including evaluation of dentition, pubertal status, and body proportions), laboratory studies, and bone age radiographs. Children with growth failure who fall into certain categories (e.g., Turner syndrome, chronic renal failure, and GHD) qualify for rhGH therapy and should be referred to pediatric endocrinologists to initiate the process. Clinicians should be aware of the possible adverse effects of rhGH therapy (including pseudotumor cerebri, slipped capital femoral epiphyses, increased insulin resistance, and scoliosis) and screen for those possibilities in patients receiving rhGH who develop worrisome symptoms.

Suggested Readings

Bondy CA. Care of girls and women with Turner syndrome: a guideline of the Turner Syndrome Study Group. *J Clin Endocrinol Metab.* 2007;92(1):10–25.

CDC Growth Charts, United States. www.cdc.gov/growthcharts. Accessed December 5, 2011.

Clayton PE. Management of the child born small for gestational age through to adulthood: a consensus statement of the International Societies of Pediatric Endocrinology and the Growth Hormone Research Society. *J Clin Endocrinol Metab.* 2007; 92(3):804–810.

Greulich WW, Pyle SI. *Radiographic Atlas of Skeletal Development of the Hand and Wrist.* Stanford: Stanford University Press; 1959.

Grimberg A, Kutikov JK, Cucchiara AJ. Sex differences in patients referred for evaluation of poor growth. *J Pediatr.* 2005;146:212–216.

Grummer-Strawn LM, Reinold C, Krebs NF; Centers for Disease Control and Prevention (CDC). Use of World Health Organization and CDC growth charts for children aged 0–59 months in the United States. *MMWR Recomm Rep.* 2010;59(RR-9):1–15. Erratum in: *MMWR Recomm Rep.* 2010;59(36):1184.

Hall SS. *Size Matters: How Height Affects the Health, Happiness, and Success of Boys—and the Men They Become.* Boston: Houghton Mifflin; 2006.

Nathan BM, Palmert MR. Regulation and disorders of pubertal timing. *Endocrinol Metab Clin N Am.* 2005;34(3):617–641, ix.

Seminara S, Rapisardi G, La Cauza F, et al. Catch-up growth in short-at-birth NICU graduates. *Horm. Res.* 2000;53:139–143.

Tanner JM, Goldstein H, Whitehouse RH. Standards for children's height at ages 2–9 years allowing for height of parents. *Arch Dis Child.* 1970; 45:755–762.

Topor LS, Feldman HA, Bauchner H et al. Variation in methods of predicting adult height for children with idiopathic short stature. *Pediatrics.* 2010;126:938–944.

WHO Infant (0–24 month) Growth Charts. www.who.int/childgrowth/standards/en. Accessed December 5, 2011.

Wilson TA, Rose SR, Cohen P, et al. Update of guidelines for the use of growth hormone in children: the Lawson Wilkins Pediatric Endocrine Society Drug and Therapeutics Committee. *J Pediatr.* 2003; 143:415–421.

Sore Throat

INTRODUCTION

Sore throat is one of the most common reasons children are brought to medical attention. Most often, this complaint is part of an upper respiratory tract infection. Because children experience an average of five to seven upper respiratory tract infections per year, health care providers must be familiar with the evaluation and treatment of sore throat. In addition, misdiagnosis or inadequate treatment of a sore throat caused by certain bacterial pathogens can result in serious complications.

 DIFFERENTIAL DIAGNOSIS LIST

Infectious Causes

- Nasopharyngitis
- Pharyngitis
- Peritonsillar abscess or cellulitis
- Retropharyngeal abscess or cellulitis
- Parapharyngeal abscess
- Tonsillitis
- Laryngitis
- Uvulitis
- Epiglottitis
- Lemierre syndrome
- Laryngotracheobronchitis (croup)
- Herpangina
- Herpetic gingivostomatitis
- Hand-foot-and-mouth disease
- Cervical adenitis (referred pain)
- Acute otitis media (referred pain)
- Dental abscess (referred pain)
- Scarlet fever
- Kawasaki disease
- Tularemia (*Francisella tularensis* infection)

Toxic Causes

- Caustic or irritant ingestions (e.g., acid, lye)

- Inhaled irritant (e.g., tobacco smoke)

Neoplastic Causes

- Leukemia
- Lymphoma
- Rhabdomyosarcoma

Traumatic Causes

- Foreign body
- Intraluminal tear
- Gastroesophageal reflux disease
- Vocal abuse (e.g., shouting)
- External neck trauma (e.g., strangulation, child abuse)

Congenital or Vascular Causes

- Branchial cleft cyst
- Thyroglossal duct cyst

Inflammatory Causes

- Autoimmune disorders
- Allergy
- Postradiation

Psychosocial Causes
- Psychogenic pain (globus hystericus)

Miscellaneous Causes
- Cyclic neutropenia
- Periodic fever, aphthous stomatitis, pharyngitis, cervical adenitis (PFAPA) syndrome
- Vitamin deficiency—A, B-complex, C
- Dehydration
- Pharyngeal irritation from breathing dry, heated air

DIFFERENTIAL DIAGNOSIS DISCUSSION
Nasopharyngitis
Etiology
Most cases of nasopharyngitis, also known as the common cold or upper respiratory tract infection, are caused by viral agents. There are more than 200 serologically different causative agents. The most common are rhinoviruses, coronaviruses, parainfluenza virus, enteroviruses (coxsackievirus A and B, echovirus, and polio virus), adenovirus, influenza virus A and B, and respiratory syncytial virus.

Clinical Features
The clinical picture typically includes fever, runny nose, sneezing, and nasal congestion with clear or purulent nasal secretions, a sore throat lasting for several days, and a self-limited clinical course of 4 to 10 days. Infection caused by group A beta hemolytic *Streptococcus* (GABHS) may present as a seromucoid rhinitis in toddlers.

Associated symptoms may include irritability, restlessness, muscle aches, cough, eye discharge, vomiting, or diarrhea, depending on the causative agent. Otitis media with effusion, laryngotracheobronchitis, or bronchiolitis may be present.

Complications are typically attributable to bacterial superinfection and include sinusitis, cervical adenitis, mastoiditis, peritonsillar and periorbital cellulitis, acute otitis media, and pneumonia.

Evaluation
The patient or parent should be asked about associated symptoms and about ill contacts at home, school, or child care. A complete physical examination should be performed, paying particular attention to the patient's overall appearance and hydration status.

Treatment
The treatment of nasopharyngitis consists of bed rest, increased intake of fluids, and the administration of acetaminophen or ibuprofen for pain and fever. Because of the risk of Reye syndrome with influenza infection, aspirin and aspirin-containing products should be avoided. Oral decongestants (e.g., pseudoephedrine), oral antihistamine agents, and phenylephrine drops may be used for children who are greater than or equal to 6 years old. Saline drops and nasal suctioning are appropriate for infants with nasal obstruction. Humidifiers and vaporizers may be useful to prevent drying of secretions.

Pharyngitis

Etiology

Most cases of acute pharyngitis are caused by viruses—most commonly, adenoviruses. Other viral causes include influenza viruses A and B; parainfluenza viruses 1, 2, and 3; Epstein–Barr virus (EBV); cytomegalovirus; human herpesvirus 6; human immunodeficiency virus; human metapneumovirus; and enteroviruses. Bacterial causes include GABHS (15% to 30% of all acute pharyngitis in children), group C streptococci, group G streptococci, *Mycoplasma pneumoniae*, *Corynebacterium diphtheriae*, *Arcanobacterium haemolyticum*, *Neisseria gonorrhoeae*, *N. meningitides*, *Yersinia enterocolitica*, *Y. pestis*, and *F. tularensis*.

Clinical Features

- **Viral pharyngitis (caused by viruses other than EBV)** is characterized by the gradual onset of a sore throat, fever, hoarseness, and halitosis (in some patients), and an erythematous throat with or without exudate. Follicular and ulcerative lesions, mild cough, rhinorrhea, conjunctivitis, diarrhea, enanthem, or exanthem suggest a viral cause. Cervical adenopathy (tender or nontender) and poor intake of solid foods and decreased appetite are seen. The clinical course is self-limited and lasts 1 to 5 days.

- **Although infectious mononucleosis is rare before 4 years of age, young children may experience pharyngitis caused by EBV.** Clinical features include fever and a sore and erythematous throat with or without exudate. Palatal petechiae, poor intake of solid foods, posterior cervical and generalized adenopathy, hepatosplenomegaly, and fatigue may be seen.

- **Many experts consider pharyngitis caused by GABHS and rheumatic fever to be uncommon in children <3 years, but GABHS has been isolated in symptomatic infants as young as 3 months.** It may present with the sudden onset of a sore throat, a fever as high as 104°F (40°C), erythematous tonsils with or without exudate, petechiae on the soft palate, and headache. Nausea, vomiting, and stomach ache are often associated symptoms. Tender, anterior cervical adenopathy, and a fine sandpaper-like rash may be noted on physical examination. Complications include acute otitis media, sinusitis, peritonsillar and retropharyngeal abscesses, acute glomerulonephritis, rheumatic fever, and suppurative cervical adenitis.

Evaluation

The parent should be asked about associated symptoms and whether the child has had contact with anyone at home or at school with a sore throat, mononucleosis, strep throat, scarlet fever, or rheumatic fever.

The tonsils, pharynx, soft palate, skin, neck, lymph nodes, liver, spleen, and pulses should be examined, and the patient's general appearance and overall respiratory status and hydration status should be assessed.

A rapid strep test, also known as a rapid antigen detection test, should be obtained, if available, for all patients with an inflamed throat on physical examination; and if the rapid strep test is negative, a throat culture for GABHS should be sent.

TABLE 72-1	Clinical Findings Useful in the Diagnosis of Streptococcal Pharyngitis

Findings that Indicate Likely Viral Pharyngitis:
- Exposure to contacts with symptoms of upper respiratory tract infection
- Cough, runny nose, or eye discharge predominate

Findings That Suggest Streptococcal Pharyngitis:
- Exposure to contacts with strep throat, scarlet fever, or rheumatic fever
- Sore throat predominates
- History of fever, headache, and stomachache
- Inflamed throat on physical examination

Findings that Indicate Likely Streptococcal Pharyngitis:
- Palatal petechiae and tonsillar exudate
- Associated headache and abdominal pain
- Fine sandpaper-like rash over the torso and other parts of the body; strawberry tongue

Treatment

The treatment for pharyngitis of any cause includes acetaminophen and ibuprofen for pain and fever (avoid aspirin), increased fluids, and the administration of nonprescription lozenges and gargle solutions to provide temporary pain relief. Gargling with salt water (1/4 tsp of salt in 8 oz of warm water) and drinking warm liquids may be soothing. In severe cases, especially with infectious mononucleosis, patients may need to be hospitalized for intravenous hydration and airway precautions. For infectious mononucleosis, short courses of corticosteroids reduce pain and swelling; however, their use should be considered only in select patients with marked tonsillar inflammation and impending airway compromise or other serious complications, such as hemolytic anemia or thrombocytopenia. Routine use of corticosteroids in the treatment of pharyngitis is not recommended. See Table 72-1 for the clinical findings useful in the diagnosis of streptococcal pharyngitis.

In patients with GABHS pharyngitis, the primary reason for treating with antibiotics is to prevent rheumatic fever, which has not been described with group C or group G streptococcal pharyngitis. Antibiotic treatment for GABHS pharyngitis shortens the course of illness, decreases the incidence of suppurative complications, and prevents transmission to others. Penicillin V, 400,000 U, 250 mg for children, and 500 mg two to three times per day for adolescents and adults, is administered orally for 10 days. Amoxicillin is often used because of its palatability. For penicillin-allergic patients, use erythromycin, 40 mg/kg/day in two to four divided doses for 10 days. Other macrolides, including 5 days of azithromycin, clindamycin, and cephalosporins, are also effective against GABHS. Tetracycline, sulfonamides, and trimethoprim-sulfamethoxazole are ineffective in treating streptococcal infections. If poor compliance with oral medication is expected, benzathine penicillin G, 600,000 U for children less than 60 lb (27 kg); 1.2 million U for larger children and adults, should be administered in a single intramuscular dose (maximum dose, 1.2 million U). Following completion of 24 hours of antibiotics, the patient may return to school or child care. Good hand washing should be encouraged, and the patient should avoid sharing food and drink containers and towels. Empirical treatment of asymptomatic contacts is not recommended.

For isolated bacterial pharyngitis that is not caused by GABHS, antibiotic treatment is not required because rheumatic fever is not a complication and the effect of treatment is unknown or minimal. Groups C and G streptococci are very sensitive to penicillin and may be treated with this medication; however, effectiveness of treatment has not been studied. Bacterial pharyngitis caused by *M. pneumoniae or C. pneumoniae* is often associated with lower respiratory tract infection, which requires treatment.

Individuals with recurrent pharyngitis may benefit from tonsillectomy as a recent systematic review showed that tonsillectomy modestly reduced the incidence of recurrent pharyngitis. Consideration for tonsillectomy should be given on an individual basis with consultation by an otolaryngologist.

Herpangina

Etiology

The etiologic agents of herpangina are viral: nonpolio enteroviruses, coxsackieviruses A and B, and echoviruses.

Clinical Features

Herpangina affects children of all ages. The typical clinical picture includes discrete, painful vesicular and ulcerative lesions on the tonsillar pillars, soft palate, uvula, and posterior pharynx; sore throat; poor appetite; and a fever as high as 105.8°F (41°C). Nausea, vomiting, and abdominal pain may be present. The course is usually self-limited and resolves within 1 week.

Evaluation

Herpangina can be differentiated from herpes simplex virus gingivostomatitis by the location of the ulcerative lesions. With herpangina, the lesions tend to be in the posterior pharynx. In herpes gingivostomatitis, the lesions are usually in the anterior oropharynx. Hydration status must be assessed.

Treatment

Herpangina should be treated with acetaminophen and ibuprofen for fever and pain. Topical analgesics may provide temporary relief. Some physicians prescribe a mixture of viscous lidocaine (2%), Maalox, and Benadryl liquid (often referred to as "Magic Mouthwash") in equal parts to be used topically. The patient should be given adequate hydration and nutrition. Severe cases, especially in young children with dehydration, may require hospitalization for intravenous fluid administration.

Peritonsillar Cellulitis and Peritonsillar Abscess

Etiology

Peritonsillar infections may result from acute tonsillar pharyngeal infection or obstruction and infection of Weber glands, located in the superior pole of the tonsillar fossae. Peritonsillar abscesses are more commonly seen in children >10 years old. Their causes are polymicrobial, involving either anaerobic or aerobic bacteria. The aerobic bacteria may include GABHS, α- and γ-hemolytic streptococci, group D streptococci, coagulase-negative staphylococci, and *Haemophilus influenzae.*

Clinical Features

The clinical features of peritonsillar cellulitis or abscess include fever, dysphagia, voice changes (e.g., "hot potato" or muffled voice), trismus, and drooling. Unilateral tonsillar or peritonsillar swelling (usually on the superior aspect of the tonsil), deviation of the uvula to the contralateral side, ipsilateral cervical adenopathy, and trismus may be seen on physical examination. Dehydration, upper airway obstruction, or aspiration of ruptured abscess contents may occur.

Evaluation

Peritonsillar cellulitis that is not associated with the drainage of pus and parapharyngeal abscess that involves inflammation of the pharyngeal wall are in the differential diagnosis for peritonsillar abscess. The patient's respiratory status and hydration status should be assessed. The patient should be encouraged to speak so the examiner can assess the quality of the voice. The pharyngeal wall and both tonsils should be thoroughly inspected for asymmetric swelling and any uvular deviation. Avoid using a tongue blade if epiglottitis is suspected.

Treatment

A pediatric otolaryngologist should be consulted to confirm the diagnosis and, possibly, to perform a needle aspiration of the abscess. Needle aspiration should be performed initially in older children and adolescents. The contents of the abscess need not be cultured except in children who are immunocompromised.

Penicillin VK (15 to 40 mg/kg/day, divided every 6 to 8 hours for 10 to 14 days) should be started for outpatient management. Aqueous penicillin G (100,000 to 250,000 U/kg/day, divided, every 4 to 6 hours, with a maximum dose of 4.8 million U per 24 hours) should be given intravenously for inpatient management. If penicillin alone is not effective, a semisynthetic penicillin or clindamycin may be added. Clindamycin (25 to 40 mg/kg/day, divided, every 6 to 8 hours for 10 to 14 days) is used for patients who are allergic to penicillin.

Acetaminophen may be administered for fever and pain management. Hydration status should be carefully monitored. Tonsillectomy may be necessary in severe cases, in patients who are unresponsive to needle aspiration and antibiotics, and in patients with a history of recurrent peritonsillar abscesses.

Retropharyngeal Cellulitis and Retropharyngeal Abscess
Etiology

Retropharyngeal infections occur in the potential space between the posterior pharyngeal wall and the prevertebral fascia. They are believed to occur as a complication of pharyngitis but may also occur following a foreign body or penetrating injury to the posterior pharynx, and as an extension of vertebral osteomyelitis.

Retropharyngeal abscesses most often occur in young children <6 years old. The etiologic agents are polymicrobial and may include GABHS, anaerobic bacteria, *Staphylococcus aureus, and Klebsiella pneumoniae.*

Clinical Features

The clinical features of retropharyngeal cellulitis and retropharyngeal abscess include a high fever, difficulty swallowing, and a severe sore throat. The patient may refuse to eat. Hyperextension of the neck; noisy, gurgling respirations, or stridor; or meningismus (caused by irritation of the paravertebral ligaments) may be present. Drooling and increased work of breathing may be seen. Complications include respiratory compromise, aspiration of the abscess contents, expansion along fascial planes to the mediastinum (resulting in mediastinitis), and erosion into major blood vessels.

Evaluation

The patient should be assessed for drooling and difficulty breathing. A bulge may be seen in the posterior pharyngeal wall. A tongue blade should be used with caution because the abscess may rupture if poked or digitally manipulated.

Treatment

An otolaryngologist should be consulted. A semisynthetic penicillin should be administered to cover penicillinase-producing *S. aureus.* Clindamycin (25 to 40 mg/kg/day, divided, every 6 to 8 hours for 10 to 14 days) is used for penicillin-allergic patients. Cardiorespiratory monitoring is recommended because of the risk of airway compromise. Acetaminophen (with or without codeine) should be administered for pain; narcotics must be used with care because of the risk of airway obstruction.

EVALUATION OF SORE THROAT

Patient History

The following aspects of the history can provide important clues to the diagnosis:

- Concurrent upper respiratory tract symptoms (e.g., cough, runny nose) suggest a viral etiology.
- Thickened secretions suggest an infectious cause.
- Similar complaints in household and other close contacts suggest an infectious etiology.
- Seasonal variation and associated allergic symptoms, such as itchy eyes, suggest an allergic cause.
- Recurrence every 3 to 6 weeks: consider cyclic neutropenia or PFAPA.
- Bleeding with injections or easy bruisability may suggest a neoplastic process.
- Change in vocal quality suggests laryngitis but may also be the muffled voice heard with peritonsillar and retropharyngeal abscesses.
- Drooling, pain, or difficulty swallowing suggests the presence of ulcerative lesions or enlarged tissue.

Physical Examination

The following should be noted on physical examination:

- The patient's general appearance and any signs of drooling or difficulty breathing (e.g., nasal flaring, stridor).
- The patient's vital signs, including temperature.
- Mouth breathing or change in vocal quality.
- Tympanic membrane erythema or a middle ear effusion suggests acute otitis media, which often accompanies nasopharyngitis.
- Nasal mucosal erythema may suggest an infectious or allergic process.
- Oral vesicular eruptions, which suggest a viral cause (e.g., herpes simplex virus, enterovirus, coxsackievirus).
- Symmetric tonsillar hypertrophy may be seen in nasopharyngitis and pharyngitis.
- Unilateral tonsillar inflammation suggests peritonsillar cellulitis or abscess or the presence of a tumor.
- Tonsillar exudates may be seen in viral and bacterial infections.
- Palatal petechiae may be seen in strep throat and mononucleosis.
- Lymphadenopathy in the posterior cervical triangle is seen in mononucleosis.
- Tender anterior cervical adenopathy is typically seen in strep throat.
- Neck swelling and tenderness, and ill appearance should raise the suspicion for complications including lymph node abscess and Lemierre syndrome.

 HINT: When palpating potential intraoral/pharyngeal abscesses, use caution. Patients may aspirate contents of ruptured abscesses.

Laboratory Studies

A rapid strep test should be done. This test, which requires vigorous swabbing of the tonsillar pillars and the posterior pharynx, identifies the presence or absence of GABHS carbohydrate by specific antisera but does not detect group C and G streptococci. Avoid swabbing the uvula because doing so may result in dilution of the sample. The rapid strep test is highly specific and sensitive. False-negative results may occur if small numbers of streptococci are present. Negative tests should always be confirmed by throat culture. A positive test indicates that GABHS are present in the pharynx.

A throat culture, considered the gold standard for the diagnosis of strep throat, should be obtained. Untreated patients with strep throat may have positive cultures for several weeks to months. Notify the laboratory if *N. gonorrhoeae, C. diphtheriae,* or fungal infection is suspected so that appropriate culture media is used.

A complete blood cell count may also be revealing. The white blood cell count may be elevated in patients with peritonsillar abscesses, retropharyngeal abscesses, and other bacterial infections. Mild anemia and mild thrombocytopenia may be seen during viral illnesses. An atypical lymphocytosis making up 10% to 25% of

TABLE 72-2	Symptoms Associated with Life-Threatening Causes of Sore Throat
Ill appearance	
Tachypnea	
Respiratory retractions	
Stridor	
Drooling	
Difficulty swallowing	
Muffled, "hot potato" voice	
Neck stiffness	

the total white blood cell count is suggestive of infection with EBV. EBV titers and monospot tests are useful for confirming EBV infection.

Diagnostic Modalities

A lateral neck radiograph should be obtained when the diagnosis of a retropharyngeal abscess is suspected. It is useful for assessing the airway caliber, the size of the adenoids and epiglottis, and ballooning of the hypopharynx. A retropharyngeal abscess appears as widening of the soft tissues immediately anterior to vertebral bodies C1–C4. Normally, the soft tissues measure less than half the width of the adjacent vertebral body. Air in the retropharynx or loss of the normal cervical lordosis should raise suspicion of a retropharyngeal abscess.

A computed tomography scan of the neck with contrast may be useful in determining the surgical treatment of retropharyngeal abscesses. It may also help differentiate retropharyngeal cellulitis from retropharyngeal abscess.

APPROACH TO THE PATIENT

First, rule out life-threatening causes of sore throat (e.g., epiglottitis; see Chapter 66, "Respiratory Distress"), peritonsillar abscess, retropharyngeal abscess, diphtheria, severe tonsillar hypertrophy, and Lemierre syndrome (see Chapter 54, "Neck Mass"). Table 72-2 lists the symptoms associated with life-threatening causes of sore throat. Oxygen should be provided if respiratory distress is noted.

The patient should be examined for evidence of a peritonsillar abscess or foreign body. If epiglottitis is suspected, use of a tongue blade should be avoided, as should other invasive procedures (e.g., placement of an intravenous catheter, phlebotomy). The patient should be immediately referred to an anesthesiologist, a critical care specialist, and an otolaryngologist. If a retropharyngeal abscess is suspected, a lateral neck radiograph should be obtained.

Figure 72-1 outlines the approach to narrowing the differential diagnosis.

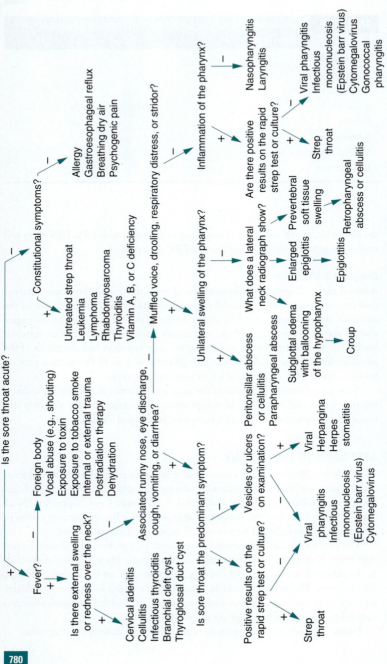

FIGURE 72-1 Approach to narrowing the diagnosis of sore throat.

Suggested Readings

American Academy of Pediatrics. Group A streptococcal infections. In: Pickering LK, Baker CJ, Kimberlin DW, Long SS, eds. *Red Book 2009: Report of the Committee on Infectious Diseases.* 28th ed. Elk Grove Village, IL: American Academy of Pediatrics; 2009:616–628.

Blakley BW, Magit AE. The role of tonsillectomy in reducing recurrent pharyngitis: a systematic review. *Otolaryngol Head Neck Surg.* 2009;140(3):291–297.

Brook I. Microbiology and management of peritonsillar, retropharyngeal, and parapharyngeal abscesses. *J Oral Maxillofac Surg.* 2004;62:1545–1550.

Cabrera CE, Deutsch ES, Eppes S, et al. Increased incidence of head and neck abscesses in children. *Otolaryngol Head Neck Surg.* 2007;136:176–181.

Candy B, Hotopf M. Steroids for symptom control in infectious mononucleosis. *Cochrane Database Syst Rev.* 2006;3:CD004402.

Gerber MA. Diagnosis and treatment of pharyngitis in children. *Pediatr Clin North Am.* 2005;52:729–747.

Luzuriaga K, Sullivan JL. Infectious mononucleosis. *N Engl J Med.* 2010;362(21):1993–2000.

Splenomegaly

INTRODUCTION

Splenomegaly may be evident in benign viral infections, serious systemic infections, hematologic diseases, neoplastic conditions, and metabolic disorders. The terms "splenomegaly" and "hypersplenism" are not interchangeable. **Splenomegaly refers to an enlarged spleen,** whereas **hypersplenism refers to a hyperfunctioning spleen that results in a reduction in the number of circulating blood cells**. Hypersplenism is usually associated with splenomegaly, but not always.

A palpable spleen tip is not necessarily pathologic. Approximately 3% of older adolescents and adults have **palpable spleens**. A palpable spleen is detected in most premature infants and up to 30% of term infants. By adulthood, the normal spleen, which is located beneath the 9th and 11th ribs, reaches dimensions of 12 cm long, 7 cm wide, and 3 cm thick. Normal spleens are soft, located at the mid-clavicular line, nontender and often only palpable on deep inspiration. Splenic tenderness or a spleen edge >2 cm below the costal margin is always abnormal. A normal-size spleen being pushed down by hyperinflated lungs may cause apparent splenomegaly.

 HINT: Percussion can be used to evaluate splenic size. To delineate the lower "tip," the examiner starts in the area of tympany in the left anterior axillary line of the mid-abdomen and percusses upward toward the splenic dullness. The upper border is defined by starting in the left midaxillary line of the midthorax and percussing downward toward the splenic dullness. Proper abdominal exam on a relaxed abdomen is critical to palpate an enlarged spleen. Begin in the left lower quadrant (an enlarged spleen may be missed by beginning in the left upper quadrant). Stand on the patient's right side and use the right hand to palpate while supporting the rib cage with the left hand.

 DIFFERENTIAL DIAGNOSIS LIST

Infectious Causes
Viral Infection
- Adenovirus
- Mononucleosis (Epstein–Barr virus [EBV] infection)
- Cytomegalovirus (CMV) infection
- Coxsackievirus
- HIV
- Rubella
- Herpes
- Hepatitis A, B, C

Bacterial Infection

- Pneumonia
- Sepsis
- Endocarditis
- Brucellosis
- Tularemia
- Splenic abscess
- Cat-scratch disease—*Bartonella* sp.
- Tuberculosis
- Syphilis
- Leptospirosis
- Rocky Mountain spotted fever (RMSF)—*Rickettsia rickettsii*
- Salmonella infection
- Streptococcal infection
- Ehrlichiosis

Other Infections

- Malaria
- Toxoplasmosis
- Babesiosis
- Histoplasmosis
- Coccidioidomycosis
- Schistosomiasis
- Trypanosomiasis

Neoplastic Causes

- Leukemia
- Lymphoma
- Lymphosarcoma
- Hamartoma
- Metastatic disease (neuroblastoma)

Traumatic Causes

- Laceration
- Hematoma
- Traumatic cyst

Metabolic or Genetic Causes
Lipid Metabolism Defects

- Gaucher disease
- Niemann–Pick disease
- Gangliosidoses
- Mucolipidoses
- Metachromatic leukodystrophy
- Wolman disease

Mucopolysaccharidoses

- Hurler syndrome
- Hunter syndrome

Hematologic Causes
Red Blood Cell (RBC) Membrane Defects

- Hereditary spherocytosis
- Hereditary elliptocytosis
- Hereditary stomatocytosis

RBC Enzyme Defects

- Glucose-6-phosphate dehydrogenase (G6PD) deficiency
- Pyruvate kinase deficiency

Hemoglobin Defects

- Sickle cell disease (SCD)
- Thalassemia

Extrinsic Hemolytic Anemias

- Autoimmune hemolytic anemia
- Erythroblastosis fetalis

Congestive Causes

- Congestive heart failure
- Constrictive pericarditis
- Chronic liver disease with portal hypertension
- Perisplenic anatomic obstructions
- Splenic vein thrombosis
- Splenic artery aneurysm
- Cavernous transformation of the portal vein

Miscellaneous Causes

- Serum sickness
- Splenic hemangioma
- Chronic granulomatous disease
- Juvenile rheumatoid arthritis (JRA)
- Systemic lupus erythematosus (SLE)
- Autoimmune hepatitis

Histiocytic Disorders

- Langerhans cell histiocytosis
- Hemophagocytic lymphohistiocytosis

- Malignant histiocytic disorders
- Beckwith–Wiedemann syndrome
- Amyloidosis

- Sarcoidosis
- Congenital splenic cyst

> **HINT:** Not all left upper quadrant masses are related to the spleen. Other conditions such as an enlarged kidney, a retroperitoneal tumor, an adrenal neoplasm, an ovarian, pancreatic, or mesenteric cyst may mimic splenomegaly on examination. Imaging such as ultrasound, computed tomography (CT), or MRI may be useful in the evaluation of a left upper quadrant mass if the history and laboratory studies are not consistent with the physical examination findings of splenomegaly.

DIFFERENTIAL DIAGNOSIS DISCUSSION
Benign Infection
Many benign infections, especially upper respiratory tract infections, can be associated with **mild, transient splenomegaly**. Adenovirus, coxsackievirus, and *Streptococcus* are commonly involved organisms.

Epstein–Barr Virus Infection (Infectious Mononucleosis)
Infectious mononucleosis is discussed in Chapter 50, "Lymphadenopathy." Of note, splenomegaly may persist for several months after resolution of mononucleosis. The splenomegaly should be resolved before the athlete returns to contact sports.

Cytomegalovirus Infection
Epidemiology
CMV is ubiquitous, and **most people are infected with the virus by adulthood**. The source is body fluids, including blood, urine, breast milk, saliva, and feces. Transmission of CMV is both horizontal (**person to person**) and vertical (**mother to child**). CMV is the most common congenital viral infection.

Clinical Features
CMV infection manifests itself differently in different hosts:

- In **neonates,** intrauterine growth retardation, microcephaly, jaundice, hepatosplenomegaly, a petechial or purpuric rash, chorioretinitis, and neurologic symptoms may be seen.
- In **immunocompetent children or adults,** infection is most commonly asymptomatic; however, patients may develop fever, malaise, anorexia, pharyngitis, headache, myalgia, abdominal pain, and hepatosplenomegaly.
- In **immunocompromised children and adults,** retinitis, pneumonitis, and enteritis are the primary manifestations.

Evaluation
Diagnosis is best made by **isolation** of the organism in body fluids (or organs) by cell culture or polymerase chain reaction. **Serologic studies** are also available.

A **CT scan of the head** may demonstrate intracerebral calcifications in patients with congenital CMV infection.

Treatment

The immunocompetent host recovers completely in a few weeks with **supportive treatment**. Immunocompromised patients are commonly treated with **ganciclovir or valganciclovir**.

Malaria

Etiology

Malaria, a disease transmitted by the *Anopheles* mosquito of the tropics and subtropics, is acquired when the host's erythrocytes are invaded by a **mosquito-borne parasite** of the genus *Plasmodium*. Four species of *Plasmodium* cause malaria: *P. falciparum, P. vivax, P. ovale, and P. malariae.* The incubation period is 1 to 2 weeks.

Clinical Features

Although constitutional symptoms are universal, the clinical presentation of malaria is often dictated by the infecting species. *P. vivax and P. ovale,* for example, are particularly associated with hypersplenism and splenic rupture.

Evaluation

Diagnosis is confirmed by **identification of the parasite** in the blood. Special stains and smears are required for optimal yield. Thick and thin blood films should be examined.

Treatment and Prevention

Treatment entails **antimicrobial therapy** (e.g., chloroquine) and **supportive** measures (e.g., management of fluid and electrolytes, RBC transfusions). Since resistance to chloroquine and other drugs is common, a multitude of **antibiotics** is used in the armamentarium against malaria (e.g., Atovaquone/proguanil, quinine, quinidine, primaquine, mefloquine, doxycycline, tetracycline, clindamycin) and may be necessary. **Chemoprophylaxis** with chloroquine, Atovaquone/proguanil, mefloquine, or doxycycline is recommended for travelers to endemic areas.

Babesiosis

Etiology

Like malaria, babesiosis is a **parasitic infection** of erythrocytes that is endemic in the coastal areas of the northeastern United States. The main reservoir of *Babesia* is the **white-footed mouse,** and the *Ixodes scapularis* tick transmits the organism. The incubation period is 1 week to several months.

Clinical Features

Symptoms include fever, chills, sweats, malaise, myalgias, nausea, and vomiting. Jaundice, dark urine, and renal failure are also possible. The clinical presentations of **babesiosis and malaria are sometimes similar**.

Evaluation

Laboratory evaluation may demonstrate hemolytic anemia and elevation of liver enzymes. The diagnosis is confirmed by **blood smears and serologic studies**.

Treatment

Patients with moderate or severe illness are treated with **clindamycin and quinine, or atovaquone and azithromycin**.

Hematologic Disorders

Hereditary spherocytosis, G6PD deficiency, SCD, and thalassemia are discussed in Chapter 40, "Hemolysis."

Lymphomas

Lymphomas—non-Hodgkin lymphoma and Hodgkin disease—are discussed in Chapter 50, "Lymphadenopathy."

Trauma

Mechanisms of injury to the spleen include motor vehicle accidents, bicycle accidents, traumatic sports injury and falls. Patients may complain of **diffuse or left upper quadrant pain**. The diagnosis is confirmed by **CT scan**.

Lacerations and hematomas are usually managed conservatively with **observation and supportive therapy**. Occasionally, **surgical splenectomy** is necessary. In rare cases, traumatic cysts are managed with aspiration, sclerosing, and surgery.

Gaucher Disease

Etiology

A **deficiency of β-glucosidase** leads to the pathologic accumulation of glucocerebroside in the reticuloendothelial system.

Clinical Features

Gaucher disease is categorized into three forms.

- **Type I, the "classic" type,** is one of the most common genetic disorders in Ashkenazi Jews. It may present at any age but usually presents in adolescence or adulthood. Its distinguishing feature is its lack of neurologic involvement.
- **Type II, the infantile form,** is characterized by slow or no achievement of developmental milestones, swallowing difficulties, and opisthotonos. Its progressive neurodegenerative course culminates in death within the first 2 years of life.
- **Type III, the juvenile form,** presents in infancy or childhood with behavioral changes, seizures, and extrapyramidal and cerebellar signs. With all three types, **splenomegaly is universal**.

Evaluation

A **bone marrow aspirate** demonstrating Gaucher cells engorged with glucocerebroside confirms the diagnosis.

Treatment

Splenectomy has been used to manage the hematologic consequences of hypersplenism. Cerezyme (Genzyme), given every 2 weeks, is effective in reversing the changes.

EVALUATION OF SPLENOMEGALY

Pertinent Patient History

- Does the patient have a history of a recent upper respiratory tract infection or any ill contacts? Benign viral infections often result in mild splenomegaly.
- What is the patient's travel history? Constitutional symptoms, in the setting of travel to a tropical area, make malaria a likely diagnosis. These same symptoms, with a history of travel to the coastal northeastern United States, suggest babesiosis.
- Is there a history of tick exposure? Ticks transmit the organisms responsible for babesiosis, RMSF, ehrlichiosis, and tularemia.
- Is there a history of exposure to any animals? Contact with cattle or other farm animals (as well as unpasteurized milk) could be the clue to brucellosis. Handling rabbits might point to tularemia as a diagnosis. Scratches from cats or kittens could lead to cat-scratch disease; toxoplasmosis is also commonly linked to interactions with cats. Leptospirosis may be transmitted through the urine of dogs, rats, or livestock.
- Is the patient immunocompromised? An immunocompromised host with splenomegaly and constitutional symptoms may have CMV infection.
- Is there a history of weight loss? Weight loss may be seen in patients with infectious mononucleosis, CMV infection, HIV, brucellosis, ehrlichiosis, malaria, or babesiosis. Oncologic processes, especially lymphoma and leukemia, must also be considered in this setting.
- What is the patient's medication history? Splenomegaly in a patient who developed a rash in response to ampicillin therapy makes mononucleosis a likely diagnosis. In patients with G6PD deficiency, exposure to medications with oxidant properties leads to hemolysis and splenomegaly. Splenomegaly in the setting of joint complaints and rash makes a drug-induced serum sickness a likely possibility.
- Is there a family history of any hematologic or immunologic disorders? Many of the hematologic disorders are inherited and a positive family history in siblings, cousins or first-degree relatives may aid in the diagnosis.
- Is there a history of trauma? The spleen is the most commonly injured intraabdominal organ.

Physical Examination

- Growth retardation in a microcephalic neonate should lead to an investigation for CMV.
- Exudative pharyngitis in combination with splenomegaly suggests mononucleosis.

- Rash of the palms and soles suggests RMSF or syphilis. The rash of RMSF is usually seen first on the wrists and ankles and may be maculopapular or petechial. A maculopapular rash is characteristic with both congenital and secondary syphilis. Bullous lesions are also common in congenital syphilis. A whole body rash with "iris" or "target" lesions suggests serum sickness. JRA and SLE also have characteristic rashes.
- Jaundice may be seen with many of the infectious processes but is more typical in the hemolytic diseases (e.g., G6PD deficiency, spherocytosis, autoimmune hemolytic anemia). Jaundice may also be present in advanced liver disease or with a biliary obstruction.
- Hepatomegaly may suggest intrinsic liver disease, a storage disease or other metabolic disorder. Splenomegaly secondary to hepatic congestion should always be considered. Prehepatic vascular lesions will cause splenomegaly without hepatomegaly (i.e., portal vein thrombosis) therefore evaluate for signs of GI bleeding or dilated abdominal veins.
- Adenopathy in combination with splenomegaly most commonly points to mononucleosis, but lymphoma should also be considered. Axillary and cervical adenopathy are the two most common sites of lymph node enlargement in cat-scratch disease. Although the examination may demonstrate evidence of feline scratches, the classic papule is usually gone by the time the node manifests.
- Abdominal pain (either diffuse or localized to the left upper quadrant) should prompt an evaluation for a traumatic cause, such as a splenic laceration or hematoma. Furthermore, one of the complications of infectious mononucleosis is splenic rupture, which can present with acute abdominal pain. The presence of fever suggests a splenic abscess.

Laboratory and Radiologic Studies

The following studies may be helpful in the appropriate clinical context:

- **"Monospot."** The mononucleosis rapid slide agglutination test for heterophil antibodies is a quick test for infectious mononucleosis, but false negatives are common in children under 6 years.
- **EBV serologies.** The definitive way to diagnose both acute and past infections at any age is through the use of EBV serologies.
- **Complete blood count.** Atypical lymphocytosis is the hallmark finding of mononucleosis. Pancytopenia is common in sepsis, AIDS, ehrlichiosis, and oncologic processes. Thrombocytopenia is seen in RMSF and babesiosis. Evidence of a hemolytic anemia (e.g., sickle cells, target cells, schistocytes, spherocytes) should prompt consideration of the common hematologic disorders (SCD, thalassemia, G6PD deficiency, and spherocytosis), as well as certain infectious diseases (e.g., malaria, babesiosis). Leukopenia and thrombocytopenia are often seen in hypersplenism, which may be associated with chronic liver disease and portal hypertension.
- **Reticulocyte count.** Reticulocytosis is the confirmatory finding in hemolytic anemias.
- **Bilirubin level and liver enzymes.** Hyperbilirubinemia is found in hemolytic anemias and may be seen in patients with intrinsic liver disease. An elevation in liver

enzymes implicates the liver as a primary or secondary source of pathology. Common causes may be infectious, neoplastic, anatomic, metabolic, traumatic, or toxic.

- **Direct antibody test.** Autoimmune hemolytic anemias are usually antibody positive.
- **Routine blood smear.** Evidence of hemolysis is also evident on inspection of the peripheral blood smear. In addition, infestations like malaria and babesiosis can often be readily identified on blood smears as long as the laboratory is made aware that these diseases are diagnostic possibilities.
- **Urinalysis.** Hemoglobinuria is a common finding in hemolytic anemias. Urinalysis abnormalities are also seen with some metabolic disorders.
- Ultrasound with Doppler is useful to evaluate the direction of portal venous flow as well as evaluate for anatomic abnormalities.

TREATMENT OF SPLENOMEGALY

Most of the diseases presenting with splenomegaly require supportive care and observation for complications.

- **Splenic rupture,** whether associated with mononucleosis or not, requires immediate surgical management.
- **Splenic abscess** is treated with intravenous antibiotics and possible surgical drainage.
- **Hemolytic anemias.** Patients with hemolytic anemias often require RBC transfusions until the hemolysis is either terminated or stable. Discontinuation of offending medications is indicated in patients with serum sickness and G6PD deficiency.

APPROACH TO THE PATIENT

- **In neonates with splenomegaly,** bacterial infection should be ruled out first. If no bacterial causes are isolated, a viral cause should be pursued aggressively. If infection is deemed unlikely, a hemolytic cause should be considered. If no hemolytic disorder can be identified, anatomic abnormalities of the spleen should be investigated.
- **In older infants and children with splenomegaly,** trauma is the first consideration. Infection and hemolysis are the next two possibilities to be considered. If these categories are eliminated, the possibility of liver disease should be investigated. If the patient has constitutional symptoms, an oncologic process is likely; rarely, a metabolic disorder also presents in this fashion.
- **Contact sports should be avoided** in patients with splenomegaly. Trauma to an enlarged spleen could result in splenic rupture and uncontrollable hemorrhage. Patients with chronic splenomegaly should be fitted for a spleen guard. These guards should be periodically evaluated to make sure the lower edge of the guard is at least 1cm below the spleen edge when the patient is standing.

Figure 73-1 outlines the approach to nonacutely ill patients with splenomegaly. Figure 73-2 outlines the approach for acutely ill patients with splenomegaly.

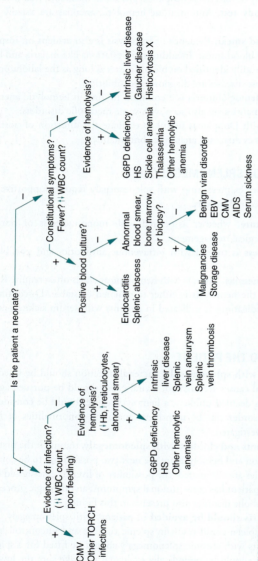

FIGURE 73-1 **Approach to a nonacutely ill patient with splenomegaly.** *CMV,* cytomegalovirus; *EBV,* Epstein–Barr virus; *G6PD,* glucose-6-phosphate dehydrogenase; *Hb,* hemoglobin; *HS,* hereditary spherocytosis; *TORCH,* toxoplasmosis, other infections, rubella, cytomegalovirus, herpes simplex; *WBC,* white blood cell count; *AIDS,* acquired immunodeficiency syndrome.

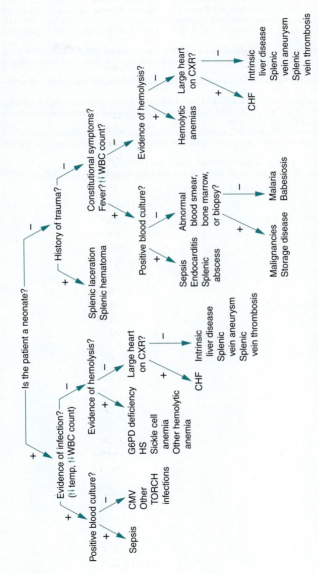

FIGURE 73-2 Approach to an acutely ill patient with splenomegaly. *CHF*, congestive heart failure; *CMV*, cytomegalovirus; *CXR*, chest radiograph; *G6PD*, glucose-6-phosphate dehydrogenase; *HS*, hereditary spherocytosis; *TORCH*, toxoplasmosis, other infections, rubella, cytomegalovirus, herpes simplex; *WBC*, white blood cell count.

Suggested Readings

American Academy of Pediatrics: Babesiosis. Brucellosis. Ehrlichiosis. Malaria. In: Pickering LK, Baker CJ, Long SS, et al., eds. *2006 Red Book: Report of the Committee on Infectious Diseases.* 27th ed. Elk Grove Village, IL: American Academy of Pediatrics; 2006:223–224, 235–237, 281–284, 435–441.

Galanakis E, Bourantas KL, Leveidiotou S, et al. Childhood brucellosis in north-western Greece. *Eur J Pediatr.* 1996;155:1–6.

Grover SA, Barkun AN, Sackett DL. Does this patient have splenomegaly? *JAMA.* 1993;270:2218–2221.

Khan SB, Alkan S, Pooley R. A 14-year-old boy with splenomegaly. *Arch Pathol Lab Med.* 2000;124: 1239–1240.

Pozo AL, Godfrey EM, Bowles KM. Splenomegaly: investigation, diagnosis and management. *Blood Rev.* 2009;23:105–111.

Scully RE. Case records of the Massachusetts General Hospital. Weekly clinicopathological exercises. Case 24-1994. A two-year-old boy with thrombocytopenia, leukocytosis, and hepatosplenomegaly. *N Engl J Med.* 1994;330:1739–1746.

Tamayo SG, Rickman LS, Mathews WC, et al. Examiner dependence on physical diagnostic tests for the detection of splenomegaly: a prospective study with multiple observers. *J Gen Intern Med.* 1993;8: 69–75.

Vane DW. Left upper quadrant masses in children. *Pediatr Rev.* 1992;13:25–31.

Woods M, Greenes D. A 16-year-old girl with epistaxis and hepatomegaly. *Curr Opin Pediatr.* 1995;7: 733–739.

Syncope

INTRODUCTION

Syncope, or the transient loss of consciousness, is a common clinical problem in children and adolescents. As many as 15% to 20% of all children will experience an episode of syncope before the end of their second decade, and the chief complaint of syncope accounts for 1% of all emergency department visits in this population. In pediatric patients presenting with syncope, neurocardiogenic syncope (NCS) must be differentiated from neurologic causes of syncope and from less common but life-threatening cardiac causes of syncope.

DIFFERENTIAL DIAGNOSIS LIST

Neurocardiogenic Syncope
Cardiac Syncope
Left Ventricular Outflow Tract Obstruction
- Aortic stenosis
- Subaortic stenosis
- Hypertrophic cardiomyopathy

Arrhythmias
- Ventricular tachycardia (VT)
- Long QT syndrome

- Bradyarrhythmias
- Sinus node dysfunction
- Conduction block

Neurologic Syncope
- Seizures
- Migraine headaches

DIFFERENTIAL DIAGNOSIS DISCUSSION
Neurocardiogenic Syncope

NCS, or the simple faint, is the most common cause of loss of consciousness in childhood. It is characterized by inappropriate vasodilatation leading to neurally mediated systemic hypotension resulting in low cerebral perfusion pressure and cerebral blood flow. This systemic hypotension stems from vagal stimulation and often is precipitated by pain, fear, excitement, positional changes, and extended periods of standing, particularly in a warm environment. In this condition, an extended period in the upright position, dehydration, a vagal trigger, or external stimuli such as pain or emotional upset increases vagal tone leading to a decreased heart rate, peripheral vasodilatation, and systemic hypotension. The child with recurrent episodes is frequently referred for cardiovascular evaluation.

Evaluation includes a detailed history, cardiovascular examination, and a 12-lead electrocardiogram (ECG). Obtaining orthostatic vital signs can also be helpful in diagnosing this problem. With the patient in the supine position, blood pressure and heart rate are recorded. The patient is then asked to stand for 10 minutes and the measurements are repeated. A drop in systolic blood pressure of ≥15 mm Hg or a rise in heart rate of ≥20 beats per minute when standing is consistent with the diagnosis of neurally mediated hypotension that may result in NCS. An **echocardiogram** may be ordered if abnormalities are noted on the ECG or cardiovascular examination. Typically, this is sufficient to rule out a serious cardiac cause. Rarely, in cases where the mechanism of syncope is believed to be NCS but symptoms are atypical, a **tilt-table test or graded exercise test** may be ordered. In the tilt-table test, the child or adolescent is placed on a table and tilted to 70 degrees while being monitored by ECG and an automated blood pressure monitor. This creates an artificial orthostatic stress that often provokes a drop in heart rate and/or blood pressure, which is diagnostic. Exercise testing can elicit similar results. Following graded exercise, testing patients are asked to stand for 10 minutes and their blood pressure and heart rate are measured. This also creates an artificial orthostatic stress that often provokes a drop in heart rate and/or blood pressure, which is diagnostic. Patients with a positive tilt-table test or graded exercise test (e.g., those with NCS) are encouraged to increase their **intake of fluids**. If syncope persists, treatment with a **mineralocorticoid** may be initiated to help expand the intravascular blood volume.

Cardiac Syncope

Cardiac syncope is the result of a sudden decrease in cardiac output, leading to systemic hypotension, decreased cerebral perfusion, and a loss of consciousness. The differential diagnosis of cardiac syncope includes left ventricular outflow tract obstruction and arrhythmia.

Left Ventricular Outflow Tract Obstruction

Anatomic causes of left ventricular outflow tract obstruction (e.g., aortic stenosis, subaortic stenosis, hypertrophic cardiomyopathy) can be considered as a single cause of cardiac syncope. All of these causes limit cardiac output, especially during exercise, and all have as part of the physical examination a systolic ejection murmur. In children with a history of syncope and a significant ejection murmur, left ventricular outflow tract obstruction should be presumed and the patient referred to a pediatric cardiologist. Although the chest radiograph or ECG may suggest left ventricular hypertrophy, echocardiography is the best method to identify and describe left ventricular outflow tract obstruction.

Treatment of symptomatic aortic stenosis includes balloon dilation valvuloplasty and/or surgical valvotomy. Subaortic stenosis is treated by surgical resection. After resection of subaortic stenosis, there is a small but finite rate of recurrence despite successful initial resection. **Hypertrophic cardiomyopathy** can be managed by the use of a β-blocker (e.g., propranolol), calcium channel blocker, and/or with surgical resection (myotomy and myomectomy).

Limited participation in competitive sports, especially those that result in isometric exercise such as football, wrestling, and heavy weight lifting, may be required in patients with unrepaired and, in some cases, repaired left ventricular outflow tract obstruction. Decisions regarding participation in sports should be made in consultation with a pediatric cardiologist.

Ventricular Tachycardia

Patients with VT (see Chapter 75, "Tachycardia") can present with a history of palpitations, chest pain, or syncope. VT presents as a wide QRS tachycardia and can be a medical emergency because this rhythm can rapidly deteriorate into ventricular fibrillation. For patients who are hemodynamically stable, an attempt at intravenous access and pharmacologic conversion to sinus rhythm should be attempted. For patients who are not hemodynamically stable or who present with mental status changes, cardioversion is the treatment of choice.

VT may be idiopathic or may result from congenital or acquired heart disease resulting in ventricular dilation or hypertrophy, right ventricular dysplasia, anomalous left coronary artery from the pulmonary artery, a suture line in the myocardium, electrolyte imbalance, or drug ingestion. Emergent evaluation of VT should include assessment and correction of electrolyte disturbances including hypocalcemia, hypokalemia, and/or hypomagnesemia. In adolescents, a toxicology screen should be sent because illegal drug abuse (e.g., cocaine) may result in ventricular arrhythmia. New-onset VT can be caused by myocardial damage secondary to a process resulting in myocarditis. Patients who have undergone corrective surgery for congenital heart disease, especially tetralogy of Fallot, are at risk for ventricular arrhythmias. Other causes of VT include congenital long QT syndrome or prolonged corrected QT interval from other causes. Patients with a suspected history of VT require evaluation by a pediatric cardiologist.

Congenital Long QT Syndrome

In patients with a history of syncope and a family history of sudden death, it is essential to rule out congenital long QT syndrome as the cause of syncope. The corrected QT interval (QTc) is calculated from the surface ECG by measuring the QT interval in seconds from the onset of the Q wave to the end of the T wave and dividing this interval by the square root of the R–R interval in seconds. The QTc is independent of heart rate and outside the infant period has an upper normal limit of 440 milliseconds.

Children with congenital long QT syndrome may have life-threatening paroxysmal episodes of VT, specifically, a form of polymorphic VT known as torsade de pointes. If a child is found to have a prolonged QTc, the entire family, including all first-degree relatives, should be screened because several inherited forms of this disease exist. Evaluation includes a 12-lead ECG, looking specifically at the QTc interval, and Holter monitoring to measure the QTc at several time points at a variety of heart rates and to assess for occult ventricular arrhythmia. Often exercise testing is used to calculate changes in the QTc during exercise. In normal patients, the QTc remains constant or shortens slightly during exercise. In patients with congenital long QT syndrome, the QTc may lengthen during exercise.

Bradyarrhythmias

Symptomatic bradycardia caused by sick sinus syndrome or complete heart block can cause cardiac syncope. This is most commonly seen in children who have undergone cardiac surgery. Patients with transposition of the great arteries who have undergone an atrial switch procedure (Mustard or Senning procedure) or patients who have had a Fontan palliation have a high incidence of both atrial tachycardia and sick sinus syndrome. Patients who have had ventricular septal defect closure or who have L-transposition of the great arteries (congenitally corrected transposition of the great arteries) may suffer from late-onset complete heart block. These patients are typically cared for by a cardiologist and have routine annual follow-up examinations that include 24-hour Holter monitoring to evaluate for these arrhythmias. Symptomatic bradycardia in patients with congenital heart disease from sinus node dysfunction or conduction block after surgical palliation may require pacemaker placement. Syncope may also result from bradycardia caused by complete heart block resulting from **inflammatory/infectious diseases** such as rheumatic fever, myocarditis, Lyme disease, or endocarditis.

Neurologic Syncope

Loss of consciousness can be seen during seizures. It is important to elicit a history of convulsions or loss of bowel or bladder control during the syncopal episode to rule out seizures as a cause for syncope. **Migraine** headaches have also been associated with syncope. Finally, dizziness and syncope may be symptoms of depression, anxiety, panic disorder, somatization, and substance abuse. Unexplained syncope is likely to have a psychiatric etiology. If there are concerns for migraine headaches or seizure activity, the patient should be evaluated by a neurologist for further diagnostics and management. Brain imaging with an MRI or recording of brain electrical activity with an EEG may be warranted.

EVALUATION OF SYNCOPE

The American Heart Association, the American College of Cardiology, and the European Society of Cardiology have created guidelines for the evaluation of syncope. These guidelines review the current evidence on the diagnosis and management of patients presenting with syncope in an attempt to improve the quality of clinical practices and utilization of heath care resources. These guidelines recommend that the essential components of evaluation of children who present with syncope include a comprehensive medical and family history, a physical examination, and an ECG. Further initial diagnostic testing, including blood work and imaging tests, are not recommended.

Patient History

In patients who present with syncope as a chief complaint, questions regarding the history should be directed toward defining the circumstances under which the child fainted and thoroughly understanding the patient's past medical and family history.

- Were there definable triggers to account for the event such as a long period of standing, dehydration, or an emotional or vagal trigger?
- Did the child have palpitations prior to syncope?
- Did the child have convulsions or loss of bowel or bladder continence during or after the syncopal event?
- Is there a family history of syncope, arrhythmias, or sudden cardiac events?
- In suspected cases of NCS, a detailed history of diet is important, specifically, how much on average the child drinks in a day.

Physical Examination

The physical examination should be directed toward cardiovascular evaluation to help rule out cardiac syncope:

- Is there a significant systolic murmur?
- Are the heart tones normal?
- Is there a gallop rhythm suggestive of cardiac dysfunction?
- In younger children, is there evidence of hepatomegaly?

Laboratory Studies

Every child with syncope should have an ECG. This test is readily available and reliable. An ECG can help delineate those children with a prolonged QTc that can be life threatening. Placement of a Holter monitor or event recorder should be performed in any child suspected of an arrhythmia as the cause of syncope. This includes the child with a history of palpitations, a history of an irregular heartbeat following syncope, or in the child with syncope during exercise. Any patient with syncope and a significant murmur should have an echocardiogram.

APPROACH TO THE PATIENT

The most common cause of syncope in children is NCS. The child with symptoms consistent with NCS should have a screening ECG but does not need further evaluation unless syncope is recurrent. In a patient without symptoms consistent with NCS, an ECG should be performed to assess the QTc. If an arrhythmia is thought to be responsible for a syncopal episode, then Holter monitoring or an event monitor should be placed to attempt to document an arrhythmia as the potential cause. The child with recurrent syncope and a positive family history of sudden death should have an evaluation by a pediatric cardiologist for long QT syndrome. In a patient with syncope that occurs during exercise, or in a child with a significant murmur, evaluation by a pediatric cardiologist is indicated, and an echocardiogram should be performed. In a patient where seizures are suspected, evaluation by a neurologist is indicated.

Suggested Readings

Brignole M, Alboni P, Benditt DG, et al. Guidelines on management (diagnosis and treatment) of syncope—update 2004. Executive summary. *Eur Heart J.* 2004;25(22):2054–2072.
Cadman CS. Medical therapy of neurocardiogenic syncope. *Cardiol Clin.* 2001;19(2):203–213.

Driscoll DJ, Jacobsen SJ, Porter CJ, et al. Syncope in children and adolescents. *J Am Coll Cardiol.* 1997;29(5):1039–1045.

Lewis DA, Dhala A. Syncope in the pediatric patient: the cardiologist's perspective. *Pediatr Clin North Am.* 1999;46(2):205–219.

Massin MM, Bourguignont A, Coremans C, et al. Syncope in pediatric patients presenting to an emergency department. *J Pediatr.* 2004;145:223–228.

Pratt JL, Fleisher GR. Syncope in children and adolescents. *Pediatr Emerg Care.* 1989;5(2):80–82.

Strickberger SA, Benson DW, Biaggioni I, et al. AHA/ACCF scientific statement on the evaluation of syncope: from the American Heart Association Councils on Clinical Cardiology, Cardiovascular Nursing, Cardiovascular Disease in the Young, and Stroke, and the Quality of Care and Outcomes Research Interdisciplinary Working Group; and the American College of Cardiology Foundation In Collaboration With the Heart Rhythm Society. *J Am Coll Cardiol.* 2006;47(2):473–484.

Strieper MJ. Distinguishing benign syncope from life-threatening cardiac causes of syncope. *Semin Pediatr Neurol.* 2005;12(1):32–38.

Tachycardia

INTRODUCTION

Tachycardia can be defined as an **atrial or** a **ventricular rate in excess of the age-related normal range**. Table 75-1 describes the upper limits of normal.

There are two primary mechanisms for tachycardia:

- **Automatic mechanisms** of tachycardia arise from a focal area within the heart due to increased automaticity. Automatic tachycardia typically displays a "warm up" and "cool down" period at the initiation and termination of tachycardia.
- **Reentrant mechanisms** of tachycardia are caused by self-perpetuating, circular electrical circuits within the heart. Reentrant tachycardia typically initiates and terminates with an abrupt change in heart rate.

Tachyarrhythmias can be separated into two main categories based on the location of the tachycardia:

Supraventricular tachycardia (SVT) is caused by mechanisms of tachycardia originating above the ventricular myocardium.

Ventricular tachycardia (VT) is caused by a mechanism originating below the bundle of His typically within the ventricular myocardium.

 DIFFERENTIAL DIAGNOSIS LIST

SUPRAVENTRICULAR TACHYCARDIA
Automatic Mechanisms of SVT

Sinus Tachycardia
Noncardiac Etiologies of Sinus Tachycardia

- Exercise
- Fever
- Anemia
- Hyperthyroidism
- Excessive catecholamines—stress, pheochromocytoma
- Arteriovenous malformation
- Drugs—therapeutic, illicit
- Seizures

Cardiac Causes
- Heart failure\Myocardial dysfunction
- Congenital heart disease
- Cardiac tamponade
- Inappropriate sinus tachycardia

Ectopic (Nonsinus) Focus of Automaticity
- Automatic (ectopic) atrial tachycardia
- Multifocal atrial tachycardia
- Junctional ectopic tachycardia

TABLE 75-1	Upper Limit of Normal for Heart Rate
Age (years)	**Upper Limit of Normal for Heart Rate (beats/min)**
Birth–1	180
1–3	160
4–7	130
7–15	120
>15	100

Reentrant Mechanisms of SVT
- Atrial flutter
- Atrioventricular nodal reentrant tachycardia (AVNRT)
- Atrioventricular reciprocating tachycardia (AVRT)

VENTRICULAR ARRHYTHMIAS
Automatic Mechanisms of VT
- Accelerated idioventricular rhythm
- Right ventricular outflow tract tachycardia

Reentrant Mechanisms of VT
- Fascicular left VT—Belhassen's Tachycardia
- Scar related reentrant VT—related to ischemia or prior cardiac surgery

Others
- Ventricular fibrillation
- Torsades de pointes—long QT syndrome, electrolyte disturbance, drug toxicity
- Catecholaminergic polymorphic ventricular tachycardia

DIFFERENTIAL DIAGNOSIS DISCUSSION
Supraventricular Tachycardia
Automatic Mechanisms of Supraventricular Tachycardia
Sinus Tachycardia
Etiology
The normal pacemaker of the heart, the sinoatrial node, is located in the superior and lateral aspect of the right atrium. Sinus tachycardia occurs when the normal pacemaker of the heart accelerates the heart rate in response to alterations in physiologic conditions. Sinus tachycardia occurs related to increased sympathetic and decreased parasympathetic tone as a normal response to increased physiologic demands (e.g., exercise, fever, anemia) and as an abnormal response to certain pathologic changes (e.g., hyperthyroidism, pheochromocytoma, arterial venous malformation). Various medications and drugs of abuse that increase sympathetic tone or mimic sympathetic output or decrease parasympathetic tone can elevate the resting sinus rate (Table 75-2). Among the common medications that increase the sinus rate are stimulants, decongestants, caffeine, and β-adrenergic agonists. The normal physiologic response to increased metabolic demands and increased sympathetic drive is to increase cardiac output. Cardiac output is augmented

TABLE 75-2	Drugs Associated with Rapid Heart Rates

Prescription Drugs
Stimulants (e.g., dextroamphetamine, amphetamine, methylphenidate hydrochloride)
β-Adrenergic agonists (e.g., albuterol)
Methylxanthines (e.g., theophylline)
Tricyclic antidepressants (e.g., imipramine)
Anticholinergic agents (e.g., atropine, scopolamine)
Nonsedating histamines (e.g., terfenadine)

Over-the-Counter Drugs
Decongestants (e.g., pseudoephedrine)
Diet aids (e.g., phenylpropanolamine)
Inhaled bronchodilators (e.g., albuterol)
Caffeine-containing products

Drugs of Abuse
Nicotine
Cocaine
Amphetamines
Alcohol
Marijuana
LSD
Phencyclidine
Amyl nitrate

either by increasing the stroke volume or the heart rate (or both). During infancy, the heart is less able to increase stroke volume; therefore, the cardiac output is primarily augmented by an increase in heart rate.

Cardiac causes for sinus tachycardia include any condition that depresses myocardial function (e.g., myocarditis, pericarditis, endocarditis) or increase cardiac output demand including cardiac lesions resulting in congestive heart failure from large left-to-right intracardiac shunts, atrioventricular valve regurgitation, or left ventricular outflow tract obstruction (aortic stenosis or coarctation of the aorta). Inappropriate sinus tachycardia occurs secondary to enhanced automaticity within the sinus node tissue itself as opposed to a secondary effect of external metabolic or pharmacologic stressors. It is a rare form of sinus tachycardia and is a diagnosis of exclusion.

Clinical Features

Patients with sinus tachycardia may be asymptomatic or minimally symptomatic with complaints of palpitations or dizziness and lightheadedness with standing. Symptoms depend on the age of the patient and the underlying etiology of the sinus tachycardia.

Evaluation

A 12-lead electrocardiogram (ECG) should be obtained for determination of P-wave axis. During sinus tachycardia, the P-wave axis is 0° to 90° and the QRS complex is narrow, unless there is associated conduction delay (e.g., bundle branch block or rate dependent aberrancy). There is typically a "warm-up" and "cool-down" periods as well as beat-to-beat variation to the heart rate, although heart rate variability is diminished in most physiologic states resulting in sinus tachycardia.

A thorough physical examination including blood pressure assessment, complete blood cell count, glucose level, thyroid function tests, and 24-hour urine catecholamine studies may be indicated for evaluation of underlying disease processes associated with sinus tachycardia. Often, observing the patient on a monitor for a short period of time helps in the diagnosis.

Treatment

Treatment of nonphysiologic sinus tachycardia is usually geared toward correction of the underlying abnormality, such as infection, anemia, or hyperthyroidism. In patients diagnosed with inappropriate sinus tachycardia, β-blockers or calcium channel blockers may be considered for rate control.

Automatic (Ectopic) Atrial Tachycardia
Etiology

Automatic (ectopic) atrial tachycardia is an automatic tachycardia that arises from the atrial myocardium at an area outside of the sinus node. It is typically identified on an ECG by an abnormal P-wave axis or P wave with a different morphology from that seen during sinus rhythm on a previous ECG. It can be difficult to distinguish ectopic atrial tachycardia from sinus tachycardia if the ectopic focus is in the high right atrium (near the sinus node) and has a normal P-wave axis. In some instances, the PR interval maybe prolonged or there maybe atrioventricular block as an indicator that there is an ectopic as opposed to sinus tachycardia. Similar to other automatic mechanisms, automatic (ectopic) atrial tachycardia typically has a "warm-up" and "cool-down" phases.

Treatment

The necessity and type of treatment for automatic (ectopic) atrial tachycardia largely depends on associated clinical findings, effects on cardiac function and the percentage of time a patient is in tachycardia. Because automatic (ectopic) atrial tachycardia is often self-limiting and resolves spontaneously, patient with infrequent episodes of tachycardia and normal cardiac function can be monitored without medications. In patients with more incessant tachycardia or with deleterious effects on cardiac function, antiarrhythmic medications and transcatheter ablation are options for tachycardia control.

Reentrant Mechanisms of Supraventricular Tachycardia
Atrial Flutter
Etiology

Atrial flutter is caused by a reentrant circuit, which is completely contained within the atrium and does not require the atrioventricular node (AN) or ventricle to sustain tachycardia. By definition, the atrial flutter circuit revolves around the tricuspid valve and uses slowed conduction through the tricuspid valve "isthmus" to propagate the tachycardia. Atrial flutter in healthy pediatric patients is rare though a similar form of tachycardia can be seen in patients with a history of atrial scar secondary to cardiac surgical repair. After cardiac surgery, lines of scar result from incisions and prior suture lines. These suture lines can be a central obstacle for an atrial reentry loop of tachycardia. Because the tachycardia does not necessarily utilize the tricuspid valve or isthmus, these tachycardias are frequently referred to as intra-atrial tachycardia. Intra-atrial tachycardia is frequently seen in patients after the Mustard/Senning operation for D-transposition of the great arteries or following the Fontan operation for single-ventricle heart disease. The atrial rate is dependent on patient size and age. In infants, flutter rates are typically between 350 and 450 beats/minute and in the adult population the atrial rate is typically between 250 and 350 beats/minute. In patients with significant atrial disease, the rate of atrial flutter can be significantly slower than is typically seen in healthy similarly aged populations. The ventricular response rate can vary based on the degree of atrioventricular block and the percent of atrial beats that are conducted to the ventricle. Classic "saw-toothed" flutter waves are typically seen in the inferior leads (II, III, and aVF) though this can be atypical in patients with a history of scar or when on antiarrhythmic medications.

Treatment
Long-term treatment involves antiarrhythmic medications or transvenous cardiac ablation. Adenosine administration can be diagnostic but will not terminate atrial flutter. Acute termination requires direct current cardioversion.

 HINT: Adenosine or vagal maneuvers may be diagnostic, in that flutter waves can often be better seen during the time period of transient atrioventricular nodal block.

Atrioventricular Node Reentrant Tachycardia
Etiology
The underlying mechanism is two electrical pathways within the AV node. One pathway typically has "slow" conduction while the other has "fast" conduction. The electrical circuit uses the slow and fast pathways to create a circular electrical loop. The entire electrical circuit is contained within the AV node and perinodal tissue and does not necessitate either atrial or ventricular activation to sustain tachycardia.

Clinical Features
Symptoms of tachycardia typically arise in early adolescence into adulthood and present during times of high sympathetic tone like exercise. The frequency and duration of the tachycardia can be affected by exogenous drugs and caffeine. Patients typically complain of palpitations that can last for minutes to hours. Patients may complain of dizziness or lightheadedness during tachycardia episodes.

Atrioventricular Reciprocating Tachycardia
Etiology
AVRT is the most common type of reentrant tachycardia seen in infants and school aged children. The underlying mechanism is an abnormal accessory pathway (electrical connection) between the atrial and the ventricular myocardium. The electrical

circuit uses the accessory pathway and the normal AV nodal pathway to create the electrical loop. Rarely a patient may have multiple accessory pathways and can use any combination of the accessory pathways and/or the AV node to create the electrical circuit. Accessory pathways can pass electrical activity from the atrium to the ventricle (antegrade), the ventricular to the atrium (retrograde) or both. Pathways that allow for antegrade electrical conduction from the atrium to the ventricle have early ventricular activation (**ventricular pre-excitation**) during sinus rhythm and present with a **delta wave** on ECG. The combination of ventricular pre-excitation and clinical tachycardia is called Wolff-Parkinson-White syndrome. An accessory pathway that allows only retrograde conduction is "concealed" and will have a normal resting ECG.

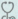 **HINT:** There are generally two epidemiologic peaks of age of presentation: infancy and school age.

Clinical Features

Patients with AVRT may be minimally symptomatic or may complain of palpitations, chest pain, or lightheadedness. Symptoms often depend on the age of the patient and the duration of the tachycardia and can present at rest or with activity. Tachycardia is difficult to recognize in otherwise healthy infants, and often not recognized until there has been an effect on cardiac function. Infants in continuous tachycardia for more than 24 to 48 hours may have cool extremities and pallor, suggesting low cardiac output. Infants often present with poor feeding or emesis. Patients with ventricular pre-excitation are at an increased risk for atrial fibrillation. If there is rapid conduction down the accessory pathway from the atrium to the ventricular during atrial fibrillation there is the potential for ventricular fibrillation induction and sudden death.

On admission, the patient's heart rate, blood pressure, and intravascular status should be assessed. A 12-lead ECG and rhythm strip during tachycardia should be obtained. It is important to answer the following questions: Is the RR interval regular? Can P waves be identified, and if so, what is the relationship to the QRS complex? How does this ECG differ from the patient's baseline ECG? **Ventricular pre-excitation** appears on the resting ECG as a short PR interval accompanied by a "delta wave" (i.e., slurring of the initial component of the QRS complex, as a result of ventricular pre-excitation).

 HINT: If the patient complains of palpitations, but no documented rhythm disturbance is seen on the 12-lead ECG, 24-hour ambulatory Holter monitoring, transtelephonic recordings, or exercise testing may be helpful.

Treatment of AVNRT/AVRT
Acute Treatment
Vagal maneuvers. Vagal maneuvers induce a parasympathetic response, which in many patients can terminate an episode of tachycardia. Common vagal maneuvers include the Valsalva maneuver, standing the patient on his head, blowing through

a restrictive straw or inducing the diving reflex by briefly placing a plastic bag with ice and water on the patient's face.

Adenosine. Adenosine causes a profound atrioventricular nodal refractoriness; blocking conduction from the atrium to the ventricle. Adenosine must be given rapidly via intravenous bolus (0.1 to 0.3 mg/kg to a maximum dose of 12 mg) while a 12-lead ECG is continuously running.

Direct current cardioversion. If the patient is hemodynamically compromised, synchronized direct current cardioversion (0.5 to 1 J/kg) is the most effective means of terminating SVT.

Transesophageal or transvenous atrial or ventricular pacing can also be effective in acute situations. These procedures should be attempted only by an experienced cardiologist.

Long-Term Treatment of Supraventricular Tachycardia

Digoxin is a potential first-line medication for atrioventricular reentrant tachycardia caused by a concealed accessory pathway or atrioventricular nodal tachycardia. The theoretical risk of potentiating antegrade accessory pathway conduction in patients with ventricular pre-excitation makes the use of digoxin in patients with pre-excitation contraindicated.

β-Blockers (e.g., propranolol, atenolol, nadolol) should be the first-line agent in all patients with ventricular pre-excitation and can be used as first line in other forms of AVRT and AVNRT. Side effects of β-blockers include fatigue, bronchospasm, hypoglycemia, and/or exercise intolerance.

Procainamide, flecainide, sotalol, and amiodarone are alternative second-line agents in the treatment of SVT and occasionally first-line medications in tachycardia that is difficult to control. Careful attention should be paid to myocardial performance, proarrhythmia, and hepatic and thyroid dysfunction depending on the choice of antiarrhythmic drug.

Transvenous catheter ablation is a potentially curative procedure. Infants and small children <15 kg are at increased procedural risk and ablation is typically used only after medication failure and significant clinical tachycardia. Patients with ventricular pre-excitation and a rapidly conducting, "high risk," accessory pathway should consider catheter ablation, even in the absence of a history of tachycardia, as the risk of the procedure may well be less than the risk of sudden death associated with atrial fibrillation.

Ventricular Tachycardia

Etiology

An episode of three or more consecutive ventricular beats at a rate defined as tachycardia for age is defined as **VT.** Ventricular rhythms at a rate slower than the age defined rate for tachycardia, but faster than the intrinsic rhythm are termed **accelerated idioventricular rhythms.**

Isolated finding. VT can be an isolated finding in children with otherwise normal hearts and is usually monomorphic and suppressed with exercise. Right ventricular outflow tract tachycardia and LV fascicular tachycardia are two forms of VT seen in otherwise healthy pediatric patients.

TABLE 75-3	Structural Heart Disease Associated with Tachycardia
Defect	**Type of Tachycardia**
Congenital Heart Disease	
Mitral valve prolapse	SVT
Aortic valve stenosis or regurgitation	VT
Ebstein anomaly of the tricuspid valve	SVT (WPW) commonly, VT less commonly
Tetralogy of Fallot	VT and SVT
Mustard/Senning repair of D-TGA	SVT (particularly atrial flutter)
Fontan repair of single ventricle	SVT (particularly atrial flutter)
Cardiomyopathy	
Hypertrophic cardiomyopathy	SVT, VT
Dilated cardiomyopathy	SVT, VT
Arrhythmogenic right ventricular dysplasia	VT (monomorphic, left bundle branch block)
Miscellaneous Causes	
Eisenmenger complex (pulmonary vascular disease and pulmonary hypertension)	VT
Cardiac tumor (atrial myxoma, rhabdomyosarcoma)	SVT, VT (depending on tumor site)

D-TGA, D-transposition of the great arteries; *SVT,* supraventricular tachycardia; *VT,* ventricular tachycardia; *WPW,* Wolff–Parkinson–White syndrome.

Structural heart defects. VT can be associated with structural heart defects (Table 75-3) and is often inducible with exercise and other catecholamine stimulation.

Torsades de pointes ("twisting of the point") is a variant of polymorphic VT in which the QRS morphology changes over time. Torsades de pointes can be associated with any of the forms of long QT syndrome (Table 75-4).

Ventricular fibrillation is rare in the pediatric population and characterized by rapid, bizarre, chaotic electrical activity without any effective cardiac output. Ventricular fibrillation may be seen in children with the long QT syndrome or cardiomyopathy, after cardiac surgery, or rarely in association with atrial fibrillation and antegrade accessory pathway conduction (ventricular pre-excitation).

Clinical Features
Symptoms generally depend on the age of the patient and the rate and duration of the VT. Patients may present with simple palpitations, syncope, signs of low cardiac output, shock, or "sudden death."

Evaluation
In a clinically stable patient, a complete history and physical examination should be performed, with particular attention to the patient's vital signs and any underlying structural heart disease. The corrected QT interval should be determined and a detailed family history regarding sudden death, history of congenital heart disease, and deafness should be taken (some syndromes are associated with long QT and deafness). A 12-lead ECG should be obtained to determine QRS duration, morphology, axis, and ventriculo-atrial relationship. If a prior ECG is available,

TABLE 75-4	Causes of Prolonged QT Interval

Congenital
Hereditary
Long QT syndrome
Brugada syndrome
Right ventricular dysplasia
Sporadic

Acquired
Electrolyte abnormalities
Hypocalcemia
Hypomagnesemia
Metabolic disturbances
    Malnutrition
    Liquid protein diets
Drugs
    Phenothiazines (e.g., haloperidol)
    Tricyclic antidepressants (e.g., imipramine)
    Nonsedating antihistamines (e.g., terfenadine)
    Class Ia antiarrhythmic agents (e.g., quinidine)
    Class III antiarrhythmic agents (e.g., amiodarone)
Central nervous system trauma
Cardiac abnormalities
    Ischemia
    Mitral valve prolapse
    Myocarditis
Intraventricular conduction abnormalities
    Bundle branch block

the two should be compared. A tachycardia originating below the bundle of His typically has a wide QRS complex, with a different QRS axis from that seen in patients in sinus rhythm though infants and children may have a relatively narrow QRS complex. Atrioventricular dissociation may be present. The ventricular rate is typically 100 to 350 beats/minute. Accelerated idioventricular rhythm ("slow VT") has the same ECG characteristics as VT, with a slower rate (80 to 120 beats/minute). Consultation with a cardiologist is indicated for all patients suspected of having ventricular arrhythmias.

Treatment

Treatment for VT, like that for SVT, is based on the underlying mechanism and any treatment should be in made in conjunction with an experience cardiologist.

VT with hemodynamic compromise. If the patient has hemodynamic compromise, synchronized cardioversion with 1 to 4 J/kg (adult: 100 to 360 J) should be used (lower energies are likely needed if biphasic shock is used), and cardiopulmonary resuscitation should be initiated. Ventricular fibrillation should be treated with emergent electrical asynchronous defibrillation and initiation of advanced cardiac life support. Treatment with amiodarone or lidocaine should be used in conjunction with electrical defibrillation. In patients with long QT syndrome and torsades de pointes a bolus of magnesium should be considered as adjunctive treatment.

Acute, asymptomatic VT. All decisions should be made under the direct supervision of an experienced cardiologist and the patient must be continuously monitored for any signs of hemodynamic compromise. If there is any evidence of hemodynamic compromise, the patient should be electrically defibrillated. In stable patients in VT, amiodarone, lidocaine, β-blocker, verapamil or other antiarrhythmic medications maybe used for control of the tachycardia depending on the underlying mechanism.

Chronic Treatment of VT. Chronic treatment of patients with VT depends on the underlying mechanism. In patients with more benign causes of VT, close patient monitoring with or without antiarrhythmics for tachycardia control are viable options. Similar to SVT, transcatheter ablation is a successful long-term treatment for most forms of benign VT.

In patients with long QT syndrome β-blockers are used as a chronic medication. β-Blockers are the only medication demonstrated to decrease the mortality rate associated with this syndrome.

Patients with structural heart disease generally undergo an electrophysiology study. Medications that maybe used, alone or in combination, include mexiletine, phenytoin, β-blockers, and amiodarone. Patients who have had an aborted sudden death episode, those deemed high risk by electrophysiology study or by patient history typically undergo implantation of a permanent implantable cardioverter defibrillator.

Suggested Readings

Batra AS, Hohn AR. Consultation with the specialist: palpitations, syncope, and sudden cardiac death in children: who's at risk? *Pediatr Rev.* 2003;24:269–275.

Campbell RM, Strieper MJ, Frias PA, et al. Survey of current practice of pediatric electrophysiologists for asymptomatic Wolff-Parkinson-White syndrome. *Pediatrics.* 2003;111:e245–e247.

Hegenbarth MA; Committee on Drugs. Preparing for pediatric emergencies: drugs to consider. *Pediatrics.* 2008;121:433–443.

Reynolds JL, Pickoff AS. Accelerated ventricular rhythm in children: a review and report of a case with congenital heart disease. *Pediatr Cardiol.* 2001;22:23–28.

Tingelstad J. Consultation with the specialist: cardiac dysrhythmias. *Pediatr Rev.* 2001;22(3):91–94.

Thermal Injuries

INTRODUCTION

Thermal injury in children involves not only the **skin,** but also the **respiratory, circulatory, immune, and central nervous systems**. Successful treatment of pediatric thermal injuries requires comprehensive assessment and management. Management of burn injury is dictated by **assessment of burn severity,** determined by the mechanism, depth, and extent of injury.

DIFFERENTIAL DIAGNOSIS LIST

- Thermal causes—direct flame burns, contact burns, scald burns
- Chemical causes
- Electrical causes
- Radiation

DIFFERENTIAL DIAGNOSIS DISCUSSION

Thermal Burns

Thermal burns are the **most common type of burns** affecting children. They may result from contact with **hot liquids** (scalds), **hot surfaces, or flames**. Scald burns tend to be more extensive but more superficial than contact burns. Flame injuries are most often associated with inhalation injuries.

Chemical Burns

Chemical burns are caused by contact with **corrosive substances**. Contact with **acids** causes **coagulation necrosis,** whereas contact with **alkali** causes **liquefaction necrosis**. Alkali burns are typically deeper and more severe than acid burns. Chemical burns require **extensive irrigation** with water or saline to remove the corrosive agent and prevent further injury.

Electrical Burns

Electrical injury results from contact with a source of electrical current or from arcing of current near the body.

Electrical injury typically produces a **depressed entry wound** and an **exit wound** that appears "blown out." With high-voltage currents (>1,000 V), the extent of the underlying deep tissue damage is typically far in excess of that suggested by the appearance of the cutaneous burn. Both low- and high-voltage currents can cause **cardiac arrhythmias,** even in the absence of visible burns.

Patients exposed to significant electrical current should have an **electrocardiogram** to monitor for arrhythmia.

> **HINT:** Alternating current is usually considered more dangerous than direct current. Alternating current, found in most households, rapidly changes direction every second, typically 60 cycles/second. When in contact with a rapidly alternating electrical current, the child's muscles may not relax and allow the child to let go, causing increased contact time and injury.

Radiation Burns

The most common type of radiation burn in children is **sunburn**. It is typically **first degree** or, rarely, **superficial second degree**.

EVALUATION OF THERMAL INJURY
Patient History

The following information should be ascertained:

- Mechanism of injury
- Duration of exposure
- If the cause of injury was fire, whether the fire occurred in a closed space
- History of loss of consciousness
- Tetanus immunization status

Physical Examination

> **HINT:** Always consider the possibility of an intentionally inflicted injury. The following features may be cause for concern: inconsistent or implausible explanation (remember to relate the reported mechanism with the developmental age of the child); the presence of other abuse risk factors; burns to typically protected areas (e.g., the dorsum of the hand or back of the neck); burns in a "stocking-glove" distribution, particularly in the absence of splash marks; burns to the buttocks or genitalia; or multiple cigarette burns.

Burns are classified according to their **depth and extent** (Table 76-1). Depth of injury is assessed on the basis of the clinical findings and is classified as **superficial** (first degree), **partial thickness** (superficial second degree), or **full thickness** (deep second degree, third degree, and fourth degree). Initially, the percentage of body surface area (BSA) involved with partial- and full-thickness burns should be estimated using the **"rule of nines"** (Table 76-2). After the patient is stabilized, a

TABLE 76-1	Classification of Burns	
Type of Burn	**Affected Skin Layer**	**Appearance**
First degree	Epidermis	Erythema, hypersensitivity
Second degree		
Superficial	Upper (papillary) dermis	Erythema, blistering intact hairs, exquisite pain
Deep	Deep (reticular) dermis	Skin may be white or mottled and nonblanching, or blistered and moist; pain may or may not be present; hairs easily pulled
Third degree	Entire dermis	Dry, white, or charred skin; leathery appearance, painless, no hair
Fourth degree	Subcutaneous tissue	Same as third degree; may have exposed muscle and bone

more detailed assessment of the extent of burns is made using a modified **Lund and Browder chart**.

The patient should be assessed for signs of **inhalation injury** (Table 76-3). Significant inhalation injury may exist in the absence of any surface burns; therefore, a high index of suspicion should be maintained in the face of a suggestive history (e.g., fire in a closed space).

> **HINT:** The presence of signs of pulmonary injury early in the course is a poor prognostic indicator.

TABLE 76-2	"Rule of Nines"		
	Percentage of BSA		
Body Part	**Infant**	**Child**	**Adolescent/Adult**
Head	18	13	9
Anterior trunk	18	18	18
Posterior trunk	18	18	18
Upper extremity (each)	9	9	9
Lower extremity (each)	14	16	18
Genitalia	1	1	1

For small burns, a rough estimate of the affected BSA can be made by comparing the burn with the size of the child's palm (which represents ~1% of the BSA).
BSA, body surface area.

	Central Nervous	
TABLE 76-3 **Signs of Inhalation Injury**		
Pulmonary	**System**	**Skin**
Tachypnea	Confusion	Facial burns
Stridor	Dizziness	Singed nasal hairs
Hoarseness	Headache	Cyanosis
Rales	Hallucinations	Cherry-red color
Wheezing	Restlessness	
Cough	Coma	
Retractions	Seizures	
Nasal flaring		
Carbonaceous sputum		

 HINT: Frank shock is uncommon in the first 30 to 60 minutes after a burn. Its presence should prompt a search for other causes of shock (e.g., abdominal trauma with occult blood loss, spinal cord injury).

Laboratory Studies

For children with minor burns, no laboratory studies are routinely needed. The following may be helpful in specific circumstances:

- **Arterial blood gases.** Arterial blood gas measurements must be interpreted with caution; normal arterial blood gases are not reassuring in the presence of clinical findings. The arterial oxygen tension (PaO_2) and the calculated oxygen saturation are unaffected, even by significant carbon monoxide poisoning. Metabolic acidosis in a patient with inhalation injury suggests the possibility of cyanide toxicity.
- **Carboxyhemoglobin level.** An elevated carboxyhemoglobin level helps in making the diagnosis of carbon monoxide poisoning, but a normal level does not exclude it, especially if there is a delay in measuring the level.
- **Blood work.** A complete blood count and blood type and cross-match may be indicated for patients with concomitant trauma or extensive burns.
- **Electrolytes, blood urea nitrogen, creatinine, and serum creatine kinase.** Baseline electrolytes, blood urea nitrogen, and creatinine may be helpful if large fluid shifts are expected for extensive burns. A serum creatine kinase level should be considered for patients with electrical injury to assess the extent of deep tissue injury and rhabdomyolysis.

TABLE 76-4	Burn Center Referral Criteria (American Burn Association Criteria)

Major Burns: Burn Center Referral

Partial-thickness burns affecting >10% of the BSA in children

Full-thickness burns

Burns involving the face, eyes, ears, hands, feet, genitalia, perineum, or major joints that may result in functional or cosmetic impairment

Associated inhalation injury

Significant chemical burns

Electrical injury

Burns complicated by underlying illness or major trauma

Diagnostic Modalities

A chest radiograph is not helpful in the initial assessment of smoke inhalation because findings are usually delayed by 24 to 36 hours. Diagnosis should be based on **clinical assessment**.

TREATMENT OF THERMAL INJURY

The appropriate treatment depends on the severity of the injury. The American Burn Association defines criteria for major burns requiring referral to a burn center (Table 76-4).

Emergency Management of Major Burns

- **First, an airway must be secured.** Concomitant trauma is common in burn patients, and cervical spine immobilization should be maintained if injury is suspected. Because rapid edema formation can make airway management difficult, intubation should be considered early in patients with evidence of significant thermal injury to the upper airway.
- **Hyperbaric oxygen therapy** should be considered if any of the following are present: a carboxyhemoglobin level >30%, neurologic symptoms (confusion and disorientation, focal deficit, history of loss of consciousness), or cardiac disturbance.
- Consider **presumptive therapy with sodium thiosulfate** (25% solution), 1.65 mL/kg given intravenously over 30 to 60 minutes, to counteract cyanide toxicity.
- **Burns covering a large surface area cause substantial fluid losses and shifts, necessitating special fluid management,** with smaller children requiring relatively greater amounts of fluid (Figure 76-1). Lactated Ringer's is recommended

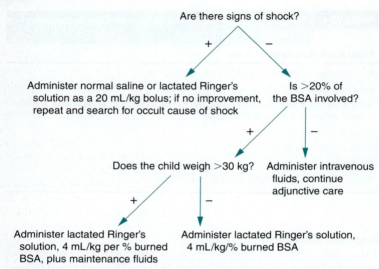

FIGURE 76-1 **Fluid replacement in a patient with major burns.** *BSA,* body surface area.

for fluid resuscitation during the first 24 hours. The amounts given in Figure 76-1 are totals for the first 24 hours: 50% of the total volume is administered over the first 8 hours after the occurrence of the burn, and the remaining 50% is administered over the subsequent 16 hours.

> **HINT:** Add maintenance fluids as well as dextrose for children <5 years or 30 kg. Monitor fluid status by maintaining urine output of at least 1 mL/ kg/hour.

- **Adjunctive care** of the patient with major burns includes the removal of all clothing from the burn areas. Adherent molten material (e.g., tar, metal) should be cooled but left in place. All burns should be irrigated with water or saline solution. Chemical burns require copious irrigation (15 to 30 minutes) with water; a small child may be placed in a sink for this purpose. Following irrigation, the burns should be covered with saline-soaked gauze or a dry sterile sheet if the burns are extensive.
- **Analgesics** (e.g., morphine, 0.05 to 0.1 mg/kg intravenously; fentanyl, 1.5 to 2 mcg/kg intranasally) should be administered early. Tetanus immunoprophylaxis should be administered as needed. Steroids and prophylactic antibiotics should be avoided. Nasogastric decompression and placement of an indwelling bladder catheter are needed for seriously injured patients.

- **Definitive wound management** should be undertaken only in consultation with the burn surgeon who will assume care of the child.

Emergency Management of Minor Burns

- **An open dressing** should be applied to small burns or burns in hard-to-dress areas. Burns should be washed with mild soap and water, and an antibacterial ointment (e.g., bacitracin polymyxin B) should be applied. No covering is needed. The wound should be washed at home and ointment reapplied two to three times daily until healed.
- **A closed dressing** is used for most burns in children. The clothing should be removed from the area, and the burn should be irrigated with water or saline solution. Chemical burns should be irrigated for 15 to 30 minutes. Analgesia (oral acetaminophen with oxycodone for small burns, intravenous morphine, or intranasal fentanyl for larger burns) should be provided, and then the burn should be washed again with mild soap and water and rinsed with saline solution. Loose or clearly nonviable tissue should be debrided with forceps. Intact blisters should be left undisturbed; ruptured bullae should be unroofed and debrided.
- Several **gauze dressings** are available, either plain or treated (e.g., Adaptic, Xeroform, Vaseline, Aquaphor). Silver sulfadiazine (1%) cream is applied to the wound surface or to the underside of the dressing, in a layer approximately 2 to 3 mm thick. Silver sulfadiazine should not be used for facial burns or if child has allergy to sulfa; bacitracin-polymyxin B ointment is an alternative. The entire wound surface is covered with the dressing, and then an outer absorbent dressing or roller gauze is applied. Silver-impregnated dressings (e.g., Acticoat, Mepilon-Ag) can also be used.
- Synthetic occlusive dressings (e.g., Biobrane, Transcyte) are increasingly being used by surgeons within the first 6 to 12 hours to decrease eschar formation, limit number of dressing changes, and expedite healing time.
- If the child has a second- or third-degree burn and her tetanus immunization status is not up-to-date, **tetanus immunoprophylaxis** should be administered.

The burn should be rechecked in 24 to 48 hours to assess for healing and signs of infection. Home dressing changes should be performed once or twice daily until healed, usually for 10 to 14 days. An analgesic (e.g., acetaminophen with oxycodone) should be provided for the first few days.

> **HINT:** Consider hospitalization or referral when there are concerns about loss of function (e.g., burns over the hands or joints), cosmetic results (e.g., large facial burns), or the risk of poor compliance with the treatment regimen. Final results depend largely on meticulous burn care.

APPROACH TO THE PATIENT

A structured algorithm for the approach to the patient with burns is presented in Figure 76-2.

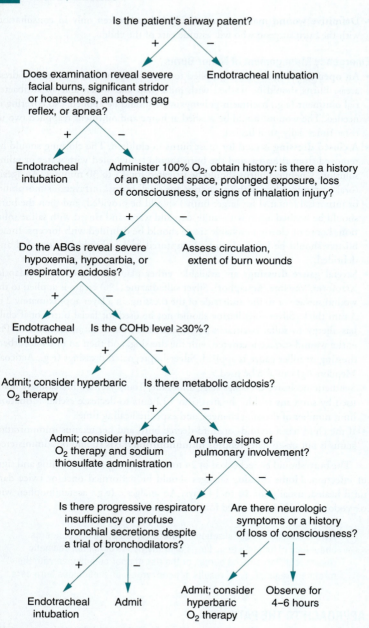

FIGURE 76-2 **Approach to the patient with major burns.** *ABGs,* arterial blood gases; *COHb,* carboxyhemoglobin; *O$_2$,* oxygen.

Suggested Readings

American Burn Association. Burn Center Referral Criteria. www.ameriburn.org/BurnCenterReferral Criteria.pdf. Accessed January 12, 2010.

Enoch S, Roshan A, Shah M. Emergency and early management of burns and scalds. *BMJ.* 2009;338:937–941.

Fidkowski CW, Fuzaylov G, Sheridan RL, et al. Inhalation burn injury in children. *Paediatr Anaesth.* 2009;19(Suppl 1):147–154.

Gomez R, Cancio LC. Management of burn wounds in the emergency department. *Emerg Med Clin North Am.* 2007;25:135–146.

Kagan RJ, Peck MD, Ahrenholz DH, et al. Surgical management of the burn wound and use of skin substitutes. American Burn Association white paper. www.ameriburn.org/WhitePaperFinal.pdf. Accessed January 12, 2010.

Mandal A. Paediatric partial-thickness scald burns: is Biobrane the best treatment available? *Int Wound J.* 2007;4:15–19.

Reed JL, Pomerantz WJ. Emergency management of pediatric burns. *Pediatr Emerg Care.* 2005;21:118–129.

Sheridan RL. Burns. *Crit Care Med.* 2002;30(Suppl 11):S500–S514.

Tibble PM, Perrotta PL. Treatment of carbon monoxide poisoning: a critical review of human outcome studies comparing normobaric oxygen with hyperbaric oxygen. *Ann Emerg Med.* 1994;24:269–276.

Urinary Frequency and Polyuria

INTRODUCTION

A perceived increase in urination is a common concern that a pediatrician may be asked to evaluate. A key task is to differentiate true polyuria from urinary frequency. **Polyuria,** defined formally as urine output 2,000 mL/1.73 m^2 over 24 hours, is usually caused by excessive fluid intake, a lack of release of antidiuretic hormone (ADH), tubular insensitivity to ADH, or an osmotic diuresis. In rare cases, it results from relief of urinary obstruction ("postobstructive dieresis") or is the polyuric phase of recovery from acute tubular necrosis. **Urinary frequency** not associated with polyuria is a common finding in children most typically caused by urinary tract infection (UTI), pollakiuria (frequent daytime urination), or chemical irritation.

 DIFFERENTIAL DIAGNOSIS LIST

Infectious Causes
- Pyelonephritis
- Meningoencephalitis
- Congenital cytomegalovirus and toxoplasmosis

Toxic Causes
- Recovery phase of acute tubular necrosis (typically caused by medications/toxins or hypoperfusion)
- Furosemide
- Aminoglycosides
- Phenytoin
- Demeclocycline
- Amphotericin B
- Vinblastine
- Cisplatin
- Lithium

Metabolic or Genetic Causes
- Inherited nephrogenic diabetes insipidus (NDI)

- Sickle cell disease
- Fanconi syndrome (e.g., cystinosis)
- Polycystic kidney disease
- Familial juvenile nephronophthisis
- Bartter syndrome
- Diabetes insipidus, diabetes mellitus, optic atrophy, and deafness syndrome
- Laurence–Moon–Biedl syndrome

Psychosocial Causes
- Primary polydipsia

Miscellaneous Causes
- Postobstructive diuresis
- Diabetes mellitus
- Idiopathic central diabetes insipidus
- Hand–Schüller–Christian disease
- Sarcoidosis
- Sjögren syndrome

Neoplastic Causes
- Craniopharyngioma
- Meningioma
- Glioma
- Metastasis—lymphoma, leukemia

Traumatic Causes
- Severe head trauma
- Hypophysectomy

Congenital or Vascular Causes
- Obstructive uropathy
- Cerebral hemorrhage

Urinary Frequency
- Cystitis
- Urethritis
- Constipation
- Pollakiuria
- Hypercalciuria
- Neuropathic bladder

DIFFERENTIAL DIAGNOSIS DISCUSSION
Central Diabetes Insipidus
Etiology
Central diabetes insipidus is urinary loss of water caused by impairment of vasopressin (ADH) production in the central nervous system (CNS) and may be **idiopathic, acquired, or inherited**. Approximately one-third of affected infants and children have the idiopathic (primary) form. Secondary causes include trauma, tumors (especially craniopharyngioma), hemorrhage, CNS infection, hypoxia, and Langerhans cell histiocytosis. The autosomal dominant form of central diabetes insipidus is rare.

Clinical Features
Children present with a **sudden onset of polyuria, nocturia, and polydipsia with a predilection for cold water**. Hypernatremia and dehydration do not occur if the thirst mechanism is intact and there is ample access to water. There are no specific abnormal physical findings in primary central diabetes insipidus.

Evaluation
Laboratory studies reveal a consistently **low urine osmolality**, but in the absence of dehydration, it is difficult to distinguish central diabetes insipidus from NDI and psychogenic polydipsia. A **water-deprivation study** is **diagnostic** for central diabetes insipidus when the serum osmolality is increased and the urine osmolality and the plasma vasopressin concentration remain decreased in the face of strict withholding of water. A brisk response, as measured by an increase in urine osmolality, to the administration of exogenous ADH is expected.

   Radiographic imaging of the head is necessary to exclude secondary causes.

Treatment
Treatment consists of replacement therapy with **desmopressin acetate,** a synthetic analogue of vasopressin administered either intranasally or orally. The dose is adjusted to the patient's needs. Hyponatremia can develop if the patient drinks

inappropriately while on therapy. **Specific treatment** is recommended **for secondary causes**.

Inherited Nephrogenic Diabetes Insipidus
Etiology
NDI is characterized by an **inability of the kidney to concentrate urine** because of insensitivity of the distal nephron to arginine vasopressin. NDI is most often found to be an acquired condition, secondary to drug ingestion (lithium, tetracycline) or systemic illness like sickle-cell disease or trait. Rarely, NDI is caused by a primary genetic mutation in the vasopressin V2 receptor or water channel protein aquaporin 2.

Clinical Features
Infants initially present with **dehydration, lethargy,** poor weight gain, or **unexplained fever**. **Older children** have **polydipsia and polyuria** with **failure to thrive,** possibly secondary to the preference of water over calorie-containing formula and foods. Recurrent episodes of dehydration and the resulting deleterious effects of rapid rehydration may affect psychomotor development.

Evaluation
A dehydrated infant with polyuria accompanied by hypernatremia is suggestive of inherited NDI. The diagnosis is **confirmed** by the presence of **hyposmolality of the urine** and the **lack of response to exogenous vasopressin** during periods of dehydration. The dehydration may need to be induced by a **water-deprivation study.** Fluids should not be restricted at home in an attempt to make the diagnosis. Serum levels of vasopressin are often normal or only slightly elevated. A **family history** of NDI is often sufficient to avoid performing this study. It is **imperative to exclude medications and systemic conditions** (e.g., sickle cell anemia, tubulointerstitial diseases) that cause an acquired form of NDI.

Treatment
Treatment consists of providing **sufficient free water** to prevent complications associated with dehydration. **Restricting sodium intake** may reduce urine output. **Thiazide diuretics** decrease extravascular volume and increase proximal tubular sodium reabsorption, reducing urine output. **Amiloride and nonsteroidal anti-inflammatory drugs,** particularly indomethacin, are also beneficial.

Primary Polydipsia
Etiology
Primary polydipsia is **water ingestion greater than** that **necessary** to maintain water balance. It may be the result of **behavioral abnormalities** (psychogenic polydipsia or compulsive water drinking) or **physiologic abnormalities** of the hypothalamus affecting the thirst mechanism (neurogenic polydipsia).

Clinical Features
Clinically, it is **difficult to distinguish primary polydipsia from diabetes insipidus**. Symptoms are similar to that seen in diabetes insipidus, although there may

not be nocturia or the desire for iced water. Because excess free water is ingested, the patient should not be dehydrated.

Evaluation

Patients with primary polydipsia may have serum sodium concentrations slightly below normal. A **water-deprivation study** may be necessary to differentiate this condition from diabetes insipidus. For safety reasons, this test should be done as part of an inpatient admission. A thorough **neurologic and psychologic examination** is recommended before labeling primary polydipsia as psychogenic in origin.

Treatment

Psychiatric counseling aimed at gradual weaning of water intake is recommended if it appears the polydipsia and polyuria are interfering with the patient's ability to function.

Urinary Tract Infection

UTI is a common disease in all stages of childhood that is important to identify because of potential long-term complications of renal scarring, hypertension and end-stage renal failure. Older children presenting with UTI may have the classic complaints of dysuria, frequency, or suprapubic, flank, or abdominal pain. In contrast, younger children, especially infants, are often well appearing with only fever as a presenting symptom (see discussion of occult UTI in Chapter 33, "Fever").

The **definitive diagnosis** of a UTI is via a positive **urine culture**. This should be done either via a midstream clean catch urine in a toilet-trained child or via bladder catheterization or suprapubic aspiration in younger children. A positive urine culture is usually defined as $>10^5$ colony-forming units (CFUs) of a single pathogen from a clean catch urine, $>10^4$ CFU from a catheter, or >100 CFU from a suprapubic aspiration. While waiting the 24 to 48 hours for a urine culture result to return, rapid tests can be used to decide whether to initiate antibiotics. **Urine dipstick** for leukocytes and nitrites has moderately good sensitivity and specificity and performs similarly to standard laboratory urinalysis. Tests with higher accuracy include **enhanced urinalysis** demonstrating >10 white blood cells/mm^3 or a positive Gram stain on uncentrifuged urine.

Empirical treatment of a UTI while waiting for culture results can be done either as an inpatient or as an outpatient. Strict criteria for admission would include age <2 months, inability to tolerate oral medication or maintain adequate hydration, inability to assure outpatient support or follow-up, or previous failure to respond to outpatient therapy.

The majority of UTIs are caused by **gram-negative bacteria** such as *Escherichia coli;* 5% to 10% of UTIs are caused by gram-positive bacteria. Increasing bacterial resistance to amoxicillin and other antibiotics has been observed, and empirical therapy may be guided by knowledge of local resistance patterns. Appropriate choices might include trimethoprim-sulfamethoxazole or cephalosporins such as cefdinir or cefixime. Quinolones are effective and safe in pediatric patients with complex medical conditions or multidrug resistance. Once culture results are available, the antibiotic regimen can be tailored to the specific sensitivity pattern.

After diagnosis of a UTI in a young child, a further workup of urinary tract anatomy may be indicated including tests such as renal ultrasound, voiding cystourethrogram, or dimercaptosuccinic acid scan. It is controversial whether the routine use of a cystourethrogram to identify **vesicoureteral reflux** after the first UTI is necessary.

Pollakiuria

Etiology

Pollakiuria, or the **sudden onset of increased urinary frequency,** may be related to stress and is seen most commonly in children 4 to 6 years of age.

Clinical Features

Children with pollakiuria present with **extraordinary urinary frequency,** voiding in low volumes as often as 15 times an hour during the day. Incontinence is absent, and affected children usually sleep through the night without awakening or wetting the bed.

Evaluation

Urinalysis and urine culture are recommended to exclude occult renal disease, diabetes mellitus, and UTI. A thorough **history** of potential **factors leading to stress** (e.g., marital discord, recent move, family illness) should be obtained.

Treatment

Reassurance and relaxation techniques are usually recommended in this self-limited condition.

EVALUATION OF POLYURIA AND URINARY FREQUENCY

Patient History

Key associated complaints include **polydipsia, nocturia, incontinence, enuresis, urgency, and dysuria**. Symptoms associated with tumors of the CNS, such as **headache or visual disturbances,** may be present. The patient may have a **family history** of NDI. Any past **history of urinary tract obstruction, acute renal failure, neurosurgery, malignancy, systemic illness, dehydration, or UTI** should be recorded, along with any **medications** recently taken. Finally, a **social history** with emphasis on stress factors should be obtained.

Physical Examination

Clinical evidence of dehydration may be present, especially in infants, if the urine output exceeds the fluids ingested. Growth parameters suggesting **failure to thrive** are seen in patients with NDI or renal insufficiency. **Ophthalmologic and neurologic examinations** must be performed to seek findings suggestive of an intracranial mass.

Laboratory Studies

- **Urinalysis, urine culture, urine osmolality, serum osmolality, and serum chemistries** (including a serum creatinine concentration) should be performed to exclude diabetes mellitus, most renal conditions, and UTI. A low urine

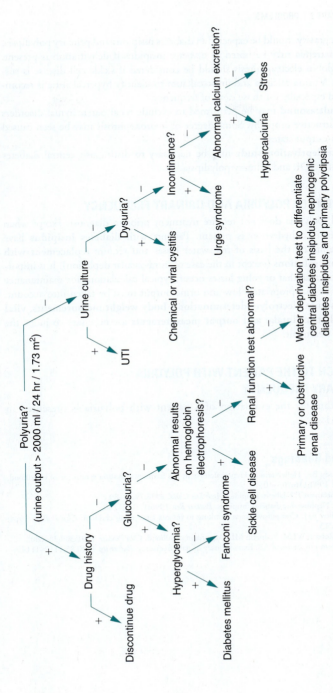

FIGURE 77-1 **Algorithm for the evaluation of polyuria and increased urinary frequency.** *CBC*, complete blood count; *ECG*, electrocardiogram; *EEG*, electroencephalogram; *EMG*, electromyelogram; *ENG*, electronystagmogram; *MRI*, magnetic resonance imaging; *NCV*, nerve conduction velocity; *UTI*, urinary tract infection.

specific gravity should be expected in diabetes insipidus and primary polydipsia. Hypernatremia may be noted in diabetes insipidus if dehydration is present. Hemoglobin electrophoresis should be considered if sickle cell disease is suspected. A urine calcium and urine calcium to identify hypercalciuria is recommended especially for those cases of frequency.

- **Renal ultrasound** may be performed to exclude renal parenchymal disorders and obstructive uropathy. Some degree of hydronephrosis may be seen caused by high-output states.

- A **water-deprivation study** may be necessary to distinguish central diabetes insipidus, NDI, and primary polydipsia.

TREATMENT OF POLYURIA AND URINARY FREQUENCY

In general, polyuria does not require treatment prior to diagnosis except when hypernatremic dehydration is present. Patients with **diabetes insipidus** have hypernatremia on the basis of free water losses and require **replacement with low-sodium solutions** (except in the case of intravascular depletion). It is important to recognize that ongoing losses occur; typical calculations for maintenance fluids will be inappropriately low and urine output must be taken into account. Frequent **serum electrolyte determinations, body weight measurements, vital signs, and strict intake and output measurements** are necessary to judge the efficacy of treatment.

APPROACH TO THE PATIENT WITH POLYURIA OR URINARY FREQUENCY

An algorithm for the evaluation of a patient with polyuria is presented in Figure 77-1.

Suggested Readings

Alon U, Warady BA, Hellerstein S. Hypercalciuria in the frequency-dysuria syndrome of childhood. *J Pediatr.* 1990;116:103–105.

Baylis PH, Cheetham T. Diabetes insipidus. *Arch Dis Child.* 1998;79:84–89.

Benchimol C. Nephrogenic diabetes insipidus. *Pediatr Rev.* 1996;17:145–146.

Horev Z, Cohen AH. Compulsive water drinking in infants and young children. *Clin Pediatr.* 1994; 33:209–213.

Leung AKC, Robson WLM, Halperin ML. Polyuria in childhood. *Clin Pediatr.* 1991;30:634–640.

Zoubek J, Bloom DA, Sedman AB. Extraordinary urinary frequency. *Pediatrics.* 1990;85:1112–1114.

Urine Output, Decreased

INTRODUCTION

Decreased urine output can be caused by either a **decrease in urine production (oliguria)** or an **obstruction to urinary flow**. Oliguria is defined as a urine output <0.5 mL/kg per hour in a child or adolescent or <1.0 mL/kg per hour in a neonate. Decreased urine output may result from prerenal, intrarenal, or postrenal factors. Oliguria may occur as the result of an **acute process** or an **acute exacerbation** of an unrecognized chronic kidney disease.

 DIFFERENTIAL DIAGNOSIS LIST

 HINT: The term **acute renal failure** has generally been replaced by a newer designation, acute kidney injury (AKI).

Prerenal
Decreased Intravascular Volume
- Dehydration (typically caused by gastrointestinal losses)
- Hemorrhage
- Inadequate fluid intake
- Sepsis (with capillary leak)

Ineffective Intravascular Blood Volume ("Edematous States")
- Hypoalbuminemia/decreased oncotic pressure
- Nephrotic syndrome
- Hepatic dysfunction

Impaired Cardiovascular Status
- Congestive heart failure
- Sepsis (with peripheral vasodilation and/or cardiac depression)

Intrarenal
Glomerular Causes
- Primary glomerulonephritis (e.g., acute postinfectious, membranoproliferative)
- Secondary GN associated with systemic disease (e.g., lupus nephritis)

Tubulointerstitial
- Acute tubular necrosis (ATN)
- Prolonged prerenal azotemia or ischemia
- Medications
- Toxins
- Pigment deposition—myoglobin or hemoglobin
- Acute interstitial nephritis (drugs, infections)

Vascular
- Hemolytic uremic syndrome (HUS)
- Renal venous or arterial thrombosis

Postrenal
Congenital or Anatomic
- Congenital obstructive uropathies (e.g., posterior urethral valves)
- Urinary stone
- Trauma
- Abdominal mass

Functional
- Acute urinary retention
- Neurogenic bladder

Others
- Syndrome of inappropriate antidiuretic hormone (meningitis, pneumonia)

DIFFERENTIAL DIAGNOSIS DISCUSSION
Prerenal Etiologies
Dehydration

Dehydration is the **most common cause** of **oliguria** in the pediatric population. The causes, clinical features, and evaluation are discussed in detail in Chapter 25, "Dehydration." Treatment is directed toward restoring intravascular volume. If dehydration is mild, **oral rehydration** may be attempted. If the patient cannot tolerate oral fluids, or if the dehydration is more severe, initial **fluid resuscitation with normal saline** should be performed, followed by oral or intravenous rehydration. In most patients, urine output improves within a few hours when these simple measures are used.

Edematous States

A variety of disorders can result in hypoalbuminemia, with resultant **decreased oncotic pressure** (e.g., nephrotic syndrome, see Chapter 62, "Proteinuria"). In these instances, there is adequate (and actually increased) total body volume, but it is not perceived so by the kidney because of the decreased oncotic pressure. This results in homeostatic responses that are identical to those of patients with dehydration, including avid salt and water retention. This is reflected in laboratory studies showing elevated blood urea nitrogen (BUN) to creatinine ratio, high urine specific gravity, and low urine sodium. Unlike dehydration, however, the treatment does not involve fluid administration (which will worsen the edema). Instead, the treatment of edematous states typically includes use of **diuretics, fluid restriction, and/or albumin** infusions based on the clinical situation.

> **HINT:** Because kidney function is preserved, prerenal azotemia is rapidly reversible if the underlying cause is corrected (e.g., restoring intravascular volume in a dehydrated patient). Intrarenal causes are not usually readily reversible.

Intrarenal Etiologies
Acute Glomerulonephritis (Typically Poststreptococcal)
See Chapter 39, "Hematuria."

Acute Tubular Necrosis

Etiology

Acute tubular necrosis is the **final common pathway of a number of renal insults,** including **prolonged prerenal ischemia, sepsis, toxicity, and pigment deposition.** ATN is a relatively common occurrence in severely ill patients in intensive care units; these patients often have multiple causes for the ATN (e.g., sepsis with hypotension plus aminoglycoside therapy).

Clinical Features

ATN traditionally has three phases:

Oliguric phase. The oliguric phase may last for days or several weeks. The hallmarks of this phase are decreased urine output and loss of renal concentrating ability, resulting in an elevated urine sodium level and a decreased urine specific gravity. As with other forms of AKI, hypertension may be present.

Diuretic phase. In the diuretic phase, urine output increases dramatically; urine sodium and water losses may be significant.

Recovery phase. In the recovery phase, urine output returns to a normal rate and concentrating ability returns.

Evaluation

The evaluation of patients with ATN is twofold: **assessing the clinical status** (including the volume and electrolyte status) and **determining the underlying cause,** which may not be immediately apparent.

Pertinent questions focus on prior medication use (especially antimicrobials such as aminoglycosides, vancomycin, and amphotericin B), recent radiocontrast dye studies, and toxin exposures (such as lead). Patients with hemoglobinuria or myoglobinuria may have a history of trauma, muscle pain, or pallor. Because prolonged ischemia from any prerenal cause can result in ATN, patients should be queried about recent gastrointestinal or blood losses.

Urinalysis in patients with ATN typically shows a low specific gravity and variable degrees of hematuria or proteinuria. The urine sodium level in the oliguric phase is usually elevated (>40 mEq/L). Specific tests as directed by the history (e.g., antibiotic levels and serum creatine kinase levels) may also be indicated.

Treatment

Treatment of ATN is similar to that of other causes of AKI. A significant number of patients with ATN, especially those with life-threatening conditions such as septic shock, require **dialysis.** ATN is not rapidly reversible because tubular damage has occurred. However, a significant number of pediatric patients, even those with prolonged oliguria, may have complete or partial recovery of renal functions.

Hemolytic Uremic Syndrome

Hemolytic uremic syndrome HUS is a syndrome of **microangiopathic hemolytic anemia, thrombocytopenia, and renal failure.** There are two main categories: **diarrheal-associated** (D+ or "typical") and **nondiarrheal-associated** (D− or "atypical"). Most cases of HUS fall into the former category.

Etiology

Diarrheal-associated HUS results from infection with Shiga-toxin-producing *Escherichia coli,* usually the strain O157:H7. Other infectious agents are also implicated in this form of HUS, including *Salmonella and Shigella* species. Infection usually results from **ingestion of contaminated foods,** especially ground beef, or from **person-to-person contact**.

Clinical Features

Patients with D+ HUS present with a **history of diarrhea, often bloody. Oliguria** often becomes evident as the diarrhea subsides. Patients also develop **pallor** and occasionally a **petechial rash. Hypertension** is common.

HUS can affect organs other than the kidney and gastrointestinal tract. Patients may have associated **central nervous system symptoms** (e.g., irritability, lethargy, and coma), **pancreatic dysfunction** (resulting in hyperglycemia), and **cardiomyopathy** (resulting in congestive heart failure).

 HINT: With the advent of improved supportive care for patients with renal failure, central nervous system complications have become the leading cause of mortality in patients with HUS.

Evaluation

Evaluation of HUS includes a careful **history** to determine exposure to contaminated foods or ill contacts.

Physical examination is directed toward **assessing volume status** as well as **neurologic status**.

Laboratory tests include serum electrolytes, BUN and creatinine levels, a glucose level, liver function tests and pancreatic enzyme measurements, urinalysis, and a complete blood count with careful examination of the smear for evidence of schistocytes and fragmented red blood cells (RBCs). Proteinuria, hematuria, and cellular casts are common urinalysis findings.

Treatment

Treatment of D+ HUS is **largely supportive**. Establishing the diagnosis early in the course of disease is essential to avoid complications (e.g., volume overload). As with other forms of renal failure, specific treatments for electrolyte abnormalities may be required. **Transfusions of packed RBCs** are given only if the hemoglobin level is <6 g/dL and should be administered slowly to avoid hypertension. **Platelet transfusions** should be avoided unless active bleeding is present. As many as 50% of patients with HUS require **dialysis. Consultation with a pediatric nephrologist** early in the course of disease is strongly advised.

Postrenal Etiologies
Posterior Urethral Valves
Etiology

Posterior urethral valves (PUVs) are the **most common cause of obstructive uropathy in infant boys**. The condition is caused by an **abnormality in urethral development** that results in the formation of mucosal folds, which act as valves, obstructing the outflow of urine.

Clinical Features

Patients usually present in the **first weeks of life** with **oliguria, poor intermittent urinary stream,** and a **distended bladder**. With the widespread use of screening antenatal ultrasounds, the majority of patients are now identified *in utero,* by the finding of **bilateral hydronephrosis** with or without oligohydramnios. **Older patients** occasionally present with **urinary tract infection** and a history of **poor urinary stream**. A **urinary concentrating defect is common** in this disorder, resulting in renal water and salt wasting. Patients with a history of severe oligohydramnios may have **pulmonary hypoplasia and respiratory distress**.

Evaluation

Specific evaluation of suspected PUV includes a **renal ultrasound** to confirm obstruction and hydronephrosis, and a **voiding cystourethrogram**. **Serum electrolytes and creatinine** should also be measured. A serum creatinine level obtained within the first 24 hours following birth is not useful as it largely reflects maternal renal function.

Urinalysis and urine culture should be obtained to assess for urinary tract infection.

Treatment

A **pediatric urologist** should be consulted if PUV is suspected. Initial treatment consists of placement of a **Foley catheter** to facilitate bladder drainage. Following bladder decompression, it is important to **monitor serum electrolytes and volume status closely**. Because of renal concentrating defects and a postobstructive diuresis, hypernatremia or hyponatremia, hyperkalemia, and metabolic acidosis may ensue. Once the electrolyte abnormalities are normalized, definitive **valve ablation** can be performed (often in the first week of life). Despite surgical correction of the obstruction, patients with PUV are at **risk for progression to chronic renal failure** due to renal dysplasia resulting from *in utero* obstruction. Therefore, **referral to a pediatric nephrologist** is recommended for patients with evidence of renal insufficiency or metabolic acidosis.

EVALUATION OF DECREASED URINE OUTPUT

Patient History

The history should be directed toward assessing the onset and severity of the oliguria, as well as determining possible causes, and includes assessment of the following:

- Fluid intake and losses (e.g., diarrhea, vomiting, and blood loss)
- History of poor feeding, pallor, cyanosis, or difficulty with exertion (may suggest underlying cardiac disease)
- History of poor growth, recent weight loss, polyuria, fatigue, or "unexplained" anemia (may suggest chronic kidney disease)
- Associated symptoms, such as macroscopic hematuria or flank pain (may suggest pyelonephritis, urolithiasis, or renal vein thrombosis)
- Toxin exposures (e.g., lead and mercury) and recent medication use (e.g., nonsteroidal anti-inflammatory agents)

- Recent illnesses and environmental exposures (e.g., recent skin or pharyngeal infection or exposure to undercooked meat)
- Results of prenatal ultrasounds (if obtained)

Physical Examination

Physical examination findings vary depending on the following causes:

- Dry mucous membranes, sunken eyes, poor skin turgor, and tachycardia suggest dehydration.
- Hypotension and poor perfusion are seen in patients with septic shock or cardiac dysfunction.
- A third heart sound (S_3) cardiac gallop may be noted if significant volume overload is present.
- Edema and hypertension are common in patients with AKI secondary to glomerular disease.
- Joint symptoms and rashes may be present in patients with systemic lupus erythematosus or vasculitic diseases.
- Patients with rhabdomyolysis have diffuse muscle tenderness, especially in the larger muscle groups of the legs and arms.
- Abdominal masses may signal an obstructing malignancy.

> **HINT:** A very distended, obstructed bladder may be mistaken for an abdominal mass.

Laboratory Studies

Initial laboratory studies in any patient with oliguria include the following:

A **serum electrolyte panel and BUN and creatinine levels** should be obtained first. If abnormal renal function is noted, calcium, phosphorus, and uric acid should also be assayed. A BUN-to-creatinine ratio >20 is suggestive of prerenal disease.

A **urinalysis** with microscopy is obligatory.

A **complete blood count** is indicated in almost all instances of AKI except in certain cases, such as medication-induced acute urinary retention.

Urine sodium level and fractional excretion of sodium (FENa). Measuring the urine sodium level is useful in determining whether the disorder is prerenal or renal in origin. A urine sodium level <20 mEq/L suggests a prerenal cause, whereas one >40 mEq/L suggests an intrinsic cause. Intermediate values of urine sodium are not diagnostic. Alternatively, a formal calculation of the FENa can be made:

$$\text{FENa} = [(\text{Urine sodium/Plasma sodium})/(\text{Plasma creatinine/Urine creatinine})] \times 100$$

FENa <1% suggests a prerenal cause, and values >2% suggest an intrinsic cause.

> **HINT:** Urinary sodium and FENa are not reliable for diagnostic purposes if diuretics were administered in the previous 24 hours.

HINT: Measurement of BUN-to-creatinine ratio and urine sodium/FENa are not useful in distinguishing among the *prerenal* etiologies because the physiologic response (sodium and water retention) is the same whether the patient has decreased intravascular volume (e.g., dehydration) or ineffective intravascular volume (e.g., congestive heart failure). The key to managing prerenal azotemia is an accurate *clinical* assessment of the patient's overall volume status, so that the appropriate therapy (e.g., fluid administration in dehydration vs. diuretics in congestive heart failure) can be instituted.

Additional laboratory studies are ordered according to the suspected cause of the renal failure, and they include laboratory investigation for past or current infection, drug levels, urine myoglobin, or serum creatine phosphokinase levels (if rhabdomyolysis is suspected). Complement levels (C3, C4) and serologies, including antinuclear antibodies and antineutrophil cytoplasmic antibodies, should be considered in all patients with suspected glomerulonephritis.

Diagnostic Modalities

A **renal ultrasound** is indicated in all cases of suspected obstruction and most cases of AKI, especially if unexplained. Additional **radiographic studies** are indicated based on the suspected cause of the AKI. A **renal biopsy** may be necessary to diagnose certain forms of glomerulonephritis and for patients with unexplained renal failure.

TREATMENT OF DECREASED URINE OUTPUT

The initial treatment for AKI from any cause is directed toward the potentially life-threatening complications of volume depletion or overload, electrolyte imbalances, and hypertension.

Volume depletion is treated with normal saline, 20 mL/kg administered as an intravenous bolus over 20 to 30 minutes and may be repeated up to two times until the patient's vital signs (heart rate and/or blood pressure) have stabilized and the patient has urinated. Rehydration can then be completed with oral or intravenous fluids. Packed RBC transfusions or cardiac inotropic agents are given if the clinical situation dictates. Normal saline should not be administered to patients with *ineffective* intravascular volume unless they also have clinical evidence of volume depletion.

Patients unresponsive to fluid administration or those who are overtly edematous may be given a diuretic challenge. Intravenous furosemide (2 mg/kg per dose) is given as a one-time dose. If a response is noticed, the dose may be repeated every 3 to 4 hours. If no response is seen, additional doses are of no benefit and may cause ototoxic and nephrotoxic side effects.

Patients with persistent oliguria should be fluid restricted to insensible losses (25% to 30% of maintenance requirements given as 5% to 10% dextrose in water) plus urine output (replaced milliliter for milliliter with a quarter to a half normal saline).

Specific therapies for electrolyte disturbances are outlined in Chapter 32, "Electrolyte Disturbances."

Check screening laboratory studies
(serum electrolytes, creatinine, BUN, CBC)

Do the history or physical examination suggest
acute retention or obstruction?

+

Place Foley catheter
Obtain renal ultrasound
Consider urology consult

−

Is the circulatory status adequate?

+

Diuretic trial; check urine sodium
if not already done

−

Trial of normal saline,
blood products, cardiac
inotropic agents as indicated

Is urine output improved?

+   **−**

Continue
diuresis

Restrict
fluids

Is the urine sodium level low?

+   **−**

Prerenal
azotemia

ATN
Intrinsic
renal disease

Urinalysis, renal ultrasound, electrolyte
management, nephrology consultation

FIGURE 78-1   Management of the patient with decreased urine output. *ATN*, acute tubular necrosis; *BUN*, blood urea nitrogen; *CBC*, complete blood cell count.

 HINT: If intravascular volume has been restored and minimal or no urine output is observed, other diagnoses should be considered, such as ATN. Continuing to administer fluid to such patients will be of no benefit and could precipitate volume overload.

APPROACH TO THE PATIENT

A structured approach to evaluation of a patient with decreased urine output is presented in Figure 78-1.

Suggested Readings

Hsu CW, Symons JM. Acute kidney injury: can we improve prognosis? *Pediatr Nephrol.* 2010;25:2401–2412.

Klahr S, Miller SB. Acute oliguria. *N Engl J Med.* 1998;338:671–675.

Lameire N, Van Biesen W, Vanholder R. Acute kidney injury. *Lancet.* 2008;373:1863–1865.

Vaginal Bleeding

INTRODUCTION

The complaint of vaginal bleeding can be concerning to parents, patients and clinicians. The differential diagnosis can be narrowed based on the patient's age and menarchal status. The clinician should maintain a high index of suspicion for pregnancy-related complications in post-menarchal patients, as these diagnoses can be life-threatening.

DIFFERENTIAL DIAGNOSIS LIST

Premenarchal Patients

Infectious Causes
- Infectious vulvovaginitis
- Genital herpes
- Condyloma acuminatum

Toxic Causes
- Exogenous estrogens

Neoplastic Causes
- Sarcoma botryoides
- Adenocarcinoma of the cervix or vagina
- Estrogen production from an ovarian cyst or neoplasm
- Hemangioma

Traumatic Causes
- Accidental trauma
- Sexual abuse
- Foreign body

Congenital or Vascular Causes
- Urethral prolapse

Miscellaneous Causes
- Vulvar skin disorders
- Neonatal withdrawal bleeding

- Precocious puberty
- McCune–Albright syndrome

Postmenarchal Patients

Infectious Causes
- Infectious vulvovaginitis
- Cervicitis
- Pelvic inflammatory disease

Neoplastic Causes

Traumatic Causes
- Accidental trauma
- Sexual abuse
- Foreign body

Metabolic or Genetic Causes
- Hyperthyroidism or hypo-thyroidism
- Hyperprolactinemia

Gynecologic Causes
- Dysfunctional uterine bleeding
- Abortion—threatened, incomplete, complete, or missed
- Ectopic pregnancy
- Polycystic ovarian disease

Hematologic Causes
- Idiopathic thrombocytopenic purpura
- von Willebrand disease

Miscellaneous Causes
- Chronic systemic illness (e.g., liver disease, connective tissue disorder)

DIFFERENTIAL DIAGNOSIS DISCUSSION
Vulvovaginitis

Vulvovaginitis is discussed in detail in Chapter 80, "Vaginal Discharge (Vulvovaginitis)." Bleeding, when present, is usually **minimal,** although a **blood-tinged discharge** is common in severe cases. *Shigella* and group A β-hemolytic streptococci are the most common causes of a bloody vaginal discharge associated with vulvovaginitis.

Vulvar Hemangiomas
Etiology

Bleeding can result following trauma to a vulvar hemangioma. Vulvar hemangiomas are common and generally **disappear as the child ages**.

Clinical Features

Patients usually present with **painless bleeding** and a **history of vulvar hemangiomas**. The bleeding is usually self-limited; however, heavy bleeding can be seen with cavernous hemangiomas, or in a child with a known or unknown bleeding disorder. Careful examination of the external genitalia identifies the source of bleeding. Vaginoscopy is not required if bleeding is limited to the external genitalia.

Treatment

When bleeding does not respond to **pressure, surgical ligation** may be required.

Trauma
Incidence and Etiology

Genital trauma is a **serious** and common cause of vaginal bleeding. The incidence is highest in children between 4 and 12 years of age. Most genital trauma results from a **straddle injury** (e.g., a child landing on the center bar of a bicycle), but **sexual abuse, accidental penetration, sudden abduction** of the lower extremities, and **pelvic fractures** must also be considered.

Clinical Features and Evaluation

- **In patients with straddle injuries** (a type of blunt trauma), a small ecchymotic area or a large vulvar hematoma may be noted. Hematomas are tender, tense, and rounded swellings that may enlarge if bleeding continues. Lacerations of the hymen or vagina may occur in association with straddle injuries; however, their presence should alert the physician to other possible sources of trauma.
- **Accidental penetration with pens and other small objects** is common in 2- to 4-year-olds. Lacerations can be superficial or deep and can extend to the peritoneal cavity. Isolated injuries to the hymen alone are rare, and careful examination of the vagina is mandatory, usually under anesthesia.
- **Lacerations of the vagina can also occur as a result of sudden abduction of the legs,** as in gymnastics or water skiing. These injuries can be difficult to

distinguish from injuries sustained secondary to sexual abuse. The paucity of other injuries helps distinguish these injuries from sexual abuse.
- **In patients with pelvic fractures,** injuries to the urinary system are more common than are vaginal lacerations. However, in complex fractures, lacerations of the vagina can be extensive, accounting for significant blood loss. A thorough examination is mandatory, including evaluation of the urinary system and rectum.

If bleeding is noted from the vagina, direct pressure should be applied to the area followed by vaginoscopy under anesthesia.

Treatment
- **Superficial abrasions and lacerations** of the vulva, if not actively bleeding, may be cleaned and left to heal.
- **Small vulvar hematomas** that are not expanding may be managed conservatively with ice packs and pressure.
- **Large or expanding hematomas** should be managed surgically with evacuation and ligation of bleeding vessels. At times, it may prove difficult to locate actively bleeding vessels. In this instance, vaginal packing should be placed and removed after several hours. Perioperative antibiotics are required.

Foreign Body
Foreign bodies placed into the vagina account for 5% of gynecologic visits in childhood. Most children **will not remember or admit** to placing an object in the vagina. The incidence is highest in children between 2 and 4 years of age. **Rolled toilet tissue** is one of the most common findings.

Clinical Features
The child presents with a history of a **foul-smelling, often bloody, vaginal discharge**. The vaginal bleeding is usually **bright red, scant, and intermittent**. A strong odor may be the most bothersome symptom.

Evaluation
On physical examination, the vagina is **erythematous** and a **foul-smelling discharge** is present. A **large foreign body may be easily palpated on rectal examination**. Smaller items (e.g., toilet tissue) may not be discerned.

Radiographic studies are of little use as most foreign bodies are not radiopaque.

Treatment
Vaginoscopy may aid in the diagnosis and removal. However, small items may be removed with **saline irrigation alone**. **General anesthesia** is frequently required for **removal of larger objects**. **Antibiotic therapy** is recommended before removing foreign bodies that may have been **in place >1 week**.

Urethral Prolapse
Etiology
Prolapse is thought to result from **increased abdominal pressure,** which could be caused by coughing or constipation. Some children are predisposed to prolapse secondary to a weakness of collagen.

Clinical Features

A **small hemorrhagic, friable mass surrounding the urethra** is the most common presentation. The bleeding associated with prolapse of the urethra is usually **painless** (because the urethra and vagina are so close that urethral bleeding may be thought to be from the vagina). The average age at diagnosis is 5 years.

The lesion can easily be **confused with condyloma acuminatum**. If the diagnosis is in question, **3% acetic acid** may be applied; condyloma acuminatum has an **acetowhite appearance**.

Treatment

If voiding is not inhibited, **local therapy** (i.e., with topical estrogen and sitz baths) may be all that is needed. The prolapse usually **resolves after 4 weeks** of therapy.

If urine retention or necrosis is present, surgical removal and catheterization are necessary.

Vulvar Skin Disorders

Most vulvar skin conditions involve the labia majora and labia minora and do not extend to the vagina or perianal area. **Seborrhea, psoriasis, and eczema** are the most common diagnoses. These lesions tend to be **pruritic**. The constant **scratching with subsequent infection** can lead to a bloody discharge similar to that seen in vaginitis. **Labial agglutination,** or labial adhesions, may also cause occasional bleeding. Adhesions occur due to lack of estrogen in the prepubertal patient. Often they are asymptomatic, but may cause irritation, bleeding (if they are traumatically separated), infections, or urinary obstruction. If the adhesions are symptomatic they may be treated with topical estrogen. If the patient is experiencing urinary symptoms, a catheter may also be necessary.

Neonatal Withdrawal Bleeding

Withdrawal of maternal estrogen after delivery causes **physiologic bleeding** in a small percentage of **newborns**. The bleeding is limited and usually **resolves within 1 week**. The parents may notice an increased blood-tinged discharge. **No treatment** is necessary unless bleeding persists for **>10 days**. At that point, a thorough examination should be performed.

Dysfunctional Uterine Bleeding

Dysfunctional uterine bleeding is defined as **any abnormal bleeding** from the uterus that is **not caused by structural abnormalities**. The average menstrual cycle has a mean interval of 28 days, with a mean duration of 4 days. The average blood loss is 30 mL/cycle, with an upper normal limit of 80 mL. A **menstrual cycle with an interval of <21 days, length >7 days, or blood loss of >80 mL is abnormal**.

Etiology

Anovulation, most commonly caused by an **immature hypothalamic-pituitary axis,** is responsible for >75% of cases of dysfunctional uterine bleeding. Without ovulation, and the resulting formation of the corpus luteum, there is no cyclic or monthly production of progesterone. The cyclic production and withdrawal of progesterone results in a normal period. Anovulation causes continuous estrogenic stimulation of the endometrium, resulting in a thick, unstable endometrium that sheds irregularly. Hypothalamic-pituitary axis immaturity can last for as many as **18 months after menarche**. McDonough and Ganett found that 55% to 82% of cycles in adolescents between menarche and 2 years after menarche were anovulatory. These percentages decreased with time.

Anovulation may also be caused by obesity, hyperthyroidism, hypothyroidism, hyperadrenalism, hyperprolactinemia, diabetes mellitus, polycystic ovarian syndrome, chronic systemic illness, substance abuse, eating disorders, physical or emotional stress, and excessive exercise.

Clinical Features

The presentation is highly variable ranging from amenorrhea to heavy irregular vaginal bleeding. Typically, a patient may experience several months of **amenorrhea followed by heavy bleeding**. The bleeding may last for weeks and be associated with cramping. Additionally, heavy menstrual bleeding with passage of clots may lead to significant pelvic pain.

Evaluation

Dysfunctional uterine bleeding is a **diagnosis of exclusion**. Organic lesions, pregnancy, and coagulation disorders must be ruled out. The history and physical examination should emphasize the **common and life-threatening conditions** in the differential, with **coagulation defects and complications of pregnancy** leading the list. If a patient is obese, hirsute, or displays signs of insulin resistance such as acanthosis nigricans, **polycystic ovarian syndrome** should be considered.

Studies helpful in the diagnosis include serum thyroid-stimulating hormone, fasting prolactin, follicle-stimulating hormone, luteinizing hormone, free testosterone, dehydroepiandrosterone sulfate, androstenedione, and 17-hydroxyprogesterone levels.

Treatment

Management of dysfunctional uterine bleeding in an adolescent **depends on the severity** of the bleeding, with the emphasis placed on stopping the bleeding and preventing recurrent episodes (Table 79-1).

- **Patients with mild bleeding** (i.e., bleeding at 20- to 60-day intervals without anemia) should be advised that the situation usually resolves after 1 to 2 years with maturation of the hypothalamic-pituitary axis and subsequent ovulation. If the patient has mild dysfunctional uterine bleeding and desires some form of contraception, a monophasic oral contraceptive may be prescribed that will provide the added benefit of regular menstrual cycles.
- **For patients with severe or recurrent dysfunctional uterine bleeding associated with anemia,** hormonal therapy is indicated. **Monophasic combined oral contraceptive pills are appropriate first-line treatment even if the patient is not sexually active**. Otherwise, progestational agents can be administered (see Table 79-1). Therapy should be continued for 6 to 8 months and then discontinued. Most patients have spontaneous maturation of the hypothalamus-pituitary

TABLE 79-1	**Treatment of Dysfunctional Uterine Bleeding**

Mild Dysfunctional Uterine Bleeding
Reassurance
Menstrual calendar
Oral contraceptives

Severe or Recurrent Dysfunctional Uterine Bleeding Without Anemia
Medroxyprogesterone acetate, 10 mg for 14 d each month
Norethindrone, 5–10 mg for 14 d each month
Oral contraceptives
Levonorgestrel-containing intrauterine system (LNG-IUS, Mirena®)—lasts for up to 5 yr
Etonogestrel implant (Implanon®)—lasts for up to 3 yr
Depot medroxyprogesterone acetate—lasts for 3 mo

Acute Anovulatory Bleeding in a Stable Patient
Oral contraceptives (35–50 mcg; one pill every 6 hr until bleeding stops)
After bleeding stops, taper oral contraceptives:
 One pill every 8 hr for 3 d
 Then one pill every 12 hr for 3 d
 Then one pill every day to complete 21 d
Continue on oral contraceptives for 3–6 mo **OR** switch to long-acting reversible progestin-only method (LNG-IUS, Implanon®, or DMPA)

Acute or Heavy Bleeding Associated with Anemia or Hypotension
Hospitalization
Transfusion if unstable
Intravenous conjugated estrogen (25 mg every 4–6 h) until bleeding stops
Begin monophasic combined oral contraceptives (35–50 mcg):
 One pill every 6 h for 3 d
 Then one pill every 8 h for 3 d
 Then one pill every 12 h for 3 d
 Then one pill every day to complete 21 d
Continue on oral contraceptives for 3–6 mo **OR** switch to long-acting reversible progestin-only method (LNG-IUS, Implanon® or DMPA)

axis with onset of regular menses after cessation of therapy. If patients continue to have irregular bleeding after stopping therapy, they must be reevaluated. In those adolescents also desiring contraception, the clinician should consider a levonorgestrel-containing intrauterine system (LNG-IUS), an etonogestrel implant (Implanon®), or Depo-Provera® (DMPA).

- **An acute episode of bleeding in a stable patient** may be treated with a 35 to 50 mg combined oral contraceptive (see Table 79-1). If the bleeding does not stop within 5 days, another cause for the bleeding, such as a coagulation disorder, must be considered. When the bleeding slows, the pills may be tapered as described in Table 79-1. The patient should be maintained on the pills for at least 3 months, or longer if sexually active. Similarly, once the acute bleeding has stopped, and if long-acting contraception is desired, the patient may choose to switch to LNG-IUS, Implanon®, or DMPA.
- **Patients who have undergone heavy bleeding leading to hypovolemia or anemia** should be hospitalized for therapy and coagulation studies. Intravenous

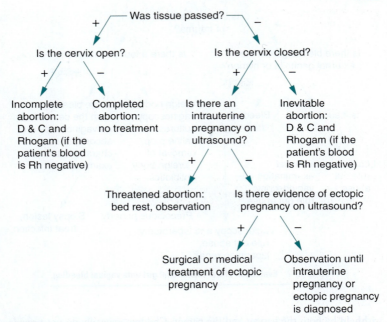

FIGURE 79-1   Evaluation of a patient with a positive pregnancy test and vaginal bleeding. *D&C,* dilation and curettage.

conjugated estrogens are given every 4 to 6 hours until the bleeding stops, usually 24 to 48 hours after initiating therapy. Once the bleeding has stopped, the patient may be started on oral contraceptives (see Table 79-1). Dilation and curettage is to be avoided in adolescents; however, when medical therapy fails, it may be necessary for diagnostic purposes. Along with dilation and curettage, hysteroscopy may be helpful in making a diagnosis.

Pregnancy

Bleeding in early pregnancy is common. In most cases, it is scant and has little clinical significance. However, bleeding may be a sign of ectopic pregnancy, which is life threatening. Therefore, pregnancy must be ruled out in all adolescent patients with bleeding, regardless of the history. Figure 79-1 illustrates the approach to a patient with a positive pregnancy test and vaginal bleeding. A gynecologic consultation is mandatory in patients who have bleeding in pregnancy.

EVALUATION OF VAGINAL BLEEDING
Patient History

The history is always helpful when evaluating children with vaginal bleeding. The physician, however, must be aware that much **information may be intentionally**

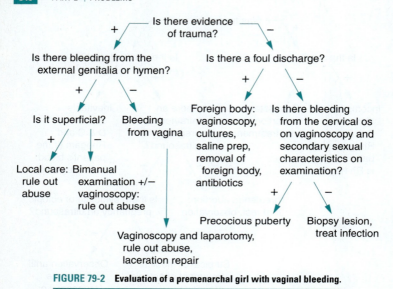

FIGURE 79-2 **Evaluation of a premenarchal girl with vaginal bleeding.**

withheld by both the patient and the parent. Children generally do not provide information regarding foreign bodies, manipulation, or sexual abuse. Likewise, parents do not often admit to sexual abuse. Whenever a child presents with vaginal bleeding, regardless of the history, other **indications of abuse must be sought** (see Chapter 69, "Sexual Abuse").

Physical Examination

A careful and thorough physical and gynecologic examination is mandatory, and may require sedation. Consultation with a **gynecologist or adolescent medicine specialist** is essential.

APPROACH TO THE PATIENT

Figure 79-2 depicts the approach to a premenarchal girl with vaginal bleeding.

Suggested Readings

Altchek A. Common problems in pediatric gynecology. *Compr Ther.* 1984;10:19–28.
Behrman RE, Kliegman RM, Nelson WE, et al. *Nelson Textbook of Pediatrics.* 14th ed. Philadelphia, PA: WB Saunders; 1992.
Carpenter SE, Rock JA. *Pediatric and Adolescent Gynecology.* Philadelphia, PA: Lippincott-Raven; 1992.
Emans JH, Goldstein DP. *Pediatric and Adolescent Gynecology.* Boston, MA: Little, Brown; 1990.
Grossman M, Dieckmann RA. *Pediatric Emergency Medicine.* Philadelphia, PA: JB Lippincott; 1991.
Hertweck SP. Dysfunctional uterine bleeding. *Obstet Gynecol Clin North Am.* 1992;19:129–149.
Reece RM. *Manual of Emergency Pediatrics.* Philadelphia, PA: WB Saunders; 1992.
Taber BZ. *Manual of Gynecologic and Obstetric Emergencies.* 2nd ed. Philadelphia, PA: WB Saunders; 1984.

Vaginal Discharge (Vulvovaginitis)

INTRODUCTION

Vulvovaginitis, a common problem for both pediatric and adolescent patients, is an entity consisting of **vaginal and vulvar irritation** associated with **vaginal discharge.** A **lack of estrogen,** which protects and toughens the skin in the genital region, renders **premenarchal girls particularly susceptible** to vulvovaginitis. **Poor hygiene,** a common problem in young girls, also contributes to the problem. Some causes of vulvovaginitis are more prevalent in adolescents (e.g., *Candida* vulvovaginitis).

DIFFERENTIAL DIAGNOSIS LIST

Infectious Causes

Bacterial Infection
- Group A β-hemolytic streptococci
- *Staphylococcus aureus*
- *Gardnerella vaginalis*
- *Streptococcus pneumoniae*
- *Neisseria gonorrhoeae, N. meningitidis*
- *Chlamydia trachomatis*
- *Shigella flexneri*
- *Yersinia enterocolitica*
- *Haemophilus influenzae*

Fungal Infection
- *Candida albicans*
- *C. glabrata*

Parasitic Infection
- *Trichomonas vaginalis*
- *Enterobius vermicularis* (pinworm)

Viral Infection
- Herpes simplex virus (HSV)

Neoplastic Causes
- Sarcoma botryoides

Traumatic Causes
- Sexual abuse
- Local irritants—bubble bath, harsh soaps, tight-fitting clothes, nylon underwear, allergy to laundry detergent or fabric softener

Congenital or Vascular Causes
- Hemangioma
- Ectopic ureter

Miscellaneous Causes
- Nonspecific vulvovaginitis
- Foreign body
- Labial adhesions
- Physiologic leukorrhea of the adolescent
- Predisposing diseases—diabetes mellitus, immunosuppression
- Systemic illness—roseola, varicella, scarlet fever, Stevens–Johnson syndrome, Kawasaki syndrome

- Dermatologic disorder—seborrhea, eczema, psoriasis, lichen sclerosis et atrophicus
- Physiologic discharge of the newborn
- Urethral prolapse

DIFFERENTIAL DIAGNOSIS DISCUSSION
Group A β-Hemolytic Streptococcal Infection

Group A β-hemolytic streptococci can cause vulvovaginitis that may be associated with a **bloody vaginal discharge**. The vulvovaginitis typically develops **7 to 10 days after an upper respiratory tract infection or sore throat. Examination reveals a beefy red vulvar erythema**. Diagnosis is via **vaginal culture**. Treatment is with penicillin VK (125 to 250 mg four times daily for 10 days) or amoxicillin.

Bacterial Vaginosis
Etiology

Bacterial vaginosis results from the **overgrowth of normal bacteria** including anaerobes, *G. vaginalis, and Mycoplasma hominis.* This overgrowth results from the imbalance between normal lactobacillus and anaerobes, which could be precipitated by changes in alkalization by sex or douches, for example. The significance of *G. vaginalis* infection or bacterial vaginosis in children is uncertain, but one should consider the possibility of sexual abuse.

Clinical Features

The patient may complain of a **vaginal discharge or a "fishy" odor after coitus or menses,** and a **gray or yellow, thin, homogeneous discharge** is noted on physical examination.

Evaluation

Using Amsel's criteria, patients must have three of the following four criteria to make the diagnosis:

- Thin, homogeneous discharge
- Clue cells seen on a saline preparation (>20% of all epithelial cells)
- A positive "whiff" test (a fishy odor noted before or after discharge is mixed with potassium hydroxide [KOH] stain)
- Vaginal secretions with a pH > 4.5

Treatment

Treatment of bacterial vaginosis is with **metronidazole,** 500 mg orally twice daily for 7 days; **metronidazole vaginal gel 0.75%,** one applicator (5 g) intravaginal at bedtime for 5 days; clindamycin **cream 2%,** one applicator (5 g) intravaginal at bedtime for 7 days; or **clindamycin,** 300 mg orally twice daily for 7 days.

Gonorrhea

N. gonorrhoeae infection is discussed in Chapter 70, "Sexually Transmitted Diseases."

Chlamydia

C. trachomatis infection is discussed in Chapter 70, "Sexually Transmitted Diseases."

Shigella Vulvovaginitis

Etiology

S. flexneri is most often responsible for this inflammation, which is **rare in children**.

Clinical Features and Evaluation

A **mucopurulent vaginal discharge** is seen; it is **bloody** in 40% to 50% of patients. Fewer than 25% of patients have associated **diarrhea**. **Vaginal culture** reveals the organism.

Treatment

The infection is treated with **trimethoprim and sulfamethoxazole,** twice daily for 7 days.

Candida Vulvovaginitis

Etiology

The most common pathogen is *C. albicans.* However, in difficult to treat cases, *C. glabrata* should be suspected. The disorder is **more common in adolescents** than in prepubescent girls.

   Predisposing factors include diabetes mellitus, recent antibiotic or steroid use, immunosuppression, pregnancy, use of oral contraceptives, and tight-fitting clothes.

Clinical Features and Evaluation

- Patients usually present complaining of intense **vulvovaginal itching, thick white discharge, and external dysuria**. On examination, vulvar and perianal **erythema,** inflammation, and excoriations may be visible. White satellite candidal plaques are sometimes noted, and thick "cottage cheese" discharge is often present. A KOH smear revealing hyphae and budding yeast confirms the diagnosis of *C. albicans, C. glabrata,* alternatively, may not be visible by KOH microscopy.

Treatment

- **In prepubescent girls,** an antifungal cream (e.g., miconazole, clotrimazole, nystatin) should be applied to the external genitalia. The applicator should not be used to avoid trauma to the hymen. If this is not successful, intravaginal nystatin liquid or gentle insertion of a vaginal suppository that has been cut in half may be prescribed. A topical steroid cream may be used to alleviate the inflammation.
- **Adolescents** should be treated with an antifungal medication (e.g., miconazole or terconazole) given as a cream or vaginal suppositories for a 3- to 7-day course. Oral fluconazole is available in a onetime dose; however, symptomatic relief may take up to 72 hours.

Trichomoniasis

Etiology

This infection is caused by *T. vaginalis,* **a protozoan**. Premenarchal girls are generally resistant to this organism because of their lack of estrogen. However, perinatal transmission can persist for up to 1 year.

Clinical Features

Some patients are **asymptomatic,** but the classic complaint is of a **gray, yellow, or green foul-smelling vaginal discharge and vaginal irritation**. The patient may note **postcoital spotting**.

Evaluation

Vulvar erythema may be seen on physical examination. Copious, **green frothy discharge** is noted in the vaginal vault. A **"strawberry red" cervix caused by punctuate hemorrhage on the surface** is classically described but not commonly seen. A **saline preparation** often reveals the **flagellated protozoa** as well as a **heavy polymorphonuclear infiltrate**. For definitive diagnosis, a culture may be sent. Because trichomoniasis is transmitted sexually, the patient should be **tested for gonorrhea and chlamydia and counseled about testing for HIV, hepatitis, and syphilis**.

Treatment

Trichomonas is a **sexually acquired pathogen;** therefore children infected with *T. vaginalis* should be **referred to agencies** familiar with evaluating children who have been **sexually abused**.

In sexually active adolescents, the preferred treatment is metronidazole in a single oral dose (2 g). Sexual partners must also be treated and abstinence encouraged until both partners are treated.

E. vermicularis Infestation (Pinworms)
Clinical Features

A typical history includes **perianal and vulvar itching,** especially at night.

Evaluation

Perianal excoriations and an **erythematous vulvar area** are seen on physical examination. **Parents** should be **asked to examine the child's anus at night using a flashlight;** it may be possible to see the worms. **Cellophane tape applied to the child's anus in the morning may** reveal **characteristic eggs**.

Treatment

Pinworm infestation is treated with **one dose of mebendazole** (100 mg), **repeated in 2 weeks**. Consideration should be given to **treating family members**.

Herpes Simplex Virus
Etiology

Precise time of infection with herpes simplex virus can be difficult to discern. Because of long latency, infection at time of childbirth may become apparent several years after delivery. Type 2 is more commonly associated with sexual transmission. **Sexual abuse must be considered.**

Evaluation

Symptoms such as **dysuria, genital erythema, and edema** are the most common complaints. The child might also experience generalized symptoms such as fatigue, adenopathy, and fever. Examination findings include clusters of vesicles.

Viral culture is important because other viruses may cause mucosal ulcers, such as coxsackievirus.

Treatment

Treatment is mostly **symptomatic**. Care must be taken to ensure that the child is voiding appropriately because the edema and pain can cause urinary retention requiring Foley catheterization. Soaking in a warm bath may ease the pain of urination. Acyclovir may be used to shorten the duration of symptoms and quicken the resolution of lesions.

Nonspecific Vulvovaginitis

Etiology

Nonspecific vulvovaginitis accounts for 25% to 70% of all cases of pediatric vulvovaginitis and is caused by an **alteration in the vaginal flora**. The most common cause of this alteration is **poor perineal hygiene**.

Clinical Features

Nonspecific vulvovaginitis is characterized by **vaginal discharge, odor, vulvar and vaginal irritation, and dysuria**.

Evaluation

The history should include the following questions:

- After a bowel movement or urination, does the child wipe her perineum from back to front?
- Does the child urinate with her knees together?
- Is the child exposed to local irritants such as harsh soaps, bubble bath, and shampoos?
- Does she wash her hair in the bathtub?
- Is the child's laundry washed with hypoallergenic soap?
- Is fabric softener (a possible local irritant) used?
- Does the child wear tight clothes (e.g., bathing suit, tights, and leotards)?
- Does the child wear white cotton underwear and use white, unscented toilet paper?

Physical examination usually reveals **vulvar erythema and inflammation**. A vaginal discharge may or may not be present. A saline wet mount reveals predominantly white blood cells (WBCs) and bacteria. A KOH smear reveals no evidence of mycotic infection. If local measures fail, vaginal yeast and bacterial cultures should be sent. Typically in patients with nonspecific vulvovaginitis, the culture reveals normal vaginal flora.

Treatment

Application of **1% hydrocortisone cream, A&D ointment, or Desitin cream** may be soothing. Patients may also take **sitz baths three times a day** (Aveeno oatmeal or baking soda may be added to the bath). The vulva should be **gently patted dry** or may be dried using a **hair dryer on the cool setting**.

If symptoms do not improve with local measures and a **predominant organism** is present on vaginal culture, an **appropriate antibiotic** can be prescribed.

If no predominant organism is identified by culture, and vulvovaginitis does not respond to local measures, **empirical antibiotic** treatment may be tried (e.g., amoxicillin, amoxicillin-clavulanate, or cephalexin for 7 to 10 days).

Prevention entails **improved perineal hygiene,** including correct voiding and wiping technique, and **avoidance of bubble baths, harsh soaps, and tight clothes**. The child should wear **white cotton underwear**.

Physiologic Leukorrhea

Etiology and Clinical Features

Physiologic leukorrhea, caused by **desquamation of epithelial cells under the influence of estrogen,** is classically described as **white, mucoid, and without odor**. It is seen in **newborns** (secondary to maternal estrogens) **and adolescents**. Sometimes it is noted months prior to the first menses.

Evaluation and Treatment

Physical examination reveals **copious white, mucoid vaginal secretions without an odor**. **Saline and KOH preparations reveal epithelial cells,** but no yeast, *Trichomonas,* or WBCs. **No treatment** is necessary.

Lichen Sclerosis

Etiology and Clinical Features

Lichen sclerosis is characterized by **vulvar pruritus and irritation**. The cause is unknown. Patients also often complain of vaginal discharge, constipation (secondary to tenesmus), and dysuria. Chronic ulcerations and inflammation may result in areas of **ecchymosis and secondary infection** of the vulva.

Evaluation

The diagnosis is generally made by the classic appearance of **whitened papules and plaques on the vulva and perineum** in a characteristic **"figure eight" or "hourglass" distribution** around the anus and introitus. Small ivory areas join to form raised patches. Some areas may contain yellow plugs in the centers. The lesion is classically described as wrinkled tissue paper. In some patients, this disorder may be difficult to distinguish from vitiligo. A **vulvar biopsy** may be necessary.

Treatment

The patient should be **referred to a dermatologist or gynecologist familiar with this condition**. Instruction in **improving perineal hygiene, including use of ointments** (e.g., A&D ointment, Desitin) and **avoidance of harsh soaps** is appropriate. **Topical steroid creams** may be of benefit.

Foreign Body

Vaginal foreign bodies are discussed in Chapter 79, "Vaginal Bleeding."

EVALUATION OF VAGINAL DISCHARGE

Physiologic discharge varies throughout a female patient's life. As an infant, maternal estrogens primarily influence the infant's physiology; therefore, her hymen is pale and thickened, and she may have a white discharge, similar to that of puberty. Withdrawal of these hormones may cause a pink or bloody discharge. After the maternal hormones clear, vaginal discharge is rare. At puberty, with the surge in hormones, the hymen again becomes pale and thicker. The vaginal mucosa produces physiologic leukorrhea.

Physical Examination

A **pelvic examination must be done slowly,** and the physician should tell the child that she or he will not hurt her. The physician must be prepared to **abandon the examination if it is too painful or traumatic for the child**. The examination should be tailored to the severity of the child's symptoms and her age; **severe symptoms require a more thorough examination**.

The child may be positioned in the **"frog leg" position, the lithotomy position** (with the aid of stirrups), or the knee-chest position. The **knee-chest** position often causes gaping of the hymen, allowing visualization of the vagina and the cervix.

The physician should **start by examining the external genitalia,** paying particular attention to the presence or absence of genital lesions and vulvar inflammation. **Having the patient cough may elicit vaginal discharge.**

A **rectoabdominal examination** is useful for detecting an **intravaginal foreign body or a pelvic mass,** and for expressing **vaginal discharge**.

The **hymen should be examined** for signs of trauma or tears and the **presence of a perforation**. If a hymenal opening cannot be visualized, placing **gentle traction on the labia majora while depressing the perineum** generally causes the hymenal opening to stretch, enabling visualization of the lower vagina.

Visualization of the **upper vagina and cervix in a premenarchal girl** can be accomplished by using one of the following methods:

- Using a pediatric otoscope, cystoscope, or vaginoscope after applying a local anesthetic (e.g., 2% viscous lidocaine) to the vulva and hymen
- Using a narrow vaginal speculum
- Using a hysteroscope

> **HINT:** When vulvovaginitis is recurrent or bloody, vaginoscopy is required to rule out a foreign body or tumor.

Laboratory Studies
Microscopic Examination

If **vaginal discharge** is present, microscopic examination of the discharge is indicated. If discharge is not present at the introitus, a **moistened** cotton swab is gently inserted into the vagina to collect a specimen. Care should be taken to **avoid touching the hymen,** which can cause discomfort. The pH of the discharge is assessed first followed by transfer of the swab into a test tube containing two to three drops of sterile saline. Preparation of saline and KOH slides are as follows:

- **Saline (wet) preparation.** Touch the saturated swab containing the specimen on a glass slide and cover with a glass cover slip. Examine the slide under a microscope for the presence of *T. vaginalis,* bacteria, WBCs, red blood cells, and clue cells.

- **KOH preparation.** Touch the swab to a small amount of 10% KOH on a glass slide. Swirl to mix the contents and perform the "whiff test." Cover the slide with a glass cover slip and examine it under a microscope for hyphae and budding yeast.

In some circumstances, it may be appropriate to obtain the following microbial studies:

- **Vaginal culture.** A bacterial vaginal culture may identify a predominant pathologic organism in premenarchal girls with nonspecific vulvovaginitis. Recurrent vulvovaginal yeast infections should be evaluated with a yeast culture.
- **N. gonorrhoeae or C. trachomatis** nucleic acid amplification techniques (**NAATs**). Several assays are available. The specimen can be obtained from a urine sample or the endocervical canal (in postmenarchal girls). In sexual abuse evaluations, some authorities recommend sequential testing (i.e., NAAT followed by culture in positive tests). Sequential testing yields fewer false-negative and false-positive results compared with either culture or NAAT alone.
- **Viral culture.** If an ulcer lesion is noted, a swab may aid in the diagnosis.

Suggested Readings

Carpenter SE, Rock JA. *Pediatric and Adolescent Gynecology.* Philadelphia: Lippincott-Raven; 1992.

Emans JH, Goldstein DP. *Pediatric and Adolescent Gynecology.* Boston: Little, Brown; 1990.

Shapiro RA, Schubert CJ, Siegel RM. *Neisseria gonorrhea* infections in girls younger than 12 years of age evaluated for vaginitis. *Pediatrics.* 1999;104(6):e72.

Sweet RL, Gibbs RS. *Infectious Disease of the Female Genital Tract.* 3rd ed. Baltimore: Williams & Wilkins; 1995.

Taber BZ. *Manual of Gynecologic and Obstetric Emergencies.* 2nd ed. Philadelphia: WB Saunders; 1984.

Vertigo (Dizziness)

INTRODUCTION

Dizziness is caused by a **distortion in spatial orientation**. The primary sensory modalities of vision, vestibular function, joint position sense, touch-pressure sense, and hearing are normally rapidly integrated by the central nervous system (CNS) into a composite sensation, keeping one aware of the body's position in space. Incorrect or insufficient sensory information or an error in integration of the perceptions produces distorted orientation, which in turn causes dizziness.

Vertigo is a sensation of spinning or rotation. Milder forms may be described as producing a rocking sensation or vague lightheadedness. Patients may describe the room spinning around them, rather than a sense that they are moving. Usually, vertigo is of sudden onset and associated with loss of balance, nausea, and nystagmus. It may also be associated with diaphoresis and pallor. The sensation can be terrifying to small children.

Vertigo can be caused by a disorder of the CNS, where primary sensory input is integrated, or peripherally, in sensory nerve dysfunction of the vestibular system.

DIFFERENTIAL DIAGNOSIS LIST

Peripheral Vertigo
- Vestibular neuronitis
- Labyrinthitis
- Benign paroxysmal positional vertigo (BPPV)
- Ménière disease
- Medications
- Head trauma

Central Vertigo
- Benign paroxysmal vertigo (BPV)
- Migraine
- Seizure
- Other

Presyncope
Disequilibrium

DIFFERENTIAL DIAGNOSIS DISCUSSION

The medical history can help refine the differential diagnosis. It is important to describe the **course** (acute, recurrent, or chronic), **precipitating events** (position change, trauma, or infection), association with **alteration of hearing** (tinnitus or hearing impairment), **drug exposure, cardiovascular disease, and family history of migraine**.

Peripheral Vertigo
Etiology and Clinical Features
Up to 85% of vertigo in children is caused by peripheral etiologies. Findings pointing to a peripheral cause include an episodic or acute course, improvement with visual fixation or holding head still, accompanying hearing complaints, and absence of other complaints worrisome for cranial nerve dysfunction (e.g., difficulty swallowing, double vision, drooling).

- **Vestibular neuronitis.** This common disorder can occur several days after an upper respiratory tract infection, most often in adolescents. There is no associated hearing loss. Vestibular neuronitis is a self-limited, postinfectious neuropathy, and symptoms generally resolve in 7 to 14 days.
- **Labyrinthitis** is a common inflammatory cause of vertigo. This also follows preceding infection, but hearing impairment is present. Furthermore, labyrinthitis often affects younger children (preschool to school age) than vestibular neuronitis. There is a positional component because vertigo worsens with movement. The course is self-limited with resolution after several days. **Acute suppurative labyrinthitis** is caused by extension of otitis media or mastoiditis. Chronic otitis media can lead to the development of cholesteatoma, which in turn can cause labyrinth damage.
- While **BPPV** is the most common cause of vertigo of peripheral origin in adults, it is a rare disorder in children. Pediatric BPPV is most often seen after head trauma. Dislodged otoliths cause aberrant vestibular input in the setting of head movement. As such, affected patients experience vertigo only with a change in head position. Symptoms are usually recurrent, with each attack lasting several weeks, and typically subside spontaneously within a year, although repositioning maneuver may lead to immediate resolution.
- **Ménière disease** is rare in children, but up to 5% of affected patients will present in childhood. It is an idiopathic disorder of the labyrinth in which there is excessive endolymph in the scala media of the cochlea. Ménière disease is characterized by recurring bouts of tinnitus, vertigo, and hearing loss.
- **Medications** that enter the CNS can cause ataxia, incoordination, and abnormal vestibular function, but vertigo is an unusual symptom in anticonvulsant and neuroleptic toxicity. Other drugs, especially aminoglycosides, can produce vertigo as a result of toxic damage to the peripheral vestibular apparatus.
- **Head trauma** may be followed by persistent vertigo. Vertigo caused by trauma-induced perilymphatic fistula is most likely to occur suddenly, and it is accompanied by hearing loss. This diagnosis should be particularly considered in cases of barotrauma. When isolated posttraumatic vertigo without hearing loss occurs, it is more likely caused by dislocation of the otoliths from the macula (see BPPV). Labyrinthine concussion can cause severe and persistent vertigo. This presents with a tendency to fall to the ipsilateral side, and symptoms often last up to 6 weeks.

Treatment
Treatment of peripheral vertigo is symptomatic. Administration of meclizine and diazepam or lorazepam may provide relief in some children; adolescents may

respond to transdermal scopolamine. Note that chronic vertigo usually self-resolves as the result of central compensation for the impaired peripheral signaling. Long-term use of symptomatic medication may impair or delay this compensation, and it may even prevent permanent recovery. Ondansetron and phenothiazines can be used to treat nausea and vomiting. Antibiotics are used to treat acute suppurative labyrinthitis; myringotomy and intravenous antibiotics are indicated for serous labyrinthitis from acute otitis media. Most patients with Méniére disease can be controlled on a low-sodium diet, with or without concomitant diuretics.

Central Vertigo
Etiology and Clinical Features
Although symptoms may be very disabling, peripheral causes of vertigo are rarely dangerous. However, vertigo of central etiology can be life threatening, particu-larly intrinsic brain tumors, which are most likely to develop in the posterior fossa of children. Historical points that help localize central vertigo are complaints sug-gesting additional cranial nerve dysfunction (e.g., double vision, difficulty swal-lowing, drooling, abnormal facial sensation), improvement with visual fixation removed (e.g., closing eyes), and lack of improvement with holding the head still. Fortunately, even most causes of central vertigo are less ominous.

- **BPV** is a common cause of vertiginous attacks, occurring mostly in toddlers and early-school-aged children. Patients report sudden onset of severe vertigo lasting only seconds, less often minutes, in duration. In younger children, this may manifest primarily as crying or falling over. Although nystagmus may be reported, it is often not noticed by observers. Pallor and diaphoresis may be prominent. Symptoms quickly resolve on their own with no postictal findings or residual impairments. Many consider BPV a migraine precursor. Although there is no associated headache, patients are more likely to have a family history of migraine and to develop migraines later in life. (Note that BPV is unrelated to BPPV, described earlier.)
- **Migraines** can occur in older children and adolescents, with a vertiginous com-ponent, and episodes lasting minutes to hours. These episodes are usually asso-ciated with a strong family history. Although dizziness and vertigo can be a part of any migraine syndrome, it is particularly prominent in **basilar migraine** in which these symptoms along with visual disturbances including diplopia and ataxia precede onset of headache. Unlike most migraines, pain may be localized to the occipital region.
- **Seizures.** Vertigo may rarely present as the only manifestation of a seizure, although generally there is some alteration in consciousness. Careful question-ing often reveals confusional attacks and automatisms or other symptoms of partial complex seizures, when vertigo is caused by epilepsy.
- **Other causes.** Other rare causes of central vertigo include stroke (lateral medul-lary syndrome of Wallenberg, with accompanying Horner syndrome), cerebel-lopontine angle tumors, neurofibromatosis type II, and demyelinating disease affecting the posterior fossa (e.g., multiple sclerosis).

Treatment

BPV rarely requires treatment because spells are brief and self-resolve. Migraine prophylaxis (e.g., cyproheptadine, topiramate) can be used in patients with frequent episodes suggesting migraine. Treatment focuses on management of the underlying cause in patients with other types of central vertigo (e.g., seizure disorder).

Presyncope

Symptoms of faintness, giddiness, or lightheadedness include **dimness of vision, "roaring" in the ears, and diaphoresis** with recovery on assuming a recumbent position. If symptoms are of **short duration and sudden onset,** the symptoms are most likely of **cardiovascular origin**. If symptoms persist, one must consider **hypoglycemia, hyperventilation,** or a **mood disturbance** (e.g., depression, anxiety).

Disequilibrium

Disequilibrium is **loss of balance** without an abnormal sensation in the head. Disequilibrium can be caused by cerebellar, peripheral nervous system, or bilateral vestibular lesions.

EVALUATION OF VERTIGO (DIZZINESS)
Patient History

An effort should be made to clarify the types of dizziness by asking the following questions:

- Was the onset of symptoms acute, recurrent, or chronic?
- Were there any precipitating events (e.g., changes in position, motion, trauma, infection)?
- What is the quality of the dizziness? For older children, it may be helpful to ask, "Describe what you feel without using the word 'dizzy'." For younger children it may be helpful to offer suggestions—like a spinning top or a swing (suggesting true vertigo), or like feeling very sleepy or confused (suggesting lightheadedness).
- Are there any associated symptoms? Hearing loss, ear pain, or tinnitus suggests inner ear or eighth cranial nerve dysfunction, whereas nausea and vomiting indicate a peripheral vestibular apparatus disorder.
- Is there a family history of cardiovascular disease, drug exposure, or a family history of migraine or ataxia?

Physical Examination

- **Ear examination.** One should look for perforations, infection, hemorrhage, or mass lesions. Blowing air into the external ear canal produces vertigo in patients with a fistula of the round or oval window of the labyrinth.
- **Neurologic examination.**
- **Oculovestibular and cranial nerve testing.** Vestibular testing should include assessment for the presence of nystagmus, changes in visual fixation, or other evidence of cranial nerve dysfunction. Many normal children have "end gaze"

(or physiologic) nystagmus with far lateral gaze in either direction. However, abnormal nystagmus includes spontaneous or induced nystagmus within a normal range of vision. Unidirectional, horizontal, or rotary nystagmus suggests a peripheral cause of vertigo. Vertical, irregular, and variable nystagmus suggests a central cause. Accompanying hearing loss suggests a peripheral cause. Older children may be asked to march in place; in the presence of a peripheral lesion of the vestibular system, the child may rotate toward the ipsilateral side.

- **Cerebellar testing.** Cerebellar testing can help clarify if there is a central component to nystagmus. Romberg testing evaluates proprioception, which might contribute to a sense of imbalance.
- **Other.** Although the neurologic examination should focus on vestibular and cerebellar function, a complete examination is needed to screen for other abnormalities. Evidence of decreased sensation, mild hemiparesis, or other neurologic deficits may indicate an underlying central lesion.
- **Orthostatic blood pressure.** Blood pressure should be recorded while lying, sitting, and standing to assess for possible orthostatic hypotension.
- **Valsalva maneuver.** The patient should be asked to squat for 30 seconds and then to stand up and strain against a closed glottis. The examiner should note whether this maneuver provokes symptoms (suggesting vasovagal syncope or near fainting).
- **Rapid deep breathing.** Reproduction of symptoms via rapid deep breathing or within 3 minutes suggests hyperventilation syndrome.
- **Hallpike maneuver.** The examiner guides the patient's head backward from a seated position to laying supine with head past the edge of the table, so that it is hanging 45 degree to one side. Vertigo with nystagmus indicates BPPV, with the nystagmus worst when the affected ear is turned down.

Laboratory Studies

Laboratory testing is guided by the presenting signs and symptoms. A **complete blood cell count and electrolyte analysis,** including glucose, blood urea nitrogen, and creatinine levels, may be obtained. **Anemia** may cause presyncopal lightheadedness. **Renal failure, hyperglycemia, and hypoglycemia** are also associated with vertigo.

APPROACH TO THE PATIENT

- Magnetic resonance imaging is indicated if there is prolonged vertigo or additional neurologic signs (Figure 81-1). One should look for evidence of a tumor or hemorrhage into the cerebellum, brainstem, or labyrinth.
- Electroencephalography is indicated when vertigo is associated with alterations of consciousness.
- Audiography is indicated when there is evidence of hearing loss, ear pain, or tinnitus.
- Electronystagmography allows one to distinguish central vertigo from peripheral vertigo.

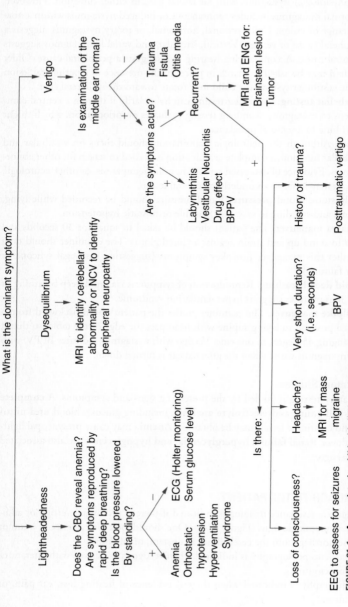

FIGURE 81-1 Approach to the child with dizziness or vertigo. *BPV,* benign paroxysmal vertigo; *CBC,* complete blood count; *ECG,* electrocardiogram; *ENG,* electronystagmogram; *MRI,* magnetic resonance imaging; *NCV,* nerve conduction velocity.

What is the dominant symptom?

Lightheadedness

Does the CBC reveal anemia?
Are symptoms reproduced by rapid deep breathing?
Is the blood pressure lowered
By standing?

+
Anemia
Orthostatic hypotension
Hyperventilation Syndrome

−
ECG (Holter monitoring)
Serum glucose level

Dysequilibrium

MRI to identify cerebellar abnormality or NCV to identify peripheral neuropathy

Vertigo

Is examination of the middle ear normal?

+
Are the symptoms acute?

+
Labyrinthitis
Vestibular Neuronitis
Drug effect
BPPV

−
Recurrent?

−
MRI and ENG for:
Brainstem lesion
Tumor

−
Trauma
Fistula
Otitis media

+

Is there:

Loss of consciousness?
EEG to assess for seizures

Headache?
MRI for mass
migraine

Very short duration? (i.e., seconds)
BPV

History of trauma?
Posttraumatic vertigo

Suggested Readings

Bacharyyatta N, Baugh RF, Orvidas L, et al. Clinical practice guideline: benign paroxysmal positional vertigo. *Otolaryngol Head Neck Surg.* 2008;139(5S4):S47–S81.

Casselbrant ML, Mandel EM. Balance disorders in children. *Neurol Clin.* 2005;23:807–829.

Drigo P, Carli G, Laverda AM. Benign paroxysmal vertigo of childhood. *Brain Dev.* 2001;23(1):38–41.

Golz A, Netzer A, Angel-Yeger B, et al. Effects of middle ear effusion on the vestibular system in children. *Otolaryngol Head Neck Surg.* 1998;119(6):695–699.

Lewis DW. Pediatric migraine. *Pediatr Rev.* 2007;28(2):43–53.

MacGregor DL. Vertigo. *Pediatr Rev.* 2002;23:10–16.

Miyamoto RC, Miyamoto RT. Pediatric neurotology. *Semin Pediatr Neurol.* 2003;10(4):298–303.

Ravid S, Bienkowski R, Eviatar A. A simplified diagnostic approach to dizziness in children. *Pediatr Neurol.* 2000;29:317.

Vomiting

INTRODUCTION

Vomiting is the expulsion of stomach contents through the mouth. In children, vomiting is one of the **most common presenting symptoms of upper gastrointestinal disease**. The degree of emesis can vary from forceful, projectile vomiting to effortless regurgitation, to unseen rumination.

 DIFFERENTIAL DIAGNOSIS LIST

Infectious Causes

- Sepsis
- Meningitis
- Urinary tract infection
- Parasitic infection—giardiasis, ascariasis
- *Helicobacter pylori* gastritis
- Otitis media
- Gastroenteritis—viral, bacterial
- Food-borne illnesses—*Salmonella and Shigella*
- Hepatitis A, B, or C
- *Bordetella pertussis* infection
- Pneumonia
- Sinusitis
- Streptococcal pharyngitis

Toxic Causes

- Drugs—aspirin, ipecac, theophylline, digoxin, opiates, anticonvulsants, barbiturates
- Metals—iron, lead
- Caustic ingestions
- Alcohol

Neoplastic Causes

- Intracranial mass lesions

Traumatic Causes

- Duodenal hematoma
- Pancreatic trauma

Congenital, Anatomic, or Vascular Causes

- Esophageal stricture, web, ring, or atresia
- Hypertrophic pyloric stenosis
- Gastric web or duplication
- Duodenal atresia
- Malrotation
- Intestinal duplication
- Hirschsprung disease
- Imperforate anus
- Superior mesenteric artery syndrome

Metabolic or Genetic Causes

- Galactosemia
- Hereditary fructose intolerance
- Other inborn errors of metabolism—amino acid or organic acid disorders, urea cycle defects, fatty acid oxidation disorders
- Diabetes
- Adrenal insufficiency

Inflammatory Causes

- Cholecystitis or cholelithiasis
- Eosinophilic enteritis
- Milk-/soy-protein allergy
- Inflammatory bowel disease
- Appendicitis
- Necrotizing enterocolitis
- Peritonitis
- Celiac disease
- Peptic ulcer
- Pancreatitis

Gastrointestinal Causes

- Gastroesophageal reflux disease (GERD)
- Eosinophilic esophagitis (EE)
- Achalasia
- Pseudo-obstruction
- Obstruction—intussusception, volvulus, incarcerated hernia
- Foreign body
- Gastric and intestinal bezoars

Psychosocial Causes

- Rumination
- Bulimia
- Psychogenic vomiting
- Overfeeding

Functional Causes

- "Cyclic vomiting" syndrome
- Gastroparesis

Miscellaneous Causes

- Pregnancy
- Central nervous system disorders— hydrocephalus, pseudotumor cerebri, migraine, motion sickness, seizure
- Renal disorders—ureteropelvic junction obstruction, obstructive uropathy, nephrolithiasis, glomerulonephritis, renal tubular acidosis

DIFFERENTIAL DIAGNOSIS DISCUSSION

H. pylori Infection

In older children and adults, *H. pylori* (a gram-negative, urease-producing bacterium) is the **major cause of gastric and duodenal ulcers**. Although the infection rate increases with age, infection with *H. pylori* is usually acquired during childhood. The overall rates of *H. pylori* infection in the United States are declining, but worldwide it remains a ubiquitous pathogen in developing nations. Furthermore, depending on socioeconomic status, rates of infection during childhood can vary from >60% in lower income homes to <15% in higher income homes.

H. pylori appears to promote disease via several mechanisms: production of urease and ammonia, adhesion to the gastric mucosa, and proteolysis of gastric mucus. All of these mechanisms result in disruption of the gastric epithelium.

Clinical Features

Complaints commonly center around **epigastric abdominal pain, vomiting, heartburn, and regurgitation**. Hematemesis can also occur.

Evaluation

Currently, **upper endoscopy with biopsy** is the gold standard for the diagnosis of *H. pylori* infection. **Serum antibodies** to *H. pylori* can be detected; however, this test carries a poor specificity because previously infected individuals may remain serum antibody positive, despite lacking clinical evidence of gastritis. Stool *H. pylori* antigen testing and the **urea breath test** may supplant the need for upper endoscopy.

Treatment

Many treatment strategies are reported in the literature, but no single therapy is 100% effective in the eradication of *H. pylori*. Currently, the recommended treatment consists of a combination of a **drug to suppress acid production** (e.g., omeprazole), **clarithromycin, and either metronidazole or amoxicillin**. In the past, the treatment of choice was a combination of bismuth subsalicylate and antibiotics (amoxicillin and metronidazole).

Gastroesophageal Reflux Disease

Etiology

Gastroesophageal reflux is the movement of stomach contents into the esophagus, past the lower esophageal sphincter. It is commonly caused by a **delay in gastric emptying** or transient **relaxation of the lower esophageal sphincter**.

Clinical Features

Many **newborns manifest inconsequential regurgitation after meals;** this condition typically resolves by 3 to 6 months of age. In the usual presentation of GE reflux, frequent small mouthfuls of stomach contents are **regurgitated in an effortless manner**. No active emesis is observed. This phenomenon is frequently referred to as "spitting" or "wet burps." Newborns with more severe reflux may also exhibit arching episodes (Sandifer syndrome) and irritability associated with feeding. Symptoms in older children include **heartburn, chest or epigastric pain, dysphagia, water brash** (a sour taste in mouth), or **globus** (the sensation that something is stuck in the throat).

In more **pathologic cases,** GERD is associated with more severe symptoms, such as weight loss, **recurrent wheezing or coughing, recurrent pneumonia** from aspiration, or **apparent life-threatening episodes**. Many times, concomitant **esophagitis** (manifested as irritability in infants) can occur. In many cases, no obvious spitting is seen, but studies clearly document gastroesophageal reflux.

Recently, an increasing number of children with symptoms of GERD were identified with EE. The presentation of EE is often very similar to GERD; however, these patients fail to respond adequately to antireflux medications. The disease is caused by **food allergy** and characterized by a severe isolated histologic esophageal eosinophilia despite aggressive acid suppression therapy.

Complications associated with GERD include **hematemesis, aspiration, and failure to thrive**.

Evaluation

GERD is primarily a clinical diagnosis, but several diagnostic tests can aid in the evaluation:

- **Contrast studies (upper gastrointestinal series)** provide information regarding the upper intestinal anatomy.
- **Upper endoscopy** is useful in assessing the degree of reflux and the presence of complications (e.g., esophagitis) and for reaching a definitive diagnosis in children.

- **Radiographic nuclear scintiscans (milk scans)** provide information regarding gastric emptying and possible aspiration.
- **24-hour pH probe** is useful when attempting to correlate acid reflux with atypical symptoms such as cough, hoarseness, or bronchospasm. An impedance probe can be used along with the pH probe to detect nonacid reflux.

Treatment
Conservative treatment includes **improved positioning** (upright and prone with head elevated 45°) after eating and while sleeping; feeding infants **thickened food; and eliminating spicy foods** and foods containing **caffeine and peppermint**.

The mainstay of medical treatment consists of **gastric acid suppression** and the use of **intestinal prokinetic agents** (e.g., metoclopramide, erythromycin). **Acid-blocking medications** (e.g., ranitidine, famotidine) are effective for preventing heartburn and for healing esophagitis. Proton pump inhibitors (PPIs) can be used for children with refractory disease. Antacids can be substituted; however, large doses must be given and the duration of action is short.

Eosinophilic Esophagitis
Etiology
EE is an **allergic (autoimmune) esophageal disorder** based on a **clinicopathologic diagnosis** that includes the presence of a large number of tissue eosinophils isolated from the esophagus.

Clinical Features
In children, EE presents with symptoms similar to those seen with GERD. These symptoms include **vomiting, regurgitation, epigastric pain, poor feeding, and failure to thrive**. Older children commonly manifest symptoms of **heartburn, water brash, nausea, and dysphagia**. It is not uncommon for adolescents to complain of **difficulty in swallowing solid foods** or have **intermittent food impactions**.

Evaluation
- **Upper endoscopy with biopsy** is required to make the diagnosis. More than 15 esophageal eosinophils must be present per high power microscopic field. GERD must be ruled out.
- Currently, there are no other useful **noninvasive tests** that can be performed.

HINT: Because patients with GERD can also manifest esophageal eosinophils, patients suspected of having EE should be treated with a PPI prior to performing upper endoscopy.

HINT: EE should be strongly considered whenever a patient presents with an unexplained esophageal food impaction.

Treatment

There are several treatment options for patients with EE. Treatments include **dilation for esophageal strictures, dietary management, and pharmacologic therapy**. **Dietary restriction** or elimination should be considered in all children with EE. Because of the difficulty in identifying the causative foods, referral to a pediatric allergist or gastroenterologist is often required. Effective medications include **corticosteroids and PPIs**. **Swallowed topical corticosteroids** act to reduce esophageal inflammation; however, when the medication is discontinued, the disease almost always recurs. **Acid blockade** is helpful in controlling secondary acid reflux; however, it should not be a primary therapy for EE.

Achalasia

Etiology

Achalasia is caused by an abnormality in the smooth muscle ganglion cells of the esophagus, which produces incomplete relaxation of the lower esophageal sphincter and poor esophageal motility. The **esophagus can become extremely dilated,** serving as a **reservoir for food,** which can be **vomited hours or days after ingestion**.

Clinical Features

Achalasia rarely develops before the **teenage years** and is present in fewer than 1 in 10,000 individuals. **Vomiting and dysphagia** are the cardinal symptoms. Patients are typically "slow" eaters and complain of food and liquids "sticking in the throat."

Choking, coughing, gagging, and aspiration pneumonias** typically occur in **infants and young children** with achalasia.

Evaluation

Although the presence of an air-fluid level in the mediastinum on the chest radiograph suggests the diagnosis of achalasia, the diagnosis is usually made using an upper gastrointestinal series or esophageal manometry:

- An **upper gastrointestinal series** reveals a dilated esophagus with a narrow, beak-like appearance at the level of the lower esophageal sphincter.
- **Esophageal manometry** reveals abnormal function of the esophageal smooth muscle.

Treatment

Balloon dilation of the lower esophageal sphincter is the usual treatment. Unfortunately, **symptoms often recur** and repeat dilations are typically necessary. Other treatments include **esophageal myotomy** and the injection of **botulinum toxin** into the distal esophageal mucosal wall.

Hypertrophic Pyloric Stenosis

Etiology

Hypertrophic pyloric stenosis is the most common **congenital abnormality** of children. It is caused by hypertrophy and hyperplasia of the smooth muscle that surrounds the gastric pylorus. The hypertrophy causes the **mucosal and submucosal tissues** to **protrude into the pyloric channel**.

Clinical Features

The incidence of pyloric stenosis is approximately 1 in 1,000; symptoms usually begin between 4 and 7 weeks of age.

Progressive, forceful, and nonbilious vomiting is the first sign of pyloric stenosis in infants. **Dehydration, weight loss, and failure to thrive** can develop. If the diagnosis is not made and the vomiting continues, infants develop a serious hypochloremic, hypokalemic **metabolic alkalosis;** an associated **jaundice** occurs in as many as 5% of infants.

Evaluation

Physical examination may reveal a palpable **"olive"** or a visible peristaltic wave in the right upper quadrant; however, in most cases, the physical examination is not diagnostic. Currently, **abdominal ultrasound** (demonstrating a thickened pyloric channel muscle layer) is the diagnostic test of choice. An upper gastrointestinal series demonstrates an elongated "double tract" of barium along the pyloric channel.

Treatment

Infants with severe dehydration and alkalosis require **fluid resuscitation**. Once the patient is stabilized, **pyloromyotomy** can be performed to correct the defect.

Malrotation

Etiology

Intestinal malrotation is **failure** of the **fetal midgut to rotate to its normal position**. The associated shortened mesenteric ligament (ligament of Treitz) may result in twisting and torsion of the intestine and its blood supply, resulting in midgut volvulus, **intestinal obstruction, and ischemic bowel**.

Clinical Features

Most affected infants present with **signs and symptoms of intestinal obstruction,** including bile-stained emesis, abdominal pain, and borborygmi; however, the symptoms can be delayed for many years.

Older children present with **intermittent vomiting and abdominal pain;** rarely, malabsorption and diarrhea are seen.

Evaluation

Radiographic contrast studies of the upper gastrointestinal tract demonstrate the positioning of the ligament of Treitz. Whenever the position of this ligament is in question, contrast should be allowed to flow into the jejunum, ileum, and cecum to define the intestinal rotation.

Treatment

Surgery is indicated to prevent the complications of malrotation, which include small bowel obstruction and midgut volvulus.

Esophageal Atresia

Etiology

Esophageal atresia occurs when the **esophagus ends as a blind tube** as a result of malformation of the tracheoesophageal septum during embryologic development.

Although many forms of esophageal atresia can occur, the most common include **proximal esophageal atresia with a distal tracheoesophageal fistula** (80% of patients), **isolated esophageal atresia** (10% of patients), and **pure tracheoesophageal fistula** (<5% of patients).

Clinical Features

Esophageal atresia is almost always **diagnosed within hours of birth**. Most commonly, the infant **coughs, chokes, and vomits** all liquids immediately. Occasionally, **aspiration pneumonia** develops.

Evaluation

The condition can be diagnosed quickly by passing a **nasogastric tube;** if the tube meets resistance at 3 to 5 in., esophageal atresia is suspected. A plain **chest radiograph** confirms the presence of a blind esophageal pouch. Pure tracheoesophageal fistulas (H-type) may be missed because the esophagus is intact. **Radiographic contrast studies** can be performed; however, very small amounts of a water-soluble contrast material should be used to prevent pulmonary edema and respiratory distress.

Treatment

Initial conservative therapy includes **upright positioning,** frequent **nasopharyngeal suctioning, and intravenous fluids**. The infant should be placed on **nothing per mouth status**.

Surgical correction is performed to reconnect the esophagus to the gastric cavity and to repair any associated fistulas. Occasionally, reconnection of the esophagus and stomach is not possible, and **colonic interposition** (i.e., using a portion of colon to connect the distal esophagus to the stomach) is required.

Patients often require long-term **antireflux medical therapy** secondary to poor esophageal motility.

Bezoars
Etiology

Bezoars are accumulations of exogenous matter in the stomach or small intestine. The various types include **trichobezoars** (hair balls), **phytobezoars** (food balls), **lactobezoars** (milk or formula in infants), and **foreign body bezoars**.

 HINT: Although lactobezoars usually occur in infants, the other types of bezoars most commonly occur in developmentally delayed individuals between 10 and 19 years of age. Bezoars are often seen in institutionalized children.

Clinical Features

Children typically present with **vomiting, abdominal distention, pain, severe halitosis, and weight loss,** and they may have a history of **pica. Patchy baldness** is often a clue to the presence of a trichobezoar. Commonly, an **abdominal mass** can be palpated in the epigastrium or left upper quadrant.

Evaluation

Plain radiographs and radiographic contrast studies may demonstrate the mass; however, **upper endoscopy** is the most useful test because it may be both diagnostic and therapeutic. Children with documented bezoars should be evaluated for **pica, iron-deficiency anemia, and lead toxicity**.

Treatment

Lactobezoars respond to **withholding oral feeding** for 48 hours. Trichobezoars require **surgical removal**. The removal of all other bezoars may be attempted **endoscopically;** however, in many cases, surgical removal is necessary.

Cholecystitis
Etiology

Cholecystitis, **inflammation of the gallbladder,** is caused by bile stasis within the gallbladder. The causes of bile stasis in children include **cholelithiasis (most common), congenital ductal anomalies, external compression of the bile duct, and trauma**.

Clinical Features

The history typically reveals **right upper quadrant pain** radiating to the back, **jaundice, rigors, and fever**. **Nausea and vomiting** occur after eating. Symptoms usually develop rapidly; however, the patient may have mild symptoms for several years.

Evaluation

Murphy sign (tenderness upon palpating the right costal margin during inspiration) can often be appreciated.

Hyperbilirubinemia, an **elevated γ-glutamyl transpeptidase** level, and **leukocytosis** may suggest cholecystitis.

Although **abdominal plain radiographs** can detect the calcified stones, **abdominal ultrasound** is warranted to detect a thickened gallbladder wall, dilated ducts, or an obstructing stone. Occasionally, **cholescintigraphy** is indicated to show abnormal filling of bile into the gallbladder (the administration of cholecystokinin can help reproduce clinical symptoms).

Treatment

Conservative therapy includes hospitalization for the administration of **intravenous fluids and antibiotics** (for patients with a high fever or clinical deterioration) and the **cessation of eating**. In some patients with acalculous cholecystitis, conservative therapy is all that is required for the resolution of symptoms; however, in most patients (and all of those with cholelithiasis), the accepted treatment is **cholecystectomy**.

Central Nervous System Disorder

Irritation of the brainstem vomiting center by brain tumors, congenital cysts, hydrocephalus, or infections can cause severe vomiting; a **neurologic cause should always be considered in a child with vomiting**.

The vomiting commonly occurs in the **early morning** and is associated with **headaches**. Other signs and symptoms include **changes in the child's**

personality, fatigue, ataxia, diplopia, nystagmus, papilledema, head tilt, and loss of vision.

Ureteropelvic Junction Obstruction
Etiology
An unusual but important cause of vomiting in children is ureteropelvic junction obstruction, a morphologic **abnormality of** the **ureteropelvic junction** that causes obstruction or restriction of urinary outflow and subsequent hydronephrosis.

Clinical Features
Children frequently present with **right- or left-sided abdominal pain and vomiting**. The pain is often **intermittent,** which makes the diagnosis difficult. Occasionally, patients also have **hematuria** or signs of a **urinary tract infection**.

Evaluation
Abdominal ultrasound usually permits diagnosis; however, because the kidneys may appear normal between episodes, the ultrasound should be performed when the child is experiencing symptoms. In rare cases, an **intravenous pyelogram** is indicated.

Treatment
Surgical correction is required.

Bulimia
Etiology
A **psychogenic cause** of vomiting should be considered in adolescents, especially adolescent girls, who otherwise appear well and have no other cause for their vomiting.

Clinical Features and Evaluation
A **careful history** should be taken, looking for evidence of **anorexia, bulimia, or laxative and ipecac abuse**. Questions should be designed to elicit information regarding diet, eating habits, self-worth, exercise, changes in menses, purging, and medication use. The diagnostic criteria for bulimia include repeated episodes of **binge eating,** regular episodes of **self-induced vomiting,** a persistently **poor self-image** (e.g., of being overweight), and a **lack of control of eating during meals**.

The **nails, teeth, and gums** should be examined for evidence of nutritional inadequacies. **Laboratory studies** may reveal electrolyte abnormalities (as a result of persistent vomiting) and provide an overview of the patient's nutritional health (e.g., albumin, calcium, phosphorus, iron stores). An **electrocardiogram** may be abnormal in severely affected patients.

Treatment
The **prevention of acute life-threatening complications** (e.g., dehydration, cardiac abnormalities, electrolyte disturbances) is the primary concern. Patients should be referred to a qualified **psychotherapist** who has expertise in the management of eating disorders.

EVALUATION OF VOMITING
Patient History
The following questions may provide insight into the cause of the vomiting:

- **Does the patient have a fever?** Fever implies infection.
- **Does the patient have a history of pica?** Pica implies bezoar.
- **Does the patient complain of heartburn, globus, water brash, or epigastric pain related to meals?** Think GERD and esophagitis.
- **If the child is an infant, does he have an unusual odor?** Unusual odors may be a sign of a metabolic disorder.
- **When does the vomiting occur?** Frequent vomiting in the morning can be a sign of pregnancy or a neurologic disorder.
- **How old is the patient?** Some causes of vomiting are more prevalent in certain age groups (Table 82-1).
- **Is the vomitus bilious or bloody?** Bile-stained vomitus points to an anatomic problem (e.g., intestinal volvulus, intussusception, incarcerated hernia).

Physical Examination
The following should be noted during physical examination:

- **Head and neck**—abnormal teeth, reflux, bulging fontanelle.
- **Abdomen**—right upper quadrant mass, signs of gallbladder disease, epigastric tenderness (suggests pancreatitis, gastritis, or esophagitis), right upper quadrant tenderness (suggests liver or gallbladder disease), borborygmi (suggests possible intestinal obstruction).
- **Rectum**—heme-positive stools (suggest mucosal disease).
- **Neurologic examination**—cranial nerve abnormalities, gait abnormalities, papilledema (suggests central nervous system disease).

Laboratory Studies
The following studies may be appropriate:

- **Complete blood count with differential**—eosinophilia suggests eosinophilic enteritis or allergic disease.
- **Erythrocyte sedimentation rate and C-reactive protein**—an abnormal erythrocyte sedimentation rate/C-reactive protein suggests inflammation, possibly of the intestine.

TABLE 82-1	Common Causes of Vomiting by Age
Infant	Anatomic obstruction, metabolic disorder, infection, GERD, allergy, overfeeding, bezoar
Toddler	Infection, medication, GERD, intussusception, foreign body, bezoar, malrotation
Child	GERD, cyclic vomiting, malrotation, infection
Adolescent	Pregnancy, bulimia, infection, ulcer, malrotation, celiac disease, pseudo-obstruction, drug abuse, pancreatitis, GERD, cyclic vomiting

GERD, gastroesophageal reflux disease.

- **Chemistry panel**—increased alanine aminotransferase, γ-glutamyl transpepti- dase, or bilirubin levels suggest gallbladder or liver disease
- **Amylase and lipase levels**—increased amylase or pancreatic lipase levels sug- gest pancreatitis
- **Antiendomysial and tissue transglutaminase antibodies**—elevation suggests celiac disease
- **Stool sample**—occult blood suggests intestinal mucosal disease; viral or bacte- rial pathogen detection

Diagnostic Modalities

The following diagnostic modalities may be appropriate:

- **Contrast radiographic studies** are integral in the diagnosis of intestinal ana- tomic abnormalities.
- **Endoscopy** may be the most important tool for the definitive diagnosis of many esophageal, gastric, and duodenal disorders.
- A **barium enema** identifies distal obstructions.
- **Abdominal ultrasound** is useful in the evaluation of liver and gallbladder dis- orders, pyloric stenosis, pancreatitis, and kidney disease.
- An **abdominal computed tomography scan** defines the anatomy of the abdominal cavity (when used with both enteral and intravenous contrast). In most patients, computed tomography provides a more specific image than ultra- sound.

Suggested Readings

Behrman RE, Kliegman RM, Jensen HB. *Textbook of Pediatrics*. 16th ed. Philadelphia: WB Saunders; 2000.

Fleisher GR, Ludwig S, Henretig FM, et al. *Textbook of Pediatric Emergency Medicine*. 4th ed. Baltimore: Williams & Wilkins; 2000.

Furuta GT, Liacouras CA, Collins MH, et al. Eosinophilic esophagitis in children and adults: a sys- tematic review and consensus recommendation for diagnosis and treatment. *Gastroenterology*. 2007;133:1342–1363.

Li BK, Sunku BK. Vomiting and nausea. In: Wyllie R, Hyams JS, Kay M, eds. *Pediatric Gastrointestinal and Liver Diseases*. 4th ed. Philadelphia: Elsevier; 2011: 88–105.

Malaty HM. Epidemiology of *Helicobacter pylori* infection. *Best Pract Res Clin Gastroenterol*. 2007;21:205– 214.

Polin RA, Ditmar MF. *Pediatric Secrets*. 4th ed. Philadelphia: Hanley & Belfus; 2005.

Sadow KB, Atabaki SM, Johns CM, et al. Bilious emesis in the pediatric emergency department: etiology and outcome. *Clin Pediatr*. 2002;41(7):475–479.

Sondheimer JM. Vomiting. In: Walker WA, Goulet O, Kleinman RE, et al. eds. *Pediatric Gastrointestinal Disease*. 4th ed. Hamilton, ON: BC Decker; 2004:203–209.

Toxicology

GASTRIC DECONTAMINATION

Administration of **activated charcoal** is the preferred method of gastric decontamination. **Whole bowel irrigation and gastric lavage** play a much lesser role in the management of the poisoned patient but may still be of benefit in selected patients. **Syrup of ipecac** is not recommended for most poisonings.

Activated Charcoal
Indications and Contraindications

Activated charcoal is indicated for all ingestions if administration can occur within 1 hour of ingestion, unless specifically contraindicated. **Contraindications** include the following:

- Compromised, unprotected airway (aspiration risk)
- Gastrointestinal bleeding or perforation
- Caustic ingestions (charcoal impedes endoscopic visualization)
- Aliphatic hydrocarbon ingestion (may promote vomiting and aspiration)

 HINT: Not all substances bind to activated charcoal (Table 83-1).

TABLE 83-1	**Agents with Limited or Uncertain Binding to Activated Charcoal**
Iron	**Caustics**[a]
Lithium	NaOH (lye)
Heavy metals	KOH
Arsenic	HCl (hydrochloric acid)
Mercury	H_2SO_4 (sulfuric acid)
Lead	**Low-molecular-weight compounds**
Thallium	Cyanide
Alcohols	**Pesticides**
Methanol	Organophosphates
Ethanol	Carbamates
Isopropanol	
Ethylene glycol	
Hydrocarbons	
Kerosene	
Gasoline	
Mineral seal oil	

[a]Administration of activated charcoal may also impede further management.

Administration

The **dose is 1 g/kg, up to 60 g total** of activated charcoal. Mixing the charcoal with **flavored syrups** and putting it in a covered cup with a straw facilitates oral administration. **Nasogastric intubation** is required in alert but uncooperative patients, but should be done with extreme caution as it increases the risk of charcoal aspiration. Patients with altered mental status should not receive activated charcoal unless their airway is first secured.

Complications

Complications of activated charcoal use include **vomiting and aspiration, constipation or obstipation, desorption of poison** from charcoal, and **late absorption** in patients with delayed gastrointestinal motility (e.g., those taking drugs with anticholinergic properties). **Death** has occurred in a child who aspirated activated charcoal mixed with a magnesium cathartic.

Whole Bowel Irrigation

Whole bowel irrigation involves **copious irrigation of the gastrointestinal tract,** via nasogastric tube, to force the poisons rapidly through the bowel before significant absorption can occur. The solution used, polyethylene glycol 3,500 MW iso-osmotic bowel solution **(GoLYTELY),** causes no significant fluid or electrolyte loss in the gut.

Indications and Contraindications

Potential indications, to date, have been limited to **agents that do not adsorb well to charcoal** or that have the potential for absorption distally in the gastrointestinal tract, such as **iron, heavy metals such as lead**, **lithium, and sustained-release**

products (e.g., many antiarrhythmics, theophylline). Other scenarios may be amenable to whole bowel irrigation as an adjunct to activated charcoal administration, such as ingestions of patch medications, and delayed presentation of high-lethality toxic ingestions. In addition, whole bowel irrigation is used to **treat body packers** (people who ingest large numbers of packets of cocaine or heroin wrapped in latex condoms). Whole bowel irrigation is **contraindicated in patients with evidence of ileus or bowel perforation**.

Administration
GoLYTELY is administered at a dose of **500 mL/hour in young children** and at a dose of **up to 2 L/hour in adolescents and adults,** usually via nasogastric tube. The patient should be sitting up during treatment. The **endpoint** for stopping whole bowel irrigation is a **clear rectal effluent and recovery from poisoning**.

Complications
The major complications reported from whole bowel irrigation are **vomiting and abdominal pain**. Further, patients should not be permitted to "drink" whole bowel irrigation as the required volume per hour cannot be achieved voluntarily and the treatment will fail.

Gastric Lavage
Gastric lavage removes 10% to 25% of ingested toxin when performed within 30 to 60 minutes of ingestion.

Indications and Contraindications
Gastric lavage may **not be useful more than 1 hour after ingestion** unless the ingested poison delays gastric emptying. It has been shown to improve outcome in patients who are comatose and receive gastric lavage **within 60 minutes**. In other patients, the potential risks of gastric lavage must be weighed heavily against its benefit.

Gastric lavage should be reserved for the **critically ill poisoning patient** or a patient who is likely to undergo rapid decompensation. **Patients who ingest liquid medicines** may benefit from nasogastric lavage if it is performed within 30 to 60 minutes.

Gastric lavage **should not be performed in patients with airway compromise before endotracheal intubation**. Other **contraindications** include the **ingestion of caustic alkaline substances** or small amounts of **acids or hydrocarbons, abnormal esophageal anatomy, and bleeding diatheses**.

Administration
Gastric lavage requires the placement of a **large-bore** (24 to 36 French) **orogastric tube** followed by **repeated infusion and withdrawal** of room temperature **normal saline** in 50- to 200-mL aliquots. Before lavage, one must **ensure a protected airway:** Position the patient on the left side with the head below the feet, and determine correct gastric tube position.

Complications
Complications include **vomiting** with pulmonary aspiration, **gastric or esophageal perforation, hypopharyngeal and airway trauma with bleeding,**

laryngospasm, and accidental tracheal intubation with inadvertent pulmonary lavage.

Syrup of Ipecac

Syrup of ipecac, derived from the ipecacuanha plant, causes vomiting by **direct gastric irritation** and through a direct central effect at the chemotactic trigger zone in the medulla. Up to 93% of patients who receive ipecac vomit within 30 to 60 minutes.

Indications and Contraindications

Indications are now limited to patients within 30 to 90 minutes after ingestion who are at substantial risk of toxicity, do not have a contraindication to ipecac administration, who will be delayed beyond 1 hour before receiving emergency care, and for whom syrup of ipecac will not delay or adversely affect definitive treatment. Except for rural residents, these guidelines severely limit the potential use of syrup of ipecac, and the American Academy of Pediatrics no longer recommends routine prescribing of syrup of ipecac as part of well child care. It is almost never used in the hospital setting.

Contraindications to ipecac use consist of **altered mental status** (lethargy, coma, seizures—either existing or impending) and ingestion of **caustic substances, aliphatic hydrocarbons, or drugs with a high likelihood of rapid serious effects** (e.g., cyclic antidepressants, antiarrhythmics, clonidine, isoniazid, lithium, alcohol). In addition, **patients who have already spontaneously vomited** will not receive any further benefit from syrup of ipecac administration.

Administration

Dose is based on age: for children **6 months to 1 year of age,** give **10 mL** (2 tsp); **1 to 12 years, 15 mL** (1 tbsp); and **>12 years, 30 mL** (2 tbsp). Give the **child 10 mL/kg of water,** up to 240 mL (8 oz), after administering the syrup of ipecac. Repeat the dose if no vomiting occurs within 30 minutes.

Complications

Complications include **excessive vomiting, Mallory–Weiss tears, pneumomediastinum, and delayed delivery** of activated charcoal or other oral antidotes. Chronic use of syrup of ipecac or inadvertent administration of the much more concentrated extract of ipecac has caused myocardial and neuromuscular toxicity.

Cathartics

Indications and Contraindications

Cathartics have **no demonstrated efficacy** in poisoning treatment. Coadministration of cathartic with activated charcoal in patients >12 years of age may prevent obstipation. Cathartics are **contraindicated** in patients with **bowel perforation, ileus, or diarrhea.**

Administration

Cathartics should only be given as a **single dose** when administered with activated charcoal; **multiple doses** of cathartics should be **avoided except as outlined in** section on "**Elimination Enhancement.**" If a cathartic is given, sorbitol **35%** is the preferred agent because it has a rapid onset of catharsis. The **dose of sorbitol 35% is 1 g/kg** (3 mL/kg).

Complications

Complications include **electrolyte imbalance and dehydration**. Sorbitol also increases the likelihood of **vomiting** when given with activated charcoal. **Death** has occurred in several patients who received 4 to 6 doses of sorbitol over 24 hours.

ELIMINATION ENHANCEMENT

Extracorporeal clearance of toxin can be achieved by administering multiple-dose activated charcoal, inducing alkaline diuresis, or by performing hemodialysis or charcoal hemoperfusion.

Multiple-Dose Activated Charcoal

Multiple doses of activated charcoal **increase the clearance of theophylline, carbamazepine, phenytoin, phenobarbital,** and some **cyclic antidepressants**. The dose is **1 g/kg with cathartic for the initial dose, followed by 0.5 to 1 g/kg of activated charcoal without cathartic every 4 hours** until the patient has nontoxic blood levels, has shown clinical improvement, and has passed charcoal-laden stool.

Alkaline Diuresis

Alkaline diuresis can **enhance the excretion of weak acids,** especially **salicylates and phenobarbital** (but not other barbiturates). This procedure promotes conversion of these drugs to their ionized form within the proximal renal tubule and prevents distal tubular resorption (ion trapping). **Sodium bicarbonate** is given **intravenously** until a urine pH greater than 7.0 is achieved. Care must be taken to **avoid fluid overload, hypernatremia, hypokalemia, hypocalcemia, and hypomagnesemia** during alkaline diuresis.

Hemodialysis

Hemodialysis can **remove toxins with low molecular weight** (200 Da), **low plasma protein binding, and low tissue binding** as expressed by the volume of distribution (Vd):

Vd (L/kg) = Dose absorbed (mg/kg)/plasma concentration (mg/L)

Hemodialysis is most effective for drugs with a Vd <1 L/kg (Table 83-2).

Hemoperfusion

Hemoperfusion **diverts the patient's circulation** through a charcoal filter where the toxin binds to an activated charcoal cartridge. Charcoal hemoperfusion is technically more difficult and less available than hemodialysis. Furthermore, ingestions of theophylline and phenobarbital, the drugs most amenable to removal with hemoperfusion, are now more typically managed using multiple-dose activated charcoal or hemodialysis.

TABLE 83-2	Toxins Removed by Hemodialysis
Toxin	**Measured Level Suggestive of Need for Hemodialysis[a]**
Acetaminophen	≥1,000 µg/mL in conjunction with antidote
Arsenic	Only with coexistent renal failure
Bromide	≥150 mg/dL and severe symptoms
Ethanol	500 mg/dL
Ethylene glycol[b]	25 mg/dL
Isopropanol	400 mg/dL
Lithium	4 mEq/L in acute overdose As needed for severe symptoms in chronic overdose
Methanol	25 mg/dL
Salicylates	100–120 mg/dL in acute overdose 60–80 mg/dL in chronic overdose
Theophylline	80–100 µg/mL in acute overdose 60–80 µg/mL in chronic overdose

[a]The decision to perform hemodialysis should be based on physical findings as well as drug levels. A repeat measure should be obtained when the drug level is elevated to ensure that a laboratory error has not occurred. In addition, units of measurement should be checked before instituting hemodialysis.
[b]Administration of fomepizole may allow for management of higher levels of ethylene glycol without hemodialysis.

 HINT: Less than 1% of all pediatric poisoning patients require hemodialysis or hemoperfusion.

APPROACH TO THE POISONED PATIENT
Stabilization
Airway, breathing, circulation, and disability must be assessed in order, and compromise in any of these areas requires prompt attention. Complete exposure of the patient occurs as part of the rapid assessment. **Vital signs,** including **temperature,** continuous **monitoring of the heart rate, respiratory rate, blood pressure, and pulse oximetry,** should be initiated. **Supplemental oxygen** in an inspired concentration of 100% should be administered.

Administration of Substrates and Antidotes
Dextrose and Thiamine
The **glucose level** should be determined in any poisoned child with a **depressed level of consciousness,** using a rapid reagent strip. Hypoglycemia suggests certain ingestants (Table 83-3) and requires correction with **0.5 to 1 g/kg dextrose** administered as an **intravenous bolus**. Children who have ingested oral hypoglycemic agents should also receive **octreotide** (Table 83-4). **Thiamine (100 mg** intramuscularly or intravenously) should precede dextrose infusion in a patient who is suspected to be **alcoholic.**

TABLE 83-3	Agents Causing Hypoglycemia in Overdosed Children

Ethanol
Salicylates
Oral hypoglycemic agents
Propranolol
Insulin

 HINT: Hypoglycemia is the one metabolic abnormality that can cause focal neurologic findings.

Naloxone

Naloxone (**2 mg** intravenously, intramuscularly, or via endotracheal tube) **reverses coma caused by opioids**. It may also help some patients who have ingested clonidine. It should be given to **any child** with a **depressed level of consciousness** because it has **few adverse effects** in this setting and may prevent the need for aggressive intervention, such as endotracheal intubation. Response to naloxone occurs within 1 to 2 minutes of administration. After 30 minutes, the naloxone will wear off and resedation may occur. **Repeated naloxone administration or continuous intravenous naloxone infusion** is often required to prevent further depressed mental status.

 HINT: Children who have ingested codeine, dextromethorphan, LAAM (long-acting acetyl morphine), oxycodone, or methadone may require up to 10 mg of naloxone to fully reverse the opioid effects.

Flumazenil

Flumazenil is a benzodiazepine antagonist that has **reversed lethargy and coma** in adult benzodiazepine overdose patients. Flumazenil **may cause seizures** in a patient who has also ingested cyclic antidepressants or in a patient with a seizure disorder controlled by benzodiazepines, and it **may cause cardiac arrhythmias** in a poisoned patient who has also ingested chloral hydrate. Other side effects include **vomiting and anxiety**. Flumazenil administration **may help differentiate benzodiazepine overdose from other causes of coma** in children.

Given its potential risks, flumazenil should **only be given to children with severe symptoms** of benzodiazepine ingestion and **only if no signs of significant cyclic antidepressant overdose** (such as widened QRS) are present and **only if the patient does not have a seizure disorder**. The currently recommended dose is **0.01 mg/kg over 1 minute up to 0.5 mg per dose** and a **total maximum amount of drug administered of 1 mg**. Response occurs within 1 minute in most cases. Resedation may occur.

Physostigmine

Physostigmine, a cholinesterase inhibitor, **reverses the central anticholinergic effects of severe agitation and seizures** caused by **antihistamines** (e.g., diphenhydramine,

TABLE 83-4	Common Poisons and Antidotes[a]	
Poison	**Antidote**	**Administration**
Acetaminophen	N-Acetylcysteine (NAC)	Loading dose 140 mg/kg, then 17 doses at 70 mg/kg/dose. Dilute 20% solution to 5%–10% with juice or soda to improve palatability
		or
		IV NAC (Acetadote) given as 150 mg/kg over 1 hr, then 50 mg/kg over 4 hr and finally 100 mg/kg over 16 hr; use recommended pediatric concentration in young children
Anticholinergics	Physostigmine	See text
Benzodiazepines	Flumazenil	See text
β-Blockers	Glucagon	1–10 mg bolus, followed by 3–6 mg/hr
Calcium channel blockers	Glucagon	As for β-blockers
	Calcium gluconate 10%	0.3–0.6 mL/kg (8–16 mEq calcium/kg)
	Insulin	Insulin bolus 1 IU/kg followed by infusion of 0.5–1 IU/kg given concomitantly with 0.25 g/kg bolus dextrose followed by D10W+ 1/2 NS of and 20 mEq/L of potassium at 0.8 times maintenance with close monitoring of glucose and potassium
Carbon monoxide	Hyperbaric oxygen	
	Sodium thiosulfate 25%[a]	See cyanide
Cyanide	Hydroxocobalamin	70 mg/kg IV over 7 min
	Sodium nitrate 3%	Dose depends on hemoglobin (see cyanide antidote kit package insert). Do not exceed recommended dosage. Do not give to patients suffering from concomitant carbon monoxide exposure
	Sodium thiosulfate 25%	Dose depends on hemoglobin (see cyanide antidote kit package insert)
Digitalis	Digitalis Fab fragments	Calculate dose based on level or dose ingested or 10 vials if acute overdose, 5 vials if chronic overdose
Ethylene glycol	Ethanol	0.6 g/kg load over 1 hr followed by 100 mg/kg/hr infusion
	Or	
	Fomepizole	15 mg/kg loading dose, then 10 mg/kg every 12 hr for four doses followed by 15 mg/kg every 12 hr until ethylene glycol level <25 mg/dL. Give fomepizole every 4 hr during hemodialysis
	Pyridoxine	2 mg/kg
	Thiamine	0.5 mg/kg

TABLE 83-4	Common Poisons and Antidotes[a] (*Cont.*)	
Poison	**Antidote**	**Administration**
Methanol	Ethanol OR	As for ethylene glycol
	Fomepizole	As for ethylene glycol
	Folate	1 mg/kg every 4 hr
Iron	Deferoxamine	5–15 mg/kg/hr IV infusion
Isoniazid	Pyridoxine	3–5 g IV or dose equal to grams of isoniazid ingested
Lead	Lead level 45–69 μg/dL	
	Dimercaptosuc-cinic acid OR	10 mg/kg PO three times daily for 5 d, then twice daily for 14 d (may be useful at lower levels)
	Calcium NaEDTA	50–75 mg/kg/d divided, every 6 hr either IM or by slow IV infusion (IV use not FDA approved)
	Lead level $70 μg/dL	
	Calcium NaEDTA And	Administer as described earlier
	British antilewisite (BAL)	3–5 mg/kg IM every 4 hr for 5 d
	δ-Penicillamine	10 mg/kg/d for 1 wk increasing to 30 mg/kg/d as tolerated, only if unacceptable adverse reactions to dimercaptosuccinic acid or calcium NaEDTA
Methemoglobin-emia	Methylene blue 1%	1–2 mg/kg (0.1–0.2 mL/kg)
Opiates	Naloxone	2 mg IV, ETT, IM; repeat as needed
Oral hypoglyce-mic agents	Dextrose	IV bolus of 0.5 to 1 grams/kg
	Octreotide	1–1.5 mcg/kg (up to 150 mcg) every 6 hr
Organophos-phates	Atropine	0.1–0.5 mg/kg initial dose with additional doses as needed to counteract bronchorrhea
	Pralidoxime	25–50 mg/kg (up to 1 g); for severe cases, consider 10–15 mg/kg/hr infusion
Phenothiazines (dystonia)	Diphenhydramine or	1–2 mg/kg IM or IV or
	Benztropine	1–2 mg/kg IM or IV

D10W, 10% aqueous dextrose solution; *ETT*, endotracheal tube; *FDA*, Food and Drug Administration; *IM*, intramuscularly; *IV*, intravenously; *NaEDTA*, sodium ethylenediaminetetraacetic acid; *NS*, normal saline; *PO*, orally
[a]Consider for possible cyanide inhalation if the patient suffers from smoke inhalation.

doxylamine, scopolamine), **certain plants** (jimson weed, deadly nightshade, and henbane), **antiparkinsonian medications, dilating eyedrops, and skeletal muscle relaxants**. Physostigmine administration has **preceded asystole and death in patients who ingested cyclic antidepressants** and should be **avoided in these patients** and in patients with asthma, gastrointestinal obstruction, or genitourinary obstruction. The dose of physostigmine for children is **0.5 to 1 mg,** given **intravenously,** slowly over 5 minutes, with **atropine immediately available** for administration should **cholinergic symptoms** develop. Response to physostigmine occurs within minutes, and beneficial effects may persist longer than expected based on physostigmine's half-life of 60 minutes.

 HINT: Given the risks of physostigmine, it should be reserved for patients with a clear central anticholinergic syndrome who display hyperthermia, seizures, or severe agitation and only if no evidence exists of cyclic antidepressant toxicity. Consultation with a medical toxicologist is strongly advised prior to giving physostigmine and can occur by calling the regional poison control center (United States, 1-800-222-1222).

Pyridoxine (Vitamin B$_6$)

Pyridoxine **stops seizures caused by ingestion of isoniazid** by reversing γ-aminobutyric acid depletion. The dose is **3 to 5 g** or the **equivalent dose of isoniazid** ingested. This dose is much larger than the therapeutic dose and requires the administration of multiple vials of pyridoxine.

 HINT: If you anticipate that it will be necessary to reverse seizures from an isoniazid ingestion, notify the pharmacy so that they can obtain an adequate supply of pyridoxine.

N-acetylcysteine

N-acetylcysteine (NAC) completely prevents **acetaminophen-induced hepatic failure** when given within 8 hours of acute acetaminophen overdose, and greatly improves prognosis even when given beyond this time window. It prevents the conversion of nontoxic acetaminophen to toxic metabolites, which cause direct hepatocellular injury. There are two formulations available: one for oral administration (Mucomyst) and the other for IV administration (Acetadote). Efficacy is comparable between the two, but there is a small risk of anaphylactoid reactions with the IV preparation. The oral formulation is given as a **140 mg/kg loading dose, followed by 70 mg/kg every 4 hours**. The IV infusion is given as **150 mg/kg over 1 hour, followed by 50 mg/kg over 4 hours, then 100 mg/kg over 16 hours,** with continued infusion as necessary at this rate. Therapy can be discontinued with the guidance of a toxicologist or Poison Control Center as the optimal length of treatment varies between patients.

Sodium Bicarbonate

Sodium bicarbonate can be a life-saving intervention in patients with **cyclic antidepressants** or other **cardiac sodium channel-blocking agents**. By altering the acid-base toxicokinetics of these agents, bicarbonate prevents seizures and narrows the QRS complex, decreasing the likelihood of ventricular dysrhythmias. In addition, alkalinizing the serum with IV bicarbonate shifts **salicylates** out of target tissues, such as brain and myocardium, and back into the serum where it can be filtered and excreted by the kidney. A reasonable starting dose is one 50 mEq ampule in adults, or **1 to 2 mEq/kg** in children through rapid IV administration. Doses may be repeated as necessary, as long as care is taken to avoid over-alkalinizing the serum (pH > 7.55).

Table 83-4 lists the most commonly used antidotes. Those who are unfamiliar with the use of antidotes should consult with a regional poison control center (1-800-222-1222) or medical toxicologist before attempting administration.

 HINT: Antidotes help in ~3% of poisonings.

Decontamination
Gastric decontamination should be carried out as described in the previous section. External decontamination of the patient requires **removal of any clothing and copious irrigation** of the skin and eyes with room-temperature normal saline solution.

 HINT: External decontamination of some poisoned patients (e.g., those who have ingested pesticide) may place health care providers at risk. Universal precautions should be used.

Supportive Care
The patient's clinical course is altered by administration of specific antidotes in only 3% of toxic exposures. **Good outcome** for the remainder of patients **depends on adherence to general principles of toxicology** and good general medical care, primarily **rapid assessment and intervention** to maintain **airway, breathing, and circulation**.

 HINT: Institution of supportive care is most important to the successful resuscitation of the poisoned patient.

Identification of the Toxin
Presumptive Diagnosis
Presumptive diagnosis of the type of agent causing poison symptoms can **guide treatment until a definitive diagnosis** is made. Many times the exact toxin is known from the outset by the history. However, with very ill children, the first history is often not the best, and one must **look for specific clues** on physical examination. **Combinations of physical findings ("toxidromes") indicate specific classes of drugs** with effects on vital signs, pupillary response, neurologic status, breath and body odors, and skin changes (Tables 83-5 and 83-6).

TABLE 83-5	Common Toxidromes in Children	

Agent	Toxidrome	
Opiates	VS:	Hypothermia, bradypnea, bradycardia, hypotension
	CNS:	Flaccid coma
	Pupils:	Miotic to pinpoint
	Other:	Extraocular paralysis, delayed GI motility
Sedatives	VS:	Hypothermia, bradypnea, bradycardia, hypotension
	CNS:	Coma, often prolonged or cyclical; nystagmus
	Pupils:	Miotic (early barbiturate)
		Dilated (late barbiturate, glutethimide)
	Other:	Delayed GI motility
Ethanol	VS:	Hypothermia, bradypnea, bradycardia
	CNS:	Coma, nystagmus
	Pupils:	Miotic
	Skin:	Flushed
	Odor:	Sickly sweet breath odor
	Other:	Hypoglycemia, increased osmolal gap
Anticholinergic agents	VS:	Hyperthermia, tachycardia, hypertension
	CNS:	Agitation, delirium, seizures
	Pupils:	Mydriatic
	Skin:	Flushed, dry, warm
	Other:	Decreased GI motility, urine retention, cardiac tachyarrhythmias
Sympathomimetic agents	VS:	Hyperthermia, tachycardia, hypertension (bradycardia if pure α-adrenergic)
	CNS:	Agitation, delirium, seizures
	Pupils:	Mydriatic
	Skin:	Diaphoretic, cool and clammy
	Other:	Increased GI motility, piloerection
Cholinergic agents	VS:	Bradycardia or tachycardia, hypotension, tachypnea with bronchospasm
	CNS:	Coma, seizures
	Pupils:	Miotic
	Skin:	Diaphoretic
	Other:	Muscle fasciculation, weakness, paralysis, salivation, lacrimation, vomiting, urinary and fecal incontinence
Serotonin syndrome	VS:	Hyperpyrexia, tachycardia, hypertension
	CNS:	Agitation, coma
	Pupils:	Mydriatic
	Skin:	Diaphoretic
	Other:	Lower extremity rigidity, myoclonus, hyperreflexia

Toxidromes represent a collection of clinical findings often associated with poisoning by a specific class of drugs. However, a poisoned child may not display all physical findings commonly associated with a specific drug or may have findings not usually associated with a specific drug. Toxidromes by themselves cannot be used to exclude or confirm ingestion of a particular drug.

CNS, central nervous system; *GI*, gastrointestinal; *VS*, vascular system.

Adapted from Henretig FM, Shannon M. Toxicologic emergencies. In *Textbook of Pediatric Emergency Medicine*. 3rd ed. Baltimore: Williams & Wilkins; 1993:750; Mofenson HC, Greensher J. The unknown poison. *Pediatrics* 1974;54:446.

TABLE 83-6	Common Causes of Toxidromes in Children

Opiates
Buprenorphine (child of a heroin addict)
Cough syrups (dextromethorphan)
Codeine
Methadone (child of a heroin addict)
Oxycodone (prescription drug abuse)

Sedatives
Benzodiazepines
Barbiturates
γ-Hydroxybutyrate (GHB, club drug)

Anticholinergic agents
Antihistamines
Antidepressant drugs[a]
Antipsychotic drugs[a]
Plants (jimsonweed, Amanita muscaria mushrooms, henbane, Atropa belladonna)
Skeletal muscle relaxants (cyclobenzaprine)

Sympathomimetic agents
Decongestants (pure α-adrenergic drugs)
Cocaine
Amphetamines
Cholinergic agents
Pesticides (organophosphate, carbamate)
Mushrooms

Serotonin syndrome
Serotonin specific reuptake inhibitors
Monoamine oxidase inhibitors
MDMA (ecstasy)

[a]Drug effects may not be primarily anticholinergic.

 HINT: The history and physical examination can provide valuable clues to the possible ingestant even when the patient does not display all the components of a toxidrome.

Bedside Tests

Bedside tests give additional information as to the poison ingested but **require definitive laboratory studies** for confirmation. A **rapid glucose reagent stick** detects the presence of hypoglycemia (see Table 83-3 for a list of the common toxic causes of hypoglycemia in children). Moreover, hyperglycemia is a useful indicator of toxicity in suspected calcium-channel blocker ingestions.

- The **ketone square on the urine dipstick** turns purple in the presence of ace- toacetic acid (nitroprusside reaction). Urinary ketones are commonly seen after ingestion of salicylates and isopropanol.

  Contrary to some teaching, using an ultraviolet light to test for **urine fluo- rescence** is not helpful in making the diagnosis of ethylene glycol poisoning. For urine to fluoresce, the product ingested must contain fluorescein, which is not present in all antifreeze or other ethylene glycol products. A negative result may be falsely reassuring.

- **Discordance between patient appearance and pulse oximetry** may suggest the presence of carboxyhemoglobin or methemoglobinemia (pulse oximetry reading appears higher than expected or normal in the presence of cyanosis). This impression should be confirmed by direct measurement of carboxyhemoglobin or methemoglobin on a venous or arterial blood sample.

Laboratory Studies

Initial studies in symptomatic poisoned patients may include **arterial or venous blood gases, electrolytes** with calculation of the anion gap (Table 83-7), **serum glucose, blood urea nitrogen (BUN) and creatinine levels, and serum osmolarity** by the freezing point depression method with calculation of the osmolar gap:

$$\text{Osmolar gap} = \text{Measured osmolarity (freezing point depression)} - [(2 \times \text{Na}) + \text{blood urea nitrogen}/2.8 + \text{glucose}/18]$$

Normally, the osmolar gap is <10 mOsm. An **elevated osmolar gap suggests** the presence of alcohols (e.g., ethanol, methanol, isopropanol, ethylene glycol).

> **HINT:** A normal osmolar gap does not exclude the potential for serious ethylene glycol poisoning.

Specific drug levels are useful when the poison shows a dose-dependent toxicity, when treatment with an antidote is contemplated, or when a specific intervention, such as extracorporeal removal, is helpful (Table 83-8).

TABLE 83-7	Poisons Causing an Abnormal Anion Gap

Increased anion gap with metabolic acidosis
Carbon monoxide[a]
Cyanide
Ethanol[a]
Ethylene glycol[a]
Iron[a]
Isoniazid
Methanol[a]
Salicylates[a]
Theophylline[a]

Decreased anion gap
Bromide
Lithium[a]
Hypermagnesemia[a]
Hypercalcemia[a]
Anion gap = $\text{Na}^+ - (\text{Cl}^- + \text{CO}_2)$

[a]Specific levels rapidly available.

TABLE 83-8	Helpful Specific Drug Levels	
Drug	**Time to Peak Blood Level (Hours Postingestion)**	**Potential Intervention**
Acetaminophen	4	NAC administration
Carbamazepine	2–4[a,b]	—
Carboxyhemoglobin	Immediate	Hyperbaric oxygen therapy
Digoxin	2–4	Fab (digoxin antibody) fragment
Ethanol	1/2–1[b]	—
Ethylene glycol	0.5–1	Ethanol infusion OR fomepizole and hemodialysis
Iron	2–4	Deferoxamine administration
Isopropanol	0.5–1[b]	—
Lead	5 wk[a]	Chelation and environmental abatement
Lithium	2–4	Hemodialysis
Methanol	0.5–1	Ethanol infusion OR fomepizole and hemodialysis
Methemoglobinemia	Immediate	Methylene blue administration
Phenobarbital	2–4	Alkaline diuresis, multiple-dose activated charcoal
Phenytoin	1–2[a]	Multiple-dose activated charcoal
Salicylates	6–12[a]	Alkaline diuresis, multiple-dose activated charcoal, hemodialysis
Theophylline	1–36[a]	Multiple-dose activated charcoal, whole bowel irrigation, charcoal hemoperfusion, hemodialysis

[a]Repeated measurement of levels is necessary because of significant variation in time to reach to peak level.
[b]The peak level is predictive of toxicity and clinical course.
Adapted from Weisman RS, Howland MA, Verebey K. The toxicology laboratory. In: Goldfrank LR, Flomenbaum NE, Lewin NA, et al., eds. *Goldfrank's Toxicologic Emergencies*. 5th ed. East Norwalk, CT: Appleton Lange; 1994:105.

The rapid urine screen for drugs of abuse and the **comprehensive drug screen ("tox screen") have limited usefulness** in the management of the poisoned child. **False-positive and false-negative drug screens** can lead to misinterpretation of the patient's signs and symptoms. **Toxicologic screening may be warranted to confirm the diagnosis of poisoning** as opposed to other conditions such as central nervous system (CNS) infection or trauma, **or if intentional ingestion or child abuse is suspected**.

> **HINT:** Results of comprehensive drug screens typically take 6 to 24 hours and rarely change immediate management of the patient.

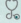

> **HINT:** Testing in the poisoned patient should progress from less specific to more specific, with emphasis on clearly identifying the presence of toxins that require antidotes or other specific procedures to prevent morbidity or mortality.

Diagnostic Modalities

A 12-lead electrocardiogram is an important adjunct in identifying seriously poisoned children. Strict attention should be paid to rhythm, QRS interval, and QT interval. Prolongation of the QRS interval (i.e., >0.10 milliseconds) indicates an increased risk of ventricular arrhythmias and commonly suggests ingestion of cyclic antidepressants, selected antipsychotics, quinidine, and type IA antidysrhythmic agents. Prolongation of the QT interval can occur with many psychotropic agents and if severe, may progress to Torsades de Pointes. Bradycardia with atrioventricular block suggests ingestion of digitalis-like agents, β-blockers, and calcium channel blockers.

- **An abdominal radiograph** allows detection of some toxic agents (e.g., iron, calcium salts, potassium salts, heavy metals [lead], chlorinated hydrocarbons). A **chest radiograph** may reveal the presence of hydrocarbon pneumonitis, a radiopaque foreign body, or acute lung injury from opioids, salicylates, and a number of other toxins. A **soft tissue neck radiograph** may help diagnose caustic airway injury.

> **HINT:** The absence of radiopaque pills or fragments does not exclude the possibility of ingestion if the film is taken after the substance (e.g., iron) has been absorbed.

Suggested Readings

Nelson LS, Lewin NA, Howland MA, et al. *Goldfrank's Toxicologic Emergencies.* 9th ed. New York: McGraw-Hill; 2010.

Olson KR (ed). *Poisoning & Drug Overdose.* 5th ed. New York: McGraw-Hill; 2006.

Shannon MW, Borron SW, Burns MJ. *Haddad and Winchester's Clinical Management of Poisoning and Drug Overdose.* 4th ed. Philadelphia: Saunders Elsevier; 2007.

Cardiology Laboratory

CHAPTER 84

Timothy M. Hoffman

BLOOD PRESSURE MEASUREMENT

Accurate measurement of the blood pressure depends on **selection of an appropriate cuff size** of a sphygmomanometer. By convention, an appropriate cuff size is a cuff with an inflatable bladder width that is at least 40% of the arm circumference at a point midway between the olecranon and the acromion. For a cuff to be optimal for an arm, the cuff bladder length should cover 80% to 100% of the circumference of the arm. Such a requirement demands that the bladder width-to-length ratio be at least 1:2. If the cuff size is too small, the blood pressure will be overestimated, and if it is too large, the blood pressure will be underestimated.

Auscultation of the diastolic component of the blood pressure exhibits **two end points, Korotkoff phases IV and V,** respectively. **In children, Korotkoff phase IV** (i.e., the point of diminution or muffling of the Korotkoff sound) is generally considered a **more accurate representation** of the diastolic pressure. Korotkoff phase V (i.e., the disappearance of the Korotkoff sounds) should be **considered the diastolic end point if it falls within 6 mm Hg of Korotkoff phase IV**.

Pulsus Paradoxus

Pulsus paradoxus, a **decrease of >10 mm Hg in the systolic blood pressure during inspiration,** may be associated with **cardiac tamponade** (e.g., as a result of pericardial effusion), **constrictive pericarditis, or severe respiratory compromise** (e.g., reactive airway disease exacerbation).

> 🫀 **HINT:** Pulsus paradoxus must not be confused with pulsus alternans (i.e., a decrease in the systolic pressure on alternate contractions that indicates left ventricular failure).

Using a sphygmomanometer, the cuff is **inflated until the pressure is 20 mm Hg above the systolic pressure**. The bladder is then **slowly deflated until the Korotkoff phase I sound is heard** independent of the respiratory cycle—this is the first data point. The slow deflation of the bladder is **continued until the Korotkoff phase I sound is noted throughout the respiratory cycle** (during inspiration *and* expiration)—the second data point. The difference in systolic blood pressure between the points is considered the reduction in systolic pressure during inspiration and is abnormal (pulsus paradoxus) if it is >10 mm Hg. Figure 84-1 depicts pulsus paradoxus schematically.

HYPEROXIA TEST

The hyperoxia test can be useful for **differentiating cardiac and pulmonary causes of cyanosis,** and it is **one of the first evaluations** performed when confronted **with a cyanotic newborn**. Cyanosis usually becomes apparent at a mean capillary concentration of at least 3.0 g/dL of deoxygenated hemoglobin, a concentration that corresponds to an oxygen saturation of 70% to 80% in the child with a normal hemoglobin level.

In infants with **cyanotic congenital heart disease (CHD)** (transposition of the great arteries [TGA] or a lesion with restrictive pulmonary blood flow [tricuspid

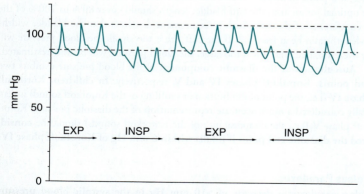

FIGURE 84-1 **Pulsus paradoxus.** *EXP,* expiration; *INSP,* inspiration. Modified with permission from Park MK. *Pediatric Cardiology for Practitioners.* 3rd ed. St. Louis: Mosby-Year Book; 1996:15.

atresia with pulmonary stenosis or atresia, pulmonary atresia or critical pulmonary stenosis with intact ventricular septum, or tetralogy of Fallot]) **and hypoxemia, the arterial oxygen tension** (PaO$_2$) is generally **<50 mm Hg** on 100% oxygen. In an infant with **cyanotic CHD** and a complete mixing lesion without restrictive pulmonary blood flow (truncus arteriosus, total anomalous pulmonary venous return, TGA with ventricular septal defect, single ventricle, hypoplastic left heart syndrome, and tricuspid atresia without pulmonary stenosis or atresia), the **PaO$_2$ is generally <150 mm Hg** in response to the administration of 100% oxygen. In an infant with a **pulmonary cause** for the cyanosis, administration of **100% oxygen increases the PaO$_2$** to a level significantly **>150 mm Hg.** In patients with **CHD,** this phenomenon is attributable to **right-to-left shunting** (i.e., the mixing of deoxygenated blood and oxygenated blood within the circulatory system). Right-to-left shunting may be either **intracardiac or extracardiac** (intrapulmonary shunting from ventilation-perfusion mismatch) (see section on "Agitated Saline Contrast Echocardiography").

BIOMARKERS

Brain natriuretic peptide (BNP) and N-terminal pro-brain natriuretic peptide (NT-proBNP) assays are used in algorithms for the diagnosis and management of acute and chronic heart failure in adults. BNP is biologically active with a half-life of 20 minutes, yet NT-proBNP is inactive with a half-life of 60 to 120 minutes. These assays should always be interpreted with caution as the results are method-dependent and comparisons amongst different laboratories may not be possible. In the pediatric age group and in patients with varying forms of CHD, there are **no absolute standards to date concerning levels of BNP or NT-proBNP**. Heterogeneous etiologies for heart failure in children as compared to adults have lead to studies that attempt to define the clinical relevance of BNP and NT-proBNP levels. In pediatrics, cardiac disease enhances natriuretic peptide expression due to hemodynamic stress and neurohormonal activation. Reference ranges are difficult to establish and are based on age, gender, and underlying pathophysiology (especially those with univentricular physiology). In light of this background, studies have suggested that BNP and NT-proBNP may be increased in concert with clinical severity amongst the following conditions: (1) hemodynamic load on either the right or the left ventricle in those with dilated cardiomyopathy, (2) excessive shunt with a patent ductus arteriosus (PDA), (3) right ventricular volume overload (e.g., s/p tetralogy of Fallot repair with resultant pulmonary regurgitation), (4) right ventricular pressure overload, and (5) with cardiac involvement in Kawasaki disease. Some studies suggest an adjunct utility of these assays in those rejecting post heart transplant, although absolute values have not been established. Similar to adult uses, longitudinal assessment may be helpful in an individual patient to monitor disease process or response to heart failure treatment. Finally, elevation of these markers may be noted in those postchemotherapy which portends the likely development of cardiac dysfunction.

> 🩺 **HINT:** Use of BNP and NT-proBNP in pediatrics must be done with the knowledge that absolute value cutoffs have yet to be established across all pathophysiologies. However, longitudinal assessment (i.e., using the patient as their own control) of the values may be helpful in determining response to treatment or severity of disease.

Troponin is a vital protein involved in the cascade leading to actin and myosin contraction. Cardiac contraction is regulated by calcium via a tropomyosin-like protein factor, which was discovered to be a complex of tropomyosin and troponin. Troponin is the calcium receptive protein and is integral in the contraction and relaxation of cardiac muscle. Troponin I and Troponin T are noted only in cardiac muscle. Troponin levels in pediatrics have been used to predict the degree of myocardial damage, either postoperatively or after use of cardiotoxic medications (including chemotherapy), and longitudinal evaluation has been helpful in predicting recovery or mortality. In neonates, troponin levels may be useful to assess the degree of cardiac damage associated with asphyxia. Troponin levels may be helpful in other disease states such as active myocarditis and determining cardiac damage to ischemia in those rare coronary anomalies noted in pediatrics.

ELECTROCARDIOGRAPHY

The electrocardiogram provides data concerning the following:

- Rate
- Rhythm
- Axes
- Intervals
- Hypertrophy
- Wave changes (Q waves and ST/T waves)

Rate

The heart rate is determined accurately by **dividing 60 by the RR interval** (measured in seconds). For example, if the RR interval is 0.4 second (10 small boxes), the heart rate is 60 divided by 0.4, or 150 beats/minute.

Rhythm

Rhythm diagnosis is beyond the scope of this chapter (see discussion in Chapter 74, "Syncope" and Chapter 75, "Tachycardia)."

Axes

The frontal axis should be determined for the **P, QRS, and T waves from the limb leads** (I, II, III, aVR, aVL, aVF). The **hexaxial reference system** (Figure 84-2) is usually used. The **normal** axes generally fall **between 0° and 90°**. The specific axis is **equal to the direction of the largest positive force on depolarization**.

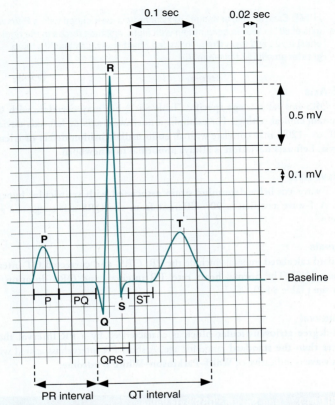

FIGURE 84-2 **Hexaxial reference system (frontal axis).** The shaded area represents the normal axis.

A cursory way to determine the frontal axis is to **note the complex that is isoelectric and locate the two planes perpendicular to it.** The **perpendicular plane with the greatest positive deflection** is indicative of the axis.

P-Wave Axis

The location of the P-wave axis **determines the origin of an atrial-derived rhythm:**

0° to 90° = high right atrial rhythm (normal sinus rhythm)
90° to 180° = high left atrial rhythm (ectopic atrial rhythm)
180° to 270° = low left atrial rhythm (ectopic atrial rhythm)
270° to 0° = low right atrial rhythm (ectopic atrial rhythm)

HINT: Classic "mirror image" dextrocardia is associated with a P-wave axis of 90° to 180° in conjunction with high amplitude forces in the right chest leads and low voltage in the left chest leads (i.e., lead V$_{4R}$ has a greater amplitude than lead V$_4$).

QRS Axis

The QRS axis value is **age specific** (Table 84-1) but **may correlate with CHD** in certain clinical settings. For example, a **northwest axis or left axis deviation** (−30° to −120°) may correlate with an **endocardial cushion defect or tricuspid atresia. Left axis deviation is always abnormal in a newborn.**

T-Wave Axis

The T-wave axis helps **determine strain associated with ventricular hypertrophy.** A T-wave axis that is **90° different from the QRS** axis suggests a strain pattern.

Intervals

Standard calculated intervals include the **PR, QRS, and corrected QT intervals** (Figure 84-3). The **normal heart rate, PR interval, and QRS duration vary with age** (Table 84-2).

PR Interval

First-degree atrioventricular block is characterized by a **PR interval that is greater than the standard** range for age. A short PR interval associated with a **delta wave** is indicative of **Wolff–Parkinson–White syndrome.**

TABLE 84-1	Age-Specific QRS Axis Values	
Age	**Mean (Degrees)**	**Range (Degrees)**
<1 d	135	60–180
1–7 d	125	60–180
8–30 d	110	0–180
1–3 mo	80	20–120
3–6 mo	65	20–100
6–12 mo	65	0–120
1–3 yr	55	0–100
3–5 yr	60	0–80
5–8 yr	65	340–100
8–12 yr	65	0–120
12–16 yr	65	340–100

Adapted with permission from Liebman J, Plonsey R, Gillette PC. *Pediatric Electrocardiography.* Baltimore: Williams & Wilkins; 1982:90.

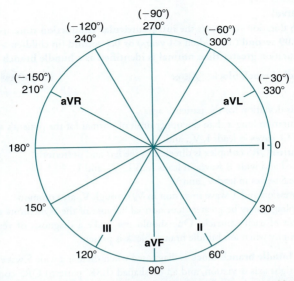

FIGURE 84-3 **A normal electrocardiogram showing waveforms and intervals.**
The standard paper speed is 25 mm/s; therefore, a single 1-mm box equals 0.04 second, and a large
(5-mm) box equals 0.20 second.

TABLE 84-2	Normal Heart Rate, PR Interval, and QRS Duration for Age					
	Heart Rate (beats/min)		**PR Interval in Lead II (second)**		**QRS Duration (second)**	
Age	**Mean**	**Range**	**Mean**	**Range**	**Mean**	**Range**
<1 d	126	95–155	0.106	0.082–0.138	0.05	0.025–0.069
1–7 d	135	100–180	0.107	0.079–0.130	0.05	0.025–0.068
8–30 d	160	120–190	0.100	0.075–0.128	0.053	0.026–0.075
1–3 mo	147	95–200	0.098	0.075–0.126	0.052	0.027–0.069
3–6 mo	139	114–170	0.105	0.078–0.137	0.053	0.028–0.075
6–12 mo	130	95–170	0.105	0.077–0.138	0.055	0.03–0.070
1–3 yr	121	95–150	0.113	0.090–0.140	0.056	0.032–0.070
3–5 yr	98	70–130	0.119	0.092–0.150	0.058	0.03–0.069
5–8 yr	86	65–120	0.124	0.094–0.155	0.059	0.035–0.075
8–12 yr	86	65–120	0.129	0.093–0.165	0.062	0.038–0.079
12–16 yr	86	65–120	0.135	0.098–0.169	0.065	0.040–0.081

Adapted with permission from Liebman J, Plonsey R, Gillette PC. *Pediatric Electrocardiography.* Baltimore:
Williams & Wilkins; 1982:96–97; Cassels DE, Ziegler RF. *Electrocardiography in Infants and Children.*
Philadelphia: Saunders; 1966:100.

QRS Interval

The QRS duration represents the **intraventricular conduction time** and is normally **<0.09 second** (in children **<4 years**) or **0.1 second** (in children **>4 years**). A QRS duration **greater than normal is identified as a bundle branch block:**

Left bundle branch block
Criteria:

- Left axis deviation for the patient's age.
- QRS duration longer than the upper limit of normal for the patient's age.
- Loss of Q waves in leads I, V_5, and V_6.
- The slurred QRS complex is directed to the left and posteriorly.
  - Slurred and wide R waves in leads I, aVL, V_5, and V_6
  - Wide S waves in lead V_1 and V_2
- ST depression and T wave inversion in V_4 through V_6 are common.
- QRS voltages may be greater than normal because of the asynchrony of depolarization of each ventricle. One should not make a diagnosis of ventricular hypertrophy when left bundle branch block is present.

Right bundle branch block is diagnosed when there is a wide S wave in leads I and V_6, right axis deviation, and an M-shaped (RSR′ pattern) QRS complex in lead V_1.

Criteria:

- Right axis deviation for the patient's age.
- QRS duration longer than the upper limit of normal for the patient's age.
- Terminal slurring of the QRS complex directed to the right and usually, but not always, anteriorly.
  - Wide and slurred S in lead I, V_5, and V_6
  - Terminal, slurred R′ in the right precordial leads (V_{4R}, V_1, and V_2)
- ST depression and T wave inversion are common in adults with right bundle branch block but not in children.
- Asynchrony of the normally opposing electromotive force of each ventricle may result in a greater manifest potential for both ventricles. Therefore, the diagnosis of ventricular hypertrophy is insecure when either right or left bundle branch block is present.

Left anterior hemiblock can be diagnosed in the setting of left axis deviation associated with right bundle branch block.

Left posterior hemiblock is manifested by marked right axis deviation and normal QRS duration. It is extremely rare in children.

QT Interval

The QT measurement is corrected for heart rate using this formula:

$$QT_c = \frac{measured\ QT\ (seconds)}{\sqrt{RR\ interval\ (seconds)}}$$

A normal **corrected QT interval (QTc) is <450 milliseconds for infants <6 months, and <440 milliseconds for children**.

Hypertrophy

Right Atrial Hypertrophy

Right atrial hypertrophy is shown on electrocardiogram when there is a **peaked P wave 3.0 mm in any lead**. This pattern is present most often in lead II and occasionally in V_1 and V_2.

Left Atrial Hypertrophy

A **P wave with a notched contour** and a duration of **<0.08 second in lead II** is diagnostic of left atrial hypertrophy. Alternatively, a **biphasic P wave in lead V_1 or V_{3R} with a terminal inverted portion** that measures 1×1 mm is diagnostic.

Right Ventricular Hypertrophy

Table 84-3 summarizes the normal measurements of R and S waves in leads V_1 and V_6 by age. Right ventricular hypertrophy can be diagnosed if any one of the following is seen:

- An R wave in lead V_1 > 98th percentile for age
- An S wave in lead V_6 > 98th percentile for age
- An upright T wave in lead V_1 in a patient >4 days
- Pure qR in leads V_{3R} or V_1

TABLE 84-3	Normal Range of Values (5th–95th Percentile) for R and S Waves in Leads V_1 and V_6			
	Lead V_1		Lead V_6	
Age	**R Wave (mm)**	**S Wave (mm)**	**R Wave (mm)**	**S Wave (mm)**
<1 d	7.0–20.0	2.5–27.0	2.3–7.0	1.6–10.3
1–7 d	9.0–27.4	4.6–18.8	2.2–13.1	0.8–9.9
8–30 d	4.2–19.8	2.5–12.8	1.7–20.5	0.6–9.0
1–3 mo	3.6–17.9	2.0–17.4	3.6–12.9	0.8–5.8
3–6 mo	6.1–16.7	2.1–11.8	5.0–15.8	0.6–4.9
6–12 mo	4.0–16.0	1.9–14.4	5.5–17.6	0.7–3.3
1–3 yr	3.6–15.0	2.2–20.5	5.0–17.5	0.6–3.4
3–5 yr	2.6–15.6	5.0–24.8	5.4–20.6	0.6–2.4
5–8 yr	2.6–13.5	5.3–21.0	7.9–20.5	0.6–2.9
8–12 yr	3.6–11.3	4.8–22.3	8.4–19.2	0.6–2.8
12–16 yr	2.1–11.1	5.5–22.3	7.9–17.4	0.7–3.1

Adapted with permission from Liebman J, Plonsey R, Gillette PC. *Pediatric Electrocardiography*. Baltimore: Williams & Wilkins; 1982:84–85.

- An RSR′ pattern in leads V_{3R} or V_1, in which the R′ portion is 15 mm greater than the R wave (in a child <1 year) or 10 mm greater than the R wave (in a child >1 year)

Left Ventricular Hypertrophy

Left ventricular hypertrophy can be diagnosed if any one of the following is seen:

- An R wave in lead V_6 > 98th percentile for age
- A narrow Q wave in lead V_5 or V_6 > 4 mm
- An R wave in lead V_1 < 5th percentile for age
- An S wave in lead V_1 > 98th percentile for age

Wave Changes

ST segment elevation >2 mm in the precordial leads may indicate pericarditis, myocardial injury, ischemia, infarction, or digitalis effect.

Tall peaked T waves may be seen in patients with hyperkalemia.

Flat T waves can occur in children with myocarditis, hypokalemia, or hypothyroidism.

CHEST RADIOGRAPH

When examining a chest radiograph, one must comment on the **cardiac size, organ situs, and the pulmonary vascular markings** (i.e., normal, increased, or decreased).

Cardiac Size

Cardiac size is determined by **estimating the cardiothoracic ratio**. The ratio is calculated by **dividing the largest diameter of the heart by the largest internal diameter of the thorax**. If the result is **>0.5, cardiomegaly** is present.

Organ Situs

Figure 84-4 depicts the normal cardiac silhouette in the anteroposterior and lateral views.

Pulmonary Vascular Markings

Pulmonary vascular markings **reflect the appearance of the pulmonary arteries and veins** on a chest radiograph **over the lung fields**.

These markings can be **increased in states of excessive pulmonary arterial flow** (e.g., ventricular septal defect, atrial septal defect, PDA), as well as in states characterized by **excessive pulmonary venous flow** (e.g., congestive heart failure, conditions characterized by pulmonary edema, or pulmonary venous obstruction). On the radiograph, **increased pulmonary vasculature is noted when cephalization occurs and the vascular shadows extend across more than two-thirds of the lung field**.

Decreased pulmonary vasculature markings are manifested radiographically as **hyperlucency of the lung field** and a **paucity of pulmonary vasculature,** as seen in patients with **tetralogy of Fallot**.

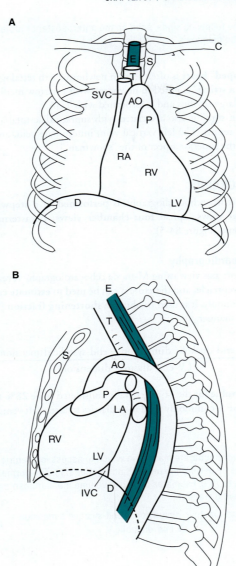

FIGURE 84-4   Normal cardiac silhouette. A. Anteroposterior view. **B.** Lateral view. *AO,* aorta; *C,* clavicle; *D,* diaphragm; *E,* esophagus; *IVC,* inferior vena cava; *LA,* left atrium; *LV,* left ventricle; *P,* pulmonary outflow tract; *RA,* right atrium; *RV,* right ventricle; *S,* sternum; *SVC,* superior vena cava; *T,* trachea. Modified with permission from Sapire DW. *Understanding and Diagnosing Pediatric Heart Disease.* East Norwalk, CT: Appleton & Lange; 1991:64.

> 🩺 **HINT:** The following signs, seen on the anteroposterior projection, offer clues to the diagnosis.

A "**boot-shaped**" **heart** is often seen in newborns with tetralogy of Fallot.

An "**egg on a string**" is noted in newborns with a narrow mediastinum owing to absence of a large thymus and is associated with TGA.

A "**snowman sign**" is also associated with supracardiac total anomalous pulmonary venous return. The left vertical vein, innominate vein, and the superior vena cava form the superior aspect of the "snowman."

ECHOCARDIOGRAPHY

In pediatric patients, echocardiography is **performed in a stepwise fashion** to obtain **subcostal views, apical four-chamber views, parasternal views, and suprasternal views** (Figure 84-5).

M-Mode Echocardiography

A parasternal short axis view using M-mode echocardiography reveals a **cross section of the left ventricle,** and therefore it can be used to **estimate cardiac dimensions**. Most commonly, it is used to obtain a **shortening fraction** (SF) calculated in the following manner:

$$SF = \frac{LV \text{ end-diastolic dimension} - \text{end-systolic dimension}}{LV \text{ end-diastolic dimension}} \times 100$$

The **normal value** for the SF is generally considered to be **28% to 40%,** independent of age. SF is commonly used in pediatrics to assess left ventricular systolic performance.

> 🩺 **HINT:** A more accurate manner in which to assess left ventricular performance is by performing an ejection fraction (EF). The normal values for EF are 54% to 75%. Estimates of EF use volume measurements calculated in the following manner:
>
> $$EF = \frac{LV \text{ end-diastolic dimension} - \text{end-systolic dimension}}{LV \text{ end-diastolic V}} \times 100$$

Doppler Echocardiography

Doppler echocardiography detects a **frequency shift** that reflects the **direction and velocity of blood flow**. Doppler echocardiography is used to detect **valvular insufficiency or stenosis and abnormal vasculature flow patterns**. The Bernoulli equation is used to assess gradients or pressure estimates depending on the flow pattern sampled. The equation can be simplified to the following:

A. Subcostal views

B. Apical views

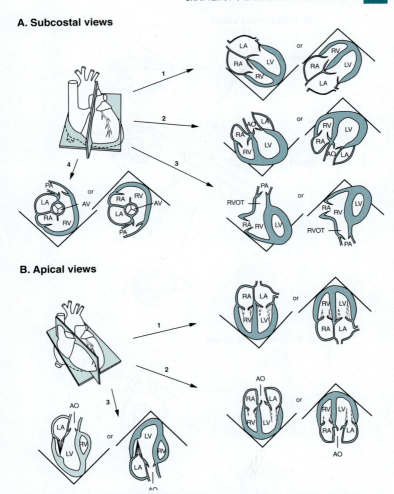

FIGURE 84-5 **Echocardiographic series.** The *numbers* represent different planes along a sweep of the echocardiographic beam. **A.** Subcostal views. **B.** Apical views. (*continued*)

C. Parasternal views

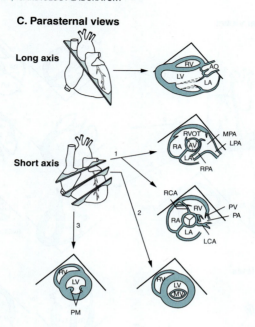

D. Suprasternal views

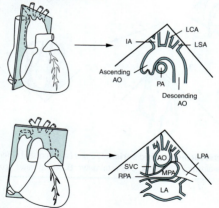

FIGURE 84-5 (*Continued*) **C.** Parasternal views. **D.** Suprasternal views. *AO,* aorta; *AV,* aortic valve; *IA,* innominate artery; *LA,* left atrium; *LCA,* left coronary artery; *LPA,* left pulmonary artery; *LSA,* left subclavian artery; *LV,* left ventricle; *MPA,* middle pulmonary artery; *MV,* mitral valve; *PA,* pulmonary artery; *PM,* papillary muscle; *PV,* pulmonary valve; *RA,* right atrium; *RCA,* right coronary artery; *RPA,* right pulmonary artery; *RV,* right ventricle; *RVOT,* right ventricular outflow tract; *SVC,* superior vena cava. Modified with permission from Park MK. *Pediatric Cardiology for Practitioners.* 3rd ed. St. Louis: Mosby; 1996:70–73.

ΔP (pressure difference across an obstructed orifice) = $4 \times V_2$ (velocity distal to the obstruction)^2. For example, if one is measuring Doppler flow across the aortic valve and V_2 is 3 m/s, using the modified Bernoulli equation would estimate the pressure gradient to be 4×3^2, which equals 36 mm Hg.

Agitated Saline Contrast Echocardiography

Agitation of saline produces 10- to 100-μm-diameter microbubbles that are absorbed by transit in the capillary bed. If a patient has a suspected right-to-left shunt (either extracardiac [intrapulmonary] or intracardiac) that cannot be detected by standard echocardiographic techniques, agitated saline contrast echocardiography may be helpful. The presence of microbubbles in the left heart after venous injection of agitated saline confirms the presence of right-to-left shunting.

The site of injection to answer specific questions must be carefully planned. For example, investigation of a potential left superior vena cava drainage pattern would be best served with an intravenous saline injection in the left upper extremity.

Extracardiac (intrapulmonary) shunts (i.e., pulmonary arteriovenous malformations) are marked by microbubbles appearing in the left side of the heart three to four cardiac cycles after injection.

Intracardiac shunts (e.g., atrial septal defect) are marked by microbubbles appearing in the left side of the heart almost immediately after their injection into the right side of the heart.

CARDIAC CATHETERIZATION

Cardiac catheterization allows **sampling of oximetric and hemodynamic data**. Figure 84-6 depicts the normal pressures and oxygen saturations for children. Cardiac catheterization, an **invasive procedure,** is often used in **conjunction with angiography** to confirm the **diagnosis and physiology** of certain **acquired and congenital heart disease**. The technique also has **therapeutic applications,** such as PDA coil embolization, coil embolization of aortopulmonary collaterals, pulmonary artery angioplasty and stent placement, and balloon valvuloplasty of semilunar valvular stenosis.

Shunts

Data obtained from cardiac catheterization can be used to calculate the **degree and direction of an intracardiac or extracardiac shunt**. The calculation is based on the **Fick principle,** using oxygen as the indicator.

The **oxygen content is equal to the dissolved oxygen** (which is usually negligible) **plus the oxygen capacity** [hemoglobin (g/dL) $\times$ 1.36 mL O_2/dL $\times$ 10] **multiplied by the oxygen saturation** (as a percentage).

Flow (Q) is the **oxygen consumption divided by the arteriovenous oxygen content difference:**

$$Qp = \frac{VO_2}{PV - PA} \quad Qs = \frac{VO_2}{AO - MV}$$

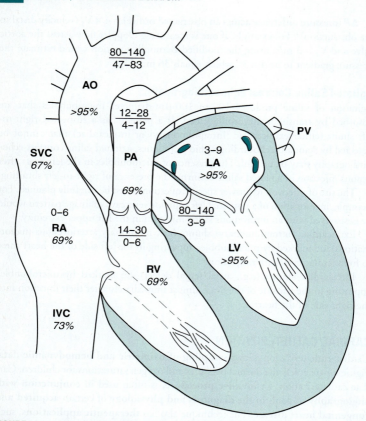

FIGURE 84-6 **Normal pressures (systolic over diastolic, in mm Hg), mean pressures, and oxygen saturations for children.** The data are based on information compiled from healthy patients between 2 months and 20 years of age. *AO*, aorta; *IVC*, inferior vena cava; *LA*, left atrium; *LV*, left ventricle; *PA*, pulmonary artery; *PV*, pulmonary vein; *RA*, right atrium; *RV*, right ventricle; *SVC*, superior vena cava.

Qp = pulmonary flow
Qs = systemic flow
VO₂ = oxygen consumption per unit time
PV = pulmonary venous oxygen content
PA = pulmonary arterial oxygen content
MV = mixed venous oxygen content
AO = aortic oxygen content

To calculate the **amount of a shunt,** one needs to **calculate the effective pulmonary blood flow** (Qp eff):

$$Qp \ eff = \frac{VO_2}{PV - MV}$$

A **left-to-right shunt** is the **pulmonary flow less the effective pulmonary flow** (Qp – Qp eff), and a **right-to-left shunt** is the **systemic flow less the effective pulmonary flow** (Qs – Qp eff).

Resistance

Systemic and pulmonary vascular resistance can also be calculated using **catheterization data.** This calculation is based on **Ohm's law** (essentially, the pressure change across the vascular bed divided by flow equals resistance):

$$Rp = \frac{PA - LA}{Qp} \quad Rs = \frac{AO - RA}{Os}$$

Rs = systemic resistance
Rp = pulmonary resistance
AO = mean aortic pressure
RA = mean right atrial pressure
PA = mean pulmonary artery pressure
LA = mean left atrial pressure

A pulmonary resistance (Rp) of ≤**3.0 Wood units** is considered within the **normal** range; however, no vascular bed is rigid, and **variations in flow can affect the result** obtained.

PART 5

Surgical Glossary

Aortopexy—procedure in which the aorta is approximated to the anterior thoracic wall; for the treatment of tracheomalacia.

Bishop–Koop procedure—resection of a dilated loop of bowel proximal to meconium obstruction, with end-to-side anastomosis between the proximal bowel and obstructed loop, combined with end ileostomy; for the treatment of meconium ileus.

bladder augmentation—procedure in which a portion of the intraabdominal gastrointestinal tract is used to increase the volume of the bladder.

Blalock-Taussig shunt—procedure in which the subclavian artery is anastomosed to the pulmonary artery; for the temporary treatment of tetralogy of Fallot.

Boix-Ochoa procedure—restoration of the intraabdominal esophageal length, repair of the esophageal hiatus, fixation of the esophagus to the hiatus, and restoration of the angle of His; for the treatment of incompetent lower esophageal sphincter.

chordee correction—procedure in which the corpus spongiosum is moved ventrally and the corpus cavernosa are approximated dorsally; for the treatment of chordee (abnormal penile curvature associated with epispadias or hypospadias).

Clatworthy mesocaval shunt—division of the common iliac veins and side-to-end anastomosis of the inferior mesenteric vein to the left renal vein; for the treatment of portal hypertension.

Cohen procedure—trigonal reimplantation of the ureter; for the treatment of vesicoureteral reflux.

colonic conduit diversion—procedure involving two stages: (1) a loop diversion using a colonic segment and (2) an end-to-side anastomosis of the colonic segment to the gastrointestinal tract.

colonic interposition—replacement of the esophagus with a colonic segment; for the treatment of esophageal atresia or stricture when gastric mobilization is not feasible.

diaphragmatic plication—surgical shortening of the diaphragm (abdominal, transthoracic, or bilateral); for the treatment of diaphragmatic eventration.

distal splenorenal shunt—see Warren shunt.

Drapanas mesocaval shunt—prosthetic graft implantation from the inferior mesenteric vein to the inferior vena cava; for the treatment of portal hypertension.

Duckett transverse preputial island flap—technique in which a flap of foreskin is used to elongate the urethra; for the treatment of hypospadias.

Duhamel procedure—resection of the aganglionic colon above the dentate line with stable anastomosis to the rectal stump; normally performed in children 6 to 12 months of age for the treatment of Hirschsprung disease (see Martin modification).

end-to-side portacaval shunt—procedure in which the portal vein is divided and anastomosed to the inferior vena cava; for the treatment of portal hypertension.

esophagectomy—resection of the esophagus, with gastric pull-up and anastomosis with the cervical esophagus; for the treatment of esophageal atresia or stricture.

Fontan procedure—procedure in which a graft is created to connect the pulmonary artery to the right atrium; for the treatment of hyperplastic right heart syndrome.

Glenn shunt—shunt from the superior vena cava to the pulmonary artery; for the treatment of tricuspid atresia or stenosis.

gridiron incision—see McBurney incision.

Hegman procedure—surgical release of the tarsal, metatarsal, and intertarsal ligaments; for the treatment of metatarsus adductus.

Heller myotomy—myotomy of the anterior lower esophagus (always accompanied by a Thal fundoplication); for the treatment of achalasia.

ileal loop diversion—resection and implantation of ureters into an isolated ileal segment, with an ileal stoma and primary anastomosis of ileum to cecum.

ileal ureter—ileal interposition between the renal pelvis and bladder when the ureteral length is insufficient for anastomosis; for the treatment of urinary obstruction.

ileocecal conduit diversion—bilateral ureteral diversion and anastomosis to an isolated ileocecal segment and cecostomy with primary anastomosis of ileum to the right colon.

Jatene procedure—arterial retransposition; for the treatment of transposition of the great vessels.

J-pouch—creation of an ileal reservoir in the distal ileum using a J-shaped configuration; used following colectomy.

Kasai procedure—resection of atretic extrahepatic bile ducts and gallbladder with Roux-en-Y anastomosis of the jejunum to the remaining common hepatic duct; for the treatment of biliary atresia or other extrahepatic obstruction.

Kimura procedure (parasitized cecal patch)—a multistep operation in which (1) a side-to-side anastomosis is made with a portion of the distal ileum and the right colon and (2) an ileoanal pull-through is performed; for the treatment of Hirschsprung disease.

King operation—resection of the knee with placement of a Küntscher rod to fix the femur to the tibia, followed by a Syme amputation for the treatment of proximal focal femoral deficiency.

Koch pouch diversion—procedure involving bilateral ureteral diversion with anastomosis to a neobladder formed from an isolated ileal segment, combined with an ileal stoma and primary anastomosis of ileum to ileum.

Ladd operation—restoration of intestinal anatomy from a malrotated state; for the treatment of intestinal malrotation.

Lanz incision—abdominal incision made in the left iliac fossa; for colostomy formation.

left hepatectomy—resection of the left hepatic lobe (medial and lateral segments).

MAGPI (meatal advancement and glanuloplasty) procedure—distal advancement of the urethral meatus and glanuloplasty; for the treatment of hypospadias.

Mainz pouch diversion—procedure involving bilateral ureteral division with anastomosis to a neobladder formed from isolated cecum and terminal ileum; combined with an ileal stoma and primary anastomosis of the ileum to the right colon.

Martin modification (of Duhamel procedure)—right and transverse colectomy with ileoanal pull-through and side-to-side anastomosis of the remaining left colon to the ileum; procedure preserves some absorptive capacity of the large bowel; for the treatment of total colonic Hirschsprung disease.

McBurney (gridiron) incision—abdominal incision from the anterior superior iliac spine to the umbilicus; used for appendectomy.

Mikulicz procedure—diverting enterostomy performed proximal to the meconium obstruction without resection; for the treatment of meconium ileus.

mini-Pena procedure—anterior sagittal anorectoplasty; for the treatment of anterior rectoperineal fistula (boys) or rectal-fourchette fistula (girls).

Mitrofanoff technique—modification of neobladder diversion procedures in which vascularized appendix is used to create the stoma.

Mustard technique—redirection of blood through an atrial septal defect using a pericardial pathway; for the treatment of transposition of the great vessels; because of associated increased turbulence, this technique is not widely used today.

Mustardé procedure—correction, using simple mattress sutures, of a prominent ear with normal or absent antihelical folds.

Nissen fundoplication—technique involving a 360° wrap of the gastric fundus around the gastroesophageal junction; for the treatment of incompetent lower esophageal sphincter; patient is rendered unable to vomit or belch.

Norwood procedure—three-stage palliative procedure including (1) atrial septectomy, transection and ligation of the pulmonary artery, "neoaorta" formation using the proximal pulmonary artery, and creation of a synthetic aorto-pulmonary shunt; (2) creation of a Glenn shunt; and (3) performance of a modified Fontan procedure; for the treatment of hypoplastic left heart syndrome.

onlay island flap—technique in which a flap of foreskin is used to elongate the urethra; for the treatment of hypospadias.

orchidopexy—testicular pull-down and attachment; for the treatment of undescended testis.

orthoplasty—surgical correction of excessive penile curvature.

parasitized cecal patch—see Kimura procedure.

Pena procedure—posterior sagittal anorectoplasty performed in children aged 1 to 6 months; for the treatment of imperforate anus.

Pfannenstiel incision—an abdominal incision used to gain access to the lower abdomen and bring pelvic organs within reach without dividing muscular tissue.

pharyngoplasty—elevation of the posterior pharyngeal wall following a primary cleft palate repair (to narrow the pharyngeal space); for the treatment of velopharyngeal incompetence.

Potts shunt—anastomosis of the descending aorta to the pulmonary artery for the permanent treatment of tetralogy of Fallot.

proximal splenorenal shunt—end-to-side anastomosis of the splenic vein to the left renal vein with splenectomy; for the treatment of portal hypertension.

pyeloplasty—resection of an atretic ureter with primary anastomosis to the renal pelvis; for the treatment of ureteropelvic junction obstruction.

Ramstedt operation—relaxation of the pyloric sphincter; for the treatment of pyloric stenosis.

Rashkind procedure—balloon atrial septostomy; for the treatment of palliation of the great vessels.

Rastelli repair—technique involving the closure of a ventricular septal defect with a patch and the creation of a conduit from the distal pulmonary artery to the right ventricle; for the treatment of transposition of the great vessels.

Ravitch procedure—procedure involving (1) creation of osteotomies between the manubrium and costal cartilages, (2) a greenstick fracture of the manubrium, and (3) the temporary insertion (for 6 to 12 months) of a stabilizing bar; for the treatment of pectus excavatum or pectus carinatum.

right colon pouch—procedure involving bilateral ureteral division with anastomosis to a neobladder (formed from an isolated segment of the right colon), combined with an ileal stoma and primary anastomosis of the ileum to the transverse colon.

right hepatectomy—resection of the right hepatic lobes (anterior and posterior segments).

rooftop (bilateral subcostal) incision—abdominal incision used to access the liver and portal structures.

Roux-en-Y anastomosis—division of the jejunum distal to the ligament of Treitz with end-to-side anastomosis of the duodenum to the distal jejunum and anastomosis of the proximal jejunum (typically) to the bile duct.

Santulli–Blanc enterostomy—modification of the Bishop–Koop procedure that involves the resection of a distal dilated bowel segment with side-to-end anastomosis to the proximal enterostomy; for the treatment of meconium ileus.

Senning procedure (venous switch)—technique involving intraatrial redirection of venous return so that systemic caval return is shunted through the mitral valve to the left ventricle and pulmonary return is brought through the tricuspid valve to the right ventricle; for the treatment of transposition of the great vessels.

side-to-side portacaval shunt—procedure in which the portal vein is anastomosed to the inferior vena cava; for the treatment of portal hypertension.

side-to-side splenorenal shunt—side-to-side anastomosis of the splenic vein to the left renal vein; for the treatment of portal hypertension.

Sistrunk operation—complete excision of a thyroglossal duct cyst.

Soave procedure—technique involving endorectal pull-through; for the correction of rectal resection.

S-pouch—creation of an ileal reservoir in the distal ileum using an S-shape configuration following colectomy.

Stamm gastrostomy—placement of an open gastrostomy tube; the opening is designed to close spontaneously on removal of the tube.

Sting procedure—subureteric Teflon injection; for the endoscopic correction of vesicoureteral reflux.

Sugiura procedure—technique that involves lower esophageal transection and primary anastomosis, devascularization of the lower esophagus and stomach, and splenectomy; for the treatment of esophageal varices.

Swenson procedure—resection of the posterior rectal wall to the dentate line (aganglionic region); for the treatment of Hirschsprung disease; technically difficult and rarely performed.

Syme amputation—amputation of the foot, calculated to bring the end of the stump above the opposite knee at maturity; for the treatment of proximal focal femoral deficiency.

Thal procedure—procedure involving a 180° anterior wrap of the gastric fundus around the gastroesophageal junction, preserving the patient's ability to vomit and belch; for the treatment of incompetent lower esophageal sphincter.

Thiersch operation—procedure in which a distal rectal segment that has prolapsed is approximated to the external sphincter muscle; for the treatment of rectal prolapse.

trisegmentectomy—resection of the right hepatic lobe and the quadrate lobe of the liver (right posterior segment, right anterior segment, and medial segment).

ureteropyelostomy—partial resection and side-to-side anastomosis of a partially duplicated ureter.

ureterocalicostomy—technique for the treatment of urinary obstruction involving division of the ureter (distal to the obstruction) and intrarenal anastomosis to the most dependent renal calyx; when the renal pelvis is insufficient for anastomosis, the lower pole of the kidney is resected.

vaginal switch operation—procedure in which the vagina is separated from the urinary tract; for the treatment of duplicated vagina.

Van Ness procedure—rotational 180° osteotomy of the femur in which the foot and ankle are brought to the level of the opposite knee; for prosthetic attachment for the treatment of femoral deficiency.

venous switch—see Senning procedure.

ventricular shunt procedure—procedure in which a silastic catheter is positioned in a lateral ventricle and tunneled subcutaneously to drain into the central venous system or peritoneal cavity; for the treatment of hydrocephalus.

Warren (distal splenorenal) shunt—procedure in which the splenic vein is anastomosed to the left renal vein; for the treatment of portal hypertension.

Waterston aortopulmonary anastomosis—procedure involving anastomosis of the ascending aorta and the right pulmonary artery; for the temporary treatment of tetralogy of Fallot.

Whipple procedure—resection of the pancreatic head, duodenum, and gallbladder with gastrojejunostomy, hepatojejunostomy, and pancreaticojejunostomy.

Syndromes Glossary

4p-syndrome—characterized by a round face, prominent nasal tip, polydactyly, and scoliosis.

5p-syndrome—characterized by macrocephaly; small mandible; long, thin fingers; short, big toes; and anorectal and renal anomalies.

13q-syndrome—typically involves malformations of the brain, heart, kidneys, and digits; usually lethal.

Aagenaes syndrome—hereditary (autosomal-recessive transmission); characterized by recurrent intrahepatic cholestasis, with lymphedema.

Aarskog syndrome—X-linked recessive disorder characterized by short stature and musculoskeletal and genital anomalies of unknown etiology. Physical features include short stature (90%), hypertelorism, small nose with anteverted nares, broad philtrum and nasal bridge, abnormal auricles and widow's peak, brachyclinodactyly (80%), broad feet with bulbous toes (75%), simian crease (70%), ptosis (50%), syndactyly (60%), "shawl" scrotum (80%), cryptorchidism (75%), inguinal hernia (60%), hyperopic astigmatism, large corneas, ophthalmoplegia, strabismus, delayed puberty, mild pectus excavatum, and prominent umbilicus. Radiographs show delayed bone age.

abetalipoproteinemia—recessive transmission; characterized by progressive cerebellar ataxia and pigmentary degeneration of the retina (starts with malabsorption of fat and progresses to ataxia); absent or reduced lipoproteins and low carotene, vitamin A, and cholesterol levels; and acanthocytosis (spiny projections on red blood cells).

acanthosis nigricans (Lawrence–Seip syndrome)—characterized by hyperpigmented lichenoid plaques in the neck and axilla; may be associated with insulin resistance.

acrodermatitis enteropathica—autosomal-recessive transmission; characterized by zinc deficiency, vesicobullous and eczematous skin lesions in the perioral and perineal areas, cheeks, knees, and elbows; photophobia, conjunctivitis, and corneal dystrophy; chronic diarrhea; glossitis; nail dystrophy; growth retardation; and superinfections and *Candida* infections.

Adie syndrome—characterized by a large pupil with little or no reaction to light; pupil may react to accommodation; and patients have hyperreflexia.

agenesis of corpus callosum—cause unknown (rarely, X-linked recessive); absence of the major tracts connecting the right and left hemispheres is usually associated with hydrocephalus, seizures, developmental delay, abnormal head size, and hypertelorism.

Alagille syndrome (arteriohepatic dysplasia)—characterized by paucity or absence of intrahepatic bile ducts with progressive destruction of bile ducts; patients have a broad forehead, deep-set eyes that are widely spaced and underdeveloped, a small, pointed mandible, cardiac lesions, vertebral arch defects, and changes in the renal tubules and interstitium.

Albers–Schönberg disease (osteopetrosis tarda, marble bone disease)—most cases are autosomal dominant, a few are autosomal recessive; patients are prone to fractures and have mild anemia and craniofacial disproportion; radiologic changes include increased cortical bone density, longitudinal and transverse dense striations at the ends of the long bones, lucent and dense bands in the vertebrae, and thickening at the base of the skull.

Albright syndrome—see McCune–Albright syndrome.

Alexander disease—unknown pathogenesis; characterized by megalencephaly in infants, dementia, spasticity, and ataxia; may cause seizures in younger children; patients become mute, immobile, and dependent; hyaline eosinophilic inclusions occur in the footplates of astrocytes in subpial and subependymal regions.

Alport syndrome—several forms are hereditary male-to-male autosomal dominant, and an X-linked form also exists; characterized by neurosensory deafness and progressive renal failure.

Anderson disease (glycogen storage disease, type IV)—caused by a defect in the glycogen branching enzyme 1, 4-α-glucan branching enzyme; characterized by hepatomegaly and failure to thrive in the first few months, progressing to liver cirrhosis and splenomegaly.

Apert syndrome (acrocephalosyndactyly)—autosomal dominant; characterized by high and flat frontal bones, underdevelopment of the middle third of the face, hypertelorism and proptosis; a narrow, high, arched palate; a short, beaked nose; and syndactyly of the toes and digits.

arthrogryposis multiplex congenita—characterized by fixed contractures of the middle joints; present at birth.

Asperger syndrome—a developmental disorder on the higher functioning end of the autism spectrum. These patients, often viewed as brilliant, eccentric, and physically awkward, fail to develop relationships with peers, have repetitive and stereotyped behaviors, usually with hand movements (see www.asperger-syndrome.org).

Bart syndrome—autosomal dominant; congenital aplasia of the skin; characterized by nail defects and recurrent blistering of the skin and mucous membranes.

Bartter syndrome—hypertrophy of the juxtaglomerular apparatus; characterized by hypokalemic alkalosis, hypochloremia, and hyperaldosteronism; patients have normal blood pressure but the renin level is elevated; may lead to mental retardation and small stature.

Beckwith–Wiedemann syndrome—characterized by hypoglycemia, macrosomia, and visceromegaly; patients have umbilical anomalies and renal medullary dysplasia.

Behçet syndrome—unknown cause; involves relapsing iridocyclitis and recurrent oral and genital ulcerations; 50% of patients have arthritis.

blind loop syndrome—stasis of small intestine, usually secondary to incomplete bowel obstruction or a problem of intestinal motility.

Bloch–Sulzberger syndrome (incontinentia pigmenti)—characterized by mental retardation; a third of patients have seizures and ocular malformations.

Bloom syndrome—autosomal recessive; characterized by erythema and telangiectasia in a butterfly distribution, photosensitivity, and dwarfism.

Blount disease (tibia vara)—characterized by irregularity of the medial aspect of the tibial metaphysis adjacent to the epiphysis; bowing starts as angulation at the metaphysis.

blue diaper syndrome—defective tryptophan absorption; characterized by bluish stains on the diapers, digestive disturbances, fever, and visual difficulties.

Brill disease (Brill–Zinsser disease)—repeat episode of typhus; caused by a *Rickettsia* infection.

bronchiolitis obliterans—begins with necrotizing pneumonia secondary to viral infection (e.g., adenovirus, influenza, measles); tuberculosis; or inhalation of fumes, talcum powder, or zinc; and involves the obstruction of small bronchi and bronchioles by fibrous tissue.

Byler disease—autosomal-recessive familial cholestasis; characterized by hepatomegaly, pruritus, splenomegaly, elevated bile acids, and gallstones.

Caroli disease—autosomal recessive; cystic dilation of the intrahepatic bile ducts; characterized by recurrent bouts of cholangitis and biliary abscesses secondary to bile stasis and gallstones.

cat's eye syndrome—autosomal dominant; characterized by ocular coloboma, down-slanting eyes, congenital heart disease, and anal atresia.

Charcot–Marie–Tooth disease (peroneal muscular atrophy)—most common cause of chronic peripheral neuropathy; characterized by foot drop, high-arch foot; patients may have stocking-glove sensory loss.

Chédiak–Higashi syndrome—autosomal-recessive disorder; involves partial oculocutaneous albinism, increased susceptibility to infection, lack of natural killer cells, and large lysosome-like granules in many tissues; patients have splenomegaly, hypersplenism, hepatomegaly, lymphadenopathy, nystagmus photophobia, and peripheral neuropathy.

Coat disease—telangiectasia of retinal vessels, with subretinal exudate.

Cobb syndrome—intraspinous vascular anomaly and port-wine stains.

Cockayne syndrome—autosomal recessive; characterized by dwarfism, mental retardation, bird-like facies, premature senility, and photosensitivity.

Cornelia de Lange syndrome—prenatal growth retardation; characterized by microcephaly, hirsutism, anteverted nares, down-turned mouth, mental retardation, and congenital heart defects.

cri du chat syndrome—characterized by growth retardation, mental deficiency, hypotonia, microcephaly, round "moon face," hypertelorism, epicanthal folds, and down-slanting palpebral fissures.

Crigler–Najjar syndrome (congenital nonhemolytic unconjugated hyperbilirubinemia)—type 1 is recessive; a deficiency of uridine diphosphate glucuronyl transferase causes a rapid increase in the unconjugated bilirubin level on the first day of life; no hemolysis occurs and patients have no conjugation activity; type 2 is autosomal dominant and characterized by variable penetrance and partial activity of uridine diphosphate glucuronyl transferase.

Cronkhite–Canada syndrome—diffuse intestinal polyps involving large and small intestine; characterized by alopecia, brown skin lesions, and onychatrophia; patients have diarrhea and protein-losing enteropathy.

Crouzon syndrome (craniofacial dysostosis)—autosomal dominant with a range of expressivity; characterized by exophthalmos, hypertelorism, and hypoplasia of maxilla; patients have oral cavity anomalies and premature closure of the external auditory meatus.

cyclic neutropenia—syndrome involving lack of granulocyte macrophage colony-stimulating factor; characterized by fever, mouth lesions, cervical adenitis, and gastroenteritis occurring every 3 to 6 weeks; neutrophil count may be zero.

de Toni–Fanconi–Debré acute syndrome—fatal; infantile myopathy with renal dysfunction; involves abnormal mitochondria and lipid and glycogen accumulation; patient has weak cry, poor muscle tone, poor suck, and lactic acidosis.

De Sanctis–Cacchione syndrome—autosomal recessive; characterized by xeroderma pigmentosum with mental retardation, dwarfism, and hypogonadism; skin is unable to repair itself after exposure to ultraviolet light; patients may have erythema, scaling bullae, crusting telangiectasia keratoses, photophobia, corneal opacities, and tumors of the eyelids.

Diamond–Blackfan syndrome (congenital hypoplastic anemia)—failure of erythropoiesis; characterized by macrocytic anemia; patients have anemia, pallor, and weakness, no hepatomegaly, elevated fetal hemoglobin, and defect in abduction with retraction of the eye on adduction.

DiGeorge syndrome—thymic hypoplasia with hypocalcemia; patients have tetany, abnormal facies, congenital heart disease, and increased incidence of infection.

Dubin–Johnson syndrome—autosomal recessive; characterized by elevated conjugated bilirubin, large amounts of coproporphyrin I in urine, and deposits of melanin-like pigment in hepatocellular lysosomes.

Dubowitz syndrome—Children with this syndrome nearly always have a history of intrauterine growth retardation involving both low birthweight and reduced length.

Eagle–Barrett syndrome (prune-belly syndrome)—characterized by deficiency of the abdominal musculature, dilation and dysplasia of the urinary tract, cryptorchidism, dilation of the posterior urethra, and a hypoplastic or absent prostate.

ectodermal dysplasia—characterized by the poor development, or absence, of teeth, nails, hair, and sweat glands; patients have hyperextensible skin, hypermobile joints, and easy bruisability.

Eisenmenger syndrome—characterized by ventricular septal defect with pulmonary hypertension.

Fabry disease—X-linked lipid storage disease; involves a defect of the ceramide trihexoside α-galactosidase; characterized by tingling and burning in the hands and feet; small red maculopapular lesions on the buttocks, inguinal area, fingernails, and lips; and an inability to perspire; patients have proteinuria, progressing to renal failure.

Farber syndrome—autosomal recessive; involves a deficiency of acid ceramidase; characterized by hoarseness; painful, swollen joints; and palpable nodules over affected joints and pressure points.

fetal alcohol syndrome—characterized by a small body, head, and maxillary bone; abnormal palpebral fissures; epicanthal folds; cardiac septal defect; delayed development; and mental deficiency.

fetal hydantoin syndrome—characterized by hypoplasia of the midface, low nasal bridge, ocular hypertelorism, and cupid bow upper lip; patients experience slow growth, may have mental retardation, cleft lip, and cardiac malformation.

Friedreich ataxia—mostly autosomal recessive; appears in late childhood or in adolescence; involves progressive cerebellar and spinal cord dysfunction; patients have high-arched foot, hammer toes, and cardiac failure.

fructose intolerance, hereditary—autosomal recessive; involves deficiency of fructose-1-phosphate aldolase or fructose 1,6-diphosphatase; characterized by vomiting, diarrhea, hypoglycemic seizures, and jaundice.

Gardner syndrome—characterized by multiple gastrointestinal polyps with malignant transformation, skin cysts, and multiple osteoma.

Gaucher disease—abnormal storage of glucosylceramide in the reticuloendothelial system; three types: (1) adult or chronic, (2) acute neuropathic or infantile, and (3) subacute neuropathic or juvenile; characterized by splenomegaly, hepatomegaly, delayed development, strabismus, swallowing difficulties, laryngeal spasm, opisthotonos, and bone pain.

Gianotti–Crosti syndrome—papular acrodermatitis and hepatitis B virus infection; usually benign and self-limited.

Gilles de la Tourette syndrome—dominant trait with partial penetrance; characterized by multiple tics (e.g., blinking, twitching, grimacing) and involvement of muscles of swallowing and respiration; patient may exhibit swearing behavior and may have learning disabilities.

Glanzmann disease—autosomal recessive; involves defective primary platelet aggregation (size and survival of platelets is normal).

Goldenhar syndrome—characterized by oculoauriculovertebral dysplasia and mandibular hypoplasia; patients have a hypoplastic zygomatic arch; malformed, displaced pinnae, and hearing loss.

Goltz syndrome—focal dermal hypoplasia; herniations of fat through thinned dermis produce tan papillomas associated with other skin defects and skeletal anomalies (e.g., syndactyly, polydactyly, spinal defects); patients also have colobomas, strabismus, and nystagmus.

Gradenigo syndrome—acquired palsy of the abducens nerve and pain in the trigeminal nerve distribution, usually occurs after otitis media; produces diplopia, ocular and facial pain, photophobia, and lacrimation.

Hand–Schüller–Christian disease—see Langerhans cell histiocytosis.

Hartnup disease—autosomal recessive defect in transport of monoamine monocarboxylic amino acids by intestinal mucosa and renal tubules; characterized by photosensitivity and a pellagra-like skin rash; patients may have cerebellar ataxia.

histiocytosis X—see Langerhans cell histiocytosis.

Hunter syndrome (mucopolysaccharidosis II)—X-linked recessive; characterized by an accumulation of heparan sulfate and dermatan sulfate, and enzyme deficiency of L-iduronate sulfatase. Can cause a variety of symptoms including mental retardation, deafness, hepatosplenomegaly, and cardiac disease.

Hurler syndrome (mucopolysaccharidosis IH)—autosomal recessive; characterized by an accumulation of heparan sulfate and dermatan sulfate, and enzyme deficiency of α-L-iduronidase. Can cause a variety of symptoms including mental retardation, deafness, hepatosplenomegaly, and cardiac disease.

hyper-immunoglobulin E (IgE)—characterized by recurrent deep tissue and skin staphylococcal infections; patients have eosinophilia and IgE levels that are 10 times greater than normal.

incontinentia pigmenti—see Bloch–Sulzberger syndrome.

Jeune thoracic dystrophy—characterized by respiratory distress, short limbs, and polydactyly; may progress to renal insufficiency.

Job syndrome—characterized by severe staphylococcal infections, chronic skin disease, and cold abscesses; patients may have elevated immunoglobulin E.

Kallmann syndrome—familial; characterized by isolated gonadotropin deficiency and anosmia.

Kartagener syndrome—characterized by sinusitis, bronchiectasis, and immotile cilia.

Kasabach–Merritt syndrome—characterized by hemangioma and consumption coagulopathy, platelet trapping, and microangiopathic hemolytic anemia.

Kleine–Levin syndrome—characterized by unusual hunger, somnolence, and motor restlessness.

Klinefelter syndrome—XXY karyotype; characterized by seminiferous tubule dysgenesis, testicular atrophy, eunuchoid habitus, and gynecomastia.

Klippel–Feil syndrome—characterized by a short neck, limited neck motion, and low occipital hairline.

Krabbe leukodystrophy—autosomal recessive; characterized by cerebroside lipidosis and lack of myelin in white matter; usually presents by 1 year of age; patients have hyperreflexia, rigidity, swallowing difficulties, and lack of development.

Langerhans cell histiocytosis—(reticuloendotheliosis) formerly called eosinophilic granuloma, Hand–Schüller–Christian disease, or Letterer–Siwe disease; patients may have a few solitary bone lesions or seborrheic dermatitis of scalp, lymphadenopathy, hepatosplenomegaly, tooth loss, exophthalmos, or pulmonary infiltrates.

Larsen syndrome—usually autosomal dominant; characterized by hyperlaxity, multiple dislocations, and skin hyperlaxity.

Laurence–Moon–Biedl syndrome—characterized by retinitis pigmentosa, polydactyly, obesity, and hypogonadism.

Lennox–Gastaut syndrome (childhood epileptic encephalopathy)—characterized by severe seizures, mental retardation, and characteristic electroencephalography pattern (i.e., generalized bilaterally synchronous sharp wave and slow wave complexes); patients have seizures starting in infancy; condition is difficult to treat; and mental retardation is common.

Lesch–Nyhan syndrome—X-linked recessive disorder; characterized by a defect in purine metabolism; patients have hyperuricemia as a result of diminished or absent hypoxanthine guanine phosphoribosyl transferase activity, choreoathetosis, compulsive self-mutilation, mental retardation, and growth failure.

Letterer–Siwe disease—component of Langerhans cell histiocytosis characterized by acute disseminated histiocytosis; patients have seborrheic-looking skin lesions, bone lesions, gingival lesions, and liver and lung infiltrates.

Lowe syndrome (oculocerebral dystrophy)—X-linked recessive; patients have congenital cataracts, glaucoma, hypotonia, hyperreflexia, severe mental retardation, rickets, osteopenia, pathologic fractures, aminoaciduria, and organic aciduria.

Maffucci syndrome—multiple enchondromata and hemangioma of the bone and overlying skin; patients have short stature, skeletal deformities, scoliosis, and limb disproportion.

Marfan syndrome—connective tissue disorder characterized by ectopia lentis; dilation of the aorta; long, thin extremities; pectus excavatum or carinatum; scoliosis; and pneumothorax.

McCune–Albright syndrome—polyostotic fibrous dysplasia; characterized by prominent skin discoloration with ragged edges; patients may have precocious puberty, hyperthyroidism, gigantism, headaches, epilepsy, and mental deficiency.

MELAS syndrome—*m*itochondrial *e*ncephalopathy, *l*actic *a*cidosis, and *s*troke-like episodes; causes seizures, alternating hemiparesis, hemianopsia, or cortical blindness; patients have lactic acidosis, spongy degeneration of the brain, sensorineural hearing loss, and short stature.

Menkes syndrome—X-linked recessive; patients have short scalp hair, hypopigmentation, hypothermia, growth failure, skeletal defects, arterial aneurysms, seizures, and progressive central nervous system failure.

Möbius syndrome—characterized by cranial nerve defects and a hypoplastic tongue or digits.

Morquio syndrome (mucopolysaccharidosis)—characterized by severe skeletal deformities, pectus carinatum, kyphoscoliosis, short neck, hypoplasia of the odontoid processes, C1 and C2 dislocation, neurosensory deafness, and aortic insufficiency.

multiple cartilaginous exostosis—characterized by bony projections near the ends of the tubular bones and ribs, scapula, vertebral bodies, and iliac crest; the exostoses become calcified and cause skeletal deformities; appears after 3 years of age.

nail-patella syndrome—autosomal dominant; characterized by dystrophic and hypoplastic nails, hypoplastic patellae and iliac horns, and malformed radial heads; may lead to nephrotic syndrome and renal failure.

Niemann–Pick disease—four types; storage of sphingomyelin and cholesterol causes hepatomegaly; patients are normal at birth but experience delayed development; 50% have a macular cherry red spot.

Noonan syndrome—normal karyotype; syndrome is characterized by cardiac lesions (atrial septal defect or pulmonic stenosis); facial changes (palpebral slant, broad flat nose); webbed neck; short stature; a high arched palate; and malformed ears.

Osler–Weber–Rendu syndrome—hereditary hemorrhagic telangiectasia; patients have telangiectasia in the skin, respiratory tract mucosa, lips, nails, conjunctiva, and nasal and oral mucosae.

Parinaud syndrome—characterized by weakness of upward gaze, poor convergence and accommodation, refractive nystagmus with upward gaze, and pupillary changes.

Patau syndrome—see trisomy 13.

Pelizaeus–Merzbacher disease—characterized by dancing eye movements, delayed motor development and spasticity, small head, poor head control, and possible optic atrophy and seizures.

Peutz–Jeghers syndrome—autosomal dominant; patients have bluish black macules around the mouth and intestinal polyposis in the small bowel.

Pickwickian syndrome—characterized by obesity and hypoventilation syndrome; patients may have respiratory arrest and restless sleep.

Pierre Robin syndrome—characterized by severe micrognathia, glossoptosis, and cleft palate.

Poland syndrome—characterized by a unilateral hypoplastic pectoral muscle with ipsilateral upper limb deficiency, syndactyly, and a defect of the subclavian artery.

Prader–Willi syndrome—characterized by hypotonia, hypomentia, hypogonadism, obesity, narrow bifrontal diameter, and hypotonia; patients may have a deletion in chromosome 15.

primary microcephaly—Facial characteristics include triangular face; small receding chin; and broad and sometimes flat nasal bridge. As the child matures, the nasal bridge appears less wide and often becomes prominent, producing a continuous line with the forehead when viewed in profile. Tip of nose is frequently wide, rounded, or prominent; hypertelorism; shortened palpebral fissure that may be slanted; ptosis; sloping and high forehead; scanty hair and eyebrows; and ear abnormalities.

progeria—characterized by premature aging, severe growth failure, atherosclerosis, alopecia, and dystrophic nails.

prune-belly syndrome—see Eagle-Barrett syndrome.

Rieger syndrome—sporadic autosomal dominant; characterized by microcornea with opacity, iris hypoplasia, anterior synechiae, hypodontia, and maxillary hypoplasia.

Riley–Day syndrome—familial dysautonomia; affects sensory and autonomic functions; patients have poor feeding, aspiration, no tears, high threshold to pain, markedly decreased reflexes, smooth tongue and impaired taste, and erratic blood pressure and temperature.

Rotor syndrome—autosomal recessive; characterized by elevated conjugated bilirubin, elevated coproporphyrin I and coproporphyrin in urine, and normal liver biopsies.

Rubinstein–Taybi syndrome—characterized by broad thumbs and toes, short stature, mental retardation, beaked nose, hypoplastic mandible, and congenital heart defect.

Russell–Silver dwarf syndrome—characterized by intrauterine growth retardation, subnormal growth velocity, triangular facies, clinodactyly, simian creases, and genitourinary malformations.

Sandhoff GM$_2$-gangliosidosis type II—characterized by deficient hexosaminidase activity leading to cherry red spot in macula, failure to develop motor skills, blindness, weakness, and seizures.

Sanfilippo type A syndrome (mucopolysaccharidosis IIIA)—autosomal recessive; characterized by accumulation of heparan sulfate, dermatan sulfate, and sulfatidase.

Sanfilippo type B syndrome (mucopolysaccharidosis IIIA)—autosomal recessive; characterized by accumulation of heparan sulfate, dermatan sulfate, and α-N-acetylglucosaminidase.

Scheie syndrome (mucopolysaccharidosis IS)—autosomal recessive; characterized by accumulation of heparan sulfate and dermatan sulfate, and an enzyme defect affecting α-L-iduronidase.

scimitar syndrome—characterized by hypoplasia of the right lung with systemic arterial supply, anomalous right pulmonary vein, and dextroposition of heart.

Seckel syndrome—characterized by intrauterine growth retardation, microcephaly, sharp facial features with underdeveloped chin, and mental retardation.

Shwachman syndrome—characterized by pancreatic dysfunction, short stature, bone marrow dysfunction, and skeletal abnormalities.

silo filler disease—acute pneumonitis caused by inhalation of nitrogen dioxide; patients have chills, fever, cough, dyspnea, and cyanosis; associated with a high mortality rate.

Smith–Lemli–Opitz syndrome—characterized by short stature, microcephaly, ptosis, anteverted nares, micrognathia, syndactyly, cryptorchidism, and mental retardation.

Sotos syndrome—characterized by cerebral gigantism, large head and ears, prominent mandible, mental retardation, and poor coordination.

Stickler syndrome—autosomal dominant; characterized by high myopia, cataract formation, and retinal detachment.

Sturge–Weber syndrome—characterized by a port-wine stain on the face at the first branch of the trigeminal nerve; patients have seizures and mental retardation.

Swyer–James syndrome—characterized by unilateral hyperlucent lung following bronchiolitis obliterans.

Tourette syndrome—see Gilles de la Tourette syndrome.

Treacher Collins syndrome—autosomal dominant with incomplete penetration; characterized by mandibulofacial dysostosis; patients have hypoplastic mandible; hypoplastic zygomatic arches; antimongoloid slant to eyes; deformities of the pinna; and a high arched palate with or without cleft palate.

trisomy 9—characterized by deep-set eyes, bulbous nasal tip, an anxious facial expression, and cleft lip.

trisomy 13 (Patau syndrome)—characterized by cleft lip, microphthalmia, postaxial polydactyly, and cardiovascular anomalies.

trisomy 18—characterized by a small face, high nasal bridge, short palpebral fissures, micrognathia, small mouth, overriding fingers, and hypoplastic nails; patients have mental retardation and intrauterine growth retardation.

tuberous sclerosis—characterized by epiloia; patients have seizures, mental deficiency, adenoma sebaceum foci of intracranial calcification, hypopigmented macules, ash leaf spots, connective tissue nevi (shagreen spots), adenoma sebaceum, and angiofibroma.

Turcot syndrome—characterized by adenomatous colonic polyposis associated with malignant brain tumors, especially glioblastomas.

Turner syndrome—characterized by gonadal dysplasia (streak gonads stem from XO karyotype), short stature, sexual infantilism, atypical facies, low hairline, webbed neck, congenital lymphedema of the extremities, coarctation of the aorta, and increased carrying angle.

Usher syndrome—autosomal recessive; characterized by retinitis pigmentosa, cataracts, and sensorineural deafness.

vanishing testes syndrome—characterized by bilateral gonadal failure with normal external male genitalia, normal 46, XY karyotype, absent testes, and no male puberty.

VATER syndrome—syndrome involving *v*ertebral defects, *a*nal atresia, *t*racheo-*e*sophageal atresia, *r*adial dysplasia, *r*enal dysplasia, and congenital heart defect.

Vogt–Koyanagi–Harada syndrome—characterized by vitiligo, uveitis, dysacousia, and aseptic meningitis.

von Gierke disease (type 1 glycogenosis)—glucose-6-phosphate dehydrogenase is absent in the liver, kidney, and intestinal mucosa; characterized by hypoglycemia under stress (e.g., fasting), hepatomegaly, and seizures.

von Hippel–Lindau disease—autosomal dominant (linked to chromosome 3); characterized by hemangioblastoma of the cerebellum and retina; patients have cystic cerebellar neoplasm with increased intracranial pressure.

Waardenburg syndrome—autosomal dominant; characterized by white forelock, heterochromic irides, displacement of the inner canthi, broad nasal root, and confluent eyebrows.

Wegener granulomatosis—necrotizing granulomatous vasculitis of the arteries and veins; involves airways, lungs, and kidneys with resultant rhinorrhea, nasal ulceration, hemoptysis, and cough; patients have hematuria caused by necrotizing vasculitis.

Werner syndrome—autosomal recessive; characterized by short stature, juvenile cataracts, hypogonadism, and gray hair in second decade.

Williams syndrome—characterized by mental retardation, hypoplastic nails, periorbital fullness, supravalvular aortic stenosis, growth delay, and stellate iris.

Wilson–Mikity syndrome—characterized by pulmonary immaturity; occurs in premature infants; patients have slow onset of respiratory distress, retractions, and apnea; may clear in several weeks.

Wiskott–Aldrich syndrome—characterized by thrombocytopenia, severe eczema, and recurrent skin infections.

Wolff–Parkinson–White syndrome—characterized by a short PR interval and slow upstroke of the QRS-delta wave; usually occurs in patients with a normal heart but also may occur in patients with Ebstein anomaly and cardiomyopathy.

Wolman disease—fatal condition characterized by primary xanthomatosis, adrenal insufficiency, vomiting, failure to thrive, steatorrhea, hepatomegaly, and adrenal calcification.

Zellweger syndrome—cerebrohepatorenal syndrome; characterized by hepatic fibrosis and cirrhosis; patients have seizures, mental retardation, hypotonia, glaucoma, congenital stippled epiphyses, and cysts of the renal cortex.

Zollinger–Ellison syndrome—characterized by islet cell tumors that produce duodenal and jejunal ulcers; patients have high gastrin levels and excessive acid secretion.

INDEX